human developmental anatomy

The National Medical Series for Independent Study

human developmental anatomy

Kurt E. Johnson, Ph.D.
*Professor of Anatomy
The George Washington University
 Medical Center
Washington, D.C.*

A WILEY MEDICAL PUBLICATION
JOHN WILEY & SONS
New York • Chichester • Brisbane • Toronto • Singapore

Harwal Publishing Company, Media, Pennsylvania

Editor: Gloria R. Hamilton

Some illustrations found in the study questions and challenge exam appear without credit lines. In these cases, the illustrations are modifications of figures used in the text, where appropriate credit is given.

Library of Congress Cataloging-in-Publication Data

Johnson, Kurt E.
  Human developmental anatomy/Kurt E. Johnson.
    p.   cm.—(The National medical series for independent study)
(A Wiley medical publication)
  Includes index.
  ISBN 0-471-62157-9 (pbk.)
  1. Embryology, Human.   I. Title. II. Series. III. Series: A Wiley medical publication.
    [DNLM: 1. Embryology—examination questions. 2. Embryology—outlines. QS 18 J67h]
QM601.J64   1988
612′ .64′ 0076—dc19
DNLM/DLC
for Library of Congress   89-2001
                                                                         CIP

©1988 by John Wiley & Sons, Inc.

Printed in the United States of America. All rights reserved. Except as permitted under the Copyright Act of 1976, no part of this publication may be reproduced or distributed in any form or by any means or stored in a data base or retrieval system, without the prior written permission of the publisher.

10 9 8 7 6 5 4 3 2 1

Dedication

This book is lovingly dedicated to my own two efforts in human development: Melissa H. Johnson and Abraham Q. Johnson.

Dedication

Contents

	Preface	ix
	Acknowledgments	xi
	Introduction	xiii
1	Introduction and General Aspects of Development	1
2	Gametogenesis	17
3	Overview of Embryonic and Fetal Periods	33
4	Fertilization, Cleavage, and Implantation	45
5	Gastrulation and Neurulation	61
6	Establishment of the Basic Body Plan and Primitive Circulation	79
7	Development of the Placenta and Fetal Membranes (Amnion and Chorion)	93
8	Development of Body Cavities, Mesenteries, and Diaphragm	115
9	Development of the Musculoskeletal System	125
10	Development of the Heart and Major Blood Vessels	145
11	Development of the Nervous System	167
12	Development of the Integument and Teeth	191
13	Development of the Digestive System	207
14	Development of the Respiratory System	225
15	Development of the Immune System	239

16	Development of the Urinary System	263
17	Development of the Male and Female Reproductive Systems	279
18	Development of the Face, Oral Cavity, and Pharyngeal Arches	303
19	Development of the Endocrine System	321
20	Development of the Eye	337
21	Development of the Ear	351
22	Normal Labor and Delivery	361
23	Etiology of Congenital Birth Defects	369
24	Medical Genetics and Related Birth Defects	385
	Challenge Exam	401
	Index	427

Preface

This book evolved from a series of handouts given to first-year medical students taking my Human Developmental Anatomy course at George Washington University Medical School. I have written a book that I hope develops the six concepts that I had in mind.

- First, I wanted to write a comprehensive yet concise description of human developmental anatomy that would help students understand concepts encountered in other anatomic disciplines. For example, I hope that my account of the development of the gastrointestinal system will make it easier for students to master the intricacies of the lesser omentum and epiploic foramen.
- Second, I wanted to write a textbook that contained information about the gross organogenesis of organ systems and also contained details of the histogenesis of certain organs, especially those whose complexities of histologic development reveal important features of the functional development of the embryo and fetus.
- Third, I wanted to write an up-to-date textbook that would contain accurate, modern descriptions of the formation of certain organ systems not covered adequately in more traditional textbooks of human embryology. For example, when this was written, no textbooks were available that contained clear, modern descriptions of the formation and development of the immune system. This book describes the functional differentiation of both the organs (lymph nodes, spleen, and thymus) and the complex and essential cellular elements of the immune system, without which no medical student can be adequately prepared for current medical practice.
- Fourth, I wanted to set the stage for complex descriptions of the development of systems by beginning each chapter with an overview of the development, followed by a brief section on the anatomy and function of the system (for those students who are learning or reviewing developmental anatomy before gross anatomy or microscopic anatomy). This is followed by a clear, concise, in-depth description of the developmental anatomy of that organ system.
- Fifth, I wanted to include material not always found in textbooks of embryology and have done so because of the obvious medical relevance of the material. Human development is a continuous process that begins with the fertilization of the ovum by a spermatozoon. (The formation of gametes themselves is also a complex developmental process.) I have rather arbitrarily chosen birth as the end of the developmental period and have considered a number of topics that are caused

by developmental defects but are not usually expressed until the immediate perinatal period. I have not covered the developmental anatomy of childhood, adolescence, or aging because that material is beyond the scope of most developmental anatomy courses.
- Sixth, I wanted to include a brief discussion of human genetics, particularly as it pertains to recurrence risks for certain congenital anomalies. This is not meant to substitute for more rigorous treatments of the subject; rather, I hope that this discussion will supply a crucial background level of knowledge so that medical students, future physicians, can understand some of the common modes of genetic transmission of anomalies and be able to give future patients information about recurrence risks should they decide to have more children after the birth of an affected child.

Most chapters contain examples of common defects found in the development of a particular system, as well as simple descriptions of the therapeutic modalities currently in use. This information is intended primarily to evoke the students' interest in the material at hand and to provide a clinical rationale for covering the subject.

Kurt E. Johnson, Ph.D.
Washington, D.C.
April, 1989

Acknowledgments

My thanks go to the following people for their generous contributions to the progress of this work. They supplied specimens of human embryos, photographs of clinical examples of congenital anomalies, and sonograms of normal and abnormal conditions.

Frank D. Allan, Ph.D.
Department of Anatomy
The George Washington
  University Medical Center
Washington, D.C.

Teresita L. Angtuaco, M.D.
Department of Obstetrics
  and Gynecology
University of Arkansas for
  Medical Sciences
Little Rock, Arkansas

Frank A. Chervenak, M.D.
Department of Obstetrics
  and Gynecology
Mount Sinai School of Medicine
New York, New York

William J. Cochrane, M.D.
Private Practice
Washington, D.C.

Mary H. McGrath, M.D.
Department of Surgery
The George Washington
  University Medical Center
Washington, D.C.

Also, it was a great pleasure to work with Diane Abeloff and Gloria R. Hamilton, whose talents as medical illustrator and editor, respectively, helped immensely in the creation of this book.

In addition, I thank the following friends and colleagues for their support and understanding friendship: Bryant D. Chomiak, M.D., of Las Vegas, Nevada; Ralph L. Kramer, M.D., of Alexandria, Virginia; and Michael H. Silver, M.D., Ph.D., of Washington, D.C.

Finally, I thank my wife, Julie M. Okkema, M.D., for her constant love and support during the development of this project.

Kurt E. Johnson

Introduction

Human Developmental Anatomy is 1 of 11 basic science review books in the *National Medical Series for Independent Study*. This series has been designed to provide students and house officers, as well as physicians, with a concise but comprehensive instrument for self-evaluation and review within the basic sciences. Although *Human Developmental Anatomy* would be most useful for students preparing for the National Board of Medical Examiners examinations (Part I, FLEX, and FMGEMS), it should also be useful for students studying for course examinations. These books are not intended to replace the standard basic science texts but, rather, to complement them.

The books in this series present the core content of each basic science, using an outline format and featuring approximately 500 study questions. The questions are distributed throughout the book, at the end of each chapter and in a challenge examination at the end of the text. In addition, each question is accompanied by the correct answer, a paragraph-length explanation of the correct answer, and specific reference to the outline points under which the information necessary to answer the question can be found.

We have chosen an outline format to allow maximum ease in retrieving information, assuming that the time available to the reader is limited. Considerable editorial time has been spent to ensure that the information required by all medical school curricula has been included and that the question format parallels that of the National Board examinations. We feel that the combination of the outline and the Board-type study questions provides a unique teaching device.

We hope you will find this series interesting, relevant, and challenging. The author as well as the staff at Harwal Publishing Company/Wiley Medical welcome your comments and suggestions.

1
Introduction and General Aspects of Development

I. CLINICAL DISCIPLINES RELATED TO EMBRYOLOGY. A knowledge of embryology is particularly important in several clinical disciplines.

  A. Obstetrics. In obstetrics and a good deal of gynecology, the "patient" is really two intimately associated individuals, mother and fetus.

    1. The mother may carry a fetus with a **congenital anomaly**.

    2. The mother may have a completely normal fetus in an **abnormal implantation site**; for example, ectopically in the uterine tubes.

    3. The **placenta** may be in an **abnormal location**; for example, across the cervical os, as in **placenta previa**.

  B. Pediatrics

    1. Many diseases in children are due to **congenital birth defects.** These may be as minor as a pigmented nevus or may be much more severe and life-threatening, as in the case of **anencephaly** (failure of development of the brain and skull).

    2. Congenital defects may also be biochemical or cellular defects. For example, a child may be born with an immunodeficiency disease, and may appear morphologically normal but may prove to be subject to repeated and potentially fatal infections soon after birth.

    3. Pediatricians often must console and counsel parents of children afflicted with congenital anomalies. A knowledge of embryology is of importance, because it allows the physician to
      a. Explain the disorder to the parents
      b. Discuss the child's prognosis
      c. Explain what may have caused the anomaly (an important point in psychological counseling)
      d. Discuss the possibility of a recurrence of the affliction in subsequent children

  C. Surgery

    1. Surgeons are frequently confronted with **normal anatomic variations** in surgical patients, and these usually have an embryologic basis. For example:
      a. Supernumerary renal arteries may arise during the development of the kidney.
      b. The ducts draining the biliary apparatus and the pancreas show several important anatomic variants due to minor differences in embryonic organogenesis.

    2. Surgeons are often called upon to correct **congenital defects**, such as a cleft lip and palate.

II. DEFINITIONS OF SOME COMMON ANATOMIC TERMS. Throughout this book, standard anatomic terms will be used constantly. Therefore, some definitions are in order. The various terms are illustrated in Figure 1-1.

  A. Anatomic adjectives. These are pairs of opposites.

    1. Superior and **inferior** refer to structures that are **above** or **below** one another. Thus, the head is superior to the rump, and the rump is inferior to the head.

    2. Cranial (rostral) and **caudal** refer to structures that are **toward the head** and **toward the rump** of the embryo, respectively. Thus, the eyes are cranial to the kidneys, and the kidneys are caudal to the eyes.

2 Human Developmental Anatomy

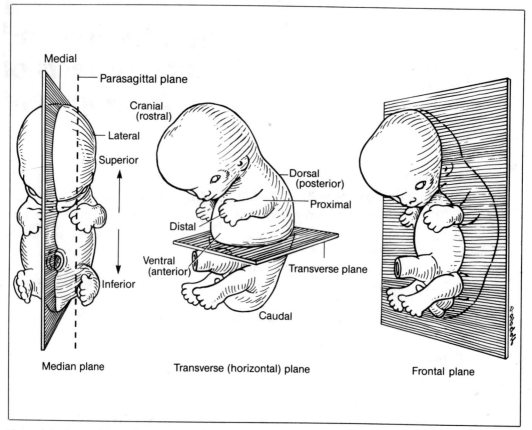

Figure 1-1. Commonly used anatomic terms as they apply to the human embryo and fetus. The principal anatomic planes of section and anatomic adjectives are indicated.

    3. Dorsal and **ventral** refer to structures that are **toward the back** or **toward the front** of the embryo, respectively. Thus, the spinal cord is dorsal to the liver, and the liver is ventral to the spinal cord. In most instances, **dorsal** and **posterior** will be synonymous; similarly, **ventral** and **anterior** will be synonymous.

    4. Proximal and **distal** refer to structures that are **toward the point of origin or attachment**, or **away from the point of origin or attachment**, respectively. Thus, the wrist is proximal to the fingers, and the fingers are distal to the wrist. The trachea is proximal to the bronchi, and the bronchi are distal to the trachea.

    5. Medial and **lateral** refer to structures that are **toward the midline** or **away from the midline**, respectively. Thus, the nose is medial to the ear, and the ear is lateral to the nose.

B. Anatomic planes

    1. The **median (midsagittal) plane** passes through the axis of bilateral symmetry of the embryo. The median plane divides the body into left and right halves. **Parasagittal planes** are parallel to the median plane but do not pass through the median plane.

    2. Frontal planes are vertical, longitudinal, and perpendicular to the midsagittal plane. The frontal plane divides the body into **anterior (ventral)** and **posterior (dorsal)** halves.

    3. Coronal planes are perpendicular to both the midsagittal and the longitudinal plane. Coronal planes pass through the body in a plane like that defined by a crown sitting on the top of the head.

    4. Transverse (horizontal) planes are perpendicular to the long axis of a structure. A transverse plane of the arm would not be parallel to a transverse plane of the trunk, because the long axes of the two structures are not parallel to one another.

    5. Longitudinal sections pass through a plane parallel to the long axis of a structure.

III. BASIC DEVELOPMENTAL CONCEPTS

A. Growth

1. **Early growth of the embryo**
   a. The human embryo begins its development as a single cell about 100 µm in diameter.
   b. At first, this single cell divides extensively without much increase in volume.
   c. Soon, however, the numbers of cells and the volume of the entire embryo begins to increase.
   d. As the embryo assimilates nutrients from the maternal circulation, its mass increases dramatically as it grows. Growth consists essentially of an increase in mass and volume of the embryo.

2. **Mechanisms of growth.** Increase in mass and volume occurs by several mechanisms.
   a. Increase in cell number by cellular proliferation, with maintenance of cell size.
      (1) Proliferation is nearly ubiquitous early in development.
      (2) In the adult, some organs (e.g., the brain) have no proliferative cells, while other organs (e.g., the basal layer of the skin) contain cells that remain proliferative throughout life.
   b. Increase in extracellular material. A bone, for example, grows larger in part by deposition of calcified extracellular matrix.
   c. Growth of cavities within the embryo. The ventricles of the brain, for example, expand during development.

B. Differentiation

1. Differentiation is the process whereby the complexity of the adult organism arises from the simplicity of the zygote.
   a. The whole human organism develops from a single cell, the **zygote**, which contains a set of chromosomes from the father and a bit of cytoplasm and a set of chromosomes from the mother.
   b. It is truly wondrous that this one cell can produce a complex organism with a brain, teeth, several kinds of muscle, a complex gastrointestinal system, and many other intricately integrated systems.

2. All this complexity springs from the incredibly diverse potential **encoded within the genome** of the cell. Differentiation is due to **differential gene activity.**
   a. The zygote contains the complete chromosomal complement of the adult organism.
   b. Further, all of the somatic cells of the organism, despite their great structural and functional differences, contain essentially the same genetic material (i.e., the same genes).
   c. Differentiation results because different portions of the genetic material become expressed to a greater extent in certain cells. That is, different genes become activated selectively.
      (1) The activation of selected genes results in the production of **cell-specific proteins** which define each differentiated cell type.
      (2) This spectrum of proteins is determined by the translation of the nuclear genetic code.

3. A differentiated cell is best described on the basis of its morphology, which in turn depends on the spectrum of proteins that it produces. Differentiated cells accumulate characteristic arrays of proteins in their cytoplasm and they also often secrete characteristic materials into their surroundings to create a tissue-specific extracellular matrix.

4. **Examples of cell differentiation**
   a. Differentiation of the embryonic **mesenchyme**, which occurs early in development, suggests the variety of cells that can result.
      (1) Mesenchyme is an embryonic connective tissue that forms during early development.
      (2) Mesenchymal cells are relatively undifferentiated when compared to the differentiated cells that arise from mesenchyme, such as **osteocytes** (cells of bone) and **chondrocytes** (cells of cartilage). Figure 1-2 shows some of the variety of cell types which arise from mesenchymal cells by differentiation.
   b. **Chondrocytes** differentiate from mesenchyme. The process exemplifies the **mechanisms of differentiation.**
      (1) An undifferentiated mesenchymal cell becomes committed to the chondrocyte pathway. As a result of this commitment, the chondrocyte begins to secrete large

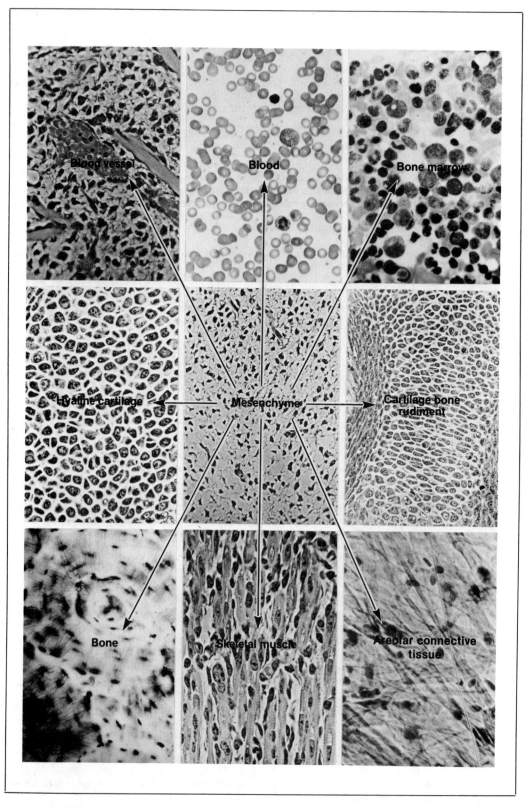

Figure 1-2. Differentiation of embryonic mesenchyme. This undifferentiated connective tissue can form many highly specialized tissues, as indicated in the figure.

amounts of several kinds of proteins and other macromolecules characteristic of cartilage, such as
- **(a)** Collagen
- **(b)** Cartilage proteoglycan
- **(c)** Hyaluronic acid
- **(d)** Glycoproteins

(2) In order to synthesize these macromolecules, a chondrocyte must first
- **(a) Differentiate** by elaborating the appropriate synthetic enzymes
- **(b)** Organize these enzymes into secretory organelles, such as the endoplasmic reticulum and the Golgi apparatus

(3) Other cells also synthesize collagen and proteoglycan, but only the chondrocyte manufactures and secretes large amounts of collagen and cartilage proteoglycan.

  c. **Skeletal muscle and cardiac muscle cells** are also derived from mesenchyme (see also Chapter 9 section VII).
   (1) Their differentiation is characterized by the synthesis and intracellular accumulation of large amounts of the **proteins characteristic of muscle cells**, including
   - **(a)** Actin
   - **(b)** Myosin
   - **(c)** Troponin
   - **(d)** Tropomyosin
   - **(e)** α-Actinin

   (2) These proteins are then arranged within the cells into organized semicrystalline arrays called **sarcomeres.** This arrangement increases the functional efficiency of the muscle proteins for generating contractions.
   (3) Muscle proteins are also found in nonmuscle cells, but they are neither found in such large quantities nor arranged into sarcomeres.

  d. **Differentiation of nervous tissue** provides an example of the **integrated function** of several differentiated cell types (see also Chapter 11 section II).
   (1) The property of excitability or response to a stimulus is one of the fundamental properties of living cells.
   (2) In man, nervous tissue has become highly differentiated to utilize this property of excitability for detection of changes in the environment, integration of different components of the body, and the complex processes of mentation.
   - **(a)** The primitive embryonic **neuroepithelium** contains a group of undifferentiated, highly proliferative cells.
   - **(b)** Among these cells is an **undifferentiated stem cell population** that continues to divide and gives rise to a series of progeny that undergo subsequent differentiation.
   - **(c)** The dividing cells of the neuroepithelium produce **neuroblasts** and **glioblasts.**
     - **(i) Neuroblasts** differentiate into a fantastic array of **neurons** (Fig. 1-3), the main functional communicating cells of the nervous system.
     - **(ii) Glioblasts** differentiate into a variety of **glial cells** that subserve a supportive function in the nervous system.

5. **Consequences of differentiation**
  a. The end result of differentiation is the production of a complex array of cell types, each with peculiar morphologic features closely related to its specialized role in the overall economy of the organism.
  b. In many instances, there is an antagonism between proliferation and differentiation.
   (1) Often, highly proliferative cells, such as those found in the embryonic neuroepithelium or in the basal layer of the skin, are undifferentiated.
   (2) Highly differentiated cells, such as erythrocytes or motor neurons in the spinal cord, usually lose the ability to proliferate.
  c. In other instances, differentiated cells (e.g., chondrocytes) continue to proliferate even after they are differentiated.
  d. Some tissues have the ability to **regenerate** and thus replace defects caused by traumatic injury. Generally speaking, regenerating cells lose their differentiated characteristics, proliferate, and then reacquire their differentiated characteristics.

C. Morphogenesis

1. Morphogenesis is a developmental process involving **changes in the morphology, or form,** of embryonic structures. During morphogenesis, new shapes arise from simpler patterns of cellular organization.

2. **Examples of morphogenesis.** During early human development, several key morphogenetic events are involved in the conversion of a **flat, two-layered (bilaminar) disk** into a

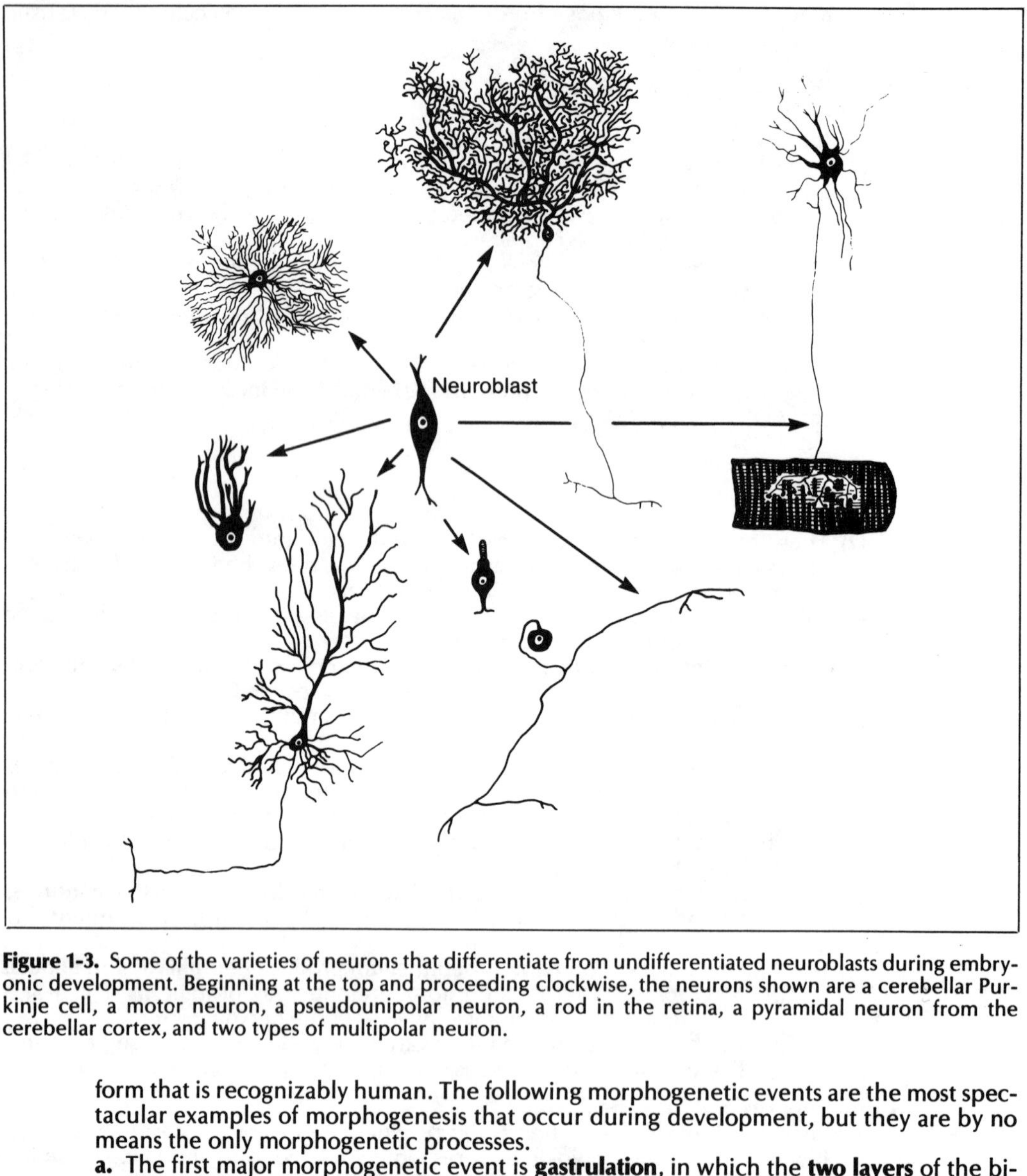

Figure 1-3. Some of the varieties of neurons that differentiate from undifferentiated neuroblasts during embryonic development. Beginning at the top and proceeding clockwise, the neurons shown are a cerebellar Purkinje cell, a motor neuron, a pseudounipolar neuron, a rod in the retina, a pyramidal neuron from the cerebellar cortex, and two types of multipolar neuron.

form that is recognizably human. The following morphogenetic events are the most spectacular examples of morphogenesis that occur during development, but they are by no means the only morphogenetic processes.
  a. The first major morphogenetic event is **gastrulation**, in which the **two layers** of the bilaminar disk become the **three primary germ layers**:
    (1) Ectoderm
    (2) Mesoderm
    (3) Endoderm
  b. The second major event is **primary embryonic induction**, during which the mesoderm causes (**induces**) the ectoderm to form the primitive central nervous system (CNS). After induction, the CNS forms by the process of **neurulation**, in which the **neural plate**, an open flattened sheet, thickens and then rolls up to form the closed **neural tube** (Fig. 1-4).
  c. During **flexion and growth of the amnion**, the initially flat embryo is converted into a **tubular structure** with the **basic vertebrate body plan.**
    (1) The laterally placed body walls grow ventrally and medially.
    (2) Next, they are brought together in the ventral midline.
    (3) A recognizable head and tail begin to appear, sculpted by growth of the head and tail folds of the amnion, respectively.
  d. The **limbs** are formed (Fig. 1-5) by a series of morphogenetic events involving cell proliferation, changes in cell shape, and even cell death. Cell differentiation also plays a key role in the development of the limbs.

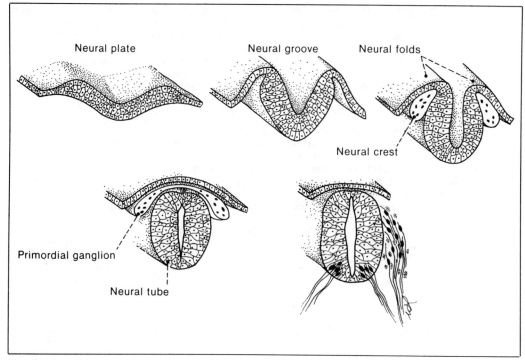

Figure 1-4. An example of morphogenesis. Formation of the cylindrical neural tube by folding and fusion of the flat neural plate. (Adapted from DeMyer W: *NMS Neuroanatomy.* Media, Pa., Harwal/Wiley, 1988, p 33.)

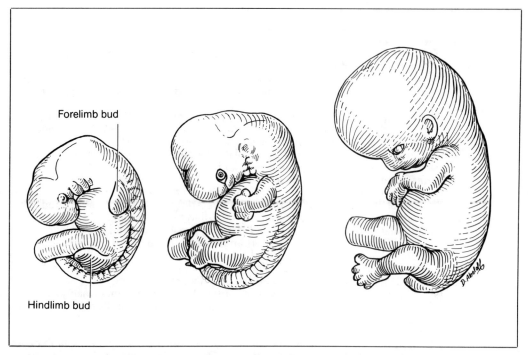

Figure 1-5. An example of morphogenesis. The limbs begin as simple swellings on the flanks. By the process of morphogenesis, involving striking changes in shape, the complex definitive limbs are sculpted from simple limb buds.

- (1) The limbs first arise on the flanks of the embryo as uncomplicated mounds of mesenchymal cells covered by an epithelium of the prospective epidermis.
- (2) **Cytodifferentiation** occurs as undifferentiated mesenchymal cells proliferate, condense, and develop into specialized cells.
  - (a) Connective tissue fibroblasts differentiate and form ligaments, tendons, and fascia.
  - (b) Chondroblasts differentiate and form chondrocytes and cartilage.
  - (c) Osteoblasts differentiate and form osteocytes and bone.
  - (d) Myoblasts differentiate and form myocytes and muscle.

3. **Morphogenesis, cytodifferentiation, and growth**
   a. In this discussion, cytodifferentiation and morphogenesis have been described as if they are unrelated processes. In fact, they usually occur simultaneously in one organ system, as outlined above for limb development.
   b. **Cytodifferentiation** sometimes involves complex **cytomorphogenesis**, as in the case of **spermiogenesis**.
      (1) As a spermatid becomes differentiated into a spermatozoon, its shape changes from a rounded, nonmotile cell into an extremely long, streamlined cell.
      (2) Moreover, the unicellular sperm is equipped with two subcellular organelles, a flagellum for movement in the female reproductive system and an acrosome for penetration of the layers surrounding the ovum.
   c. Similarly, **growth** is often an important component of **morphogenesis**.
      (1) Intense cell division takes place in the epiphyseal plate during development of a long bone, such as the femur.
      (2) Intense cell division occurs nearly everywhere in the development of the central nervous system.
      (3) In areas where there are differences in the rates of cell division, bulges and folds form, giving shape to the newly developing structure.

D. Inductive epithelial–mesenchymal interactions during organogenesis

1. The induction of the central nervous system during neurulation (see section III C 2) is only one of many instances in which tissues interact and induce morphogenesis in one another. **Reciprocal inductive interactions** between an embryonic epithelium and associated mesenchymal cells also play a major role in the formation of many organs, a process known as **organogenesis**.
2. **Examples of reciprocal inductive interactions**
   a. **Formation of the lungs**
      (1) The epithelial components of the airways of the lungs form from an **endodermal diverticulum** of the foregut, which grows and branches extensively, penetrating into the surrounding undifferentiated mesenchymal tissue. The **mesenchymal tissue** induces the growth, branching, and differentiation of this endodermal diverticulum.
      (2) By **reciprocal interaction**, the respiratory diverticulum induces the surrounding mesenchymal cells to differentiate into connective tissue, cartilage, smooth muscle, and blood vessels characteristic of the respiratory system.
      (3) If either component failed to stimulate the other in a reciprocal fashion, no lungs would form. **Pulmonary agenesis** would result.
   b. **Formation of the metanephric kidney**
      (1) The epithelial rudiment of the kidney, the **ureteric bud**, is an epithelial diverticulum of the mesonephric duct. The ureteric bud is closely associated with an undifferentiated mass of mesenchyme called the **metanephric blastema**.
      (2) Stimulated by the metanephric blastema, the ureteric bud branches extensively and differentiates into the ureters and collecting tubules of the kidney.
      (3) Stimulated by the ureteric bud, the metanephric blastema develops into the nephrons, which consist of the glomeruli, Bowman's capsule, and the rest of the convoluted and straight renal tubules that actually produce urine.
      (4) As with the lung, no kidney would form if there were an abnormality of the interaction between ureteric bud and metanephric blastema. **Renal agenesis** would result.
   c. **Limb development**
      (1) An intricate epithelial–mesenchymal interaction also occurs during limb development. This has been demonstrated by experimental manipulations of the ectoderm and mesodermally derived mesenchyme in developing limbs.
         (a) The vast bulk of the tissues in a limb, namely the bones, cartilages, ligaments, tendons, and muscles, are all derived from **limb bud mesenchyme**.

- (b) If the ectoderm from a forelimb is combined with the mesenchyme from a hindlimb, the experimental limb will develop as a hindlimb.
- (c) The experiments show that the **ectodermal component** of the developing limb is also crucial for normal development.
- (d) The most distal portion of the limb bud is covered by a group of cells known collectively as the **apical ectodermal ridge (AER)**.
- (e) If the AER is surgically removed from a developing limb and not replaced, the proximal portions of the limb will develop but the more distal portions will fail to develop.
- (f) If two AERs are transplanted into a limb, then two distal portions of that limb will form.
- (g) If the AER from a hindlimb is transplanted into a forelimb where the forelimb AER has been removed, then a composite structure will develop that has proximal forelimb structures and distal hindlimb structures.

(2) Clearly then, the **mesenchymal elements** of the limb bud are essential for the formation of much of the substance of the limb, while the **apical ectodermal ridge** is essential both for the continued development of the mesenchymal elements of the limb bud and for the kinds of mesenchymal elements which are actually formed.

d. Many **other structures** are also formed by reciprocal inductive interactions between an embryonic epithelium and associated mesenchymal cells. Examples are:
(1) Teeth, hair, and nails
(2) Mammary glands
(3) Salivary glands and pancreas

IV. FUNCTIONAL ANATOMY OF THE MALE REPRODUCTIVE SYSTEM

A. **Gross anatomy** (Fig. 1-6)

1. The **testes** are paired structures contained in an outpocketing of the body wall, the **scrotum**.
2. Each testis is drained by a convoluted duct called the **epididymis (ductus epididymidis)**, which in turn drains into the **ductus deferens (vas deferens)**.

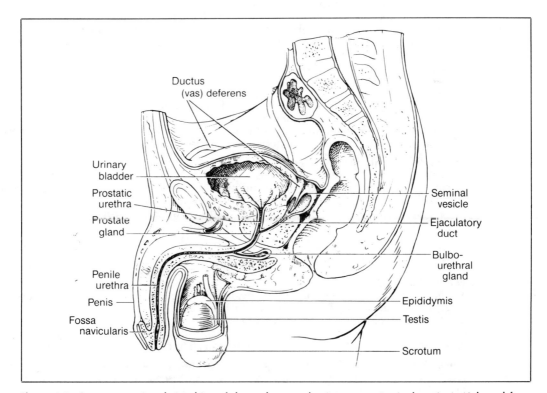

Figure 1-6. Gross anatomic relationships of the male reproductive system (sagittal section). (Adapted from Abeloff D: *Medical Art: Graphics for Use*. Baltimore, Williams and Wilkins, 1982.)

3. Each ductus deferens extends from the epididymis to the ejaculatory duct.
   a. The ductus deferens travels toward the body wall in the spermatic cord, passes through the inguinal rings, and enters the body wall proper. Next, it loops over the ureters and passes downward and medially.
   b. Just before entering the prostate gland, the ductus deferens is dilated into an **ampullary portion**, and just below this dilation there is a diverticulum of the ductus deferens, the **seminal vesicle**.
   c. The ductus deferens penetrates the **prostate gland** and is connected to the prostatic urethra by an **ejaculatory duct**.
4. The **prostatic urethra** drains into the **penile urethra**.
5. The **prostate gland** is a mass of fibromuscular tissue at the base of the bladder.
   a. The prostate gland is pierced by the ejaculatory ducts and the urethra.
   b. The urinary and reproductive systems come together at the prostate gland and share a common excurrent duct, the **urethra**.
6. The **penis** is a part of the male reproductive system and the male urinary system.

B. Functional microscopic anatomy

1. **The testes. Spermatogenesis**, the production of male gametes, occurs in the testes for the entire adult life of the male.
   a. The testis is surrounded by a tough connective tissue capsule known as the **tunica albuginea**.
   b. On the posterior aspect of the testis is the **mediastinum testis**.
      (1) Here, connective tissue elements, blood vessels, nerves, and lymphatic vessels enter the organ.
      (2) The connective tissue elements penetrate deep into the testis from the capsule, forming septa which divide the testis into a series of lobules. Each lobule contains many tortuously coiled seminiferous tubules.
   c. The **seminiferous tubules** are lined by a complex, unique epithelial layer of **Sertoli cells** with the spermatogenic cell lines embedded in them.
      (1) The **spermatogenic cells** are, successively, spermatogonia, primary spermatocytes, secondary spermatocytes, spermatids, and spermatozoa.
      (2) Spermatogenesis is described in detail in Chapter 2, section V.
   d. Between the seminiferous tubules are the interstitial **Leydig cells**, which produce large quantities of the steroid male sex hormone **testosterone**. In the adult male, testosterone is required for the maintenance of several activities:
      (1) Male secondary sexual characterisitcs
      (2) Spermatogenesis
      (3) Libido
   e. The seminiferous tubules connect to **tubuli recti**, which then empty into an anastomosing network of channels known collectively as the **rete testis**. The channels of the rete testis in turn are connected to the epididymis by **efferent ductules**. All of these passages are lined by cells designed to propel spermatozoa into the epididymis.
2. **The epididymis and ductus deferens**
   a. The epididymis and ductus deferens are lined by tall columnar cells with nonmotile cilia (**stereocilia**) that are part of a pseudostratified epithelium. There are smooth muscle cells in the walls of the epididymis and ductus deferens.
   b. Several **functions** are thought to be associated with these two structures.
      (1) Propulsion of spermatozoa toward the prostate
      (2) Modification of secretions of testes
      (3) Maturation of spermatozoa
      (4) Production of some components of semen
3. **The seminal fluid**
   a. The urethral orifice near the urinary bladder is surrounded by a complex network of glands that secrete their contents into the urethra.
   b. Most of the volume of the seminal ejaculate is the result of the secretory activity of the prostate gland.
   c. The seminal vesicles produce the remaining small fraction of the seminal fluid.
4. **The bulbourethral glands (Cowper's glands)** are located along the penile urethra in close proximity to the prostate gland. They produce a clear, viscous lubricating fluid produced during sexual arousal.

5. **The penis**
   a. The penis is an erectile organ with two major **functions**:
      (1) The introduction of semen into the female reproductive tract during sexual intercourse
      (2) The elimination of urine from the body
   b. The penis has three columns of **erectile tissue**, the paired dorsal **corpora cavernosa** and a single ventral midline **corpus spongiosum** which carries the urethra.
      (1) These three bodies are bound together by a tough fibrous connective tissue capsule, the **tunica albuginea**, and they are covered with thin skin with unusually rich sensory innervation.
      (2) During erection, the blood flow into the venous sinuses in the erectile tissue is far greater than the outflow, causing the erectile tissue to fill with blood and become tumescent. When the inward blood flow decreases and the outward drainage increases, tumescence is lost.
   c. The **penile urethra** is lined by a mixture of either stratified columnar epithelium or pseudostratified epithelium proximally and by stratified squamous epithelium distally, at the **fossa navicularis** (a dilation just proximal to the penile meatus) and at the penile meatus.

V. FUNCTIONAL ANATOMY OF THE FEMALE REPRODUCTIVE SYSTEM

A. **Functional gross anatomy**
   1. **The key organs of the female reproductive system** (Fig. 1-7)
      a. The **ovaries** are paired organs dedicated to the production of ova. In the postpubertal female, the ovary is the site of active oogenesis until menopause.
      b. The **oviducts (uterine tubes, fallopian tubes)** convey ova and pre-embryos toward the uterus, and spermatozoa toward the distal parts of the tubes.

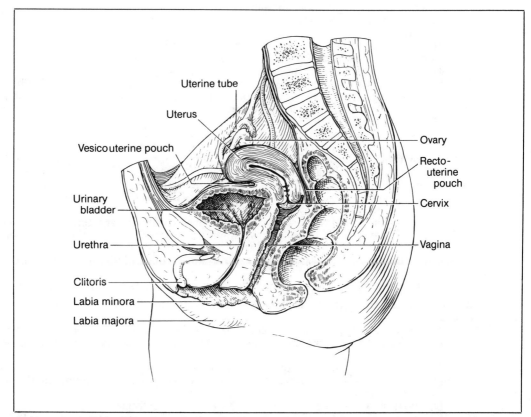

Figure 1-7. Gross anatomic relationships of the female reproductive system (sagittal section). (Adapted from Abeloff D: *Medical Art: Graphics for Use*. Baltimore, Williams and Wilkins, 1982.)

c. The **uterus** is the site for implantation of the pre-embryo and for the subsequent embryonic and fetal development.
d. The **cervix** is a narrow passageway between the vagina and the uterus.
e. The **vagina** is both an entryway and an exit for the female reproductive system.
   (1) Spermatozoa are deposited here and make their way into the uterine tubes via the cervix and uterus.
   (2) After a fetus (or the menstrual flow) is expelled from the uterus, it passes through the cervix and vagina and out of the body.
f. The female **external genitalia** consist of the **clitoris**, the **labia minora**, and the **labia majora**. These organs function during sexual activity, and the labia also serve partially to close or to enshroud the vagina.

2. **Important mesenteries and ligaments in the female reproductive system**
   a. The **broad ligament**, a peritoneal fold, suspends the uterus and attaches it to the body wall. It also divides the pelvis into an anterior vesicouterine pouch and a posterior rectouterine pouch.
   b. The **suspensory ligament** of the ovary is also a peritoneal fold. It attaches to the tubal extremity of the ovary, covering the ovary and suspending it from the body wall.
   c. The **ovarian ligament** attaches the ovary to the superior lateral margin of the uterus.
   d. The **mesovarium** is a fold of the broad ligament which encloses both the ovary and the ovarian ligament.
   e. The **mesosalpinx** is the mesentery which suspends the uterine tubes. It runs laterally away from the body of the uterus along the superior border of the broad ligament.

B. **Functional microscopic anatomy**

1. **The ovaries**
   a. The ovaries have three **coverings**.
      (1) Both ovaries are covered by **peritoneal folds**.
      (2) On the surface of the ovary is a **mesothelial covering**. It is a simple cuboidal epithelium called the **germinal epithelium**.
      (3) The **capsule** of the ovary is a thin connective tissue capsule known as the **tunica albuginea**.
   b. The ovary has a **hilus** near its attachment to the suspensory ligament where it receives blood vessels, nerves, and lymphatic vessels.
   c. The ovary is divided into a **medulla** and a **cortex**.
      (1) The **medulla** is the central portion of the ovary. It is occupied by twisting blood vessels and a connective tissue stroma consisting of dense aggregates of fibroblasts, which also occupies much of the cortex.
      (2) The **cortex** surrounds the medulla.
         (a) The cortex contains stromal fibroblasts and ovarian follicles in various stages of development and **atresia** (i.e., programmed degeneration).
         (b) **Ovarian follicles** consist of a follicular epithelium composed of **granulosa cells**, surrounded by a basement membrane. Within the epithelium of each follicle is a developing **oocyte** (see Chapter 2, section IV C).
         (c) Just peripheral to the follicle are the **theca interna** (a rich capillary plexus) and the **theca externa**.
            (i) The **thecal cells** are differentiated stromal cells and are **steroidogenic**: they are involved in estrogen synthesis prior to ovulation and they differentiate into thecal lutein cells of the corpus luteum after ovulation.
            (ii) The network of capillaries conveys the estrogen into the systemic circulation.
         (d) The outer boundary of the ovarian cortex comprises the **tunica albuginea**.

2. **The oviducts [uterine (fallopian) tubes].** The oviducts extend from the uterus toward the ovaries.
   a. Moving distally, away from the uterus and toward the ovary, the **lumen** of the uterine tube becomes larger and its **mucosa** develops into a series of folds of increasing complexity.
   b. The uterine tube has several different **segments**.
      (1) The **interstitial uterine tube** attaches the tube to the uterus and penetrates the wall of the uterus.
      (2) The **isthmus** attaches the interstitial portion to the ampulla.
      (3) The **ampulla** is more dilated than the isthmus and has more complex mucosal folds. **Fertilization** is thought to occur in the ampullary portion of the uterine tubes.
      (4) The **infundibulum** is the dilated, funnel-shaped portion at the terminal end of the

ampulla. The mucosal folds in the infundibular portion are labyrinthine in their complexity.
  (5) The distal portion of the infundibulum opens into the peritoneal cavity near the ovary and has many fingerlike projections called **fimbria**.
c. All regions of the uterine tube have certain **histologic similarities**.
  (1) The outer layer of the uterine tubes, the **serosa**, consists of a simple squamous mesothelium and a thin layer of connective tissue.
  (2) Beneath the serosa is the **tunica muscularis**, consisting of several layers of smooth muscle cells. **Peristaltic waves** of smooth muscle contraction are thought to be important in three ways:
    (a) For placing the tubes in close proximitiy to the ovary during ovulation
    (b) For distal sperm transport
    (c) For proximal transport of the ovum and conceptus after fertilization
  (3) The **mucosa** lining the lumen of the uterine tube consists of a simple columnar epithelium with a majority of ciliated cells and a few tall secretory cells. The **cilia** aid in transporting the ova and the conceptus proximally toward the uterus.

3. **The uterus**
  a. The **wall of the uterus** contains three **subdivisions**.
    (1) An outer **perimetrium** is covered in most places by a mesothelium and a thin connective tissue capsule.
    (2) A middle **myometrium** consists of several thick coats of smooth muscle cells interwoven with stromal fibroblasts and many blood vessels that are branches of the uterine artery.
    (3) An inner **endometrium** consists of a simple columnar endometrial epithelium composed predominantly of secretory cells, with a small number of interspersed ciliated cells. The endometrium also has a connective tissue stroma, the **lamina propria**, beneath the epithelium, and contains many deep glandular clefts.
  b. **Endometrial layers and the menstrual cycle**
    (1) The endometrium has two layers.
      (a) The **superficial layer** is called the **functionalis** because it grows, sloughs, and reforms with each menstrual cycle (the sloughing of the functionalis and loss of blood occurs during **menstruation**). This layer varies in thickness from as much as 7 mm just before the onset of the menses to as little as 1 mm just after menstruation.
      (b) The **deep layer** of the endometrium is called the **basalis**. It is not sloughed during menstruation. The new functionalis which forms after the menses are completed is derived from the basalis.
    (2) The endometrium undergoes **cyclic changes** during the **menstrual cycle**. These can be divided into two distinct **phases**.
      (a) The **follicular phase** begins after the menses are completed.
        (i) The functionalis grows increasingly thicker, under the influence of ovarian **estrogen** derived from the growing follicle.
        (ii) Endometrial glands grow in length and complexity during this phase.
      (b) The **secretory phase** is initiated by formation of the corpus luteum after ovulation, and prepares the endometrium for potential pregnancy.
        (i) After **ovulation** and the formation of the ovarian **corpus luteum**, the endometrial glands begin to secrete substances that are thought to nourish the developing conceptus.
        (ii) The corpus luteum secretes **progesterone**, which is required for maintenance of the secretory phase.
      (c) If **no fertilization** occurs, the lack of hormonal stimulation from a developing conceptus causes a regression of the corpus luteum and a loss of progesterone to support the endometrium, leading to **menstruation** as the functionalis breaks down and is expelled from the body.

4. **The cervix**
  a. The upper portion of the cervical canal has a simple columnar epithelium with glands that secrete cervical mucus.
  b. The lower portion of the cervix has a stratified squamous epithelium that is continuous with the vaginal epithelium.

5. **The vagina**
  a. The vagina is lined by a stratified squamous epithelium. It is richly vascularized but lacks glands.
  b. During sexual arousal, vascular transudates contribute to fluids lubricating the vagina.

STUDY QUESTIONS

Directions: Each question below contains five suggested answers. Choose the **one best** response to each question.

1. Embryonic mesenchyme can differentiate into all of the following cell types EXCEPT

(A) chondrocytes
(B) osteocytes
(C) fibroblasts
(D) motor neurons
(E) adipocytes

2. All of the following statements about anatomic relationships of body parts make proper use of anatomic terms EXCEPT

(A) the fingers are distal to the elbow
(B) the umbilicus is ventral to the spinal cord
(C) the nose is medial to the ears
(D) the foot is inferior to the head
(E) the bronchi are proximal to the trachea

Directions: The groups of questions below consist of lettered choices followed by several numbered items. For each numbered item select the **one** lettered choice with which it is **most** closely associated. Each lettered choice may be used once, more than once, or not at all.

Questions 3–9

For each functional or morphologic description of components of the female reproductive system below, choose the appropriate lettered structure in the accompanying diagram.

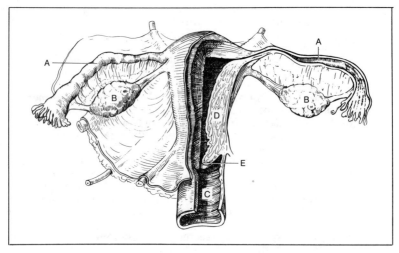

(Adapted from Abeloff D: *Medical Art: Graphics for Use.* Baltimore, Williams and Wilkins, 1982.)

3. This component contains structures that secrete progesterone after ovulation

4. This component contains a mucosa that deteriorates after ovulation if fertilization does not occur

5. This component contains a luminal lining where ciliated cells outnumber secretory cells

6. This component is covered by a simple cuboidal epithelium

7. This component is lined by a stratified squamous epithelium but lacks glands

8. This component contains a zone where there is a transition from simple columnar epithelium to stratified squamous epithelium

9. This component contains the site where fertilization normally occurs

Questions 10–15

For each functional or morphologic description of components of the male reproductive system below, choose the appropriate lettered structure in the accompanying diagram.

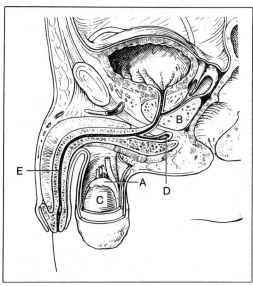

(Adapted from Abeloff D: *Medical Art: Graphics for Use*. Baltimore, Williams and Wilkins, 1982.)

10. This component contains a duct lined by a pseudostratified epithelium where some cells have stereocilia. In histologic section, this structure looks like a honeycomb of channels but actually consists of a highly convoluted tubule.

11. This component contains many testosterone-secreting cells

12. This component produces most of the volume of the ejaculate

13. This component produces a clear, viscous lubricant during sexual arousal

14. This component contains a luminal epithelium that is stratified squamous, stratified columnar, or pseudostratified in its different parts

15. This component conveys spermatozoa from the testis to the ductus deferens

ANSWERS AND EXPLANATIONS

1. The answer is D. *(III B 4)* Embryonic mesenchyme is largely derived from the intraembryonic mesoderm. It is a loose areolar connective tissue characteristic of the embryo prior to the differentiation of mesenchymal derivatives such as cartilage, bone, fat, and tendons. Embryonic mesenchyme can differentiate into cartilage, which contains chondrocytes; bone, which contains osteocytes; tendons, which contain fibroblasts; and fat, which contains adipocytes. Motor neurons are derived from the neuroepithelium, which is an ectodermal derivative.

2. The answer is E. *(II A)* There is often some confusion about the use of the terms proximal and distal. Proximal means nearest to the point of origin of an organ system or nearest to the trunk. Distal is the opposite of proximal. Thus, for example, the shoulder is the point of origin of the upper limb. Therefore the elbow is proximal to the fingers, which are distal to the elbow. In the respiratory system, the nasopharynx can be considered to be the point of origin of the trachea, bronchi, and lungs. Thus, the trachea is proximal to the bronchi, which are distal to the trachea. Inferior and superior mean below and above. Dorsal and ventral mean toward and away from the back. Medial and lateral mean toward and away from the plane of bilateral symmetry.

3–9. The answers are: 3-B, 4-D, 5-A, 6-B, 7-C, 8-E, 9-A. *(V B)* The diagram accompanying the questions shows the anatomic relations of the various organs in the female reproductive tract. The ovaries (B) contain ovarian follicles surrounded by stromal thecal cells. Follicular and thecal cells are involved in estrogen synthesis before ovulation and in progesterone synthesis once the follicle has been converted into a corpus luteum after ovulation. The ovaries are coated by a simple cuboidal (germinal) epithelium that is continuous with the simple squamous epithelium lining the rest of the peritoneal cavity. The uterine tubes (A) are lined by an epithelium consisting of many ciliated cells and a few secretory cells. Their walls have several layers of smooth muscle. The uterine tubes convey ova from the ovary to the uterus. Fertilization occurs in the uterine tubes (ampullary portion), and implantation occurs in the endometrium of the uterus (D). If no fertilization occurs, the corpus luteum regresses, progesterone levels fall, and the endometrium (the uterine mucosa) is sloughed during menstruation. The uterus is connected to the vagina (C) by the cervix (E). There is an epithelial transition in the cervical canal. Near the uterus, the cervical canal is lined by a simple columnar epithelium, whereas near the vagina it is lined by a stratified squamous (unkeratinized) epithelium much like that found in the vagina. The vagina (C) lacks glands. Fluid transudates are released from engorged blood vessels during sexual arousal.

10–15. The answers are: 10-A, 11-C, 12-B, 13-D, 14-E, 15-A. *(IV B)* The diagram accompanying the questions shows the anatomic relationships of the different components of the male reproductive system. The testes (C) contain the seminiferous tubules, where spermatogenesis occurs. Between the seminiferous tubules are the testosterone-secreting Leydig cells. Testosterone is required for spermatogenesis and maintenance of male secondary sexual characteristics. The epididymis (A) is a single, highly convoluted duct that conveys spermatozoa from the testes to the ductus (vas) deferens. Its luminal epithelium is a tall columnar pseudostratified epithelium equipped with apical stereocilia. There are many smooth muscle cells in the wall of the epididymis. The prostate gland (B) lies at the base of the bladder. It has many glands that contribute a secretion product that makes up most of the volume of the ejaculate. The bulbourethral (Cowper's) glands (D) lie at the base of the penis and secrete a clear, viscous lubricant which aids penetration of the vagina during sexual intercourse. The penis (E) contains the penile urethra, which is lined by a pseudostratified or stratified columnar epithelium proximally and a stratified squamous epithelium distally, in the fossa navicularis.

2
Gametogenesis

I. INTRODUCTION

A. The purpose of sexual reproduction

1. Most living systems in the natural universe contain sexually dimorphic adult organisms whose most important biologic function is sexual reproduction; that is, they are dedicated to producing the next generation of individuals.
2. Sexual reproduction involves the exchange of genetic material for **two simultaneous purposes**:
   a. Perpetuating individuals similar to the parental generation
   b. Providing the advantages that accrue to the species by mixing diverse genetic material
3. This dual purpose immediately creates a problem for the individual organism, namely, how to perpetuate the parental similarity while at the same time reducing inbreeding in a population.
   a. Extensive **inbreeding** can increase the frequency of deleterious recessive mutations. **Diversity** no doubt ensures the genetic health and perhaps the cultural health of the human race.
   b. Presumably, innate drives among young adults to breed with representatives of different groups of humans, as well as culturally determined incest taboos, represent a manifestation of a primal urge to avoid the degeneration of a population.

B. Cardinal features of gametogenesis

1. **Preservation of chromosome number**
   a. Sexual reproduction involves the merging of two **gametes**, ovum and spermatozoon, in the earliest stages of the development of a new individual.
   b. The **somatic cells** throughout an adult organism are, by and large, diploid; that is, the cells contain **two complete sets of chromosomes** and thus two complete copies of the genetic material characteristic of the organism.
   c. If gametes were also diploid, there would be a doubling of the chromosome number with each generation. Therefore, a mechanism has evolved for dividing the genetic material in two, namely, the **reduction division of meiosis**.
      (1) **Meiosis**, a process restricted to the germ cell lines of adults, provides a way for germ cells to divide, and thereby increase in number, while simultaneously reducing their number of chromosomes by half.
      (2) Meiosis results in the creation of **haploid gametes from diploid germ cells** in the gonads (testes in males and ovaries in females). Each haploid gamete contains **one-half the number of chromosomes** in the diploid cell.
   d. During fertilization, **two haploid gametes** unite to form a **single diploid zygote**, thus **conserving the diploid chromosome number** from generation to generation.

2. **Ensuring genetic diversity**
   a. There is another important aspect of meiosis, namely, the **exchange of genetic material** between homologous chromosomes, which eventually results in **variability in the progeny** of a single pair of parents.
   b. Furthermore, gametogenesis involves, in addition, the production of specialized, **sexually dimorphic gametes** that are truly different. The morphologic differences between the gametes in males and females reflect anatomic and functional differences of these two different cells.

3. Consequently, at fertilization, a male and a female haploid gamete create a single diploid zygote containing a complete set of chromosomes, half of them paternal and the other half maternal.
   a. This single diploid cell then begins the spectacular developmental history which eventually culminates in the formation of a new, reproductively mature, adult organism.
   b. This adult organism begins again the cycle of sexual reproduction, with its population of diploid cells in the gonads that undergo meiotic divisions, leading to the production of gametes with half of the diploid number of chromosomes.

C. **Behavior of sex chromosomes in gametogenesis**
   1. Female and male gametes show **morphologic differences**.
      a. In higher mammals, including humans, the **female** of the species produces only one kind of gamete. Each ovum bears a haploid set of somatic chromosomes (autosomes) and one kind of sex chromosome, the X chromosome.
      b. In contrast, the **male** produces spermatozoa of two different kinds. The spermatozoa all have a haploid set of autosomes but 50% have an X chromosome and 50% have a Y chromosome.
   2. The **genetic sex** of the organism is determined at fertilization.
      a. At fertilization, theoretically there is an equal chance that an X-bearing ovum will encounter either an X-bearing sperm cell or a Y-bearing sperm cell. (In actuality, there is a slightly greater chance that a Y-bearing sperm will fertilize, perhaps because the Y chromosome contains less DNA than the X chromosome.)
         (1) When an ovum is fertilized by an X sperm, an XX female zygote is formed.
         (2) When an ovum is fertilized by a Y sperm, an XY male zygote is formed.
      b. Thus, male and female zygotes are alike with respect to their content of autosomes but differ with respect to their content of sex chromosomes.
   3. The phenotypic and behavioral traits associated with "maleness" or "femaleness" are determined later in development (see Chapter 17).

II. MITOSIS AND MEIOSIS

A. **How mitosis differs from meiosis**. Both mitosis and meiosis are concerned with the **conservation of chromosome number**. Meiosis and mitosis are similar in some features but are also fundamentally different.
   1. **Mitosis** is the mechanism for **conserving chromosome number from cell to cell**.
      a. Mitosis takes place in all **somatic cells** during periods of growth. During mitosis, the diploid number of chromosomes exists before mitosis begins.
      b. In mitosis there is a replication of chromosomes followed by nuclear and cytoplasmic division.
      c. Early in mitosis, chromosomes are doubled so that there is a temporary **tetraploid state**. Then centromeres divide, chromosomes separate, and each daughter cell receives a diploid set of chromosomes.
      d. The end result of mitosis is to create numerous identical **diploid daughter cells** from diploid mother cells.
   2. **Meiosis** is the mechanism for **conserving chromosome number from generation to generation**.
      a. Meiosis is a process restricted to the **germ cell lines** of adults. During meiosis, cells divide twice with only one round of DNA replication, resulting in the formation of **haploid cells**.
      b. The end result of meiosis is to create numerous **haploid gametes** from diploid germ cells.

B. **Primordial germ cells and gamete formation**
   1. Certain diploid somatic cells in the embryo differentiate into **primordial germ cells**. These cells are the precursors of the gametogenic cell lines in the body.
   2. After migrating to the gonads, the primordial germ cells undergo many rounds of mitotic cell divisions, producing myriads of diploid **spermatogonia** in the testis or **oogonia** in the ovary.
   3. The spermatogonia and oogonia differentiate into a large diploid collection of **primary spermatocytes** and **primary oocytes**, in the male and female, respectively.

4. **Meiosis** begins in the primary spermatocytes and primary oocytes.
   a. At the end of meiosis, **each primary spermatocyte** has been converted into **four haploid spermatozoa**, and **each primary oocyte** has been converted into **one haploid ovum** and, usually, **three polar bodies**.
   b. As will be seen in sections IV and V, there are other substantial differences in the details of the meiotic process in males and females.

III. THE PHASES OF MEIOSIS. The process of meiosis involves two meiotic divisions (Fig. 2-1).

   A. **The first meiotic division (meiosis I)**
   1. The first meiotic division has an extended **prophase** period with five distinct phases.
      a. **Leptotene phase**: Chromosomes begin to condense and shorten.
      b. **Zygotene phase**: Homologous chromosomes pair precisely and DNA is duplicated.
         (1) Equivalent stretches of each homologous chromosome come into close association, while the chromosomes continue to condense. Next, there is a duplication of DNA without centromere division.
         (2) This phase results in the attainment of a tetraploid amount of DNA and a tetraploid number of chromatids. The chromosomal number is still diploid, but each chromosome has two **chromatids**. These double chromosomes are called **bivalents**.
      c. **Pachytene phase**: Chromosomes continue to condense, and **chiasmata** become evident. The chiasmata are points of **genetic exchange (crossing over)**. At a chiasma, chromatids trade homologous portions, resulting in new genetic combinations.

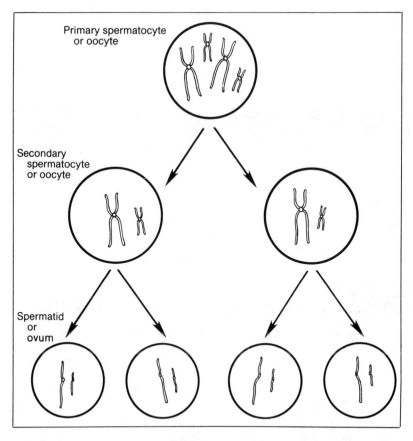

Figure 2-1. The basic principles of meiosis. The primary oocyte or spermatocyte enters prophase I to begin meiosis. The first meiotic division (meiosis I) creates the secondary oocyte or spermatocyte. The second meiotic division (meiosis II) creates the spermatid or the ovum and polar body. During the first meiotic division (meiosis I), there is no centromere division. During the second meiotic division (meiosis II), the chromatids divide at centromeres.

d. **Diplotene phase**: The paired chromosomes appear to move apart a bit, although they remain attached at chiasmata. Meanwhile, further condensation and shortening of chromosomes occurs.
   e. **Diakinesis:** There is further chromosomal condensation. At the end of diakinesis, the nuclear envelope disintegrates and **prophase I ends**.
  2. **Metaphase I** begins at the end of prophase I.
   a. A **spindle** forms and, just as in mitosis, a **metaphase (equatorial) plate** appears.
   b. In contrast to mitotic metaphase, meiotic metaphase I involves **no centromere division**.
  3. **Anaphase I**: The bivalents separate and are distributed to daughter cells, the nuclear envelopes begin to reassemble, and the chromosomes become less coiled.
  4. **Telophase I**: Cytokinesis (division of the cytoplasm) occurs and nuclear envelopes reform.
  5. There is now a brief resting **interphase**, followed by the second meiotic division.

 B. **The second meiotic division (meiosis II)**
  1. **Prophase II**: The chromosomes again condense and shorten, and the nuclear envelope disintegrates for a second time.
  2. **Metaphase II**: The chromosomes align themselves on the metaphase plate for the second time. It is at this point that **centromeres divide**, committing one half of each chromosome to each daughter cell. It is thus at this point that the haploid DNA content of each germ cell has been established.
  3. **Aanaphase II**: Separation of chromosomes occurs.
  4. **Telophase II**: Cytokinesis (division of cytoplasm) and reassembly of the nuclear envelope complete the process of meiosis.

IV. FEMALE GAMETOGENESIS (OOGENESIS)

 A. **The reproductive cycle and ovulation**
  1. In mammals, the female invariably produces a relatively small number of ova. These haploid gametes are specially designed to support early development.
  2. In humans, the **menstrual cycle** is a monthly **reproductive cycle** during which an **ovum** normally is shed at random from one or the other ovary.
   a. During the physiologic reproductive period of a woman, beginning with **menarche** roughly at age 13 and ending with **menopause** at about age 50, a single ovum is normally produced in each 28-day menstrual cycle, giving a total of 400 to 500 ova per lifetime.
   b. **Multiple ovulation** can occur and sometimes leads to the formation of multiple embryos (dizygotic twins, for example).
   c. The fertility drugs used in some cases of anovulatory infertility can result in the production of many ova and multiple gestations.
 B. **Specifics of female gametogenesis.** The **production of ova** is a long, drawn-out process. It begins before birth, stops in mid-process, and only resumes years later, after menarche.
  1. **Production of oogonia and oocytes**
   a. The developing ovary is colonized by **primordial germ cells** prior to birth. These diploid cells proliferate by numerous mitotic divisions.
   b. The primordial germ cells differentiate into **oogonia**. These also increase in number by mitotic divisions, and then begin to differentiate into **primary oocytes**.
   c. Meiosis begins in the primary oocytes soon after their formation. However, the oocytes are **arrested** in the early part of meiotic **prophase I**: They undergo a round of DNA synthesis, and chromosome pairing takes place, but meiosis does not proceed further until years later.
   d. Meanwhile, oogonia continue to proliferate and form additional primary oocytes. At about the middle of the gestation period, the fetal ovary contains millions of oogonia and primary oocytes.
   e. Even before birth, however, some oogonia and primary oocytes begin to undergo regressive changes known as **atresia**, so that at birth there are approximately 1 million primary oocytes, and no oogonia, in the ovary.
   f. Only about 400 to 500 of these primary oocytes will ever undergo a complete maturation resulting in the release of an ovum from the mature ovary. (1 per month X 12

months X 40 years = 480 ova in a woman's lifetime). All of the rest undergo slow atresia and disappear from the ovary gradually over the life of the female.

2. **Completion of meiosis in females**
   a. The **primary oocyte**, arrested in meiosis at **prophase I** during embryonic life, remains in that state until the female reaches adulthood. **After menarche**, at each menstrual cycle, only one oocyte (or only a few) leaves the dormant state and continues the process of gametogenesis. Thus, some oocytes remain dormant for as long as 50 years.
   b. The **oocyte** resumes its development just prior to **ovulation**.
      (1) At this time, only **meiosis I** is completed, with the formation of a **first polar body** and a **secondary oocyte** (Fig. 2-2).
      (2) If **fertilization** occurs, the secondary oocyte is stimulated to complete **meiosis II**, with the formation of a **second polar body** and a **haploid ovum**. The nucleus of the ovum that forms after fertilization is known as the **female pronucleus**.
   c. **Cytokinesis** is unequal in oogenesis, so that the first polar body is small while the secondary oocyte is large and receives most of the cytoplasm of the primary oocyte. Similarly, the second polar body is small, leaving most of the ooplasm in the ovum.
   d. The **first polar body may or may not divide** after it is formed. If it divides, an ovum and **three polar bodies** will be produced. If the first polar body fails to divide, an ovum and only **two polar bodies** will be produced.

C. **Follicular development**

1. **Follicle formation and growth** (Fig. 2-3)
   a. In the ovarian cortex, each developing oocyte is surrounded by a layer of **follicular epithelial cells**, a **basement membrane** for the follicular epithelium, and a layer of **thecal cells**.
   b. In **primordial follicles**, the follicular epithelium is a single squamous layer of cells. Under the influence of the pituitary gonadotropic hormones [primarily **follicle-stimulating hormone (FSH)**], the follicular epithelial cells (**granulosa cells**) begin to elongate and to proliferate, forming a multi-layered structure, the **primary follicle**.

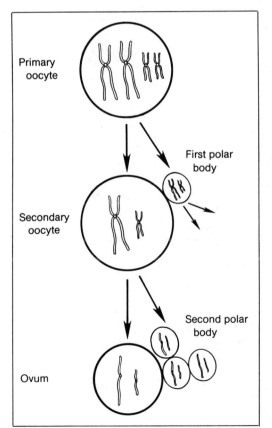

Figure 2-2. Cytokinesis (division of the cytoplasm) is unequal during oogenesis. The first meiotic division creates a secondary oocyte and a first polar body. The first polar body in the figure is dividing, but this does not always happen. The second meiotic division, which occurs only after fertilization, results in the formation of a haploid ovum and a second polar body.

c. The granulosa cells continue to proliferate, and the entire follicle grows in volume. The granulosa cells now begin to secrete a glycoprotein-rich fluid, **liquor folliculi**, into the spaces between cells. This fluid accumulates in a growing cavity known as the **antrum**.
d. Once an antrum of liquor folliculi is formed, the follicle is known as a **secondary follicle**. Within the mature follicle, the ovum is surrounded by a group of granulosa cells called the **cumulus oophorus**.

2. **Events at ovulation**
    a. As the follicular epithelial cells continue to proliferate and secrete large volumes of liquor folliculi, the follicle grows rapidly and moves toward the surface of the ovarian cortex.
    b. Now, due to a surge in **luteinizing hormone (LH)**, secreted from the pituitary gland, **ovulation** occurs.
        (1) The mature follicle ruptures through the germinal epithelium of the ovarian cortex, releasing the ovum from the ovary.
        (2) The ovum is released inside a **protective covering** (Fig. 2-4).
            (a) During folliculogenesis, granulosa cells immediately adjacent to the ovum secrete an extracellular matrix known as the **zona pellucida**.
            (b) The follicular epithelial cells adjacent to the zona pellucida send long processes through it and make direct contact with the surface of the ovum.
            (c) In addition, granulosa cells from the cumulus oophorus form an outer covering, the **corona radiata**.
            (d) Thus, at ovulation, the ruptured follicle releases a structure consisting of the ovum and its polar body, along with some of the attached liquor folliculi, all lying within the zona pellucida and the outer corona radiata.
    c. The ovum and its surrounding adnexa are released from the ovarian follicle into the **peritoneal cavity**. From here, they make their way into the **uterine tubes**.
        (1) The **structures surrounding the ovum** add considerable volume to the ovum and

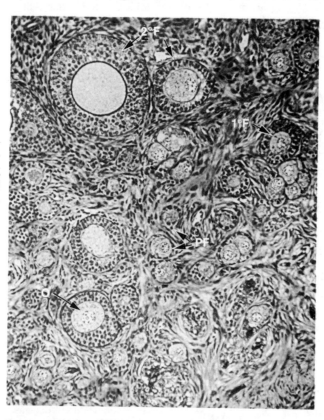

Figure 2-3. The ovarian cortex, showing follicles at various stages of development. (Light micrograph) *PF*, primordial follicle; *1° F*, primary follicle; *2° F*, secondary follicle; *S*, connective tissue stroma; *ZP*, zona pellucida; *O*, oocyte, with a nucleus (*N*) and a nucleolus (*Nu*).

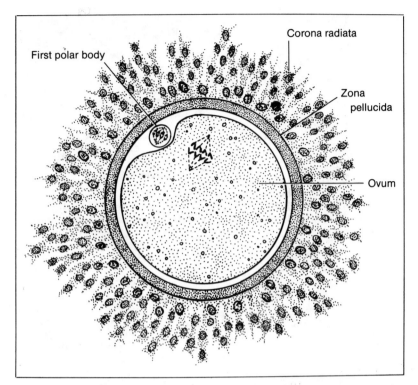

Figure 2-4. The ovum as it is released at ovulation, with its associated first polar body and surrounding zona pellucida and corona radiata.

   probably ensure that it will be trapped by cilia of the fimbriae on the uterine tubes and swept into the female reproductive tract.
   (2) **Fertilization** is thought to occur in the ampullary portion of the uterine tubes.
  d. Ovulation takes place at the middle of the menstrual cycle and is usually accompanied by a transient increase in body temperature and, in some women, by a mildly painful sensation called mittelschmerz.
  e. The growing follicles secrete large amounts of **estrogen**. After ovulation, the follicular remnants are converted into a **corpus luteum**, which secretes **progesterone**.

V. MALE GAMETOGENESIS

A. Prepubertal phase
1. In the male embryo, **primordial germ cells** migrate to the developing testis and divide many times, producing large numbers of **spermatogonia**. In the developing **seminiferous tubules** (Fig. 2-5), the spermatogonia become intercalated among supporting **Sertoli cells**.
2. **Before puberty**, the seminiferous tubules contain Sertoli cells and spermatogonia but no evidence of advanced spermatogenesis.
3. **Just prior to puberty**, the spermatogonia begin to differentiate into **primary spermatocyctes**.
4. Spermatogonia persist throughout life and remain as a mitotic stem cell population, giving rise to myriads of primary spermatocytes.

B. Spermatogenesis after sexual maturation
1. Spermatogenesis begins at puberty and continues until death, so that over a normal lifetime many billions of spermatozoa are produced. A normal ejaculate contains 50 million to 300 million spermatozoa. However, sperm motility, survival, and transport in the female reproductive tract are relatively inefficient, so that only a few spermatozoa ever reach a waiting ovum.

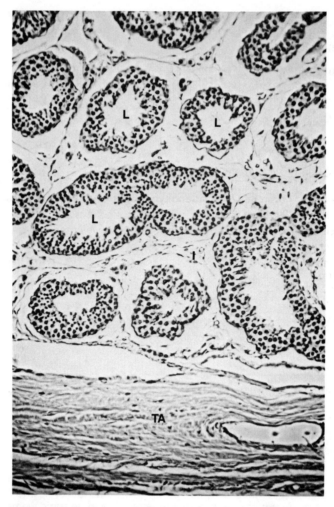

Figure 2-5. The testis, showing the lumina (L) of the seminiferous tubules, the Leydig-cell interstitial tissue (I) between seminiferous tubules, and the tunica albuginea (TA), a thick connective-tissue capsule. (Light micrograph)

2. **Meiosis in males**
   a. **At puberty**, primary spermatocytes enter into **meiosis I**, duplicating their chromosomes by a round of DNA synthesis. Prophase I, which lasts so long in the female, is very brief in the male. Rapidly, the primary spermatocyte produces two **secondary spermatocytes**, as meiosis I is completed.
   b. Secondary spermatocytes have a diploid amount of DNA per cell and a haploid number of chromosomes and centromeres. However, each chromosome contains two chromatids.
   c. Each secondary spermatocyte now undergoes **meiosis II**. Its centromere divides, leading to the formation of two **spermatids**. Spermatids are haploid in all respects.
3. **Spermiogenesis**
   a. Spermiogenesis is the portion of spermatogenesis in which the the spermatids undergo cytomorphogenesis to become mature **spermatozoa**.
      (1) During spermiogenesis, the rounded haploid spermatids are rapidly converted into streamlined, flagellated spermatozoa.
      (2) Spermatozoa are equipped for two **functions**:
         (a) Transit through the female reproductive tract
         (b) Penetration of the corona radiata and zona pellucida at fertilization

b. Specifics of spermiogenesis
   (1) The spermatid **nucleus** becomes highly condensed and streamlined.
   (2) The spermatid centrioles migrate to one pole of the nucleus and elaborate a long **flagellum** for propelling the spermatozoon.
   (3) The spermatid mitochondria form a **spiral sheath** around the flagellum, where they supply energy in the form of adenosine triphosphate (ATP) for flagellar motility.
   (4) The spermatid Golgi apparatus is converted into an **acrosome**, which forms a cap over the nucleus at the end opposite to the flagellum. The acrosome contains many hydrolytic enzymes and thus resembles a cellular lysosome.
   (5) Excess cytoplasm is shed as a **residual body** which is phagocytosed by the Sertoli cells.

VI. HORMONAL CONTROL OF GAMETOGENESIS

A. **Gonadotropic hormones.** The **adenohypophysis** of the pituitary gland produces two gonadotropic hormones.
   1. **Follicle-stimulating hormone (FSH)** stimulates development of the ovarian follicular cells (Fig. 2-6) and has an influence on Sertoli cells as well.
   2. **Luteinizing hormone (LH)** stimulates ovulation and the formation of the ovarian corpus luteum in the female (see Fig. 2-6), and stimulates testosterone production by the testicular Leydig cells in the male. LH is sometimes called interstitial-cell–stimulating hormone (ICSH) in the male.

B. **Steroidal sex hormones**
   1. **Estrogen** is secreted by the developing follicles. It stimulates the development of endometrial glands.
   2. **Progesterone** is secreted by the corpus luteum and causes secretory activity of the endometrial glands.

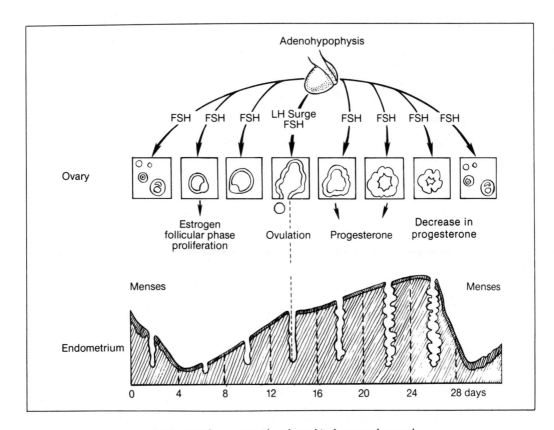

Figure 2-6. The menstrual cycle and its hormonal control.

3. **Testosterone** is secreted by the Leydig cells. It is required for the maintenance of spermatogenesis, development of male secondary sexual characteristics, and libido.

C. **Feedback control mechanisms**
1. A negative feedback loop controls sex steroid secretion.
   a. When sex steroids are at high levels, they cause a suppression of pituitary gonadotropic hormone secretion.
   b. When sex steroids are at low levels, the feedback inhibition stops, so that gonadotropins are released.
2. **Birth control pills** contain synthetic steroids that suppress gonadotropin release and thus suppress ovulation.

D. **Hormone secretion by the developing conceptus**
1. Once fertilization has initiated development, the conceptus forms a trophoblastic precursor of the placenta. This part of the pre-embryo secretes a glycoprotein hormone, **chorionic gonadotropin** (abbreviated as **hCG** because it is called human chorionic gonadotropin when given as a drug).
2. This hormone stimulates and maintains the functional activity of the corpus luteum for continued progesterone secretion.
   a. **With hCG stimulation**, the corpus luteum continues to produce progesterone and the endometrium is supported.
   b. **Without hCG stimulation**, the corpus luteum regresses, stops producing progesterone, and endometrial support is lost. Menstruation ensues rapidly.

VII. ABNORMALITIES OF HUMAN GAMETOGENESIS

A. **Abnormalities in morphology**
1. **Abnormal spermatogenesis**
   a. Abnormal spermatogenesis can produce poorly formed spermatozoa.
      (1) These spermatozoa may have poor motility due to defects in microtubules or other poorly understood causes.
      (2) They may have misshapen or double heads.
   b. Spermatozoa may be morphologically normal but produced in insufficient numbers (**oligospermia**).
2. **Abnormal oogenesis**
   a. Hormonal deficiencies can cause anovulatory menstrual cycles, in which no ovum is produced.
   b. For poorly understood reasons, there may be production of abnormal ova which can not be fertilized.
   c. The production of multiple ova is abnormal in a sense, since only one ovum per menstrual cycle is the rule.

B. **Abnormalities in chromosomal number (nondisjunction)**
1. During meiosis I, paired bivalents separate from one another; that is, they **disjoin.** When a bivalent fails to separate normally, the condition is known as **nondisjunction** (Fig. 2-7).
2. Nondisjunction can occur in ova or in spermatozoa. There are two **consequences of nondisjunction**:
   a. Production of a gamete with **two copies of a single chromosome**.
      (1) Fertilization of such an ovum by a normal spermatozoon results in **trisomy**. Trisomy also occurs if the fertilized ovum is normal and the sperm cell has the two copies of the chromosome.
      (2) Trisomies are discussed in detail in Chapter 23, section II, and Chapter 24, section VI. **Examples of trisomies** include:
         (a) Trisomy 21 (Down syndrome)
         (b) Trisomy 18 (Edwards syndrome)
         (c) Trisomy 13 (Patau syndrome)
   b. Production of a gamete with **no copies of a single chromosome**.
      (1) Fertilization of such an ovum by a normal spermatozoon results in **monosomy**. Monosomy also occurs if the fertilized ovum is normal and the sperm cell has no copies of the chromosome.
      (2) Turner syndrome (written as 45, X) is an example of monosomy due to nondisjunction. Other monosomies have been described but they are usually lethal prior to birth.

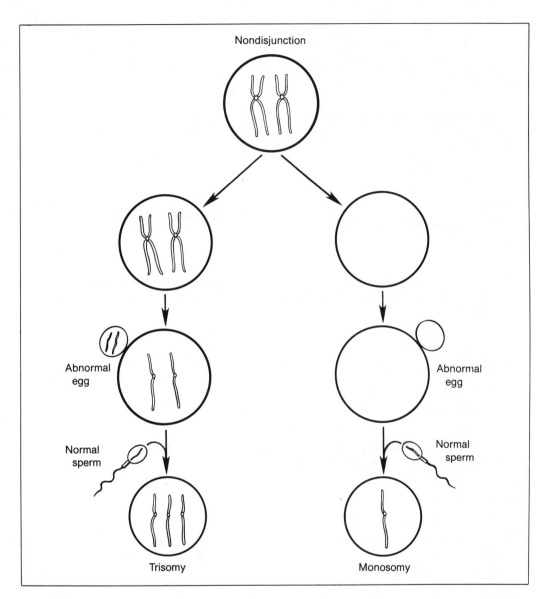

Figure 2-7. Nondisjunction during gametogenesis, occurring in this case in the oocyte. The unequal distribution of the chromosomes can result in either trisomic (*left*) or monosomic (*right*) zygotes after fertilization by a normal haploid gamete, in this case the sperm cell.

STUDY QUESTIONS

Directions: Each question below contains five suggested answers. Choose the **one best** response to each question.

1. Which of the following would have a haploid number of chromosomes and a haploid DNA content?

   (A) Primary spermatocyte
   (B) Primary oocyte
   (C) Secondary oocyte
   (D) First polar body
   (E) Spermatid

2. Which of the following organelles in a spermatid will contribute to the formation of the acrosome?

   (A) Mitochondria
   (B) Microtubules
   (C) Endoplasmic reticulum
   (D) Golgi apparatus
   (E) Nuclear envelope

3. Which of the following cellular structures in an ovulated ovum is derived from the granulosa cells of a developing follicle?

   (A) First polar body
   (B) Second polar body
   (C) Corona radiata
   (D) Zona pellucida
   (E) Female pronucleus

4. All of the following cell types are derived from primordial germ cells EXCEPT

   (A) the corona radiata
   (B) the ovum
   (C) the first polar body
   (D) the second polar body
   (E) the spermatid

5. How many secondary oocytes are normally produced during the reproductive life of a human female?

   (A) 4,000,000
   (B) 400,000
   (C) 40,000
   (D) 4000
   (E) 400

Directions: Each question below contains four suggested answers of which **one or more** is correct. Choose the answer

- A if **1, 2, and 3** are correct
- B if **1 and 3** are correct
- C if **2 and 4** are correct
- D if **4** is correct
- E if **1, 2, 3, and 4** are correct

6. Primary follicles contain which of the following?

(1) Gametes in meiosis I
(2) Gametes which complete meiosis II prior to ovulation
(3) One or several layers of granulosa cells
(4) An antrum

7. Characteristics of ovulation include which of the following?

(1) Ovulation involves rupture of a secondary follicle
(2) Ovulation occurs after a surge of luteinizing hormone
(3) Ovulation precedes an increase in progesterone secretion
(4) Meiosis is completed before ovulation

8. True statements concerning the menstrual cycle include which of the following?

(1) The menses occur after a decrease in progesterone secretion
(2) Endometrial glandular development is caused by an increase in estrogen secretion
(3) Endometrial glandular secretion is caused by an increase in progesterone secretion
(4) A missed period (lack of menses) is caused by increased hCG secretion by the conceptus

9. Nondisjunction can cause which of the following?

(1) Trisomy
(2) Monosomy
(3) A missing Y chromosome
(4) Down syndrome

10. True statements concerning spermatogenesis include which of the following?

(1) It can occur in a normal 6-year-old male
(2) It can occur in a normal 70-year-old male
(3) Primordial germ cells are present in the 70-year-old male testis
(4) Spermatogonia are present in the 6-year-old male testis

Directions: The group of questions below consists of lettered choices followed by several numbered items. For each numbered item select the **one** lettered choice with which it is **most** closely associated. Each lettered choice may be used once, more than once, or not at all.

Questions 11-15

For each description below of a component of the seminiferous epithelium (shown in the accompanying micrograph), choose the type of cell that it best describes.

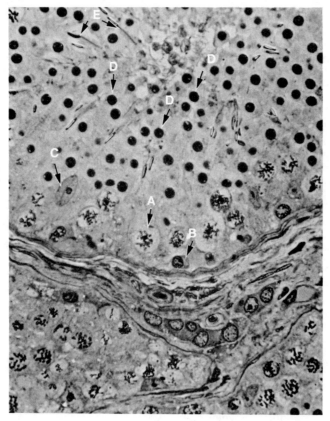

11. A diploid proliferative cell which forms secondary spermatocytes immediately after it completes meiosis I

12. A diploid cell which is the immediate product of a primordial germ cell

13. A haploid cell which has completed spermiogenesis

14. A haploid cell which is the immediate product of a secondary spermatocyte

15. A diploid cell which is not part of the spermatogenic cell line

ANSWERS AND EXPLANATIONS

1. The answer is E. *(III B; IV B 2; V B 2; Fig. 2-1)* Primary oocytes and primary spermatocytes have not yet completed the first meiotic division. Therefore, they both have a diploid number of chromosomes and a tetraploid DNA content. The secondary oocyte and the first polar body have completed meiosis I and thus have a haploid number of double chromosomes (bivalents) and therefore a diploid amount of DNA. Only the spermatids have completed meiosis II and therefore have a haploid chromosome number and a haploid amount of DNA. Spermatids are then converted into spermatozoa during spermiogenesis.

2. The answer is D. *(V B 3 b)* Mitochondria assemble in a spiral around the flagellum and provide adenosine triphosphate for flagellar motility. Microtubules contribute to the flagellar axoneme. The endoplasmic reticulum is sparse in the spermatid and disappears during formation of spermatozoa. The Golgi apparatus assembles the acrosome, a modified lysosome containing hydrolytic enzymes for penetration of the structures surrounding the ovum. The nuclear envelope of the spermatid persists as a nuclear envelope surrounding the nucleus of the spermatozoon.

3. The answer is C. *(IV B 2, C)* The first and second polar bodies are cells produced by the unequal divisions of the primary and secondary oocyte during meiosis I and meiosis II, respectively. The corona radiata consists of a collection of follicular epithelial cells that remain attached to the ovum and its surrounding zona pellucida. The zona pellucida is an extracellular matrix secretion product of follicular epithelial cells; it surrounds the ovum and serves as an attachment site for the granulosa cells that make up the corona radiata. The female pronucleus is the nucleus of the ovum that forms after fertilization. It will fuse with the male pronucleus derived from the spermatozoon to produce a diploid zygote nucleus.

4. The answer is A. *(II B; IV C; V B 2)* The cells of the corona radiata are not part of the gametogenic cell line. They come from follicular epithelial cells with a supportive function during oogenesis. The oogonia and all of its products, namely the primary oocyte, secondary oocyte, polar bodies, and ovum, are formed from the primordial germ cells. In the male, primordial germ cells form spermatogonia, which in turn differentiate into primary and secondary spermatocytes, spermatids, and finally spermatozoa.

5. The answer is E. *(IV A 2 a)* Under normal circumstances, ovulation occurs once each month for approximately 400 months between menarche and menopause. Meiosis I is not completed until just before ovulation. The ovulated oocyte is a secondary oocyte. Meiosis II is not completed until after fertilization; the stimulus for the completion of meiosis II is penetration of the secondary oocyte by the spermatozoon.

6. The answer is B (1, 3). *(IV B 2, C)* Primary follicles contain primary oocytes, which are arrested in the first meiotic prophase. Meiosis I is completed just before ovulation but meiosis II is not completed until after fertilization. The single layer of cuboidal follicular cells in a primary follicle multiply to form many layers, but the follicle has no antrum. Once an antrum forms, it is a secondary follicle.

7. The answer is A (1, 2, 3). *(IV C, VI A, B)* At ovulation, a large secondary follicle ruptures through the surface of the ovary, partly due to a surge in the production of luteinizing hormone by the pituitary. After ovulation, the remnants of the follicle become converted into a corpus luteum which secretes progesterone. Meiosis is not completed until after fertilization, when the second polar body is formed.

8. The answer is E (all). *(VI A, B, D; Fig. 2-6)* Prior to ovulation in the middle of the menstrual cycle, the developing follicle produces estrogen, which stimulates endometrial glandular development. After ovulation, the corpus luteum secretes progesterone, which stimulates endometrial glandular secretion. If fertilization occurs, the trophoblast of the conceptus begins to produce chorionic gonadotropin (hCG). This glycoprotein hormone stimulates the corpus luteum to continue its secretion of progesterone, and thus the menses do not occur and the conceptus becomes established in the wall of the endometrium.

9. The answer is E (all). *(VII B)* Nondisjunction means that paired bivalents do not separate during meiosis I. As a result, gametes are produced with either two copies or no copies of a given chromosome, rather than the proper one copy of that chromosome. At fertilization, the former event results in trisomy and the latter event results in monosomy, when the abnormal gamete combines with a normal gamete. Down syndrome is an example of a trisomy (of chromosome 21) which is caused by nondisjunction. Turner syndrome is an example of monosomy in which one sex chromosome is missing.

10. The answer is C (2, 4). (*V A, B*) Spermatogenesis begins at puberty and continues until death under normal conditions. Prior to puberty, the seminiferous tubule contains spermatogonia and Sertoli cells but no primordial germ cells. After puberty, the spermatogonia begin to produce primary spermatocytes, which progress to secondary spermatocytes, spermatids, and finally spermatozoa.

11–15. The answers are 11-A, 12-B, 13-E, 14-D, 15-C. (*V B*) The light micrograph accompanying the questions shows the seminiferous epithelium of an adult male. It contains many diploid spermatogonia (B) which proliferate and form diploid primary spermatocytes (A). During meiosis I, the primary spermatocytes become tetraploid after DNA synthesis and then divide to form secondary spermatocytes. During meiosis II, these secondary spermatocytes form haploid spermatids (D). The spermatids undergo spermiogenesis to form mature spermatozoa (E), which are also haploid cells. The Sertoli cells (C) form a continuous epithelial layer of diploid cells that are not part of the spermatogenic cell line. Sertoli cells support spermatogenic cells.

3
Overview of Embryonic and Fetal Periods

I. INTRODUCTION

A. It is difficult to describe the events that occur during the development of a new human being, because so many things are occurring simultaneously. Therefore, this chapter outlining the overall events of pre-embryonic, embryonic, and fetal development (Fig. 3-1) is intended to provide a chronologic frame of reference for the details described in the chapters that follow.

B. The meaning of conceptus. It is often convenient to refer to the entire developing system as a **conceptus**, which is the name given to all of the products that result from a successful fertilization or conception. Thus, conceptus is a collective term for both embryonic and extraembryonic structures.

  1. During the embryonic period, the conceptus includes the embryo and the amnion, chorion, and developing placenta.
  2. During the fetal period, conceptus includes the fetus, chorioamnionic membrane, umbilical cord, and placenta.

C. A word about dates

  1. An obstetrician, in assessing the duration of a pregnancy, calculates the **gestational age** from the date of the **last menstrual period (LMP)**.
     a. Thus, obstetricians speak of a 20-week pregnancy taken from the LMP.
     b. Using this system, human gestation covers 40 weeks from LMP to delivery.
  2. The embryologist, in contrast, calculates age from the **time of fertilization**, which is the actual time of conception. Fertilization occurs about 2 weeks after the LMP.
     a. Thus, the fetus in a 20-week LMP pregnancy is actually about 18 weeks old, counting from conception.
     b. Using this system, which is the one used in this book, human gestation covers 38 weeks from fertilization to delivery.

II. OVERVIEW OF THE EMBRYONIC PERIOD

A. Pre-embryonic period. The **first two-week period**, from fertilization to the end of the second week, is often called the pre-embryonic period.

  1. **During the first week**, the conceptus is **cleaving**, to become first a **morula** (a berrylike ball of cells) and then a **blastocyst** (a fluid-filled ball) with an embryoblast (inner cell mass) and a trophoblast (Fig. 3-2); it is also beginning to **implant** in the maternal endometrium.
  2. **During the second week**, implantation continues, and an amnion, yolk sac, and chorion form. The **bilaminar disk stage** is reached (see Fig. 3-2): the pre-embryo is a flat, disk-like structure with **two primary germ layers**, an ectoderm and an endoderm.

B. Embryonic period proper. The embryonic period covers **weeks 3 through 8**. During the embryonic period, the **major morphogenetic and organogenetic events** occur. The developing organism takes on its vertebrate shape, and the major organ systems are established, although these must later undergo considerable further development. It is during the embryonic period that the developing organism is particularly sensitive to teratogenic agents such as microorganisms and chemicals.

34 *Human Developmental Anatomy*

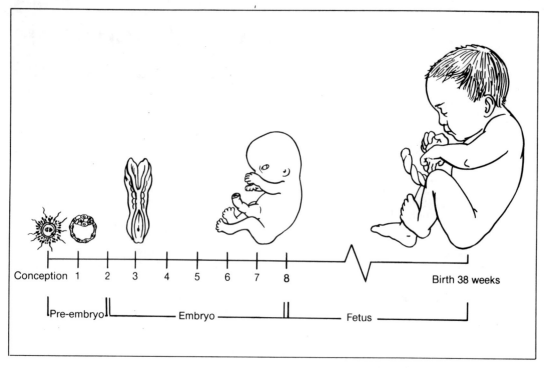

Figure 3-1. The periods of human development.

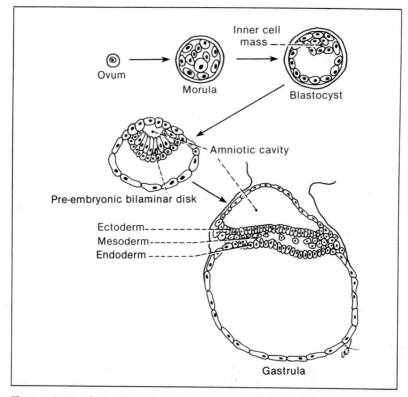

Figure 3-2. Development of the fertilized ovum into a morula, a blastocyst, a two-layered (bilaminar) pre-embryonic disk and into the trilaminar gastrula. (Adapted from DeMyer W: *NMS Neuroanatomy*. Media, Pa., Harwal/Wiley, 1988, p 32.)

1. **Events during week 3**
   a. **Overview.** During this week of rapid change, the disk-like conceptus lengthens and becomes tube-like, and the primordial nervous system, skeleton, and circulatory system appear.
   b. The **events of this week** are as follows.
      (1) Gastrulation and **neurulation** occur.
         (a) In **gastrulation**, the bilaminar disk becomes a **trilaminar gastrula**, with **three primary germ layers**, ectoderm, mesoderm, and endoderm (Fig. 3-3).
         (b) In **neurulation**, a **neural plate** forms in the ectoderm and then curls up and fuses to form the **neural tube**, the precursor of the central nervous system, along the midline of the lengthening pre-embryo.
      (2) Late in week 3, **somites** begin to appear on either side of the neural tube. These paired blocks of mesodermal cells are the precursors of somatic structures—dermis, skeleton, and skeletal muscle.
      (3) The primitive **circulatory system** arises and begins to transport blood.
      (4) There is extensive development in the **chorion** and numerous **villi** begin to appear on the chorionic surface.

2. **Events during week 4**
   a. **Overview.** During the fourth week the embryo grows from 2 mm long to 4 mm long. External form changes dramatically as **flexion** creates a recognizable head and tail, and miniature **limb buds** appear. The embryo now clearly is a vertebrate, but primate or human characteristics only become evident much later, when facial features develop.
   b. In the fourth week, the following events occur.
      (1) **Definitive body form** is established by flexion and growth of the folds of the amnion.
      (2) The primitive **gut tube** is formed in this process, as is the **intraembryonic coelom**, a cavity that is the precursor of the body cavities.
      (3) **Eye and ear rudiments** are laid down, and the **pharyngeal arches** appear.
      (4) Formation of somites is nearly complete, and limb buds first arise.
      (5) **Cardiac morphogenesis** is extensive, so that a prominent cardiac bulge is now visible ventrally (see Fig. 3-4).
      (6) Chorionic villi are bathed in maternal blood, and **maternal-fetal exchange** of blood gases, nutrients, and wastes is established.

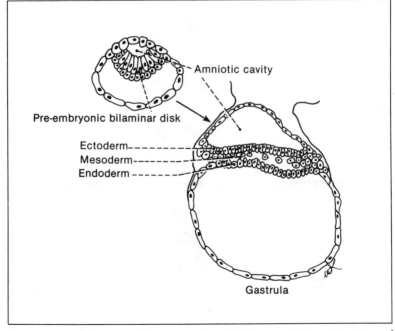

Figure 3-3. Development of the pre-embryonic bilaminar disk into the trilaminar gastrula. (Adapted from DeMyer W: *NMS Neuroanatomy*. Media, Pa., Harwal/Wiley, 1988, p 32.)

3. **Events during week 5** (Fig. 3-4). During the fifth week, the embryo increases in length from 4 mm to 8 mm. Changes in this week appear less dramatic because they involve growth of already-formed structures. In the fifth week, the following events occur.
    a. The **head** grows rapidly due to the high rate of growth of the brain and skull. The lens vesicles become visible, and prominent nasal pits form in the head region. The second pharyngeal arch (hyoid arch) begins to grow caudally over the more caudal arches.
    b. **Limb buds** elongate and become expanded distally. The forelimbs develop more rapidly than the hindlimbs, so that by the end of the fifth week, the forelimb has a hand plate and the hindlimb is paddle-shaped.

4. **Events during week 6** (see Fig. 3-4). During this week, the embryo grows from 8 mm long to 14 mm long.
    a. Marked changes occur in the **head**: pigment in the retina becomes visible, and auricular hillocks arise on either side of the first pharyngeal groove.
    b. The **cervical flexure** becomes more pronounced, so that the head now rests directly on the growing cardiac prominence.
    c. The **forelimbs** have a distinct wrist and five digital rays, while the **hindlimbs** have only a foot plate and still lack digital rays.
    d. The **liver** and the **midgut** begin to grow extensively.
    e. The **trunk** has straightened out somewhat by the end of the sixth week.

5. **Events during week 7** (see Fig. 3-4). During this week the embryo grows from 14 mm long to 20 mm.
    a. The **head** continues to grow very rapidly. Eyelids become visible and the auricular hillocks fuse into a single auricle. The crown of the skull has a prominent vascular plexus. The face begins to take on a humanoid appearance, although the eyes are placed more laterally than they will be later in development.
    b. The **limbs** project more ventrally. The forelimb has a well-defined elbow and wrist, with distinct digits connected by flaps of skin. The hindlimbs have an ankle and toe rays.

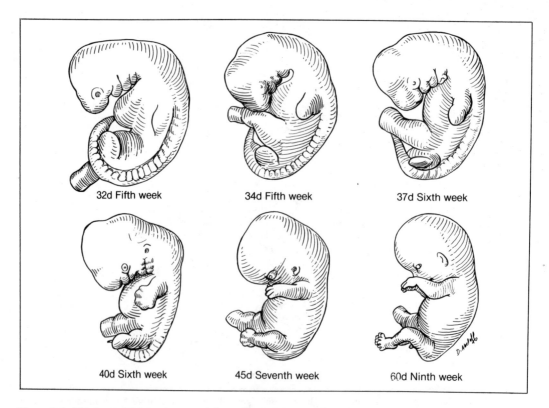

Figure 3-4. Human embryos and a 9-week fetus showing some of the salient features of changes in the external morphology. These are not drawn to proportional scale.

c. Rudiments of the **nipples** appear on the ventral thorax.
d. The enlarging **liver** mass causes a physiologic **herniation of the midgut loop** into the umbilical cord.

6. **Events during week 8** (see Fig. 3-4). The embryo increases in length from 20 mm to 30 mm in this last week of the embryonic period. It is interesting to note that although the embryo continues to grow rapidly, the rate of increase in growth is decreasing. For example, in the fifth week the embryo increases in length by 100%, whereas in the eighth week there is only a 50% increase.
   a. The growth rate of the **head** has slowed with respect to the rest of the body, so that the head is no longer such a prominent feature of the body.
   b. The **face** becomes more human in appearance as the eyes migrate into the frontal plane.
   c. The webs between the digits disappear, first leaving distinct **fingers** and then distinct **toes**.
   d. The **trunk** elongates and the last remnants of the tail disappear.
   e. The **external genitalia** are beginning to exhibit slight differences in the two sexes, but they are still essentially alike.
   f. The **herniation of the midgut loop** into the cord is still extensive.

III. OVERVIEW OF THE FETAL PERIOD

A. The fetal period covers **weeks 9 through 38** inclusive. It is a period when the fetus grows extensively.

   1. Most organ systems have formed prior to the fetal period, but they undergo extensive growth and considerable functional maturation so that the fetus will be capable of survival outside the uterus.
   2. The fetus is much less sensitive to teratogenic agents than is the embryo. However, the central nervous system is still sensitive to various teratogens because its development continues through the fetal period.

B. **Size changes during the fetal period**
   1. **Determination of size and development**
      a. Determining the developmental state of an embryo or fetus is usually based largely on its **length**.
         (1) The early embryo, before flexion has occurred, is measured for its greatest length, that is, the distance between the cranial and caudal ends.
         (2) Once the basic body plan has been established, the length from the crown of the head to the base of the buttocks is usually measured. This so-called **crown–rump length** is a reliable measure of the age of the embryo, assuming that normal development has occurred.
         (3) Once the limbs begin to develop, the **crown–heel length** can be measured.
      b. Naturally, **other criteria** such as the development of limbs or facial characterisitics are also helpful in determining the true age of the fetus.
   2. The most striking feature of the fetal period is the **absolute increase in length and weight** (Fig. 3-5). At 9 weeks, the fetus has a crown–rump length of 50 mm and it weighs about 8 g. By term, the fetus has a crown–rump length of 360 mm and a weight of 3400 g. Figure 3-6 shows changes in length and weight during the fetal period.
   3. Another striking feature of the fetal period is the relatively **slow growth of the head** and the relatively more **rapid growth of the rest of the body** (see Fig. 3-5). At 9 weeks, the head alone represents nearly 50% of the entire length of the fetus. At term, the head represents only 25% of the entire body length. In an adult, the head represents only 10% to 15% of the entire length of the body.

C. **Morphologic changes during the fetal period**
   1. **Events during the third month**
      a. During this period, the fetus grows rapidly and the tail is completely resorbed.
      b. The volume of the **peritoneal cavity** increases. Consequently, the intestinal loops that formerly were herniated into the umbilical cord are drawn back into the peritoneal cavity, and the prominence of the hepatic bulge decreases.
      c. In the **head**, the eyes move into the frontal plane and the ears come to lie on the same level with the mandible. The forehead is prominent. The eyelids grow together and fuse.

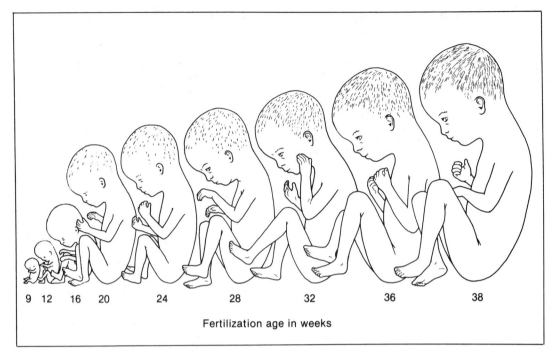

Figure 3-5. Changes in the relative size of the fetus throughout the fetal period. (Reprinted with permission from Moore K: *The Developing Human*, 3rd ed. Philadelphia, Saunders, 1982, p 93.)

  d. Fine **hair** appears over the body; the hairs are known collectively as **lanugo** (the Latin word for down).
  e. **Sexual dimorphism** in the external genitalia and gonads is now clearly defined.
  f. The **forelimbs** are now completely formed, even to small fingernails, and they are approximately their normal size in relation to the rest of the body. The **hindlimbs** are proportionately smaller and less well developed, with smaller nails.
2. **Events during the fourth month**
  a. The **gonads** continue to differentiate.
  b. Extensive **ossification** occurs in the skeleton, so that bones are now visible on x-ray films. **Hair follicle** formation is extensive.
  c. The growth rate, formerly rapid, now slows during the fourth and fifth months.
3. **Events during the fifth month**
  a. **The hindlimbs** now become completed and assume their normal proportions with respect to the rest of the body (Fig. 3-7).
  b. **Fetal movements** now become strong enough to be detected by the mother as **quickening**.
  c. The **skin** is now completely covered by lanugo, which helps to hold a protective layer of sebaceous gland secretions and dead desquamated cells. This **vernix caseosa** helps to protect the fetal skin from the damaging effects of being constantly bathed in amniotic fluid.
  d. The **testes** are formed and begin their descent into the scrotum. They have distinct seminiferous tubules but have not yet differentiated a spermatogenic epithelium. The **uterus** is also formed during the fifth month.
  e. **Brown fat** begins to accumulate around the neck, around the sternum, and across the back over the shoulders.
    (1) Brown fat has a rich blood supply and contains numerous **multilocular adipocytes**, each with many fat vacuoles and an abundance of mitochondria.
    (2) Brown fat is important for the regulation of fetal **body temperature**, since body heat can be generated by oxidation of the fatty acids stored in brown fat. Normal adults have very little brown fat.

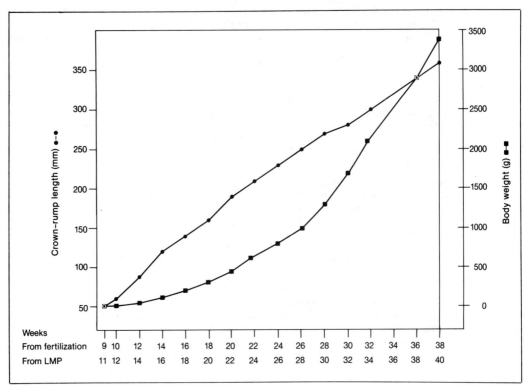

Figure 3-6. Graph showing the increase in crown–rump length (*circles*) and weight (*squares*) during the fetal period. Note that there is a linear increase in length but an exponential increase in weight. *LMP*, last menstrual period.

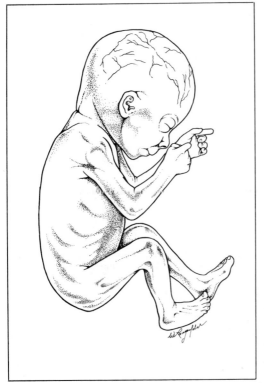

Figure 3-7. A human fetus at 17 weeks. (Redrawn from Moore K: *The Developing Human*, 3rd ed. Philadelphia, Saunders, 1982, p 99.)

4. **Events during the sixth month**
   a. The fetus has now reached almost its full term length but not its full weight.
      (1) Weight will continue to increase considerably, largely due to the later accumulation of subcutaneous white fat.
      (2) **White adipose tissue** is still sparse, so the fetus does not look chubby like a newborn does. Because of the absence of subcutaneous fat, the skin is loose and quite wrinkled.
   b. In the **lungs**, surfactant-secreting alveolar cells begin to differentiate.
      (1) **Surfactant** is a mixture of phospholipids (lecithin), proteins, and polysaccharides.
      (2) It reduces the surface tension of the water layer coating the alveolar surface of the lungs and thus assists in inflating the lungs.
   c. It is possible for a 6-month fetus to survive outside the uterus, although pulmonary immaturity makes this survival difficult.

5. **Events during the seventh month**
   a. **Pulmonary maturation** continues and now it is relatively easier for a premature infant to survive. However, survival of such a premature infant is by no means guaranteed without the assistance of the technologic advances that have been made in perinatology in the recent past.
   b. **Subcutaneous fat** deposition is marked during the seventh month. Consequently, the fetal skin becomes smoother and the fetus takes on its characteristic chubbiness.

6. **Events during the eighth and ninth months** (Fig. 3-8)
   a. **Weight gain** is extensive during the eighth and ninth months, due largely to further accumulation of subcutaneous fat.
   b. The diameter of the abdomen grows until it is equal to the diameter of the head at 9 months and greater than the diameter of the head at term.
   c. The fetal period is now completed and the fetus is ready for delivery into the extrauterine environment, ready to become an air-breathing, semi-independent entity.

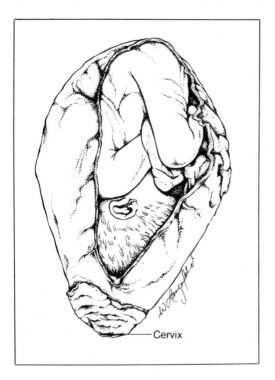

—Cervix

Figure 3-8. A human fetus at 29 weeks. (Redrawn from Moore K: *The Developing Human*, 3rd ed. Philadelphia, Saunders, 1982, p 101.)

STUDY QUESTIONS

Directions: Each question below contains five suggested answers. Choose the **one best** response to each question.

1. All of the following statements concerning the fourth month of gestation are true EXCEPT

    (A) it is not possible to distinguish the two sexes based on the morphology of the external genitalia at this stage
    (B) skeletal ossification is extensive
    (C) the growth rate is extensive
    (D) hair follicle formation progresses
    (E) the gonads become differentiated so that the testis and ovary are histologically different from one another

2. All of the following statements concerning the embryonic period are true EXCEPT

    (A) the major organ systems are established during this period
    (B) sensitivity to teratogens is higher than in the fetal period
    (C) the lanugo first appears
    (D) gastrulation and neurulation occur during this period
    (E) the limb buds first appear

3. All of the following statements concerning the third month of gestation are true EXCEPT

    (A) overall growth is rapid
    (B) the tail bud elongates
    (C) the eyes move to the frontal plane
    (D) the sex of the fetus can be determined
    (E) herniated gut loops return to the peritoneal cavity

4. All of the following statements concerning the fifth month of gestation are true EXCEPT

    (A) quickening is absent
    (B) the vernix caseosa is present
    (C) the testes begin their descent
    (D) brown fat begins to accumulate around the shoulders
    (E) hindlimb morphogenesis is largely completed

5. All of the following statements concerning the third week of gestation are true EXCEPT

    (A) the intraembryonic mesoderm is established
    (B) neural crest cells arise
    (C) the neural groove closes
    (D) chorionic villi disappear
    (E) neural folds fuse

6. All of the following statements concerning the fourth week of gestation are true EXCEPT

    (A) flexion occurs
    (B) the communication between intraembryonic and extraembryonic coeloms expands
    (C) the basic body plan is established
    (D) many somites appear
    (E) limb morphogenesis begins

7. All of the following statements concerning the fifth week of gestation are true EXCEPT

    (A) hindlimb growth outstrips forelimb growth
    (B) the head expands rapidly
    (C) lens vesicles become visible
    (D) nasal pits become visible
    (E) the third and fourth pharyngeal arches are overgrown by the second arch

8. All of the following statements concerning the sixth week of gestation are true EXCEPT

    (A) rudiments of the external ear become visible
    (B) an external manifestation of retinal development is evident
    (C) the hindlimbs lack digital rays
    (D) the liver grows extensively
    (E) the head grows away from the cardiac prominence

9. All of the following statements concerning the seventh week of gestation are true EXCEPT

(A) auricular hillocks fuse to form an auricle
(B) nipples begin to form on the thorax
(C) midgut loops are pulled back into the peritoneal cavity
(D) the liver enlarges
(E) the embryo grows from 14 mm to 20 mm

10. All of the following statements concerning the eighth week of gestation are true EXCEPT

(A) the rate of growth in length is the same as in the fifth week
(B) this is the last week of the embryonic period
(C) the eyes migrate to the frontal plane
(D) fingers and toes appear
(E) the external genitalia are alike in both sexes

11. All of the following statements concerning the sixth month of gestation are true EXCEPT

(A) the fetus has reached less than 50% of its full fetal weight
(B) surfactant-secreting cells differentiate in the lungs
(C) extrauterine life is possible after the sixth month
(D) the fetus has reached only 30% of its ultimate fetal length
(E) the skin is loose and wrinkled due to a paucity of white fat

12. All of the following statements concerning the seventh month of gestation are true EXCEPT

(A) surfactant secretion is well established
(B) pulmonary maturation occurs
(C) extrauterine survival is more difficult than at 8 months
(D) fat deposition slows and then ceases
(E) fetal skin becomes smoother than it was at 5 months

Chapter 3 — Overview of Fetal and Embryonic Periods

ANSWERS AND EXPLANATIONS

1. The answer is A. *(III C 1, 2)* Sexual dimorphism of both the external genitalia and the gonads is present but subtle during the eighth week of gestation. This difference becomes marked during the third month. Skeletal ossification first appears during the fourth month and bone growth is rapid. Overall growth of the fetus is still rapid during the fourth month. Hair follicles first appear in the third month and they continue their rapid development in the fourth month.

2. The answer is C. *(II B; III C 1 d)* The embryonic period is the time when the major organ systems are established. Consequently, this is a developmental period of great sensitivity to teratogens. In the fetal period there is a decrease in sensitivity to teratogens because the cardinal feature of this period is growth rather than organogenesis. Gastrulation and neurulation occur during the first week of the embryonic period (week 3 of development) and the limb buds first appear during the second week of the embryonic period (week 4 of development). The lanugo does not appear until the first month of the fetal period (month 3 of development).

3. The answer is B. *(III C 1)* During the third month, the growth rate of the fetus is prodigious. The tail bud, however, becomes completely resorbed and disappears. There is substantial morphogenesis of the face, including movement of the eyes into the frontal plane and closure and temporary fusion of the eyelids. The volume of the peritoneal cavity expands, allowing the gut loops to be withdrawn into the peritoneal cavity. Sexual dimorphism is complete by the third month.

4. The answer is A. *(III C 3)* During the fifth month, fetal movements become strong enough to be detected by the mother as quickening of the fetus. The vernix caseosa is a cheesy accumulation of dead epidermal cells and sebaceous gland secretions on the fetal epidermis. It serves to protect the fetal skin from the deleterious effects of bathing in amniotic fluid. Brown fat, which consists of multilocular adipocytes, is accumulated during the fifth month, especially around the neck, sternum, and shoulders. The testes have poorly differentiated seminiferous tubules and have begun their descent into the scrotum. The hindlimbs also assume their normal shape and proportions, completing their morphogenesis and positional change, although the hindlimbs will continue to grow in size until the end of puberty.

5. The answer is D. *(II B 1)* Gastrulation and neurulation occur during the third week. Gastrulation involves converting the pre-embryonic bilaminar disk into a trilaminar gastrula with ectoderm, mesoderm, and endoderm. Immediately after gastrulation is completed, neurulation begins: A neural plate forms, followed by the neural groove, which then closes up into a neural tube. Meanwhile, the dorsal neural folds form neural crest cells which migrate out from the neuroepithelium and are dispersed throughout the embryo. The chorionic villi become more numerous and grow branches to establish an increasing interfacial area between the maternal blood supply and the embryonic tissue.

6. The answer is B. *(II B 2)* The most dramatic change of the fourth week is the establishment of the basic body plan. Head and tail flexion and the growth of the amnion sculpts the flat embryo into a typical vertebrate body plan. The lateral body walls move medially and ventrally, thus reducing the communication between the intraembryonic and extraembryonic coeloms. Somite formation is also very substantial during this week. In addition, the limb buds arise as modest hillocks of the tissue on the flanks of the embryo.

7. The answer is A. *(II B 3)* All during development, the forelimbs are more advanced than the hindlimbs. For example, the forelimb buds appear before the hindlimb buds do; also, digital rays appear first in the forelimb. During the fifth week the head expands as a result of rapid growth of the brain and skull. The lens vesicles and nasal pits also form. The second pharyngeal arch (the hyoid arch) also begins to grow caudally and starts to cover the third and fourth pharyngeal arches.

8. The answer is E. *(II B 4)* During the sixth week, there are marked changes in the head. For example, the cervical flexure forms, causing the head to lie directly upon the cardiac prominence. In addition, the outer layer of the optic cup, a retinal precursor, differentiates to pigmented epithelium. This pigmentation is visible externally. The auricular hillocks (precursors of the external ear) also arise on the cranial and caudal borders of the first pharyngeal cleft. Digital rays appear in the forelimbs, but do not appear until later in the hindlimbs. The liver and midgut also undergo extensive growth. The volume of the liver expands, in part because it is becoming increasingly important as a hematopoietic center.

9. The answer is C. *(II B 5)* At seven weeks, the overall growth rate is still rapid as the embryo increases in length from 14 mm to 20 mm. The head growth is also rapid. Auricular hillocks fuse to form a single external ear or auricle. The eyelids and nipples also become visible. The liver enlarges extensively due to growth and active hepatic hematopoiesis. Also, the midgut loops elongate extensively, while the peritoneal cavity grows more slowly. As a result, the midgut loop undergoes the beginning of physiologic herniation into the extraembryonic coelom. The midgut loop remains herniated until the third month, when it is withdrawn back into the peritoneal cavity.

10. The answer is A. *(II B 6)* The length of the embryo increases by 100% in week 5 but only by 50% in week 8. The embryonic period covers weeks 3 to 8 inclusive. After week 8, the fetal period begins. The face becomes more human-like in the eighth week; for example, the eyes migrate from a lateral position into the frontal plane. Digital rays disappear as a result of programmed cell death, leading to the formation first of fingers and then of toes. The external genitalia are essentially alike in the eighth week, but by the twelfth week (third month) they are clearly differentiated in the two sexes.

11. The answer is D. *(III C 4)* By the end of the sixth month, the fetus has attained more than 50% of its ultimate fetal length. In contrast, it has attained only about 25% of its full fetal weight. Much of the increase in weight after the sixth month is due to the deposition of unilocular adipocytes as subcutaneous white fat. As this subcutaneous fat accumulates, the skin becomes smoother and less wrinkled, and the fetus appears more rotund. Fetal lung maturation begins in the sixth month due to the differentiation of surfactant-secreting type II cells in the alveolar epithelium. The surfactant secreted by these cells allows normal pulmonary inflation and respiratory function. Once type II cells have differentiated in substantial numbers, the fetal lungs are mature enough to allow extrauterine survival.

12. The answer is D. *(III C 5)* The lungs are capable of supporting extrauterine life during the sixth month. During the seventh month, pulmonary maturation continues by the formation of many more type II cells and many more pulmonary alveoli. This process continues even after birth. Extrauterine survival is possible at 7 months although less likely than at 8 months. Fat deposition is one of the chief hallmarks of the late fetal period, including the seventh month. As subcutaneous fat accumulates, the skin becomes smoother and the fetus appears chubbier.

4
Fertilization, Cleavage, and Implantation

I. **OVERVIEW:** From secondary oocyte to implanted conceptus (Fig. 4-1)

   A. **Gamete transport in the female reproductive tract**

   1. After **sperm** enter the female reproductive tract during intercourse, they must travel through the cervical mucus and enter the uterus. Next, the sperm must traverse the uterus and enter the uterine tubes.

   2. Meanwhile, the **ovum** is swept into the uterine tubes by the ciliary action of the uterine fimbriae, and is then transported proximally toward the uterus.

   B. **Sperm–egg interaction**

   1. When sperm and ovum meet, the sperm's acrosome cap releases its contents of hydrolytic enzymes, allowing the sperm to penetrate the layers surrounding the ovum.

   2. Sperm and egg membranes fuse and the male genetic material enters the egg cytoplasm.

   3. The paternal and maternal genetic material contained in **haploid pronuclei** then fuse to form a **diploid zygote nucleus.**

   C. **Fertilization**

   1. Fertilization begins when the gamete membranes fuse and ends when their pronuclei unite to form a single diploid zygote.

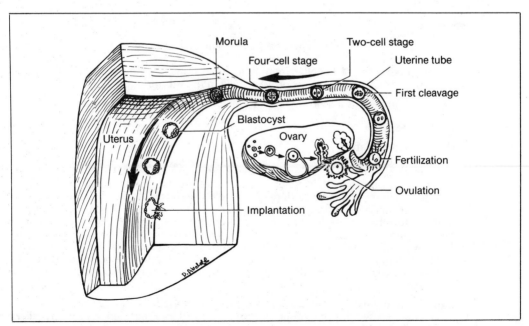

Figure 4-1. The progress of an ovum from its follicular origin through ovulation, fertilization, cleavage, and transport of the conceptus to implantation in the endometrium.

2. This union marks the beginning of the development of a new potential human being.
   a. Questions about whether the zygote is "alive" or "viable" are questions for clergy and ethicists.
   b. Practically speaking, the conceptus is alive and developing after fertilization but is not capable of independent survival outside of the uterus until after the sixth month of pregnancy. Even then, extraordinary support measures are required for the continued survival of such a premature fetus.

D. Cleavage
1. Soon after fertilization occurs, the zygote begins to divide by mitosis into increasing numbers of cells called **blastomeres**. Despite the increase in cell number, however, the volume of the conceptus remains constant, because the size of each cell decreases.
2. After several cleavages, the conceptus has become a ball of cells called the **morula**.
3. Next, a cavity called the **blastocoele** forms inside, and the conceptus now becomes a **blastocyst**.

E. Implantation
1. The blastocyst hatches from the zona pellucida and attaches itself to the wall of the endometrium.
2. The blastocyst invades the wall of the endometrium and **implants** itself in the uterus.
3. Implantation signals the beginning of an intimate interaction between the maternal blood supply and the developing conceptus.

II. SPERM AND EGG TRANSPORT IN THE FEMALE REPRODUCTIVE TRACT

A. Sperm transport
1. **Semen** is a complex mixture of secretions from the testes, the seminal vesicles, and the prostate gland. Minor components are also derived from the periurethral glands and the bulbourethral glands.
2. The semen deposited in the vagina during intercourse liquifies almost immediately, presumably allowing spermatozoa to escape from the ejaculate.
3. The spermatozoa leave the vagina, and **flagellar activity** propels them through the cervical mucus.
4. **Peristaltic contractile waves** in the uterus and uterine tubes are important for distal transport of spermatozoa.
   a. Semen is rich in **prostaglandins** which stimulate uterine and tubal smooth muscle contraction.
   b. The importance of flagellar motility in tubal transport is unclear. In animal studies, dead spermatozoa are transported distally in the uterine tubes.
5. **Sperm cell motility** is important for penetration of the layers surrounding the ovum.

B. Ovum transport
1. **The ovum at ovulation**
   a. The ovum and associated structures released at ovulation have been described in Chapter 2, section IV C 2. To recapitulate, when a mature ovarian follicle ruptures, the secondary oocyte, with its polar body, zona pellucida, corona radiata, and some of the attached liquor folliculi are all released from the ovary into the peritoneal cavity.
   b. The associated structures add considerable volume to the ovum (Fig. 4-2) and assist in its capture by the uterine fimbriae and transport along the female reproductive tract.
   c. In addition, the **zona pellucida** serves as an attachment site for granulosa cells of the corona radiata, while the cells of the **corona radiata** may play some protective and nutritive role for the ovum when it travels through the female reproductive tract.
   d. Spermatozoa must make their way through these outer layers before fertilization can be accomplished.
2. **Transport of the ovum from ovary to uterine tube ampulla**
   a. The ovum is swept from the peritoneal cavity and into the uterine tubes by **ciliary action** of the fimbriae.
      (1) The infundibulum of the uterine tubes nearly engulfs the ovary at ovulation.

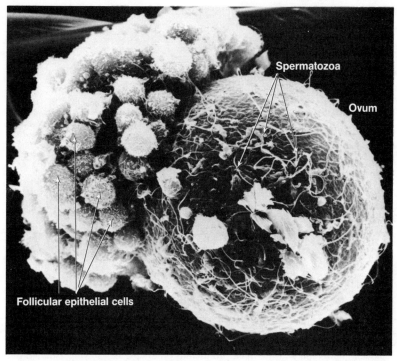

Figure 4-2. A fertilized human ovum. Note the numerous spermatozoa attached to the zona pellucida which surrounds the ovum. Many follicular epithelial cells *(left)* are also attached to the zona pellucida. This human ovum was fertilized in vitro but never transferred because it failed to cleave. (Scanning electron micrograph)

        Smooth muscle contractions increase in intensity around the time of ovulation and the uterine tubes move over the surface of the ovaries.
      (2) The structures released along with the ovum, in particular the **liquor folliculi** and the **corona radiata**, probably increase the likelihood that the ovum will be picked up in the uterine tubes.
    b. The cilia lining the tubal mucosa beat proximally so that the captured ovum is swept into the uterine tubes and toward the uterus.
  3. The combined actions of smooth muscle contraction and ciliary beating bring the sperm and egg together in the ampullary portion of the uterine tubes, where fertilization is thought to occur.

III. FERTILIZATION

  A. **Penetration of structures surrounding the ovum**
    1. The spermatozoal **acrosome** aids the sperm in penetrating the layers around the ovum. The acrosome is a highly modified lysosome, derived from the Golgi apparatus during spermiogenesis. It consists of a membrane-bound sac of hydrolytic enzymes and is completely enclosed within the plasma membrane of the sperm cell.
    2. As the sperm cell approaches the egg, the **acrosome reaction** occurs (Fig. 4-3).
      a. The acrosomal membrane fuses with the plasma membrane of the sperm cell.
      b. The enzymes within the acrosome are released into the milieu surrounding the sperm and egg.
    3. **Acrosome contents and their functions**
      a. **Hyaluronidase** is a hydrolytic enzyme.
        (1) It lyses the glycosaminoglycans in the extracellular matrix holding the cells of the corona radiata together. As the coronal cells become more loosely associated, sperm cells can propel themselves inward toward the zona pellucida.
        (2) Hyaluronidase may also be involved in breaking down the zona pellucida.
      b. **Neuraminidase**, also a hydrolytic enzyme, removes neuraminic acid (sialic acid) from

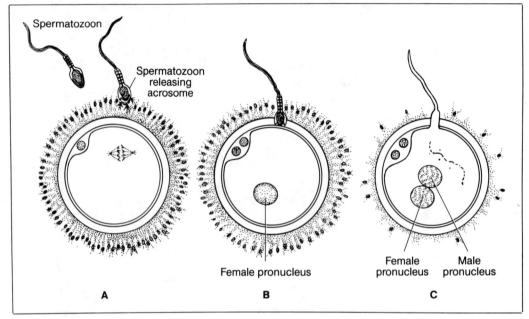

Figure 4-3. The events of fertilization summarized. Spermatozoa approach the egg and discharge their acrosomal contents. After penetrating the corona radiata and the zona pellucida, the sperm cell membrane fuses with the egg cell membrane and the male pronucleus enters the egg's cytoplasm. Note that a second polar body has formed as a result of fertilization.

glycoproteins. In experimental studies, a neuraminidase-treated zona pellucida cannot be penetrated by sperm cells. Thus, the acrosomal neuraminidase may aid in preventing more than one sperm from entering an ovum (polyspermy).
   c. **Zona lysins** are proteolytic enzymes that are capable of degrading the zona pellucida, perhaps easing the passage of sperm cells through to the ovum.
   4. Once the sperm cell has penetrated the corona radiata and zona pellucida, its unit membrane fuses with the unit membrane surrounding the egg cytoplasm. This triggers the phenomenon of fertilization.
B. **Events of fertilization.** When the membranes of sperm and ovum unite, the following events occur (see Fig. 4-3):
   1. **Shrinkage of the egg** to create a small **perivitelline space** between the ovum and the zona pellucida
   2. The **zona reaction** and subsequent **block to polyspermy**
   3. **Injection of the sperm nucleus** and middle piece (a source of mitochondria to supplement egg mitochondria) into the egg cytoplasm
C. **Consequences of fertilization**
   1. **Completion of meiosis II in the ovum** occurs soon after fertilization. The **second polar body** is formed and now resides in the perivitelline space along with the first polar body (see Fig. 4-3).
   2. The **diploid chromosome state** is reestablished in the zygote.
      a. Once the ovum completes meiosis II and the male genetic material enters, the egg cytoplasm contains a haploid male pronucleus and a haploid female pronucleus.
      b. The two pronuclei unite, in a process known as **syngamy**, forming a single **diploid zygote nucleus**.
         (1) The zygote nucleus has 22 autosomes and an X chromosome from the female pronucleus, and 22 autosomes and either an X or a Y chromosome from the male pronucleus.
         (2) Thus, the **total chromosomal complement** is either 44 autosomes plus two Xs (in potential females) or 44 autosomes plus an X and Y (in potential males), for a total number of 46.

3. The **initiation of cleavage** by mitotic divisions of the zygote is also a direct consequence of fertilization.

IV. CLEAVAGE AND BLASTOCYST FORMATION

A. Cleavage

1. **Blastomere stage**
   a. During cleavage, the zygote divides into a series of increasingly smaller cells known as **blastomeres** (Fig. 4-4).
      (1) Each blastomere contains a diploid number of chromosomes, since cleavage divisions are mitotic divisions.
      (2) The cytoplasm of the ovum is divided into smaller and smaller packets. The cell number increases, but the volume of the embryo remains constant because cells become smaller and smaller with each division.
   b. As it divides, the developing conceptus moves toward the uterus (see Fig. 4-1). It floats freely in the lumen of the uterine tube, still enclosed within the zona pellucida.
   c. The interval between fertilization and first cleavage is about 30 hours in humans. Subsequent divisions occur more rapidly.

2. **Morula stage** (Fig. 4-5; see also Fig. 3-2). Once the conceptus becomes a cluster of many cells, it is called a **morula** (the Latin word for mulberry).
   a. This stage is reached about 3 days after fertilization. At this time, the conceptus is entering the uterine cavity from the uterine tubes (see Fig. 4-1).
   b. Between individual blastomeres there are fluid-filled spaces, and these begin to coalesce into a central **cavity** called the **blastocoele** (see Fig. 4-6).

B. Blastocyst formation and hatching

1. When the blastocoele begins to form, the conceptus has become a **blastocyst** (Fig. 4-6).

2. Once the conceptus reaches the uterine cavity, the **zona pellucida** becomes thinned. On the fourth day after fertilization, with the blastocyst now floating freely in the uterine lumen, the zona pellucida breaks down completely. This process is known as **blastocyst hatching**.
   a. Without dissolution of the zona pellucida, the blastocyst would be unable to attach itself to the endometrium or to grow during implantation.
   b. After blastocyst hatching, the embryo is free to increase in volume and mass.

C. Differentiation in the blastocyst

1. Until the blastocyst stage, the developing conceptus seems to be little more than a simple ball of cells. Recent studies with mice have shown that blastomeres do undergo a certain

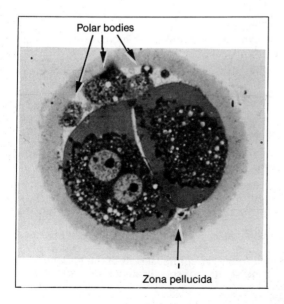

Figure 4-4. Two-celled human embryo surrounded by a zona pellucida. Note that three polar bodies are also enclosed within the zona pellucida. (Light micrograph)

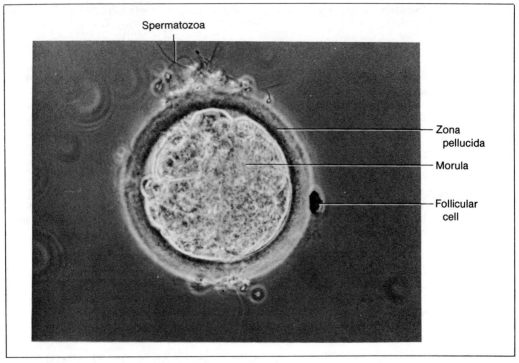

Figure 4-5. Human morula surrounded by a zona pellucida; follicular cells and spermatozoa are still attached. (Phase-contrast light micrograph)

amount of differentiation, but anatomically there appears to be little difference between early blastomeres.

2. In the blastocyst, however, **morphologic differentiation** becomes evident. A mass of cells called the **embryoblast**, or **inner cell mass**, develops at one pole, closely surrounded by an outer epithelial layer called the **trophoblast** (see Fig. 4-6).
   a. The **inner cell mass** contains cells destined to make up most of the bulk of the **embryo and fetus**. Some cells of the inner cell mass are also thought to contribute to the **amnion**, one of the extraembryonic membranes.
   b. The **trophoblast** cells are destined to form most of the **extraembryonic membranes**, most importantly the bulk of the **placenta**.

3. On the fifth day after fertilization the blastocyst has a diameter of about 300 μm, about three times greater than the diameter of the zygote. Most of the increase in volume is due to the accumulation of blastocoele fluid.

4. The blastocyst now **attaches** to the wall of the endometrium, signaling the beginning of the process of implantation.

V. IMPLANTATION

A. Blastocyst attachment and early implantation (Fig. 4-7)

1. Soon after entering the uterine cavity, and following blastocyst hatching, the blastocyst attaches to the endometrial epithelium.
2. There is probably a well-developed **recognition system** that ensures a correct initial interaction between blastocyst and endometrium.
   a. Normally, the blastocyst attaches firmly to the body of the uterus, most often at a superior and posterior site.
   b. The blastocyst attaches at its embryonic pole; that is, with the inner cell mass nearest the endometrial epithelium. Attachment occurs initially between certain trophoblastic cells of the conceptus and the tall columnar epithelial cells of the endometrium.
   c. Some authors suggest that the blastocyst attaches specifically to the endometrium in close association with a blood vessel.

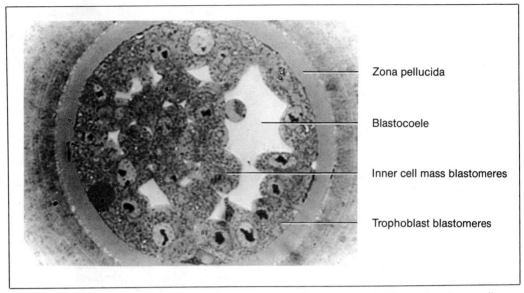

Figure 4-6. Rabbit early blastocyst. The zona pellucida is still intact. A trophoblast and an inner cell mass (embryoblast) have differentiated, and the blastocoele is also apparent. (Light micrograph)

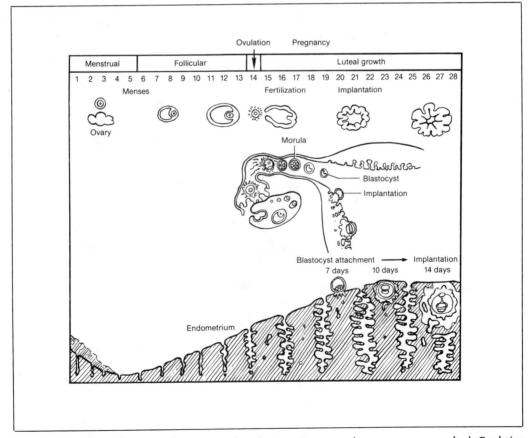

Figure 4-7. Diagram illustrating the menstrual cycle in an instance where pregnancy resulted. Ovulation occurred on day 14 of the cycle, and fertilization occurred just 1 day after. Implantation occurred 6 days later. By day 28, endometrial invasion and differentiation of the chorionic gonadotropin–producing syncytiotrophoblast were in progress.

52　*Human Developmental Anatomy*

   (1) However, the endometrium is full of glands after ovulation and has an extremely rich blood supply in the form of dense anastomosing networks of capillaries.
   (2) Given the richness of the blood supply in the endometrial stroma, it seems unlikely that the blastocyst could find an attachment site anywhere and not be close to a blood vessel. Wherever a blastocyst attaches, blood vessels and glands will not be very far away.
 3. **Abnormal implantation** may result in an **ectopic pregnancy** (see Chapter 7 section IX A). Normally, the zona pellucida probably prevents blastocyst attachment to the epithelial lining of the uterine tubes.

B. **Formation of the syncytiotrophoblast**
 1. During early implantation, the trophoblast differentiates into two distinct areas (Fig. 4-8).
    a. The **inner layer** of the trophoblast, lying next to the inner cell mass and blastocoele, forms into a **cytotrophoblast.**
       (1) These cells constitute a highly proliferative epithelium, with nuclei containing prominent nucleoli, and cytoplasm with many mitochondria, much rough endoplasmic reticulum, and a well-developed Golgi apparatus. Glycogen granules and free ribosomes are also a prominent cytoplasmic feature.
       (2) The cells rest on a well-developed basement membrane.
    b. The cytotrophoblastic cells undergo repeated mitotic divisions, and soon after dividing they fuse with one another to form a superficial **syncytiotrophoblast.**
       (1) The cells of this layer contain nuclei that never divide.
       (2) The cytoplasm is filled with membrane-bound vesicles of many different sizes.
       (3) The syncytiotrophoblast is covered on its outer surface by many **microvilli.**
 2. The syncytiotrophoblast is an **invasive** cell layer.
    a. Soon after contacting the endometrial epithelium, it begins to secrete proteolytic enzymes which destroy the endometrial epithelium, basement membrane, and underlying connective tissue stroma. Uterine glands and blood vessels are also destroyed.
    b. Presumably, these degraded components are used for the early nutritive support of the developing conceptus.

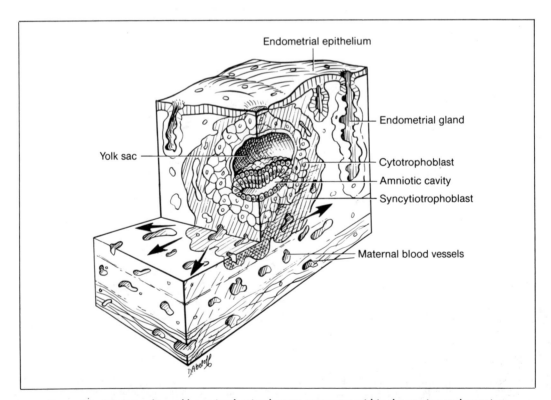

Figure 4-8. Structures formed by an implanting human conceptus within the uterine endometrium.

3. The syncytiotrophoblast is also actively **migratory.** It projects filopodia and other locomotory structures deep into the endometrium as advancing areas of syncytiotrophoblast carry the conceptus into the wall of the uterus.
4. As the conceptus burrows into the uterine wall, the cytotrophoblast cells continue to proliferate and fuse, forming increasing amounts of syncytiotrophoblast.
   a. Adjacent epithelial cells in the wall of the uterus begin to grow over the implantation site. Clotted blood and cellular debris also accumulate over the implantation site.
   b. Eventually, endometrial epithelial cells completely cover the conceptus at the implantation site, entirely surrounding it with maternal tissue.
   c. This type of **interstitial implantation** is peculiar to humans and a few other mammals.

C. **Blood supply of the syncytiotrophoblast**
1. The invading conceptus is growing very rapidly and has a great need for nutrients and gas exchange.
2. The endometrial stroma is rich in blood vessels.
3. During invasion, the walls of the maternal capillaries are broken down by invasive cytoplasmic processes of the syncytiotrophoblast. Maternal blood leaks from the capillaries and bathes the surface of the syncytiotrophoblast.
4. This direct bathing of the conceptus in maternal blood persists throughout pregnancy, beginning at implantation and continuing throughout the entire period when the definitive placenta functions as the maternal–fetal interface. The human placenta is called a **hemochorial placenta** because the maternal blood directly bathes the chorionic surface.

D. **Further development of the syncytiotrophoblast**
1. The surface area of the syncytiotrophoblast begins to expand rapidly, as irregular **microvilli** project from the surface and deep **surface invaginations** begin to form.
2. Sections through the syncytiotrophoblast also reveal spaces, or holes, in it. These **lacunae** may simply represent surface invaginations cut in unusual angles, or they may actually be isolated cavities that lack direct communication with the maternal blood supply at the time of formation. The lacunae develop and begin to fuse with one another and with surface invaginations.
3. The net result of the advance of processes and the development of lacunae is a rapid **increase in the surface area** of the syncytiotrophoblast, providing an increased area for the maternal–fetal interface that nourishes the embryo.

E. **Consequences of implantation**
1. The embryo becomes completely surrounded by maternal tissue because human implantation is **interstitial.**
2. An intimate relationship between growing conceptus and the maternal blood supply is established. This respresents a precursor of the more complex placenta that will form as the nutrient and gas exchange requirements of the growing embryo and fetus increase.

VI. **DEVELOPMENT OF THE INNER CELL MASS.** While the syncytiotrophoblast is leading the way for the implanting conceptus, the inner cell mass is beginning to develop into a complex **pre-embryonic structure with two layers.**

A. **Formation of the amniotic cavity**
1. At first, the inner cell mass is a simple cluster of cells surrounded by the trophoblast.
2. By the eighth day after fertilization, this situation has already begun to change. On the side of the conceptus facing the endometrium and opposite the blastocoele, a new cavity, the **amniotic cavity**, appears among the cells of the inner cell mass (see Fig. 4-8).
3. The amniotic cavity is a closed vesicle lined everywhere by cells.
   a. The cells of the floor of the amniotic cavity are derived from the embryoblast or inner cell mass. There is some controversy concerning the origin of the cells lining the roof of the amniotic cavity.
      (1) The cells of the roof of the amnion are probably also derived from the cytotrophoblast, although some authors believe that parts of the amnion are derived from the embryoblast rather than the trophoblast.

(2) It is not possible to resolve these controversies without experimental studies.
  b. The **cells lining the roof of the amniotic cavity** are extremely attenuated squamous cells.
  c. The **cells lining the floor of the amniotic cavity** are tall columnar epithelial cells that are arranged in a roughly circular, disk-like layer called the **epiblast.** Once gastrulation (the next stage of development) has been completed, the epiblast gives rise to:
     (1) Ectoderm
     (2) Intraembryonic mesoderm
     (3) Perhaps some endoderm as well (there is controversy here)

B. **Formation of the yolk sac**
  1. Besides the amniotic cavity, a second cavity, the **yolk sac**, forms (see Fig. 4-8).
  2. The yolk sac develops from the blastocoele. Certain cells in the inner cell mass begin to migrate along the inner aspect of the wall of the blastocyst cavity. Eventually, they form a continuous sheet of cells, making the wall of the yolk sac.
  3. The yolk sac wall is lined by **two cell layers**:
     a. The outer cell layer is derived from the wall of the blastocyst or trophoblast and is properly called **cytotrophoblast.**
     b. The inner cell layer, facing the cavity of the yolk sac, is derived from the inner cell mass.

C. **Formation of the bilaminar disk—the pre-embryo itself**
  1. Adjacent to the epiblast (which lines the amniotic floor), the cells lining the yolk sac form a low columnar or cuboidal epithelium known as the **hypoblast.**
  2. The epiblast and hypoblast are thus two epithelial layers sandwiched together at the junction of the amniotic cavity and the yolk sac.
  3. Together the **epiblast** and **hypoblast** make up the **pre-embryo proper.** All of the embryonic and fetal tissues will arise from this **bilaminar disk stage.**

VII. DEVELOPMENT OF EXTRAEMBRYONIC MESODERM, CHORION, AND YOLK SAC

A. **Development of the trophoblast.** While the bilaminar disk is forming from the inner cell mass, a tremendous development also occurs in the trophoblast.
  1. Besides the contribution that the cytotrophoblastic layer makes to the syncytiotrophoblast (see section V B), the cytotrophoblast also contributes to the development of the extraembryonic mesoderm and the chorion.
     a. Soon after implantation has begun, cytotrophoblastic cells lining the blastocoele proliferate into a reticular meshwork which completely surrounds the amniotic cavity and yolk sac. This meshwork comes to lie between the pre-embryo and a shell of cytotrophoblast and syncytiotrophoblast.
     b. There are numerous spaces between cells in this meshwork, and as these spaces begin to fuse with one another, they eventually coalesce and form a single large cavity known as the **extraembryonic coelom.**
  2. The extraembryonic coelom eventually surrounds the pre-embryo except at the place where the amniotic cavity faces the implantation site.
     a. Because the coelomic cavity does not form here, in effect the pre-embryo is suspended from the chorionic shell by a **connecting stalk.** Thus, the pre-embryo is suspended by the connecting stalk within a cavity inside the chorion.
     b. This connecting stalk later becomes the **umbilical cord.**

B. **Extraembryonic mesoderm formation**
  1. The extraembryonic coelom is lined by extraembryonic mesodermal cells. The extraembryonic mesoderm has **two layers.**
     a. The **somatopleuric extraembryonic mesoderm** layer lines the inner aspect of the chorion.
     b. The **splanchnopleuric extraembryonic mesoderm** layer covers the outer aspect of the amniotic cavity and the yolk sac.
  2. The splanchnopleuric and somatopleuric layers are continuous with one another at the connecting stalk; that is, the somatopleuric layer is **reflected** onto the splanchnopleuric layer at the connecting stalk.

3. The area of the splanchnopleuric layer that lies over the yolk sac appears to exert a constricting influence, so that part of the yolk sac is pinched off and carried outward to the chorionic shell, leaving behind a smaller **definitive yolk sac**.

C. Relationships between connecting stalk, amnion, and chorion

1. At this point in the bilaminar disk stage (day 14), the conceptus now shows the following features:
    a. The pre-embryo is suspended by the connecting stalk (the future umbilical cord) from a complex, multilayered chorion.
        (1) The **chorion** is lined by somatopleuric extraembryonic mesoderm and covered by cytotrophoblast and syncytiotrophoblast.
        (2) The **amnion** is also covered by somatopleuric extraembryonic mesoderm.
        (3) The **yolk sac** is covered by the splanchnopleuric extraembryonic mesoderm, which is a continuation of the somatopleuric extraembryonic mesoderm. It is also lined by hypoblast derivatives.
    b. Inside the closed chorionic vesicle, two other closed cavities confront one another:
        (1) The amniotic cavity
        (2) The yolk sac
    c. At the junction between these two cavities, there are two thickened cell layers, which together constitute the **blastoderm**:
        (1) The epiblast
        (2) The hypoblast
2. The **future destiny** of these structures is as follows:
    a. The **epiblast and the hypoblast** are destined to form the **embryo**, which then will become the **fetus**.
    b. The **connecting stalk** will become the **umbilical cord**.
    c. The **amniotic cavity** will expand and the **amnion** will grow down around the embryo, completely enclosing it and coating the umbilical cord.
    d. The **chorion** will sprout numerous **villi**, which will develop into the **placenta** at later stages.
    e. Also, the amnion and chorion will eventually fuse.
3. This is how a human fetus comes to reside in a closed sac (the fused chorion and amnion) that is filled with fluid (the amniotic fluid) and suspended from the placenta by an umbilical cord conveying blood between the placenta and the fetus.

VIII. FORMATION OF THE OROPHARYNGEAL AND CLOACAL MEMBRANES. Two final important events occur in the bilaminar disk stage of the embryo.

A. Formation of the prochordal plate and oropharyngeal membrane

1. At the future head end of the embryo, certain hypoblast cells become a good deal more columnar than their neighbors. They form an ovoid group of cells called the **prochordal plate**.
2. The prochordal plate defines the future cranial–caudal axis of the pre-embryo and the future axis of bilateral symmetry of the embryo.
3. The prochordal plate lies at the future cranial end of the embryo and will form part of the **oropharyngeal membrane (buccopharyngeal membrane)**, a transient structure which closes the opening of the oral cavity for a time and then disintegrates.
4. The prochordal plate is so named because it lies anterior to the notochord, a structure that forms during gastrulation, and because it precedes the formation of the notochord.

B. Formation of the cloacal membrane

1. At the caudal extremity of the bilaminar disk, a **cloacal membrane** forms. The cloacal membrane temporarily closes the caudal end of the gut.
2. Eventually the cloacal membrane also disintegrates, so that the caudal portion of the hindgut communicates with the outside world.

IX. IN VITRO FERTILIZATION (IVF) AND EMBRYO TRANSFER

A. Purpose of in vitro fertilization

1. Some couples suffer from infertility despite normal ovulation and normal endometrial

function, and despite sperm cells with normal function. In some cases, for example, this happens because the woman has a uterine tube abnormality or the man has oligospermia.
2. **IVF** has been developed as a way to allow women to bear their own children in such cases. As proof that IVF can overcome infertility in some cases, there is the fact that thousands of babies have been born as a result of IVF.

B. **Methods of in vitro fertilization**
1. Obtaining ova is the first step of IVF.
   a. Usually, multiple ovulation is induced by the use of drugs that stimulate supernumerary ovulation.
   b. The resulting eggs are recovered surgically by means of a suction device inserted through a small incision in the abdomen, using a fiberoptic device for monitoring the retrieval.
   c. More recently, a transvaginal route has been developed for egg recovery.
2. The unfertilized eggs are then placed in a Petri dish on appropriate tissue culture media. Next, the eggs are inseminated with sperm from the father and are incubated to allow fertilization.
   a. Cleavage begins in some or all of the eggs, and their development is monitored microscopically.
   b. Some fertilized eggs will not develop properly and these are discarded.
3. Of the eggs that do develop normally, as many as four are transferred to the uterus by means of a long cannula inserted through the cervix and into the uterus.
4. Currently, about 20% to 25% of all transfers result in a valid pregnancy. This low success rate will probably improve as clinicians become more experienced with this new technique.

C. **Negative aspects of in vitro fertilization**
1. IVF is expensive and time-consuming for the patient and often does not work.
2. IVF also exposes the mother and the fetus to risks that they would not otherwise encounter.
   a. Multiple pregnancies can result, since multiple eggs are transferred. Multiple pregnancies increase the likelihood of a complicated pregnancy for the mother and fetuses. Spontaneous abortions are also more common after IVF.
   b. Congenital birth defects may result from the procedure, although experience is proving this worry to be less of a concern than initially thought. As more and more IVF babies are born, the incidence of congenital anomalies in IVF babies is proving to be similar to that seen in babies derived from natural conceptions.

STUDY QUESTIONS

Directions: Each question below contains five suggested answers. Choose the **one best** response to each question.

1. All of the following statements about fertilization are true EXCEPT

(A) it initiates development of the organism
(B) it reestablishes the diploid chromosome number
(C) it stimulates formation of the first polar body
(D) it prevents polyspermy
(E) it results in formation of a male pronucleus

2. All of the following statements about in vitro fertilization (IVF) are true EXCEPT

(A) it is used in cases of blocked uterine tubes
(B) it is used in cases of oligospermia
(C) the transfer from in vitro to uterus takes place during cleavage
(D) several conceptuses are normally transferred
(E) eggs and sperm are transferred separately into the female reproductive tract

3. The human embryo in the blastocyst stage shows all of the following characteristics EXCEPT

(A) it has more cells than a morula-stage embryo
(B) it has syncytiotrophoblastic cells
(C) it has an inner cell mass destined to form the bulk of the embryo
(D) it has a trophoblast which will differentiate into a cytotrophoblast
(E) it can be surrounded by a zona pellucida

4. All of the following events take place during the first week after fertilization EXCEPT

(A) sarcomere formation
(B) cell differentiation
(C) cytokinesis
(D) DNA synthesis
(E) secretion of proteolytic enzymes

5. Which of the following chemical compounds is responsible for degrading the extracellular matrix of glycosaminoglycan macromolecules surrounding cells of the corona radiata?

(A) Neuraminidase
(B) Zona lysins
(C) Hyaluronidase
(D) Proteolytic enzymes
(E) Prostaglandins

Questions 6–10

Match each of the descriptions below with the type of extraembryonic mesoderm that it best describes.

(A) Somatopleuric extraembryonic mesoderm
(B) Splanchnopleuric extraembryonic mesoderm
(C) Both
(D) Neither

6. Derived from the cytotrophoblast

7. Lines the extraembryonic coelom and coats the inner aspect of the chorionic vesicle

8. Lines the extraembryonic coelom and coats the outer aspect of the amniotic cavity and yolk sac

9. Forms mesodermal derivatives in the embryo proper

10. Forms a continuous layer of cells which reflect onto one another at the connecting stalk

Questions 11–15

For each description of a component of the blastocyst below, choose the appropriate lettered structure in the accompanying micrograph.

11. This structure is the precursor of the cytotrophoblast and syncytiotrophoblast

12. This structure is secreted by follicular epithelial cells and degenerates prior to implantation

13. This structure is the precursor of the yolk sac cavity

14. This structure forms the bulk of the embryo proper

15. This structure forms the chorion which later sprouts villi and becomes the placenta

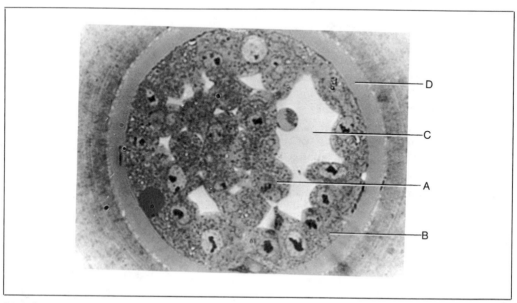

Questions 11–15

ANSWERS AND EXPLANATIONS

1. The answer is C. (*III B, C*) Fertilization results in the completion of meiosis in the female gamete. The second polar body is not formed until after fertilization has been initiated. The first polar body is formed at ovulation. Fertilization introduces a male set of chromosomes into the egg in the form of a male pronucleus, and thereby creates a diploid chromosome complement. Fertilization also prevents polyspermy, and initiates the process of development.

2. The answer is E. (*IX A, B*) In vitro fertilization (IVF) has been developed recently to aid clinicians in overcoming certain kinds of infertility. IVF can overcome either blocked uterine tubes or oligospermia. Eggs and sperm are mixed in a Petri dish, and of those conceptuses showing normal cleavage patterns, up to four are transferred into the uterus. Successful pregnancy is verified by testing for the presence of chorionic gonadotropin (hCG), secreted by the developing conceptus, and the pregnancy is allowed to continue just liked a natural conception.

3. The answer is B. (*IV A, B, C; V B*) The morula has fewer cells than the blastocyst. The cavity of the blastocyst, the blastocoele, forms by coalescence of extracellular fluids between morula blastomeres (cells). The blastocyst is differentiated into an inner cell mass (precursor of the embryo) and a trophoblast (precursor of the extraembryonic membranes). After blastocyst hatching from the zona pellucida, the trophoblast differentiates into a cytotrophoblast and a syncytiotrophoblast. The former gives rise to a proliferative cell population. Fused cytotrophoblastic cells form the syncytiotrophoblast, an invasive syncytial layer around the cytotrophoblast.

4. The answer is A. (*IV A, B, C; V B 2*) Sarcomeres are components of differentiated striated muscle cells. Their formation does not begin until after the second week of development. Cell differentiation probably begins as early as the late cleavage stages and has certainly happened by the time the inner cell mass and trophoblast have formed from the morula. DNA synthesis and cytokinesis, or cell division, occur at a furious pace from fertilization all throughout the embryonic and fetal periods, as there is a rapid increase in cell number during development. Proteolytic enzymes are involved in breakdown of the zona pellucida and in destruction of maternal tissue during syncytiotrophoblast implantation and invasion.

5. The answer is C. (*II A 4; III A*) Neuraminidase releases sialic acid from glycoprotein components of the zona pellucida and is thought to prevent polyspermy. Proteolytic enzymes are responsible for aiding spermatozoa to penetrate the zona pellucida, and zona lysins are proteolytic enzymes. Hyaluronidase degrades glycosaminoglycans such as hyaluronic acid and chondroitin sulfate. Prostaglandins are hormones present in semen. They stimulate peristalsis of the uterus and uterine tubes.

6–10. The answers are: 6-C, 7-A, 8-B, 9-D, 10-C. (*VII A, B*) The somatopleuric extraembryonic mesoderm and splanchnopleuric extraembryonic mesoderm are both derived from the cytotrophoblast, a derivative of the trophoblast. These mesodermal cell layers both line the entire extraembryonic coelom. The somatopleuric layer also coats the inner aspect of the chorionic shell, whereas the splanchnopleuric layer coats the amniotic cavity and the yolk sac. The two layers are continuous with one another at the connecting stalk. Both contribute to extraembryonic mesoderm but neither layer forms intraembryonic mesoderm, which is derived solely from the epiblast during gastrulation.

11–15. The answers are: 11-B, 12-D, 13-C, 14-A, 15-B. (*IV B, C*) The blastocyst consists of a trophoblast (B) and an inner cell mass, or embryoblast (A). The trophoblast forms a continuous epithelial layer around the entire blastocyst. Later it differentiates into the cytotrophoblast and syncytiotrophoblast, which are primarily responsible for the formation of the placenta. The inner cell mass forms most of the embryo proper during later development. The zona pellucida (D) surrounds the entire conceptus. It is an extracellular matrix secreted by the follicular epithelial cells during oogenesis and disintegrates during blastocyst hatching so that the blastocyst can attach to the endometrial epithelium during implantation. The blastocoele (C) is a fluid-filled cavity in the blastocyst. It later becomes the yolk sac cavity.

5
Gastrulation and Neurulation

I. INTRODUCTION

A. Overview of development during the gastrulation period

1. The gastrulation period begins at the end of the second week of development.
   a. By this time, a pregnant woman will note that her typical menses are absent. This will be the first outward sign of her pregnancy.
   b. In the wall of her uterus, the conceptus, with a pre-embryo in the bilaminar disk stage, has completed its implantation.
2. From the beginning of the third week until the end of the eighth week, the developing individual can properly be referred to as an **embryo**.
3. During the third week, a complex series of morphogenetic cell movements occur as the pre-embryo becomes a **gastrula**.
   a. During **gastrulation**, the two layers of the bilaminar disk stage are converted into the **three primary germ layers** (see Chapter 3, Fig. 3-3):
      (1) **Ectoderm**
      (2) **Mesoderm**
      (3) **Endoderm**
   b. During gastrulation, **other events** occur as well:
      (1) The embryo elongates somewhat in the cranial–caudal direction and shows a marked expansion of the blastoderm in the cranial end.
      (2) The **notochord** is formed.
   c. The three primary germ layers are formed by invagination, cell migration, and cell proliferation.

B. Overview of development during the neurulation period (weeks 2.5 to 3.5)

1. Once the three primary germ layers are formed, the underlying **chordamesodermal inductor** of the central nervous system (i.e., the notochord and paraxial mesoderm) brings about a change in parts of the overlying ectoderm.
   a. Ectodermal cells thicken into a **neural plate**, and soon after this they curl up into a **neural groove**.
   b. Later, the long **neural folds** along the edges of the neural groove move toward one another in the midsagittal plane, eventually forming the **neural tube** (see Chapter 1, Fig. 1-4).
2. Just before the neural folds fuse to form a closed neural tube, **neural crest cells** emigrate from the neuroepithelium and are dispersed throughout the entire body of the embryo (see Chapter 19, Fig. 19-4). Neural crest cells represent a pluripotent cell line which becomes a wide variety of highly differentiated cell types, including melanocytes and Schwann cells, to name but two examples.
3. At the same time that neurulation is taking place, other fundamental morphogenetic changes are also occurring. These will be described in Chapter 6.

II. FORMATION OF INTRAEMBRYONIC MESODERM

A. General considerations

1. To understand gastrulation, one must think of moving groups of cells and be able to imagine these movements as they occur in three dimensions.

62 Human Developmental Anatomy

2. This description will be viewing the morphogenetic cell movements from above the epiblast, looking down on it from inside the amniotic cavity.

B. Invagination in the epiblast

1. By the end of the third week, the pre-embryo has become a **blastoderm** with the following features:
    a. The pre-embryo is a **bilaminar (two-layered) disk.** It has:
        (1) An upper **epiblast** at the floor of the amniotic cavity
        (2) A lower **hypoblast** at the roof of the yolk sac
    b. The **cranial pole** of the blastoderm has been determined by the formation of the prochordal plate and a slight lateral expansion of the cranial portion of the blastoderm.

2. **Formation of the primitive streak** is the next change in the blastoderm.
    a. The **primitive streak** (Fig. 5-1) is formed at the caudal extremity of the epiblast, away from the prochordal plate.
        (1) In vertebrate embryos, a structure known as the **blastopore** is the site where invagination of the chordamesodermal mass occurs.
        (2) Avian and mammalian pre-embryos are flat rather than round. Consequently, they form a linear structure similar to the blastopore known as the **primitive streak.** The primitive streak is the location where cells leave the epiblast and begin to form the **notochord** and **intraembryonic mesoderm**—that is, the chordamesodermal mass.
    b. At first, the primitive streak appears as an area with many cells crowded together. This can be seen in human embryos at 15 days after fertilization.
    c. The primitive streak is an area of intense activity.
        (1) Cells in the primitive streak are dividing.
        (2) At the same time, cells from the lateral reaches of the epiblast are migrating medially toward the primitive streak along the midline of the embryo.
        (3) Thus, cells are constantly being added on to the primitive streak at the caudal end as it grows and moves in a cranial direction (Fig. 5-2).

3. The **intraembryonic mesoderm** forms by **invagination** at the primitive streak.
    a. Once cells from the epiblast move medially **to** the primitive streak, they invaginate **through** the primitive streak and then continue to move laterally away from it (Fig. 5-3) as they become intraembryonic mesoderm.
    b. The cells moving away from the primitive streak travel between the epiblast and the hypoblast. In fact, during their migration they probably use the epiblast or hypoblast as their substratum for locomotion, and they probably travel by means of locomotory organelles, such as long filopodia and broad flat lamellipodia, extended from their cell margins.
    c. Migrating cells have an innate tendency to move into open spaces, and thus the migrating mesodermal cells spread out away from the primitive streak.

4. **Formation of the cardiac primordium**
    a. Some mesodermal cells leave the medial primitive streak and migrate cranially and laterally as two separate sheets of cells on either side of the primitive streak (see Fig.

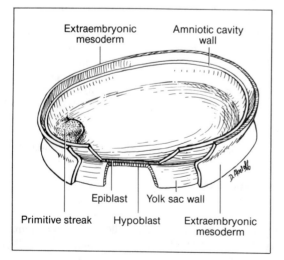

Figure 5-1. Structure of a late bilaminar disk embryo just at the beginning of gastrulation. The primitive streak is a mere accumulation of cells at the caudal pole of the blastoderm.

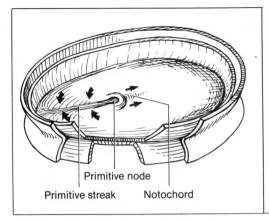

Figure 5-2. Structure of an early gastrula. The primitive node (also called Hensen's node and the primitive knot) is the site of notochord formation. Caudal to it lies the primitive streak, the site of invagination. The morphogenetic cell movements of gastrulation occur primarily in the epiblast and among the intraembryonic mesodermal cells. *Arrows* indicate the direction of cell movements.

5-3). When these sheets of cells reach the region of the prochordal plate, they move cranially around the plate and fuse medially and cranially to it.
   b. The group of cells located cranial to the prochordal plate represents the **cardiac primordium**, while the prochordal plate represents the primordium of the **oropharyngeal membrane**.
5. **Later development of the intraembryonic mesoderm**
   a. The intraembryonic mesoderm eventually forms an intermediate layer of cells interposed between ectoderm and endoderm except at the cranial oropharyngeal membrane and the caudal cloacal membrane. In these two locations, ectoderm and endoderm are in direct contact.
   b. During a later stage of development, the cardiac primordium is tucked under the ventral aspect of the embryo by the growth of the head fold of the amnion (see Chapter 6, section IV).
   c. As the intraembryonic mesoderm migrates to the outer boundaries of the blastoderm, it eventually meets up with and fuses with the splanchnopleuric and somatopleuric extraembryonic mesoderm.
   d. In the caudal extremes of the primitive streak, some mesodermal cells migrate out of the embryo into the connecting stalk and add to the extraembryonic mesodermal cells contained there.

III. NOTOCHORD FORMATION AND THE COMPLETION OF GASTRULATION

   A. **Formation of the notochord**
   1. The **primitive node (Hensen's node; primitive knot)** is a mass of cells that forms at the cranial extremity of the primitive streak (see Figs. 5-2 and 5-3). A depression forms in the center of this node.
   2. A tubular group of cells, lying only in the midline, grows cranially from the primitive node to form the **notochord**.
      a. A cavity, the **notochordal canal**, runs down the center of the notochord. This cavity communicates with the amniotic cavity at the primitive node.
      b. The notochord grows cranially (Fig. 5-4) until it meets the prochordal plate, and then notochord and plate become firmly attached.
      c. The notochord also contacts the endodermal layer lining the yolk sac and fuses with it in such a way that the lumen of the notochordal canal opens into the yolk sac.
      d. Thus, for a time there is a direct communication between the amniotic cavity and the yolk sac. This continuity, however, lasts only briefly. It is soon interrupted by a secondary invagination of the notochord.
   3. As the length of the embryo increases, the notochord folds up into a tubular structure again, and the endodermal layer fuses over the notochord.
   4. With the completion of the notochord, gastrulation is finished.

   B. **Consequences of gastrulation.** There are three major results from gastrulation:
   1. A **triploblastic embryo**, the **gastrula**, has been established, containing the **three primary germ layers** (ectoderm, mesoderm, and endoderm) and a **notochord**.

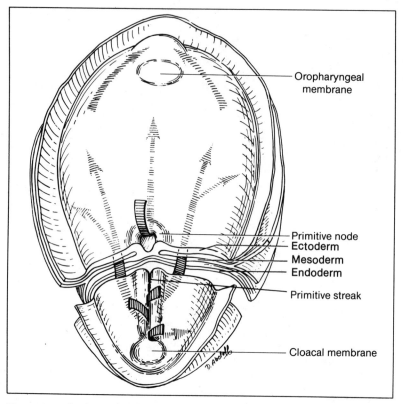

Figure 5-3. The human embryo at mid-gastrula stage. The morphogenetic cell movements of gastrulation are in full progress. *Arrows* indicate the direction of cell movements: the intraembryonic mesodermal cells invaginate through the primitive streak and then migrate laterally, while the notochord invaginates through the primitive node and then travels cranially in the midline, toward the oropharyngeal membrane.

    2. The **central nervous system (CNS) primordium** in the ectoderm is juxtaposed with the **CNS inductor.**
        a. The **CNS primordium** consists of the flattened midline ectodermal layer over the notochord and the paraxial intraembryonic mesoderm lateral to the notochord.
        b. The **CNS inductor** consists of the notochord itself plus the paraxial intraembryonic mesoderm. This **chordamesodermal mass**—notochord plus paraxial mesoderm—plays a fundamental role in establishing the basic structural plan of all vertebrate embryos.
    3. The anterior, posterior, cranial, and caudal orientations and the **axis of bilateral symmetry** of the embryo have all been established.

IV. NEURULATION. The process of neurulation, which forms the future CNS, begins on about day 18 and is largely completed by day 21 or day 22.

  A. Induction of the nervous system
    1. Prior to neurulation, the CNS is represented by the flattened ectodermal layer lying over the notochord in the midline and the paraxial intraembryonic mesoderm lying lateral to the notochord (see Fig. 5-4).
    2. The **neural plate** now forms cranially to the primitive node, from a thickened area of the overlying ectoderm.
        a. The neural plate subsequently becomes expanded somewhat in its cranial portion but remains less broad in its caudal portion (Fig. 5-5).
        b. The **cranial portion** ultimately forms the **brain** and the **caudal portion** forms the **spinal cord.**
    3. The ectoderm is **induced** to form neuroectoderm by the underlying notochord and paraxial mesoderm. This has been shown by experimental studies performed in amphibian and avian embryos.

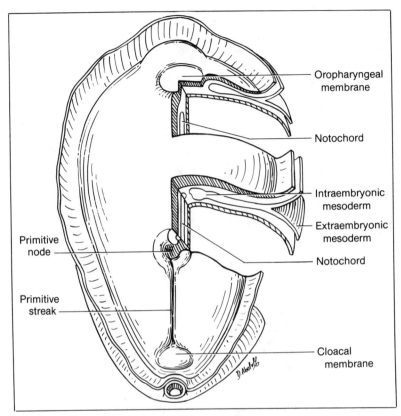

Figure 5-4. The relations between intraembryonic mesoderm and notochord during gastrulation. Note the continuity between the intraembryonic and extraembryonic mesoderm at the lateral edges of the blastoderm.

  a. During **primary embryonic induction**, the process which establishes the central nervous system primordium, the neuroectoderm is committed to form into a tubular structure whose walls become the walls of the brain and spinal cord. The cranial neural plate becomes the brain, and the caudal neural plate becomes the spinal cord.
  b. If the caudal notochord and paraxial mesoderm are transplanted under the cranial neural plate, they will induce the formation of a structure like the spinal cord, rather than the brain.
  c. Similarly, cranial notochord and paraxial mesoderm, transplanted under the caudal neural plate, induce a brain rather than a spinal cord.
 4. These studies indicate a crude regional specificity of the inductive interaction between chordamesoderm and neuroectoderm.
 5. Moreover, the inductive interaction is **reciprocal**. The neural tube, once induced by chordamesoderm, reciprocates by causing the notochord and paraxial mesoderm to form vertebral arches and vertebral bodies in intimate protective association with the developing neural tube.

B. **Formation of the neural tube**
 1. The neural plate, once induced, rapidly begins to curl up upon itself, at first forming an indented **neural groove** (see Fig. 5-5).
 2. A **neural fold** then forms on each side of the neural groove (Fig. 5-6).
 3. The neural folds actively come together, touch, and fuse with one another.
    a. The fusion of the neural groove begins in the cervical region and then progresses cranially and caudally from this point (see Fig. 5-6).
    b. As the dorsal lips of the neural groove move toward one another, and just before they fuse, **neural crest cells** are formed.

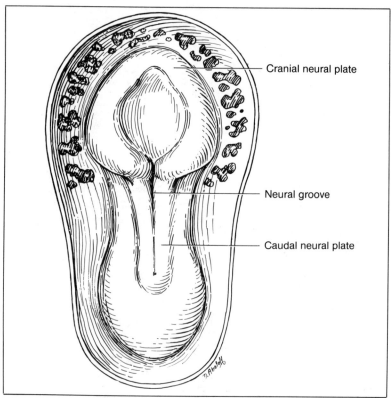

Figure 5-5. The embryo during the early phases of neurulation. Note the cranial expansion of the neural plate. This will become the brain, while the more narrow caudal portion of the neural plate will form the spinal cord. In the mesoderm surrounding the cranial neural plate are blood islands that will become the heart and great vessels.

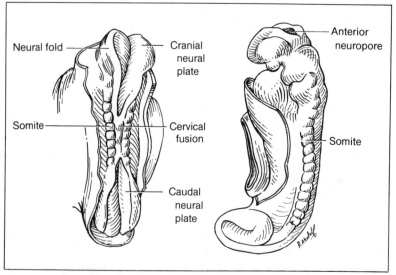

Figure 5-6. The human neurula from the dorsal *(left)* and lateral *(right)* aspects. Note that the first fusion of the neural folds occurs in the cervical region and then proceeds cranially and caudally, ultimately to form the neural groove, which becomes the neural tube. Note also the paired somites, representing a portion of the intraembryonic mesoderm formed during gastrulation, which are visible on either side of the central nervous system.

c. The edges of the neural folds are continuous with the non-neural ectoderm covering the remainder of the surface of the embryo. Once the free edges of the ectoderm fuse, there is a complete surface ectodermal layer over the tubular nervous system. The **definitive neural tube** has now formed.
   (1) For a time, the neural tube has an **anterior and a posterior neuropore**, where the neural tube remains open to the amniotic cavity at both ends.
   (2) Eventually, these neuropores are overgrown by surface ectoderm so that the nervous system comes to lie completely enclosed in the epidermis covering the body.
4. The essentially tubular character of the nervous system, albeit highly modified, persists throughout life.
   a. The brain parenchyma faces on centrally placed cavities, the **ventricles** of the brain. These are remnants of the lumen of the neural tube.
   b. Similarly, a **central canal** communicates with the brain ventricles and runs the entire length of the spinal cord. This is also a persistent remnant of the lumen of the embryonic neural tube.
   c. Interestingly enough, a primitive epithelium persists as the lining of this cavity. The **ependymal layer** here is a simple columnar epithelium which once resided on the upper surface of the neural plate, prior to neurulation.

V. DERIVATIVES OF THE PRIMARY GERM LAYERS AND THE NOTOCHORD

A. **General considerations.** Derivatives of the three primary germ cell layers are outlined here as though they were discrete structures. Obviously, however, in the human body these structures combine to form the various organ systems, as will be discussed at the end (see section V G).

B. **Ectodermal derivatives.** The ectoderm is the first of the three primary germ layers. It forms most of the nervous system tissues and coverings of the body. Ectodermal derivatives include:
   1. The bulk of the **central nervous system**
      a. The brain and spinal cord, including all CNS neurons and most glial cells (except mesodermally derived microglia)
      b. The sensory epithelial structures, including:
         (1) The retina
         (2) The organ of Corti
         (3) The vestibular apparatus
         (4) The olfactory epithelium
      c. Neural crest derivatives (see section V C)
   2. The entire **surface covering** of the body
      a. The epidermis of the skin
      b. Epithelial components of structures associated with the skin, including:
         (1) Sweat glands and sebaceous glands
         (2) Mammary glands
         (3) Hair and nails
      c. The lining of the anterior part of the oral cavity, in this capacity giving rise to:
         (1) Epithelial components of some salivary glands
         (2) The enamel layer of teeth
         (3) The covering of the tongue, the lining of the anterior oral cavity, the gingival and labial epithelium
         (4) The adenohypophysis (which arises from Rathke's pouch, an ectodermal diverticulum)
      d. The lining of the outer part of the anal canal and coverings of the external genitalia
      e. The lining of the external auditory meatus
   3. **Ocular structures** (in addition to the retina)
      a. The anterior corneal epithelium
      b. The epithelial covering of the eyelids and associated glands
      c. The lacrimal glands
      d. The lens
      e. The pupillary sphincter and dilator muscles

C. **Neural crest derivatives.** The ectodermally derived, pluripotent neural crest cells migrate far and wide just prior to fusion of the neural folds, eventually to become a variety of cells with special functions. Thus, neural crest cells become:

1. Many elements in the **nervous system**, including:
   a. Neurons and satellite cells in dorsal root ganglia
   b. Schwann cells, which myelinate peripheral neurons
   c. Ganglionic neurons of the autonomic nervous system
   d. Parts of the pia–arachnoid meninges surrounding the brain and spinal cord

2. Elements of the **endocrine system**, including:
   a. The adrenal medulla (which closely resembles autonomic ganglia)
   b. The calcitonin-secreting parafollicular cells (C cells) in the thyroid gland
   c. Hormone-secreting enterochromaffin cells in the gastrointestinal and respiratory system, such as:
      (1) Gastrin-secreting G cells of the pylorus
      (2) Amine precursor uptake and decarboxylation cells (APUD cells) of the gastroenteropancreatic (GEP) system

3. The pigment-producing **melanocytes**, the cells responsible for the production of melanin granules in the skin and hair follicles

4. Some **tissues in the head and neck** (formed as the neural crest cells migrate into the pharyngeal arches and then differentiate), including:
   a. Cartilage in the head and neck
   b. The dentin-secreting odontoblasts in developing teeth

5. There is some experimental evidence that neural crest cells also contribute to the endocardial cushions in the developing heart and to the developing thymus gland, although these origins are yet to be firmly established.

D. **Mesodermal derivatives.** The second primary germ layer forms the vascular tissues and most of the connective tissues and muscles in the body. Mesodermal derivatives include:

1. **Connective tissues.** Many of the general and special connective tissues arise from an embryonic connective tissue called **mesenchyme**.
   a. **General connective tissues**
      (1) The lamina propria and connective tissue of mesenteries
      (2) Ligaments and tendons
      (3) Fascia and aponeuroses
   b. **Special connective tissues**
      (1) Cartilage and bone (except that formed from the neural crest in the head and neck)
      (2) Blood cells and bone marrow
      (3) Adipose tissue
      (4) Reticular and elastic tissue

2. The entire **cardiovascular system**, including:
   a. The heart
   b. All blood vessels
   c. All lymphatic vessels

3. All **muscles** of the body (except the pupillary muscles, which are ectodermal derivatives); thus, mesodermal muscles include:
   a. Cardiac muscle
   b. Smooth muscle
   c. Skeletal muscles

4. Most of the **urogenital system** (portions are endodermal—see section V E 2 c); mesodermal derivatives include:
   a. The kidneys and ureters
   b. The gonads and gonadal ducts
   c. Parts of the bladder

5. Most of the **immune system**, including, as well as the bone marrow:
   a. Lymphocytes
   b. Macrophages and brain microglia
   c. Granular leukocytes
   d. The lymph nodes, spleen, and part of the thymus

E. **Endodermal derivatives.** The third primary germ layer originates as a simple epithelial layer derived from the hypoblast. The epithelial lining of the pharyngeal pouches is endodermally derived since the pouches form as diverticula (outpocketings) of the foregut. Later, the endoderm forms the epithelial lining of every organ that arises from the primitive gut tube or from diverticula of the gut tube.

1. **Derivatives of the gut tube itself**
   a. The epithelial lining of the pharynx, esophagus, stomach, small and large intestines, rectum, and upper anal canal
   b. The epithelial cells lining the lumina of the lungs, liver, pancreas, and biliary apparatus
2. **Derivatives of outpouchings from the gut tube**
   a. **Derivatives of the epithelial lining of the pharyngeal pouches** form the epithelial cells of the following:
      (1) The auditory tube (eustachian tube) and lining of the middle ear cavity
      (2) The palatine tonsils
      (3) The parathyroid glands
      (4) The thymus gland
   b. **Other derivatives of foregut diverticula** include the following:
      (1) The epithelium of the thyroid gland
      (2) Some of the salivary glands
   c. The **urogenital sinus** forms as a diverticulum from the embryonic **hindgut**. Later it forms the lining epithelium of the following:
      (1) The urinary bladder
      (2) The lower part of the vagina
      (3) The urethra

F. **Notochord derivatives**
   1. The notochord is present in the central portion of vertebral bodies when they first form but it later degenerates and disappears.
   2. The notochord persists in the adult only as the **nucleus pulposus** of the intervertebral disks.

G. **Mixed germ layer derivation of many organs**
   1. Most organs in the body are formed from rudiments derived from different primary germ layers. Thus, the parenchyma (i.e., the organ-specific functional cells) may be derived from **ectoderm** or **endoderm**, but the organ will also have **mesodermal components** in the form of blood vessels and connective tissue elements. These are derived from splanchnic mesoderm which surrounds the organ as it grows.
   2. **Specific examples**
      a. All **gastrointestinal organs** have an epithelial lining derived from endoderm, and connective tissue, blood vessels, and smooth muscle derived from mesoderm. The autonomic ganglia in the wall of these organs are derived from ectoderm by way of the neural crest.
      b. The **lungs** have an epithelial lining derived from endoderm, and connective tissue, blood vessels, cartilage, and smooth muscle all derived from mesoderm.
      c. The **skin** has an epidermis from ectoderm and a dermis from mesoderm.
      d. The **teeth** have enamel produced by ectodermally derived ameloblasts, dentin produced by odontoblasts, which are neural crest derivatives, and pulp cavities derived from mesoderm.
      e. The **liver** and **pancreas** have parenchymal cells derived from endoderm, but connective tissue elements and blood vessels derived from mesoderm.
      f. Most of the **brain** consists of ectodermally derived neurons and glia, but the blood vessels and microglia are derivatives of the mesoderm.

VI. **NEURAL TUBE DEFECTS.** Neural tube defects are the most common type of neurologic birth defects. These congenital anomalies are characterized by structural abnormalities that develop during the formation of the central nervous system and associated bony structures. They are due to abnormal fusion of the neural folds or to failure of the normal reciprocal inductive interaction between the neural tube and the vertebral bodies. (See Chapter 23, section I B, and Chapter 24, section VII, for discussions of the genetic and epidemiologic aspects of neural tube defects.)

A. **Types of neural tube defects and associated skeletal defects**
   1. Neural tube defects range widely in severity.

a. The **most severe forms** are **posterior rachischisis**, in which the entire nervous system fails to close, and the more common **anencephaly**, in which the brain fails to close.
  (1) In **anencephaly**, there is a complete failure of fusion in the central nervous system cranial to the cervical fusion point.
  (2) In the anencephalic fetus (Fig. 5-7), the brain and the overlying bones of the membranous neurocranium fail to form. The maldeveloped brain is essentially open onto the surface of the body, and the vault of the skull, which is normally induced by the developing brain, never forms.
b. **Spina bifida** encompasses a broad class of congenital anomalies in which some portion of the spinal cord fails to close; the neural arches of the vertebral bodies fail to form in the area of the neural tube defect.
  (1) Spina bifida may be caused not only by the primary failure of neural tube formation due to inductive abnormalities but also by a secondary reopening of the neural tube because of a defect in the fusion mechanisms.
  (2) This lesion can take a variety of forms, with varying degrees of severity.
  (3) The **least severe form** (and the least severe neural tube defect) is **spina bifida occulta.**
    (a) In this defect, only the vertebral arch is missing; otherwise the central nervous system is functionally intact. The meninges are intact and the spinal cord is securely buried in the recess of the vertebral arch.
    (b) Spina bifida occulta often occurs in the lumbosacral region and is commonly covered by a small tuft of hairy skin over the lesion site.
  (4) In **more severe forms** of spina bifida, not only do the neural arches fail to develop, but also the neural tube fails to close.
    (a) Parts of the spinal cord lie open on the surface of the body, and nervous tissue differentiation is severely compromised.
    (b) Several vertebrae may be involved, and there can be defects in the spinal cord or even a **meningocele.**
      (i) In this condition, a conspicuous sac of meninges covered by an attenuated layer of skin bulges onto the surface of the body.
      (ii) If the meningeal sac also includes neural tissue herniated into it, then the condition is called **meningomyelocele** (or **myelomeningocele**).

2. Neural tube defects show a wide variation in frequency among different ethnic groups. In the United Kingdom, neural tube defects occur in about 1% of all live births. They occur with a frequency of 0.05% in West Africa.

3. Neural tube defects vary widely in their **clinical consequences.**

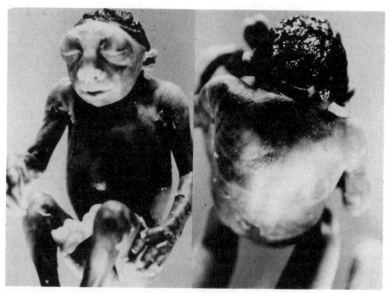

Figure 5-7. A fetus born with anencephaly, an example of a severe neural tube defect. The vault of the skull and the meninges have not formed, and a large mass of degenerate cerebral tissue is exposed on the surface of the head.

a. Both **posterior rachischisis** and **anencephaly** are incompatible with life.
b. In the patient with **meningocele** or **meningomyelocele**, neurologic signs are usually encountered.
c. Children with **spina bifida** live a life of variable quality, depending on the severity of the lesion.
   (1) In most cases, there are no neurologic signs associated with **spina bifida occulta**.
   (2) In **more severe forms** of spina bifida, as a general rule, the larger the number of vertebrae involved and the more cranial the level of the lesion, the worse the prognosis for the patient is.
      (a) Spina bifida can result in paralysis at and below the level of the defect, or bladder and bowel incompetence.
      (b) Lumbar spina bifida can be corrected surgically, and the patient will have normal or even superior mental development but severe physical handicaps. Children afflicted with small lumbosacral lesions may suffer motor impairment of the lower limbs and may have bowel and bladder control problems, but they can go on to live a reasonably normal life.

B. **Diagnosis of neural tube defects in utero**
   1. When neural tube defects occur, the open nervous system often leaks α-**fetoprotein** into the amniotic fluid.
      a. This protein can make its way from the amniotic fluid into maternal serum.
      b. Since α-fetoprotein is not found in adult blood, its presence in maternal serum can be used to test for a neural tube defect. In the United Kingdom, **maternal serum α-fetoprotein (MSAFP)** screening is done routinely in many pregnant women. Such screening is also currently available in the United States.
   2. If a woman's MSAFP level is elevated above a certain critical limit, another blood sample is tested. Two consecutive elevated readings suggest that the pregnant woman has a significantly increased probability of carrying a fetus with a neural tube defect.
   3. At this point, the parents may elect to have **amniocentesis** performed to sample α-fetoprotein levels in the amniotic fluid. This procedure is aided considerably by ultrasonographic imaging techniques. Amniotic fluid samples, once gathered, can also be tested for abnormalities in fetal chromosome composition.
   4. If the amniotic fluid α-fetoprotein levels are significantly elevated, a second ultrasonographic investigation can be performed to look for a neural tube defect. In many cases, the nature and extent of a neural tube defect, if present, can now be determined (Figs. 5-8, 5-9, and 5-10).

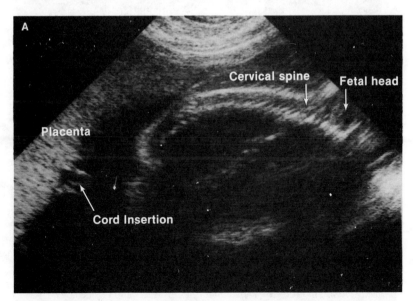

Figure 5-8. Sonograms of a normal fetus *(A)* and an anencephalic fetus *(B)*. (Courtesy of Teresita L. Angtuaco, M.D., Assistant Professor, Department of Obstetrics and Gynecology, University of Arkansas for Medical Sciences, Little Rock.)

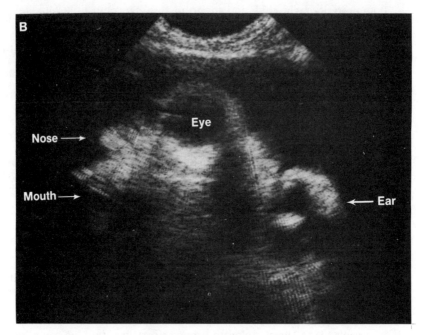

Figure 5-8. Continued.

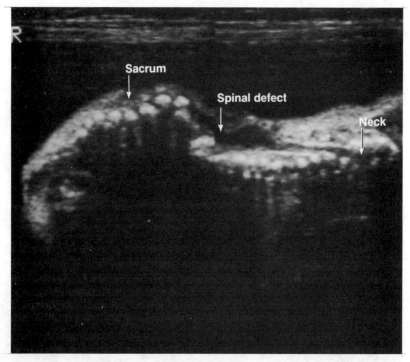

Figure 5-9. Sonogram of a fetus with spina bifida. (Courtesy of Teresita L. Angtuaco, M.D., Assistant Professor, Department of Obstetrics and Gynecology, University of Arkansas for Medical Sciences, Little Rock.)

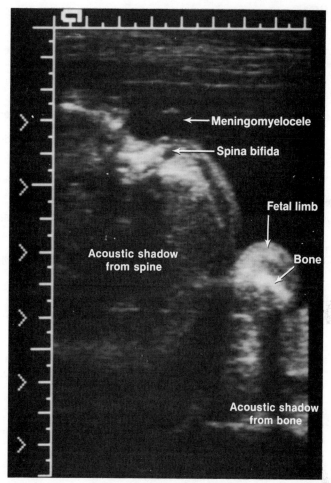

Figure 5-10. Sonogram of a fetus with meningomyelocele. (Courtesy of Teresita L. Angtuaco, M.D., Assistant Professor, Department of Obstetrics and Gynecology, University of Arkansas for Medical Sciences, Little Rock.)

- a. An anencephalic fetus or one with another extensive neural tube defect will not live after birth and the parents may elect to terminate the pregnancy.
- b. If ultrasonography reveals a less severe neural tube defect, such as a meningomyelocele in the lumbosacral region (see Fig. 5-10), the defect is compatible with life, although the newborn child will require extensive surgery to correct the defect and may be physically handicapped for life.
- c. With the information provided by ultrasonography, the parents can choose whether or not to terminate the pregnancy.
    - (1) If they elect to continue the pregnancy, they will at least be able to prepare themselves emotionally for the birth of a child with a severe congenital defect and associated neurologic problems.
    - (2) Whichever they elect, the medical technology brought to bear on the case has given them new information on which to base their ethical decisions.

STUDY QUESTIONS

Directions: Each question below contains five suggested answers. Choose the **one best** response to each question.

1. All of the following structures are ectodermal derivatives EXCEPT

   (A) the neural retina
   (B) the adenohypophysis
   (C) the dermis of the skin
   (D) the stratum corneum of the skin
   (E) hair follicles

2. All of the following structures are mesodermal derivatives EXCEPT

   (A) the pupillary dilator and sphincter muscles
   (B) skeletal muscle
   (C) cardiac muscle
   (D) smooth muscle surrounding the gut tube
   (E) the kidneys

3. All of the following structures are endodermal derivatives EXCEPT

   (A) thyroid follicular epithelial cells
   (B) thyroid parafollicular epithelial cells (C cells)
   (C) pancreatic acinar cells
   (D) pancreatic islet tissue
   (E) epithelial lining of the urinary bladder

4. All of the following cell types are derived from the same primary germ layer EXCEPT

   (A) fibroblasts in the tendons
   (B) chondrocytes in hyaline cartilage
   (C) osteocytes in the tibia
   (D) odontoblasts in teeth
   (E) adipocytes in white fat

5. Which of the following neural tube defects has the best prognosis for life after birth?

   (A) Posterior rachischisis
   (B) Low lumbar spina bifida occulta
   (C) Anencephaly
   (D) Meningomyelocele
   (E) Meningoencephalocele

Directions: Each question below contains four suggested answers of which **one or more** is correct. Choose the answer

    A if **1, 2, and 3** are correct
    B if **1 and 3** are correct
    C if **2 and 4** are correct
    D if **4** is correct
    E if **1, 2, 3, and 4** are correct

6. Mesodermal derivatives include which of the following structures?

   (1) Epithelium at the lumen of the esophagus
   (2) Epithelium in the renal nephron
   (3) Epithelium at the lumen of the penile urethra
   (4) Epithelium at the lumen of a blood vessel

7. Ectodermal derivatives include which of the following structures?

   (1) Schwann cells
   (2) Neurons in the cerebrum
   (3) Anterior epithelium of the cornea
   (4) Neural retina

8. Neural crest derivatives include which of the following structures?

   (1) Oligodendroglia
   (2) Microglia
   (3) Ameloblasts
   (4) Adrenal medullary cells

9. True statements concerning neurulation include which of the following?

   (1) The chordamesoderm induces the overlying ectoderm to form the neural plate
   (2) Neurulation precedes gastrulation in humans
   (3) Fusion of neural folds that become the brain occurs after fusion of neural folds that form the cervical spinal cord
   (4) Neural crest cells leave the neuroepithelium after the neural tube begins to differentiate into brain and spinal cord

10. True statements concerning neural tube defects include which of the following?

    (1) Anencephalic fetuses usually die soon after birth
    (2) Amniotic fluid α-fetoprotein is usually elevated when there is an open spinal cord present in the fetus
    (3) Maternal serum α-fetoprotein is usually elevated when the mother carries an anencephalic fetus
    (4) Ultrasonography is not useful for diagnosis of neural tube defects

Directions: The group of questions below consists of lettered choices followed by several numbered items. For each numbered item select the **one** lettered choice with which it is **most** closely associated. Each lettered choice may be used once, more than once, or not at all.

Questions 11–15

For each description of components of the gastrula below, choose the appropriate lettered structure shown in the accompanying diagram.

11. This structure persists in the adult as the nucleus pulposus

12. This structure forms the kidneys and most skeletal muscle

13. This structure is the site of invagination and cranial extension of the notochord

14. This structure forms the epithelial lining of the stomach and duodenum

15. This structure forms the spinal cord after primary embryonic induction has occurred

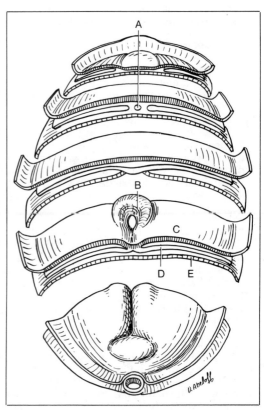

ANSWERS AND EXPLANATIONS

1. The answer is C. *(V B, G 2 c)* Ectoderm gives rise to all neural tissue, including that found in the brain, the spinal cord, and the neural retina. The adenohypophysis arises from Rathke's pouch, an evagination of the oral ectoderm. The epidermis of the skin, including the stratum corneum, forms from ectoderm. In contrast, the dermis of the skin, which is a dense irregular connective tissue, forms from the mesoderm. Hair follicles are also ectodermal derivatives.

2. The answer is A. *(V B 3 e, D)* The pupillary muscles form from the optic cup, an outgrowth of the wall of the brain. Thus, they are the only muscle cells in the body that are ectodermally derived. All other muscle cells, including skeletal muscle cells, cardiac muscle cells, and smooth muscle cells, are mesodermally derived. The entire kidney is also mesodermally derived.

3. The answer is B. *(V C 2 b, E)* Thyroid parafollicular epithelial cells are neural crest derivatives. Thyroid follicular epithelial cells form from the thyroid diverticulum, which forms as an evagination of the floor of the endodermally lined oral cavity. The acinar and endocrine cells of the pancreas both arise from the pancreatic buds, which are endodermally derived diverticula of the gut tube. The epithelial lining of the urinary bladder comes from the urogenital sinus, which is a hindgut diverticulum.

4. The answer is D. *(V C 4 b, D)* Odontoblasts secrete the dentin layer of teeth. They are neural crest derivatives. All of the other cell types listed in the question are found in adult connective tissues. As such, they are all mesodermal derivatives. In addition, the mesoderm forms dermal fibroblasts, muscle cells, and loose areolar connective tissue of the mesenteries and lamina propria, among other cell types.

5. The answer is B. *(VI A 3)* In posterior rachischisis, the entire central nervous system fails to close. In anencephaly, the brain portion of the neural tube does not close. Both conditions are incompatible with life after birth. In meningomyelocele (which involves the spinal cord) and meningoencephalocele (which involves the brain), there are defects in bone over affected areas, as well as herniation of neural tissue and meninges into skin-covered sacs. In both cases, prognosis is poor because there can be profound neurologic deficits. In low lumbar spina bifida occulta, the mildest form of neural tube defect, only the bony portion of vertebral bodies is affected. There is no neurologic involvement, and therefore the prognosis is good.

6. The answer is C (2, 4). *(V D, E)* The mesoderm forms all of the cardiovascular system, including blood; therefore, the endothelium at the vascular lumen is mesodermally derived. The mesoderm also forms most of the urogenital system, including all of the definitive kidneys. The epithelial lining of the lumen of the esophagus is an endodermal derivative, since the entire gastrointestinal tract is endodermally derived. The urogenital sinus forms as a diverticulum of the hindgut and later gives rise to the urethral epithelium. Thus, the epithelium of the penile urethra is endodermally derived.

7. The answer is E (all). *(V B)* The ectoderm forms the entire outer surface covering of the body, including the epidermis and the anterior epithelium of the cornea. The ectoderm also forms the neural crest and the central nervous system after neurulation has occurred. Thus, all neurons in the brain are ectodermal derivatives, and the neural retina, which is a portion of the central nervous system, and Schwann cells, which are neural crest derivatives, also ultimately come from the ectoderm.

8. The answer is D (4). *(V B, C, G 2 f)* Of the structures listed in the question, only the adrenal medulla contains cells that are derived from the neural crest, which also forms neurons in the autonomic nervous system. Oligodendroglial cells form myelin in the central nervous system and are derived from ectodermal neuroepithelium. Microglia are part of the mononuclear phagocyte system and arise from mesodermally derived monocytes, as do many other phagocytic cells in the body such as macrophages and Kupffer cells in the liver. The ameloblasts form the enamel layer of the teeth and are ectodermally derived. In teeth, the odontoblasts, which form dentin, are neural crest derivatives.

9. The answer is B (1, 3). *(IV A, B)* The chordamesoderm is indeed the main inductor of the central nervous system during neurulation. Neurulation occurs after gastrulation, when the inductor of the nervous system is formed. Fusion of the neural folds occurs first in the cervical region, and then cranial and caudal to this fusion point. Before fusion of the neural folds, however, the neural crest cells leave the neuroepithelium and migrate to many different locations in the body. Subsequently, they express their pluripotentiality and form many different kinds of cells.

10. The answer is A (1, 2, 3). *(VI A, B)* The nervous system cranial to the cervical fusion point is open to the surface of the body in an anencephalic fetus, and there is gross abnormality in the development of the brain and skull. Anencephalic fetuses invariably die soon after birth. Because of the open neural tube, α-fetoprotein leaks out into the amniotic fluid and from there makes its way into the maternal blood stream. When either maternal serum or amniotic fluid α-fetoprotein is elevated above critical limits, there is a strong chance that a fetus with a neural tube defect is present. The extent and level of the defect can often be determined by ultrasonography. In addition, other congenital defects such as omphalocele can also cause an elevation of α-fetoprotein. These various structural defects can be diagnosed by ultrasound.

11–15. The answers are 11-A, 12-D, 13-B, 14-E, 15-C. *(III A, B; V)* In the diagram of the gastrula, the primitive node *(B)* is regressing caudally, and as it does so, the notochord *(A)* extends out from it and grows in a cranial direction. The notochord undergoes regressive changes and disappears everywhere except in the nucleus pulposus of the intervertebral disks. The ectoderm *(C)* forms most of the central nervous system and many surface covering structures, including the epidermis of the skin, the anterior covering of the cornea, and the lining of the oral cavity and lower anal canal. Ectoderm also forms the neural crest and all of its derivatives. The mesoderm *(D)* forms connective tissues, the cardiovascular system, and much of the urogenital system. The endoderm *(E)* forms the epithelial lining of many organs, including the gastrointestinal tract, lungs, liver, pancreas, and thyroid gland.

6
Establishment of the Basic Body Plan and Primitive Circulation

I. INTRODUCTION

A. General considerations

1. Once gastrulation has established the primary germ layers, other complex morphogenetic events, including neurulation, ensue immediately.
   a. These processes overlap one another considerably, and there is a cranial to caudal progression of events. For example, while neurulation is occurring in the cranial portion of the embryo at 2.5 weeks, the following events are taking place:
      (1) **Somites** are forming craniocaudally along either side of the midline axis (Fig. 6-1).
      (2) **The primitive node** is regressing.
      (3) **Notochord** formation is still occurring in the caudal end of the embryo.
   b. Moreover, these different morphogenetic events are integrated with one another. Often, one event even causes another event; an example is the induction of neurulation discussed in Chapter 5, section IV.

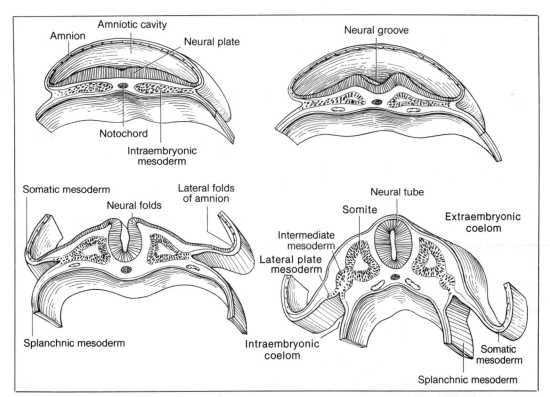

Figure 6-1. Morphogenesis of the intraembryonic mesoderm. Intraembryonic mesoderm becomes partitioned into somites, intermediate mesoderm, and lateral plate mesoderm. Note that these changes take place simultaneously with neurulation and the formation of the lateral folds of the amnion.

2. There is considerable temporal overlap in these processes, and they are discussed separately only for convenience.

B. **Overview of events.** During the third and fourth weeks of development, gastrulation and neurulation are completed, a primitive circulation is established, and the body is sculpted into a vertebrate form with a recognizable head and tail.

1. **Subdivision of mesoderm and beginnings of the circulatory system**
   a. During the third week of development, the intraembryonic mesoderm becomes subdivided into **somites, intermediate mesoderm,** and **lateral plate mesoderm.**
   b. The **primitive circulatory system**, including the heart, blood vessels, and blood cells, all form from mesenchyme and blood islands that arise spontaneously throughout the intra-and extraembryonic mesoderm. The end result of this process is the formation of a primitive circulatory system linking embryo and chorionic villi via blood vessels in the connecting stalk.

2. **Formation of body folds**
   a. Also occurring at this period are the extensive **folding** that occurs in the embryo and the **growth of folds of the amnion.**
   b. This process molds the essentially flat embryo into a rounded structure in which the **basic vertebrate body plan** is clearly recognizable.

3. **The beginning of organogenesis**
   a. By the end of the fourth week, miniature precursors of the **forelimbs and hindlimbs** are also beginning to appear and the most complex portion of the embryonic period, **organogenesis**, is in full swing.
   b. The major organ systems are formed during the period of organogenesis, even though most systems continue to undergo extensive growth and functional differentiation throughout the fetal and postnatal period.
      (1) For example, the **lungs** are functionally mature at birth but they continue to grow extensively after birth.
      (2) Similarly, all of the **neural cells** present in the adult are found in the newborn child, but considerable myelination occurs after birth.

II. CHANGES IN INTRAEMBRYONIC MESODERM

A. **Somite formation**
   1. The **intraembryonic mesoderm** forms by invagination at the primitive streak during gastrulation (see Chapter 5 section II B 3 and Fig. 5-3).
   2. Soon after its formation, the paraxial intraembryonic mesoderm begins to subdivide into a series of paired, segmentally arranged structures, the **somites** (Fig. 6-2; see also Fig. 5-6).
      a. The pairs of somites develop along either side of the notochord, increasing rapidly in number as new somites form in a cranial to caudal sequence.
      b. The number of somite pairs that have formed is useful in determining the developmental stage of the embryo.
         (1) The first somite pair appears about 20 days after fertilization.
         (2) Three somite pairs are visible by day 21.
         (3) By day 30, there are 30 to 35 pairs.
         (4) Additional somites form later in development, but they are not visible externally and are therefore of little use in determining the developmental stage.
      c. Eventually, 42 to 44 pairs of somites form; these are grouped regionally, and most are represented in adult vertebral bodies. There are:
         (1) 4 occipital pairs
         (2) 8 cervical pairs
         (3) 12 thoracic pairs
         (4) 5 lumbar pairs
         (5) 5 sacral pairs
         (6) 8 to 10 coccygeal pairs

B. **Development of the somites** (days 20 to 30)
   1. At first, somites are solid blocks of cells, but soon they develop a central cavity, the **myocoele**, which later disappears.
      a. The inner somite cells, medial to the myocoele, constitute a **sclerotome**, which later develops into parts of the axial skeleton (e.g., vertebral structures, ribs) and associated ligaments.

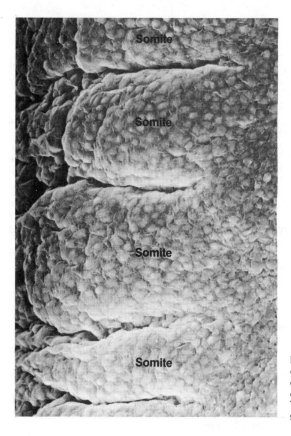

Figure 6-2. Somites in the thoracic region of a human embryo. Each somite is a block of mesodermally derived cells lying beneath the surface ectodermal covering of the embryo (precursor of the epidermis). The cells visible are individual cells of the covering surface ectoderm. (Scanning electron micrograph)

    b. The outer somite cells, lateral to the myocoele, constitute a **dermomyotome**, which later divides to form dermal connective tissues and muscles associated with body segments.

  2. The **metameric, or segmental, arrangement** provided by the somites persists in the thoracic and abdominal regions of the human body, but elsewhere becomes highly distorted by the development of the head and limbs.

C. The intermediate mesoderm and lateral plate mesoderm

  1. The intermediate mesoderm and lateral plate mesoderm develop at about day 22, soon after the intraembryonic mesoderm forms during gastrulation.
    a. The **intermediate mesoderm** forms lateral to the somites.
    b. The **lateral plate mesoderm** forms lateral to the intermediate mesoderm.

  2. Initially, the somites are connected laterally to a bit of intermediate mesoderm, which in turn is connected on its lateral border to the lateral plate mesoderm.

  3. Soon, however, during flexion (see section IV), at about day 25, the body is rolled into a structure which appears round in cross section. In this process, the somites segregate from the intermediate mesoderm and lateral plate mesoderm.

  4. The **intermediate mesoderm** later develops into much of the urogenital system and related structures.

  5. Changes in the **lateral plate mesoderm** take place soon after it forms (day 22).
    a. The lateral plate mesoderm first develops cystic vesicles throughout. These vesicles fuse with one another to create a cavity, the **intraembryonic coelom**.
      (1) Early in development, the intraembryonic coelom is a single cavity that runs around the cranial end and down the sides of the embryo. However, it represents the precursor of the **internal body cavities**, such as:
        (a) The pericardial cavity

(b) The pleural cavities
(c) The peritoneal cavity
    (2) The intraembryonic coelom develops an **epithelial lining**. This mesodermally derived simple squamous epithelium gives rise to the **mesothelium**, which lines the pericardial, pleural, and peritoneal cavities and coats most of the visceral organs that eventually grow into the intraembryonic coelom.
  b. With the formation of the intraembryonic coelom, the lateral plate mesoderm is divided into two layers:
    (1) An upper **somatopleuric layer (somatic mesoderm)**, which gives rise to body wall structures such as connective tissue and muscles
    (2) A lower **splanchnopleuric layer (splanchnic mesoderm)**, which gives rise to the connective tissue and muscle in the walls of numerous visceral organs such as the trachea and stomach
6. The intraembryonic coelom is in direct communication with the extraembryonic coelom. Also, the intraembryonic mesoderm and extraembryonic mesoderm are continuous with one another (see Figs. 6-1 and 6-6). Thus, an imaginary molecule on a fantastic voyage could travel along the inner aspect of the chorion, down the outer wall of the connecting stalk, over the outer surface of the amnion, and into the intraembryonic coelom.

III. DEVELOPMENT OF THE PRIMITIVE CIRCULATION

A. **Formation of blood cells (erythropoiesis) and blood vessels (angiogenesis)**
  1. Almost as soon as they form, the intraembryonic mesoderm and extraembryonic mesoderm begin to form blood vessels and blood cells.
  2. Blood vessel formation (angiogenesis) begins first in the yolk sac and then in the embryo, connecting stalk, and chorion.
  3. **Formation of blood islands (angiogenetic cell clusters)**
    a. Blood islands are first seen at 2.5 weeks. They appear spontaneously as isolated cell clusters, initially restricted to the yolk sac and allantois, a diverticulum of the yolk sac. The blood islands are most prominent in the yolk sac mesenchyme lying between the endodermal layer and the splanchnic mesoderm (Fig. 6-3).
    b. These groups of cells arise by differentiation of cells from the splanchnopleuric extraembryonic mesoderm in the yolk sac and chorion and the splanchnopleuric intraembryonic mesoderm in the embryo.

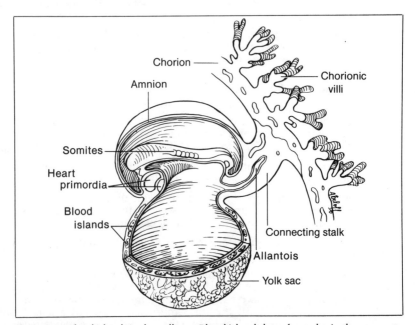

Figure 6-3. Blood islands in the yolk sac. Blood islands later form also in the connecting stalk, chorionic shell, and body of the embryo. These individual blood islands later coalesce into a closed circulatory system.

4. Primitive erythropoiesis
   a. Blood islands consist of groups of basophilic cells called **hemocytoblasts**.
   b. Initially, some hemocytoblasts become more acidophilic as they begin to synthesize **hemoglobin** and become differentiated into **primitive erythroblasts**, the precursors of erythrocytes (week 3.5).
   c. The erythroblasts accumulate substantial quantities of cytoplasmic hemoglobin and undergo marked nuclear pyknosis without nuclear extrusion, to become **primitive erythrocytes** (Fig. 6-4), the precursors of circulating blood cells designed to carry oxygen and carbon dioxide.
       (1) Hemocytoblasts have large euchromatic nuclei and prominent nucleoli. Thus, **primitive erythrocytes** are **nucleated cells**.
       (2) The **definitive erythrocytes** of later embryonic and adult life undergo nuclear extrusion during their development and are thus **cells without nuclei**.
   d. Blood cell formation begins in the **yolk sac**, but later, during fetal life, it shifts in turn to the **liver** and finally to the **bone marrow**.

5. Formation of blood vessels
   a. As the hemocytoblasts in blood islands are differentiating into the precursors of erythrocytes, the **mesenchymal cells** surrounding blood islands are becoming spontaneously arranged into a flattened endothelial layer forming closed **vesicular sacs**.
   b. These sacs next meet with one another and fuse, forming **primitive blood vessels** (week 2.5 on). Simultaneously, the endothelial layer sends out sprouts which grow away from the sacs to establish new blood vessels.
   c. All of these disjointed vascular channels spontaneously become joined together to form a **network of blood vessels** in the yolk sac, the allantois, the chorionic shell, the connecting stalk, and throughout the intraembryonic mesoderm.

B. Early formation of the heart. Cardiogenesis is fundamentally similar to angiogenesis. Similarly, the blood vessels and the heart share certain microscopic anatomic features.

   1. At neurulation, lying cranial to the oropharyngeal membrane is the **cardiogenic area**.
      a. This horseshoe-shaped area is in the splanchnopleuric intraembryonic mesoderm, in close association with the cranial intraembryonic coelom.
      b. From here, the heart and great vessels of the heart form.

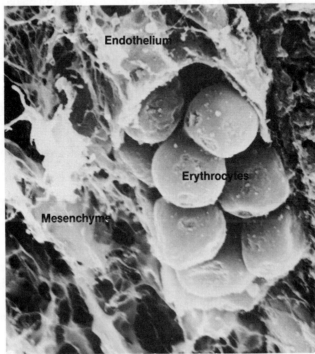

Figure 6-4. Primitive erythrocytes within a primitive blood vessel of a human embryo. Mesenchymal cells differentiate into endothelial cells and nucleated primitive erythrocytes. (Scanning electron micrograph)

2. In the cardiogenic area, at a very early stage of development (by week 3.5), paired **heart tubes** and contractile **cardiac myocytes** make their appearance.
   a. The **heart tubes** form from blood islands, which are prominent in the cardiogenic area.
   b. The paired heart tubes form on either side of the embryo in a manner similar to the formation of other vascular channels.
   c. Some **mesenchymal cells** in the cardiogenic area differentiate into endothelial cells, while others surround these cells and begin to form the contractile **cardiac myocytes**.
3. While the heart tubes are differentiating, anastomosing **networks of blood vessels** are forming, and these link the primitive vessels, heart tubes, and yolk-sac blood vessels into a complete, closed circulatory system.

C. **Functional considerations**
   1. By the end of the third week, a **fully functional cardiovascular system** has already formed.
      a. Naturally, this system will undergo dramatic developmental changes before and after birth as the hemodynamic parameters of the fetal–maternal unit change (see Chapter 10).
      b. Nevertheless, it is clear that the primitive circulatory system already performs the rudimentary functions of **gas exchange** and **nutrient transport** long before other embryonic systems have begun to function in their normal physiologic capacities.
   2. There are several reasons for the early functional development of the circulatory system in human embryos.
      a. There is little nutritive substance in the yolk sac. As a result, the embryo needs maternal nutrients. These must be transported from the developing placenta by a circulatory system; diffusion alone would not bring sufficient nutrients to the embryo.
      b. The embryo develops within a closed shell of chorionic tissue imposed between the embryo and the maternal blood supply. Therefore, the embryo must establish a circulatory system quickly to rid itself of metabolic wastes and to carry maternally derived oxygen and nutrients from the chorionic villi to the embryo.
   3. While the circulatory system is forming, there is simultaneously a substantial development of **chorionic villi** on the surface of the chorion (see Chapter 7, section III).
      a. These serve to increase the surface area of the embryo–maternal interface, in order to provide embryonic nutrition and gas and waste exchange.
      b. Some of the chorionic villi persist, and these, along with maternal decidual tissue, will eventually form the placenta (see Chapter 7, section III E).

IV. FORMATION OF BODY FOLDS: FLEXION

A. **Overview of flexion.** Until the end of neurulation, the embryo is a disk-like structure. This flat plate now curls into a cylindrical shape by folding laterally. In addition, head and tail folds of the amnion help in the formation of the cranial and caudal ends of the embryo.
   1. Soon after neurulation has finished, growth in the length of the neural tube exceeds growth of the rest of the body. This causes the cranial brain and caudal spinal cord to overgrow the rest of the body.
   2. In addition, rapid growth of the brain, combined with growth of the head and tail folds of the amnion (Fig. 6-5), causes structures that once were found cranial and caudal to the body of the embryo to become rotated and tucked under the ventral surface of the body.
   3. At the same time, lateral body folds are growing ventrally and toward the midline, sculpting the flat embryo into a tubular embryo (see Fig. 6-6). The amnion also grows down around the embryo and over the connecting stalk.

B. **Head flexion**
   1. Prior to flexion, a mass of mesoderm known as the **septum transversum** (see Fig. 6-5) lies cranial to the extraembryonic coelom, heart tubes, and oropharyngeal membrane.
      a. All of these structures are aligned in that order along the craniocaudal axis, and all lie cranial to the developing brain.
      b. This relationship is the exact opposite of the relationship found in the adult.
   2. The forebrain grows rapidly over these structures, causing the head fold of the amnion to curl over, at about day 25 (see Fig. 6-5).
      a. This curling process eventually rotates all of the cranial structures through 180° on an axis of rotation perpendicular to the craniocaudal axis of the embryo.

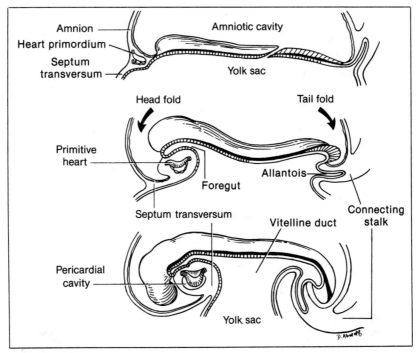

Figure 6-5. Formation of the head and tail folds of the amnion during flexion. Note the rotation of the cardiac primordium during formation of the head fold, the change in caudal relationships during formation of the tail fold, and the beginning of a passageway between the gut and the yolk sac.

  b. As a result, the septum transversum (a precursor of much of the diaphragm) comes to lie caudal to the heart tubes, the intraembryonic coelom (now the pericardial cavity), and the oropharyngeal membrane.
  c. This arrangement is much more like that found in the adult.
 3. As this flexion occurs, bilateral **pericardioperitoneal canals** form, maintaining the connection between the pericardial and peritoneal portions of the intraembryonic coelom (see Chapter 8, section II B).

C. Tail flexion
 1. In the caudal portion of the embryo, the tail fold of the amnion begins to expand and curl under as the caudal neural tube overgrows the rest of the embryonic body.
 2. While both tail fold and caudal neural tube are growing, a diverticulum of the yolk sac, the **allantois**, projects into the connecting stalk.
 3. Before tail flexion, the allantois is at the tail end of the embryo. The allantois lies caudal to the cloacal membrane, which in turn lies caudal to the remnants of the primitive streak, and this in turn lies caudal to the caudal end of the neural tube.
 4. As the caudal neural tube (now becoming the primitive spinal cord) overgrows the body and as the tail fold of the amnion curls under the embryo, the allantois, primitive streak, and cloacal membrane all become rotated and shifted under the embryo.
 5. Eventually (about day 25), the cranial to caudal order of these structures is reversed. The allantois now resides cranial to the cloacal membrane, which is cranial to the primitive streak, which is cranial to the caudal end of the spinal cord (see Fig. 6-5).

D. Lateral flexion and related changes
 1. At the same time that the embryo is curving in the craniocaudal plane, the **lateral folds of the amnion** are growing, causing the sides of the embryonic body to move ventrally and medially. The sides eventually meet (at about day 25 to 30) and fuse in the ventral midline, forming the body wall (Fig. 6-6).

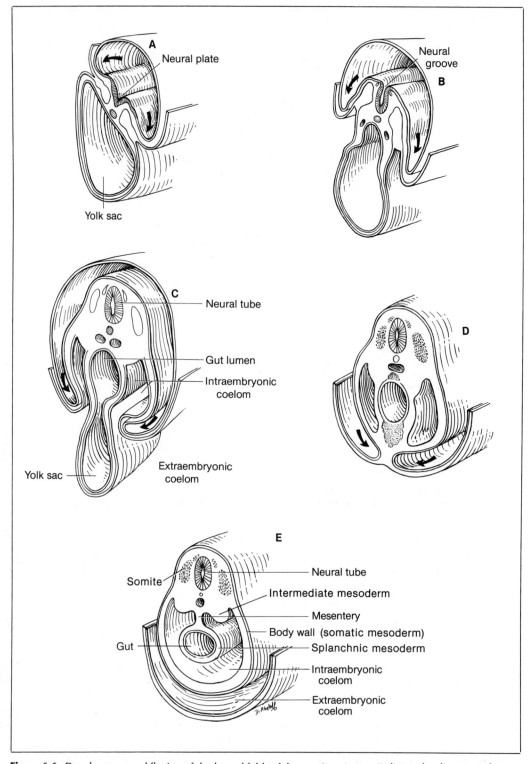

Figure 6-6. Development and flexion of the lateral folds of the amnion. *Arrows* indicate the direction of tissue growth. Note how the lateral folds of the amnion are involved in sculpting the lateral body walls to establish the basic vertebrate body plan. Note also the initial communication between the extraembryonic and intraembryonic coeloms, and between the gut lumen and the yolk sac (C).

2. With the lateral folding of the embryo, **other important changes** take place.
    a. The **primitive gut** begins to form.
        (1) The communication between the primitive gut cavity and the yolk sac becomes progressively restricted until it is little more than a narrow passageway, the **vitelline duct**.
        (2) The anterior (cranial) portion of the gut tube communicates with the vitelline duct via the **anterior intestinal portal**, and the posterior (caudal) portion of the gut tube communicates with the vitelline duct via the **posterior intestinal portal**.
        (3) By about day 25, the gut tube has been divided into **three regions**.
            (a) The **foregut** extends from the oropharyngeal membrane to the anterior intestinal portal.
            (b) The **midgut** lies between the anterior and posterior intestinal portals.
            (c) The **hindgut** extends from the posterior intestinal portal to the cloacal membrane.
        (4) The midgut thus communicates directly with the yolk sac for a time (see Fig. 6-6).
    b. The **umbilical cord** begins to take shape by about day 25 to 30.
        (1) As the **amnion** grows down around the embryo, it also grows down around the **connecting stalk**.
        (2) Eventually, the umbilical cord, which forms from the connecting stalk, is coated on the outside (facing the amniotic cavity) by a layer of amnion.
    c. The amnion later expands and meets the inner layer of the **chorion**. Here it fuses with the chorion, obliterating the extraembryonic coelom.

STUDY QUESTIONS

Directions: Each question below contains five suggested answers. Choose the **one best** response to each question.

1. All of the following statements concerning flexion are true EXCEPT

   (A) the lateral folds of the amnion grow dorso-laterally
   (B) the head fold carries the septum transversum ventrally and caudally
   (C) the tail fold carries the allantois ventrally and cranially
   (D) the growth of the head fold changes the position of the heart relative to the mouth
   (E) the lateral folds of the amnion restrict the diameter of the communication between the midgut and the yolk sac

2. All of the following statements concerning early development of the heart are true EXCEPT

   (A) angiogenesis and cardiogenesis are fundamentally similar
   (B) the primitive cardiogenic area arises caudal to the stomodeum
   (C) vascular and cardiac endothelium are continuous layers and share the same embryonic origin
   (D) the heart undergoes positional changes and morphogenesis during flexion
   (E) the heart begins to beat before 5 weeks of development

Directions: Each question below contains four suggested answers of which **one or more** is correct. Choose the answer

   A   if **1, 2, and 3** are correct
   B   if **1 and 3** are correct
   C   if **2 and 4** are correct
   D   if **4** is correct
   E   if **1, 2, 3, and 4** are correct

3. True statements concerning blood islands include which of the following?

   (1) They arise first in the chorion
   (2) Many form in the wall of the yolk sac
   (3) There is little erythropoiesis in them
   (4) They contribute to the development of the heart

4. Somite derivatives include which of the following?

   (1) Vertebral bodies
   (2) Vertebral ligaments
   (3) Intercostal muscles
   (4) Dermal connective tissue fibroblasts

5. The intermediate mesoderm forms which of the following structures?

   (1) Vertebral bodies
   (2) The kidneys
   (3) The limb buds
   (4) The gonads

Directions: The groups of questions below consist of lettered choices followed by several numbered items. For each numbered item select the **one** lettered choice with which it is **most** closely associated. Each lettered choice may be used once, more than once, or not at all.

Questions 6–10

For each description of components of an early human embryo, choose the appropriate lettered structure shown in the accompanying diagram.

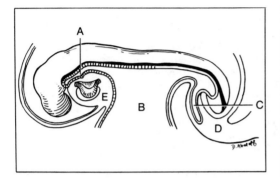

6. This structure becomes progressively restricted in diameter as flexion proceeds but persists as a connection between the yolk sac and the midgut

7. This structure lies anterior (cranial) to the anterior intestinal portal and forms the lumen and epithelial lining of the esophagus and stomach

8. This structure begins cranial to the heart but moves caudal to it, and makes a major contribution to the diaphragm

9. This structure becomes vascularized early in development and later forms the umbilical cord

10. This structure is a diverticulum of the yolk sac; it degenerates later in development, leaving no adult derivatives

Questions 11–15

For each description of components of the early human embryo, choose the appropriate lettered structure shown in the accompanying diagram.

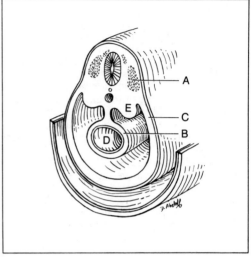

11. This structure gives rise to most of the urogenital system

12. This structure forms vertebral bodies and dermal connective tissues

13. This structure forms ribs and intercostal muscles

14. This structure eventually is the lumen of the gastrointestinal tract

15. This structure forms the smooth muscle and connective tissue in the gastrointestinal tract

ANSWERS AND EXPLANATIONS

1. The answer is A. *(IV B, C, D)* Flexion is a major morphogenetic process that converts a flat embryo into one having the basic vertebrate body plan. The amnion grows extensively and causes flexion. Lateral, head, and tail folds of the amnion all are important for establishing the basic body plan. The lateral folds grow ventrally and medially and bring the lateral body walls ventrally and into the midline. As they do so, they restrict the diameter of the vitelline duct, which connects the midgut to the yolk sac. The head fold growth and head flexion bring the septum transversum and heart from a position cranial to the oral cavity to a position caudal to the oral cavity. Similarly, tail fold growth and tail flexion bring the allantois cranially and ventrally, so that it eventually comes to lie cranial to the anus.

2. The answer is B. *(III B)* The cardiogenic area originates in angiogenetic cell clusters (blood islands) located in a portion of the intraembryonic mesoderm cranial to the stomodeum, a double layer of epithelium that lies at the cranial pole of the embryonic disk and forms a membrane covering the opening of the oral cavity. Cardiogenesis and angiogenesis are fundamentally similar processes. Both vascular and cardiac endothelium are a continuous simple squamous epithelium which arises from mesenchymal cells in the mural portions of blood islands. During head flexion, the head fold of the amnion grows and carries the heart primordium caudally and ventrally. The growth of the folds of the amnion also brings paired heart tubes together so that they can fuse in the ventral midline, an important event in early cardiac morphogenesis. The heart is the first organ to attain physiologic function during embryonic development. It begins to beat and propel blood in the embryo as early as the middle of the third week of gestation.

3. The answer is C (2, 4). *(III A, B)* Blood islands are collections of mesodermally derived mesenchymal cells. They have mural cells devoted to angiogenesis and central cells devoted to hematopoiesis. They arise first in the wall of the yolk sac and soon after appear in the embryo, connecting stalk, and chorion. These primitive blood islands sprout branches and their vesicles fuse with one another. This process leads to the formation of a closed circulatory system, including the heart tubes and primitive, nucleated erythrocytes.

4. The answer is E (all). *(II B)* The somites are paired mesodermal derivatives lying just lateral to the neural tube. Each somite becomes divided into a sclerotome and a dermomyotome. The sclerotome forms vertebral bodies, the bony neural arches of vertebrae, ribs (modified vertebral processes), and also the ligaments interconnecting the vertebrae. The dermomyotome becomes further subdivided into a dermatome and a myotome. The dermatome forms the dermal connective tissue (with fibroblasts) of a body segment. The myotome forms segmentally arranged body musculature such as the intercostal muscles.

5. The answer is C (2, 4). *(II B, C)* The intraembryonic mesoderm becomes divided into somites, intermediate mesoderm, and lateral plate mesoderm. Somites form vertebral bodies. Intermediate mesoderm forms the pronephros, mesonephros, and metanephros (precursors of adult kidneys), the gonads, and the gonadal ducts. The lateral plate mesoderm forms splanchnic mesoderm and somatic mesoderm, which later develop into structures such as gut smooth muscle and body wall connective tissue, respectively.

6–10. The answers are: 6-B, 7-A, 8-E, 9-D, 10-C. *(V B, C 2, D 2)* The diagram accompanying the questions is a sagittal section of a human embryo during flexion. The foregut *(A)* extends from the anterior intestinal portal to the oropharyngeal membrane, and becomes part of the oral cavity, esophagus, stomach, and upper portion of the duodenum. The septum transversum *(E)* is a mass of mesenchyme that becomes the bulk of the diaphragm and the connective tissue and capsule of the liver. The septum transversum initially lies at the far cranial end of the embryo, but curves caudally during flexion, coming to lie caudal to the heart. The vitelline duct *(B)* is a narrow communication between the midgut and the yolk sac. The allantois *(C)* is a yolk sac diverticulum which degenerates later in development. The connecting stalk *(D)* joins the embryo proper to the chorionic shell and forms the umbilical cord later in development.

11–15. The answers are: 11-E, 12-A, 13-C, 14-D, 15-B. *(II A 2 c, B 1, C 4, 5 b; V D 2 a)* The diagram accompanying the questions gives a three-dimensional and sectional view of an early human embryo as the lateral folds of the amnion are expanding and molding the lateral body walls. The somites *(A)* are derived from intraembryonic mesoderm established during gastrulation. They have a sclerotome, which forms vertebral bodies and intervertebral ligaments, and a dermomyotome, which forms segmentally arranged dermal connective tissue elements and muscles. The intermediate mesoderm *(E)* lies adjacent to the somites and forms the bulk of the urogenital system, namely the kidneys, ureters, gonads, and gonadal ducts. The lateral plate mesoderm becomes divided into a lower splanchnopleure, or splanchnic mesoderm *(B)*, and an upper somatopleure, or somatic mesoderm *(C)*. The former gives rise to muscles and connective tissues in the wall of visceral organs such as the stomach, lungs, and liver, while the latter gives rise to body wall tissues such as bones and muscles. The gut tube, which becomes the lumen of the gastrointestinal tract *(D)*, is initially continuous with the lumen of the yolk sac, but as flexion proceeds this continuity becomes progressively narrowed until only a small vitelline duct connects the gut tube and the yolk sac.

7
Development of the Placenta and Fetal Membranes (Amnion and Chorion)

I. OVERVIEW OF HUMAN PLACENTATION

A. General description of human placentation

1. In humans, the embryo and later the fetus develops in a shell of tissue derived from both a maternal source (the uterine endometrium, part of which becomes the **decidua**) and a collection of conceptus-derived structures including the **chorion** and **amnion** (the **fetal membranes**).

2. Part of the decidua and part of the chorion become highly modified to create the **placenta**.
   a. The placenta is a thick disk with a dense network of blood vessels.
   b. It is attached to the umbilical cord and firmly anchored to the uterine wall.
   c. The human placenta is a **hemochorial placenta**, in which maternal blood bathes fetal chorionic villi directly.
      (1) However, blood does not pass directly between mother and fetus.
      (2) Rather, nutrients, oxygen, and other substances diffuse or are transported across a thin **maternal–fetal barrier** that separates the two circulations.

B. Functions of the placenta

1. The primary function of the placenta is to serve as an **organ for exchange** between the conceptus and the mother.
   a. Nutrients and oxygen from maternal blood enter the fetal circulation, to be used for fetal growth and development.
   b. Wastes and carbon dioxide leave the fetal circulation and enter the maternal circulation.

2. In addition, the placenta and the trophoblast are the **source of hormones** that are essential for maintaining a maternal physiologic condition appropriate for continued development of the conceptus.

II. REVIEW OF IMPLANTATION (see Chapter 4, sections V and VII)

A. Evolution of the trophoblast

1. The blastocyst cavity forms as the conceptus becomes divided into an inner cell mass and a trophoblast.
   a. The **inner cell mass** becomes the embryo proper.
   b. The **trophoblast** becomes the extraembryonic structures.

2. The trophoblast becomes divided into two layers:
   a. An inner **cytotrophoblast** composed of dividing **discrete** cellular elements
   b. An outer **syncytiotrophoblast** composed of a **syncytium** of **fused** cytotrophoblastic cells

B. Implantation in the endometrium

1. The **syncytiotrophoblast** is an **invasive layer** that erodes maternal tissue as it advances during implantation.

2. During its invasion, the surface of the syncytiotrophoblast becomes highly irregular, as deep invaginations and microvilli appear.

3. As the conceptus burrows into the endometrium, the endometrial epithelium heals completely over the implantation site, so that the conceptus becomes completely surrounded by maternal tissue (Fig. 7-1). This type of implantation is characteristic of humans and is called **interstitial implantation**.

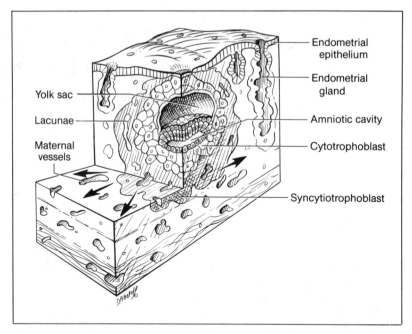

Figure 7-1. Human conceptus during implantation. Cells of the cytotrophoblast divide and fuse to form the syncytiotrophoblast, an invasive structure that facilitates the implantation of the conceptus. The endometrial epithelium has almost completely healed over the implantation site.

C. The chorionic shell

1. Soon after implantation, the pre-embryo, with its amniotic cavity and yolk sac, dangles freely in the extraembryonic coelom, suspended from the outer chorionic shell by a **connecting stalk** (Fig. 7-2).
2. The chorionic shell has three **components.**
   a. Innermost is **somatopleuric extraembryonic mesoderm**, which is formed directly from the cytotrophoblast.
   b. In the middle is the **cytotrophoblast**, the original layer.
   c. Outermost is the **syncytiotrophoblast** which, like the somatopleuric extraembryonic mesoderm, is formed from the cytotrophoblast.

III. ORIGIN AND DEVELOPMENT OF VILLI

A. Development of early villi

1. During implantation, the surface of the **syncytiotrophoblast** becomes highly irregular.
   a. It becomes indented by deep surface **invaginations.**
   b. **Microvilli** also appear on its surface, as elongated tongues of syncytiotrophoblast force themselves through the endometrial stroma. These elongated protrusions lack cytotrophoblastic cells in their core, and in transverse section they appear as a solid mass of syncytial cytoplasm.
2. The modifications in the surface of the syncytiotrophoblast have two results.
   a. The **surface area** of the maternal–fetal interface increases dramatically.
   b. **Lacunae** form in the syncytiotrophoblast and maternal blood pours into these surface invaginations and blind-ending cavities.

B. Development of chorionic villi.
While the early circulatory system is forming in the embryo (see Chapter 6, section III), there is simultaneously a substantial development of chorionic villi on the surface of the outer chorion, marking the beginning of the **villous stage** of placental development.

1. **Primary villi**
   a. Villi first appear as blunt projections from the outer chorionic surface.

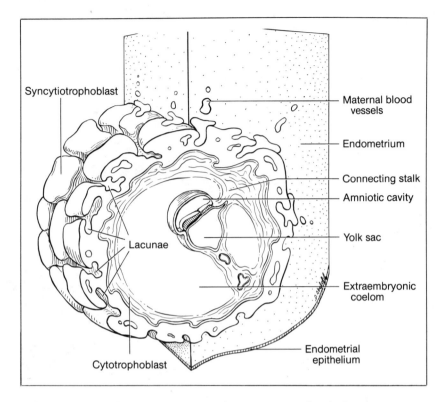

Figure 7-2. Human conceptus once implantation is completed. The conceptus is completely surrounded by maternal tissue, which has been cut away to show the syncytiotrophoblast. The surface of the syncytiotrophoblast is becoming more complex and villi are beginning to form. The embryo is located between the amniotic cavity and the yolk sac. It is attached to the chorionic shell by the connecting stalk, which will later become the umbilical cord.

    b. These projections from the syncytiotrophoblast continue to grow away from the chorionic shell. As they do so, cytotrophoblastic cells migrate into them.
        (1) Once **cytotrophoblastic cells** have invaded the advancing tongues of syncytiotrophoblast, the projections are referred to as **primary villi**.
        (2) Primary villi cut in transverse section show a core of cytotrophoblast surrounded by a shell of syncytiotrophoblast (Fig. 7-3A).

2. Secondary villi
    a. The primary villi continue to elongate and as they do so, their cores become invaded by mesenchymal cells derived from extraembryonic mesoderm in the chorionic shell.
        (1) Once villi have this **mesenchymal core**, they are called **secondary villi**.
        (2) Secondary villi cut in transverse section show a core of mesenchyme surrounded by an inner shell of cytotrophoblast and an outer shell of syncytiotrophoblast (Fig. 7-3B).
    b. The mesenchymal cells eventually will form the connective tissue stroma of the chorionic villi.

3. Tertiary villi
    a. Secondary villi continue to grow, further elongating and sending out branches.
    b. As they do so, they become invaded by fetal blood vessels which migrate in from the extraembryonic mesoderm. Other blood vessels arise in situ by mesenchymal cell differentiation.
        (1) Once villi have **blood vessels**, they are called **tertiary villi**.
        (2) Tertiary villi cut in transverse section have capillaries and mesenchymally derived connective tissue in their core and are surrounded by shells of cytotrophoblast and syncytiotrophoblast (Fig. 7-3C).
    c. Tertiary villi first make their appearance in the fourth week of development.

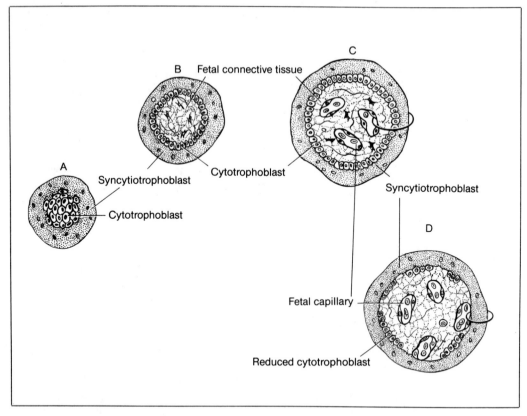

Figure 7-3. Cross sections of human chorionic villi, showing the stages of development. *A,* Primary villus; *B,* secondary villus; *C,* tertiary villus; *D,* a villus at term. Note that by the time of birth the cytotrophoblast has all but disappeared.

C. Development of a cytotrophoblastic shell and cytotrophoblastic cell columns

1. The **chorion** develops from the extraembryonic mesoderm, which forms both connective tissue and blood vessels of the chorion as well as a **cytotrophoblastic shell**, also a part of the chorion.
2. The name **"villus"** implies that chorionic villi have free distal ends. In reality, the earliest villi formed do not have free distal ends. Primitive primary villi are joined at their distal tips by syncytiotrophoblastic bridges.
3. As mesenchyme and blood vessels invade the villi, cytotrophoblastic cells seem to break through the syncytiotrophoblastic layer and unite to form a continuous outer layer of cytotrophoblast which is associated with the remnants of the once continuous syncytiotrophoblast.
4. This outer layer of cytotrophoblast forms the **cytotrophoblastic shell** and **anchoring villi (cytotrophoblastic cell columns).**
   a. The **anchoring villi** are masses of cytotrophoblast covered by syncytiotrophoblast (Fig. 7-4).
   b. They serve to interconnect the inner and outer layers of cytotrophoblast.
   c. At first, these anchoring cell columns do not become invaded by blood vessels and mesenchyme.
   d. The anchoring villi send out large numbers of **branch villi** that project from them into the intervillous space filled with maternal blood.
5. The **cytotrophoblastic shell** confronts maternal tissue, and the inner layer of cytotrophoblast becomes the **chorionic plate** of the definitive **placenta**.
6. The formation of the cytotrophoblastic shell divides the syncytiotrophoblast into two distinct populations of cells:
   a. A **continuous layer** lining the intervillous space which is interrupted only by maternal

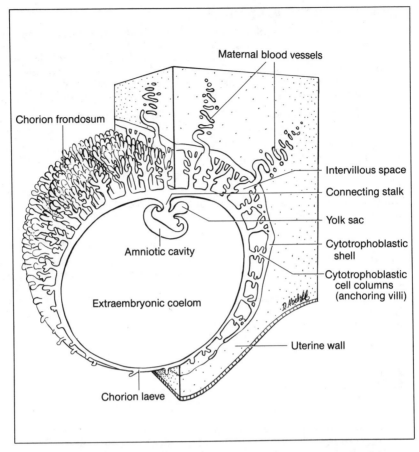

Figure 7-4. Chorionic development progressing toward the formation of a placenta. The chorionic surface shows an area with extensive villous development (chorion frondosum) and an area with few villi that is relatively smooth (chorion laeve). A cytotrophoblastic shell with cytotrophoblastic cell columns has also formed; these become the chorionic shell and anchoring villi, respectively.

blood vessels penetrating the cytotrophoblastic shell and emptying blood into the intervillous space.
  b. A **discontinuous layer** between the shell itself and the maternal decidual tissue.
7. **True villi**, with free distal ends, arise along the cytotrophoblastic cell columns projecting into the intervillous space.

D. Later development of villi and changes in the chorion
  1. The cytotrophoblastic shell first forms around day 21. At this stage, the entire chorion is covered by villi.
      a. Some of the villi are finger-like protrusions and others look more like seaweed, with collateral branches and many bifurcations.
      b. This proliferation of villi serves to increase the surface area of the chorion for increasing embryonic gas and waste exchange.
  2. Later, some of the chorionic villi disappear, leaving a smooth **chorion laeve**, while other villi persist, leaving a **chorion frondosum** (see Fig. 7-4).
      a. By the beginning of the second month of gestation, villi begin to degenerate on the side of the chorion toward the uterine cavity. As a result, this side of the chorion becomes smooth, forming the **chorion laeve** (the Latin word for smooth).
      b. On the deepest implantation side of the chorion, villi persist and continue to proliferate, forming the **chorion frondosum**. The chorion frondosum, along with maternal decidual tissue, will eventually form the **placenta**.

E. Progress toward the definitive placental morphology

1. In essence, the **definitive placenta** now consists of a chorionic plate connected to a cytotrophoblastic shell by anchoring villi.
   a. The **chorionic plate** has numerous anchoring villi projecting from its surface.
   b. The **cytotrophoblastic cell columns (anchoring villi)** are the columns of connective tissue covered by cytotrophoblast and syncytiotrophoblast which interconnect the chorionic plate to the outer cytotrophoblastic shell (see section III C 4).
2. The anchoring villi have numerous **branch villi** which project away from the anchoring villi into the intervillous space.
3. Because a hemochorial placenta is formed in the human, the chorionic villi are bathed directly in maternal blood. Maternal blood vessels penetrate the cytotrophoblastic shell and empty directly into the intervillous space (see Fig. 7-4).
4. In many instances, islands of syncytium break off from the syncytiotrophoblast. These **multinuclear giant cells** can be found in maternal blood vessels draining the placenta and in the systemic maternal circulation as well.

F. The maternal–fetal barrier consists of several structures separating maternal and fetal blood.

1. In the fourth week of development, when tertiary villi first make their appearance, an oxygen molecule in maternal hemoglobin would need to cross several structures on its way to the fetal hemoglobin molecule:
   a. Maternal erythrocyte membrane
   b. Maternal blood
   c. Syncytiotrophoblast
   d. Cytotrophoblast
   e. Cytotrophoblast basement membrane
   f. Villous connective tissue
   g. Fetal capillary basement membrane
   h. Fetal capillary endothelium
   i. Fetal blood
   j. Fetal erythrocyte membrane
2. As the placenta grows, the nature of the barrier between maternal and fetal blood also changes. This barrier becomes reduced in several different ways:
   a. The cytotrophoblast, by continuously dividing and fusing to form the syncytiotrophoblast, in effect proliferates itself out of existence, so that it is no longer present as a barrier to diffusion.
   b. The connective tissue stroma becomes more spongy.
   c. Fetal blood vessels migrate from the center of villi toward the periphery, displacing intervening connective tissue elements.
3. The end result of these changes is a barrier between fetal and maternal blood that is often only a micrometer or less in thickness.

IV. CELL BIOLOGY OF THE TROPHOBLAST

A. Origin of the syncytiotrophoblast

1. The detailed morphology of the maternal–fetal barrier first became understood through the use of the electron microscope. Prior to that, there was considerable debate about the relationship between various structures in the placenta.
2. Pulse-chase labelling experiments clearly demonstrated that the syncytiotrophoblast is a **syncytium** and that cytotrophoblastic nuclei become syncytiotrophoblastic nuclei by cell fusion.
   a. A short incubation in tritiated thymidine (pulse) was followed by longer incubation in unlabeled media (chase).
   b. Autoradiography then showed that radiolabeling decreased in the cytotrophoblastic nuclei and increased in syncytiotrophoblastic nuclei, proving the syncytial nature and origin of the latter.

B. Ultrastructure of the syncytiotrophoblast

1. **Transport structures**
   a. **Microvilli** are numerous on the surface of the syncytiotrophoblast.
      (1) The microvilli form a **brush border** similar to that found in other epithelial layers

specialized for transport, as in the small intestine and in renal proximal convoluted tubules.
- (2) They represent an increase in cell surface area to increase the efficiency of transepithelial transport.
- b. **Membrane-bound vesicles and vacuoles** honeycomb the syncytium.
  - (1) These give the cytoplasm of the syncytiotrophoblast a foamy appearance in the light microscope.
  - (2) The electron microscope reveals that this appearance is due to myriads of small vesicles and vacuoles, each bounded by a membrane.
  - (3) These are transport structures that convey various materials in both directions across the placenta. For example, immunoglobulins are transported from maternal to fetal blood; progesterone and chorionic gonadotropin are transported from the placenta to maternal blood.
2. **Structures for synthesis and secretion of proteins and steroids** (see also Chapter 19, section VII)
   - a. The syncytiotrophoblast has many free **ribosomes** for the synthesis of proteins for internal utilization.
   - b. The syncytiotrophoblast also has abundant **rough endoplasmic reticulum** for the synthesis of proteins destined for secretion. The placenta secretes several **protein hormones**, including:
     - (1) Chorionic gonadotropin (hCG), a glycoprotein
     - (2) Human placental lactogen
   - c. The syncytiotrophoblast also has a well-developed **Golgi apparatus** for packaging secreted proteins and for glycosylation of hormones such as hCG.
   - d. The syncytiotrophoblast also has an abundance of **smooth endoplasmic reticulum** and **mitochondria** with tubular cristae, features commonly found in steroid-secreting cells. The placenta secretes a large amount of **steroid hormone**, most notably progesterone.
3. **Desmosomal anchors**
   - a. Adjacent cytoplasmic masses of syncytiotrophoblast are interrupted by clefts where membranous boundaries are juxtaposed.
     - (1) In these clefts, there is a zone of **intersyncytial adhesion** where numerous **desmosomes** hold the masses together.
     - (2) In addition, the syncytial masses are anchored to the underlying cytotrophoblastic cells (**Langhans' cells**) by means of other desmosomes.
   - b. The cytotrophoblastic cells are anchored to the basement membrane of the trophoblast by **hemidesmosomes**.

V. THE DECIDUA.
The decidua is the endometrial lining of the uterus that becomes greatly modified during pregnancy. It takes its name from the fact that it is shed along with the placenta and fetal membranes during delivery.

A. The decidual cell reaction
1. While implantation and the early growth of chorionic villi are progressing, cells of the endometrial connective tissue stroma are undergoing a modification, known as the **decidual cell reaction**, to differentiate into decidual cells.
2. Certain features of this decidual cell differentiation are quite clear, although the exact mechanism of the process is poorly understood at the present time.
   - a. Decidual cells probably differentiate from stromal fibroblasts.
   - b. Progesterone secreted by the ovarian corpus luteum seems to play a role in decidual cell differentiation.
3. **Characteristics and functions of decidual cells**
   - a. Decidual cells have the following **features** (Fig. 7-5):
     - (1) They are large cells with prominent nuclei.
     - (2) Each nucleus has diffuse nuclear chromatin and a large nucleolus.
     - (3) The cytoplasm is rich in lipid vacuoles and glycogen granules.
   - b. Research is needed to clarify the **function** of decidual cells.
     - (1) Inspection of the early implantation site shows that the decidual cell layer surrounds the implanting conceptus. In this regard, some authors speculate that the decidual tissue **limits the invasiveness of trophoblastic tissue.**
     - (2) Decidual cells may play some role in **preventing maternal immunologic recognition** of the conceptus (see Chapter 15, section VII).
     - (3) Decidual cells may also **secrete nutritive or trophic substances** for the growing trophoblast.

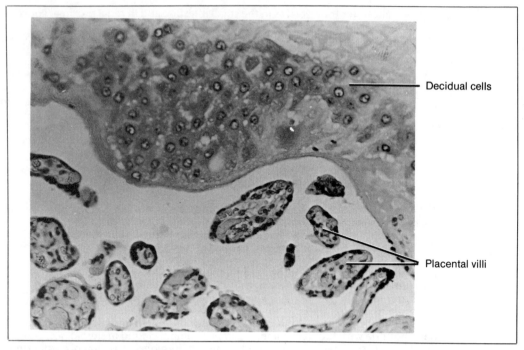

Figure 7-5. Decidual cells and villi in the human placenta at term. (Reprinted with permission from Johnson KE: *Histology: Microscopic Anatomy and Embryology.* New York, John Wiley, 1982, p 324.)

- **B. Components of the decidua** (Fig. 7-6)
    1. Decidual cells form a continuous layer in the endometrium that completely surrounds the implanting conceptus and extends around the entire endometrium and into the uterine tubes.
    2. The early decidua has three **regions.**
        a. The **decidua basalis** is the portion of the decidua directly adjacent to the conceptus at the implantation site.
        b. The **decidua capsularis** is the portion that surrounds the implanting conceptus on the side opposite the decidua basalis.
        c. **The decidua parietalis** lines the rest of the uterine lumen.
    3. The **decidua vera** is formed later from the composite decidua capsularis and decidua parietalis. These come together and fuse when the growth of the conceptus obliterates the uterine lumen.

VI. STRUCTURE OF THE DEFINITIVE PLACENTA AND PLACENTAL CIRCULATION

- **A. Basic components and morphology of the definitive placenta**
    1. The placenta becomes recognizable as a separate morphologic entity early in the fourth month of pregnancy.
    2. The definitive placenta has a fetal and a maternal component.
        a. The **fetal component** is derived from the chorion frondosum.
        b. The **maternal component** is derived from the decidua basalis.
    3. **Structural subdivisions of the definitive placenta** (see Fig. 7-7)
        a. The **decidual plate** is the **maternal surface** of the placenta.
            (1) Numerous branches of the uterine arteries form the **maternal spiral arteries**, which penetrate the decidual plate and enter the intervillous space.
            (2) These maternal arteries fill the intervillous space with maternal blood.
        b. The **chorionic plate** is the **fetal surface** of the placenta.
            (1) The **fetal villi** project into the placenta from the chorionic plate.
            (2) The **anchoring villi** cross the placenta and attach to the decidual plate, while the ends of the **branching villi** remain free in the blood-filled intervillous space.

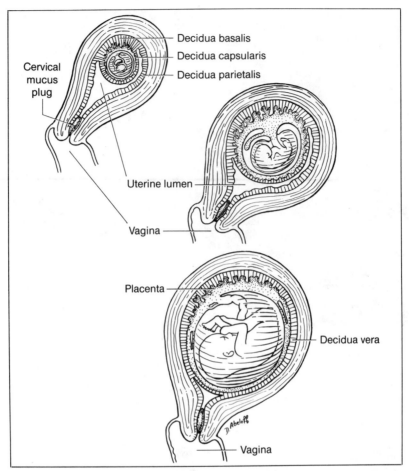

Figure 7-6. Development of the decidua. The decidua basalis, at the implantation site, and the decidua capsularis, surrounding the rest of the conceptus, fuse as the conceptus grows, to become the decidua vera. The decidua basalis and the chorion contribute to the formation of the placenta.

    c. There is a **junctional zone** of the placenta where decidual cells and syncytiotrophoblast are mixed together. This junctional zone is particularly rich in **syncytial giant cells**.
    d. As the placenta grows, **decidual septa** grow toward the chorionic plate, but they never fully reach it. These placental septa divide the placenta into a number of lobulated **cotyledons**.

B. Placental circulation (Fig. 7-7)
    1. Circulation of maternal blood. The total volume of maternal blood in the placenta is only about 150 ml but it is replaced several times each minute.
        a. Maternal blood **enters the placenta** under **high pressure.**
            (1) Just before the maternal spiral arteries enter the intervillous space, their lumina sharply decrease in diameter. This occurs because the endothelial cells lining the distal spiral arteries are tall columnar cells rather than low squamous cells.
            (2) As a result of this sudden decrease in diameter, blood is injected at high pressure into the intervillous space.
        b. The streaming fountain of oxygen-rich maternal blood pours **into the intervillous space**, where it bathes numerous **placental branch villi.**
        c. The **decidual septa** form a series of baffles that compartmentalize the blood flow in the intervillous space.
            (1) After passing over the villi, the blood is reflected from the chorionic plate.
            (2) As the blood travels along the inner aspect of the chorionic plate, it suddenly encounters the decidual septa, which **deflect the blood** so that it flows back toward the decidual plate along the decidual septa.

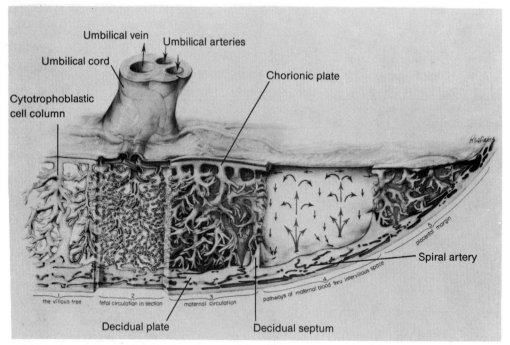

Figure 7-7. A composite diagram of the mature placenta, showing its structure and the circulation of maternal and fetal blood. *1,* The villous architecture; *2,* fetal circulation; *3,* maternal circulation, showing spurts of blood entering the intervillous space; *4,* pathways of maternal blood; *5,* the placental margin. (Adapted from Ramsey EM, Harris JWS: Comparison of uteroplacental vasculature and circulation in the Rhesus monkey and man. *Cont Embryol* 38:61–70. Washington, DC, Carnegie Institution of Washington, 1966, p 70.)

      d. Finally, the maternal blood drains into **endometrial veins**.
  2. Circulation of fetal blood
      a. Oxygen-poor fetal blood flows toward the placenta through the two **umbilical arteries**. These branch extensively soon after entering the placenta, supplying oxygen-poor blood to the **villous arterioles and capillaries**.
      b. An extensive network of **venules** drain the villi and carry oxygen-rich fetal blood into the single **umbilical vein**.

VII. PLACENTAL TRANSPORT

A. Oxygen transport

1. The most important function of the placenta is to serve as a respiratory organ for the fetus. Interruption of fetal blood flow to the placenta by constriction of the umbilical cord or of maternal blood flow to the placenta by **placental abruption** (detachment) for as little as a few minutes can be fatal to the fetus.

2. Oxygen and carbon dioxide can diffuse readily in both directions across the fetal–maternal interface.
    a. The oxygen tension in maternal blood is higher than in fetal blood, and so **oxygen** diffuses **toward fetal blood**.
    b. Carbon dioxide tension in fetal blood is higher than in maternal blood, and so **carbon dioxide** diffuses **toward maternal blood**.

3. Fetal hemoglobin also has a greater affinity for oxygen than adult hemoglobin at physiologic pH.

4. Because of the **Bohr effect**, any factor that increases the carbon dioxide tension in maternal blood will decrease the oxygen-carrying capacity of maternal blood. This may account for the well-known phenomenon of lower birth weights and lower perinatal survival rates for infants born to mothers who smoke cigarettes.

B. Water and electrolyte transport

1. **Passive diffusion** is responsible for the transport of the following electrolytes across the placenta:
   a. Water
   b. Sodium
   c. Potassium
   d. Chloride
2. **Facilitated diffusion** is thought to be responsible for the transport of the following electrolytes across the placenta:
   a. **Calcium.** Calcium accumulates in the fetus (e.g., for ossification of developing bones) at the expense of maternal calcium, which is removed from the maternal skeleton.
   b. **Phosphate.** Phosphate accumulates in fetal blood, suggesting that there is an energy-dependent transport mechanism for this anion.

C. Active transport of nutrients

1. **Glucose** is transported by facilitated diffusion involving stereospecific carrier molecules in the placenta. The maternal serum glucose concentration is less than the fetal serum glucose concentration. This difference may well be due at least in part to placental glucose utilization.
2. **Amino acids** probably also cross the placenta by active transport. This is supported by five lines of evidence:
   a. Fetal serum amino acid levels are greater than maternal serum amino acid levels.
   b. Fetal serum amino acid levels can be saturated experimentally by increasing maternal serum amino acid levels.
   c. Simultaneous infusion of two different amino acids into maternal serum can result in a decreased rate of transport of each amino acid into fetal serum.
   d. L-Amino acids are transported more rapidly than D-amino acids.
   e. Inhibitors of adenosine triphosphate (ATP) synthesis also inhibit amino acid transport across the placenta.

D. Transport of serum proteins

1. Most maternal serum proteins are transported across the placenta at an exceedingly low rate.
2. Maternal serum **immunoglobulin G (IgG)** is transported intact into fetal serum at a high rate.
   a. The mechanism of transport is **receptor-mediated.**
      (1) IgG molecules are bound to the syncytiotrophoblast by specific receptors.
      (2) They are then engulfed by receptor-mediated endocytosis and are transported across the placental barrier without being degraded by lysosomes.
   b. The **function** of this transport is to provide the fetus with **passive immunity** to antigens that the mother has been exposed to but that the fetus can not be exposed to because it is developing in a sterile uterine cavity.
3. Other maternal immunoglobulins, such as IgM, are not transported across the placenta.
4. Most **fetal serum proteins** are synthesized de novo from amino acids in the fetal system.

E. Transport of hormones and bilirubin

1. Many **endocrine hormones** are also synthesized de novo in the fetus under control of the fetal pituitary.
   a. In anencephalic fetuses, development of the pituitary gland is abnormal, causing a lack of adrenocorticotropic hormone (ACTH).
   b. The result is fetal adrenal hypoplasia, even though there are normal levels of ACTH in the maternal blood.
2. **Steroid hormones** pass freely across the placenta.
   a. Thus, steroid treatment of a pregnant woman may have undesirable effects in the fetus.
   b. For example, birth control pills taken by pregnant women will cause masculinization in the developing genital system of the female fetus. Therefore, it is essential to establish that a patient is not pregnant before administering oral contraceptives.
3. **Unconjugated bilirubin** is transported freely across the placenta. **Conjugated bilirubin** (e.g., bilirubin glucuronide) is transported very slowly.

a. Thus, conjugated bilirubin in the maternal blood does not reach the fetus, but unconjugated bilirubin in fetal blood passes rapidly into maternal blood.
b. Prior to birth, **fetal bilirubin** is transported across the placenta, conjugated in the maternal liver, and excreted in maternal bile.
c. The ability to conjugate bilirubin is undeveloped in the fetal liver and is still immature in the neonatal liver.
d. Consequently, transient jaundice is quite common in newborn infants.

VIII. **THE UMBILICAL CORD.** The umbilical cord conveys the umbilical blood vessels between the fetus and the placenta.

A. **Development and vasculature**
1. The umbilical cord forms from the connecting stalk.
2. Early in development, there are two umbilical veins and two umbilical arteries. Due to changes in the great veins (see Chapter 10, section VI D), one of the umbilical veins disappears, leaving two umbilical arteries and one umbilical vein. The diameter of each umbilical artery is less than that of the umbilical vein.
   a. The two **umbilical arteries** carry **deoxygenated blood from the fetus** to the placenta.
   b. The single **umbilical vein** carries **oxygenated blood** from the placenta **to the fetus**.

B. **Histologic structure**
1. The umbilical vessels have unusually thick walls with an abundance of smooth muscle.
2. The vessels are surrounded by loose connective tissue called **Wharton's jelly**.
   a. Wharton's jelly is a loose areolar connective tissue consisting of fibroblasts and having an extracellular matrix particularly rich in the glycosaminoglycan **hyaluronic acid**.
   b. Wharton's jelly gives the umbilical cord a rubbery, gelatinous character, making it unlikely that twists or turns in the umbilical cord will result in constriction of the life-giving umbilical blood vessels.
3. The outer surface of the umbilical cord is coated with a thin layer of amniotic epithelium which is continuous with the fetal belly skin at the umbilicus.

IX. **ABNORMALITIES OF PLACENTATION**

A. **Abnormal implantation sites.** The placenta normally forms in the upper portion of the wall of the uterus. Any implantation in a different location is considered to be an abnormal implantation site.
1. **Ectopic pregnancy**
   a. An ectopic pregnancy is one in which the implantation site lies outside the fundal cavity of the uterus.
      (1) An implantation in a uterine tube, in the cervical canal, on the ovary, or at any site outside the female reproductive tract would thus be an ectopic pregnancy.
      (2) The relative frequencies of different sites of ectopic pregnancies are shown in Table 7-1.
   b. The incidence of ectopic pregnancy varies from 1 in 80 pregnancies to 1 in 250 pregnancies, depending upon the population under consideration.
      (1) Those populations with a high incidence of chronic gonococcal infections and other pelvic inflammatory disease will also have a high incidence of ectopic pregnancy.
      (2) This is due to the fact that these bacterial diseases cause scarring of the uterine tubes and compromise their role in transport of the conceptus from the uterine tubes to the uterine cavity.
   c. In an ectopic pregnancy, both the placenta and the fetus lie outside the uterine cavity.
   d. The most common type of ectopic pregnancy is a **tubal pregnancy** (95% of all cases).
      (1) An ectopic pregnancy is not clinically different from a normal pregnancy in its early phases.
      (2) Once the conceptus grows and causes distension of the uterine tubes, the patient may report abdominal pain.
      (3) If the uterine tube ruptures, there can be life-threatening bleeding into the abdomen.
      (4) Ultrasonography can locate the gestational sac in the uterine tubes. Rarely, a normal implantation and an ectopic twin are found (Fig. 7-8).
   e. Ectopic pregnancies are removed surgically.

Table 7-1. Relative Frequencies of Different Types of Ectopic Pregnancies

Implantation Site	Incidence (% of All Ectopic Pregnancies)
Distal third of uterine tubes	41%
Middle third of uterine tubes	37%
Proximal third of uterine tubes	12%
Fimbria alone	5%
Fimbria and ovary	2%
Ovary alone	1%
Abdominal cavity	<1%
Interstitial uterine tube	<1%
Uterine cornua	<1%
Cervix	<1%
Other sites	<1%

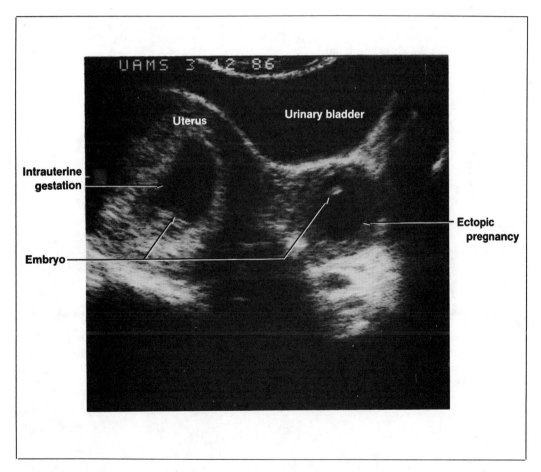

Figure 7-8. Sonogram of a normal intrauterine gestation *(left)* and a simultaneous ectopic pregnancy *(right).* (Courtesy of Teresita L. Angtuaco, M.D., Assistant Professor, Department of Obstetrics and Gynecology, University of Arkansas for Medical Sciences.)

2. Placenta previa
a. In placenta previa, the placenta forms to a greater or lesser extent **across the cervical os** (Fig. 7-9).
b. This is a common complication of pregnancy, occurring in 1 in 200 obstetrical patients.
c. In placenta previa, the fetus develops normally within the uterine cavity.
d. The placenta spanning the cervical os makes delivery of the fetus difficult.

B. Trophoblastic disease.
The placenta can undergo malignant transformation, as when it forms a hydatidiform (hydatiform) mole or a choriocarcinoma.

1. Hydatidiform mole
a. In this condition, a conceptus forms in which the embryo has died or is completely lacking and the placental villi fail to become vascularized.
b. Hydatidiform moles occur in about 1 in 2000 pregnancies in the United States; they are more common in the Orient.
c. Because the **trophoblast survives** the embryo, masses of edematous and swollen villi form, covered by syncytiotrophoblast. The uterine lumen becomes filled with these grape-like vesicles.
d. The proliferating trophoblast secretes **chorionic gonadotropin**, and the high hCG serum levels aid in diagnosis. Sonography may demonstrate the absence of an embryo.
e. Hydatidiform moles that do not abort spontaneously must be removed surgically. Most moles are benign, but about 15% invade and destroy the myometrium, a condition known as **invasive mole** or **chorioadenoma destruens**. Invasive moles sometimes metastasize to other parts of the body.

2. Choriocarcinoma
a. In this disease, uncontrolled **proliferation of cytotrophoblastic cells** results in disorganized masses of invasive tissue. There is rapid **metastasis** to many other organs, including the lungs and brain.
b. The tumor secretes large amounts of chorionic gonadotropin, an aid in diagnosis.
c. Recent advances in chemotherapy have allowed obstetricians to improve the formerly poor survival rates.

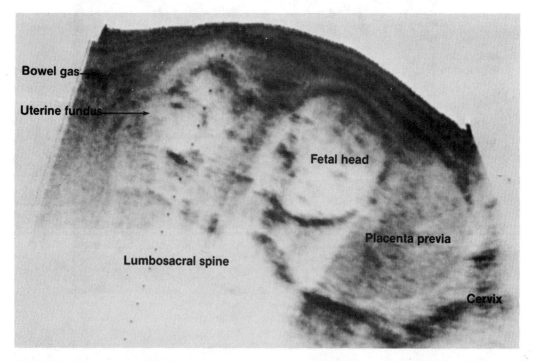

Figure 7-9. Sonogram of a complete placenta previa. Note that the placenta lies directly over the cervical canal. (Courtesy of Teresita L. Angtuaco, M.D., Assistant Professor, Department of Obstetrics and Gynecology, University of Arkansas for Medical Sciences.)

X. MULTIPLE PREGNANCIES

A. General considerations

1. Under normal circumstances, only a single ovum is released each month from one or the other ovary. When this single ovum becomes fertilized, normally a single conceptus results.
2. Natural multiple pregnancies, 90% of which are twins, arise when multiple ova are fertilized or when a fertilized ovum divides into two developing systems. Multiple pregnancies can be diagnosed by sonography (Fig. 7-10).

B. Twins.
Twinning occurs when two fetuses form. There are two types of twins, dizygotic and monozygotic.

1. **Dizygotic twins** result when two ova are released and are fertilized in one cycle. Dizygotic twins represent about 70% of all twins.
   a. Since they arise from **two separate ova** fertilized by **separate spermatozoa**, dizygotic twins may be the same sex or different sexes. They are no more alike than siblings born one at a time.
   b. Dizygotic twins have two separate chorionic sacs, two separate amniotic sacs, and usually two separate placentas. In some instances, they share a single large fused placenta (Fig. 7-11).
2. **Monozygotic twins** result when a single fertilized ovum divides into two separate developing systems. Monozygotic twins represent 30% of all twins.
   a. Because monozygotic twins arise from **cleavage of a single ovum**, they are alike in all their genetically determined characteristics. In this sense, they are **identical.**
      (1) Monozygotic twins are alike in the following ways:
         (a) Sex
         (b) Hair and eye color
         (c) Facial characteristics
         (d) Fingerprint patterns
         (e) Histocompatibility antigens
         (f) All other biochemical traits known to have a strictly genetic basis
      (2) Personality traits are even alike in monozygotic twins, even in cases where they have been separated at birth and raised in different environments.

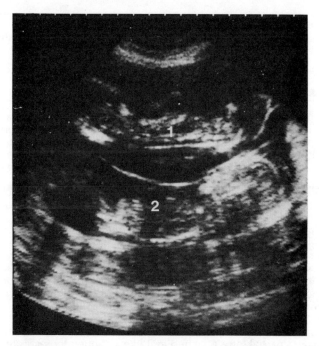

Figure 7-10. Sonogram of twin human embryos (marked 1 and 2) in utero. (Courtesy of William J. Cochrane, M.D., Washington DC.)

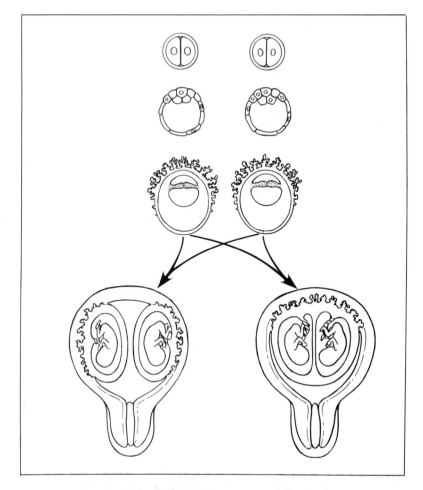

Figure 7-11. Formation of dizygotic twins. Dizygotic twins are formed by fertilization of separate ova. The twins can have either separate placentas *(left)* or a single shared placenta formed by fusion of separate placentas *(right)*.

  b. Although genetically identical, however, monozygotic twins may be slightly **different phenotypically** because of developmental differences in the uterine environment. For example, one twin may be larger than the other at birth because of differences in blood supply or placental morphology during gestation.
  c. Monozygotic twins are of several different **subtypes**, depending on the stage at which the conceptus divided (Fig. 7-12).
   (1) Diamnionic, dichorionic monozygotic twins divide at the morula stage, before the inner cell mass and trophoblast have formed. These twins have separate amnionic sacs and chorionic sacs.
   (2) Diamnionic, monochorionic monozygotic twins divide at a stage when the inner cell mass has differentiated from the trophoblast, but before the amnion has formed. They have separate amnionic sacs but are enclosed within a single chorionic sac.
   (3) Monoamnionic, monochorionic monozygotic twins result from division of the blastoderm after the amnion has formed. These twins share both a single amnionic sac and a single chorionic sac.
  d. Conjoined twins will result if there is an **incomplete division** of the blastoderm. They may be joined at the head, abdomen, or thorax. In some instances, a complete fetus will have a partial fetus attached to it like an appended parasite. This phenomenon is called **unequal conjoined twins**.

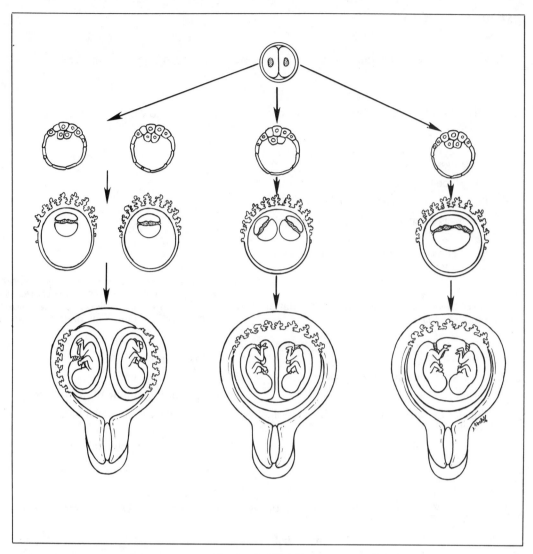

Figure 7-12. Formation of monozygotic twins. Monozygotic twins are formed by division of a single fertilized ovum into two separate developing systems. Monozygotic twins can be diamnionic and dichorionic *(left)*, diamnionic and monochorionic *(middle)*, or monoamnionic and monochorionic *(right)*, depending on the time when the conceptus splits into two separate entities.

C. Multiple pregnancies of higher number

1. Multiple pregnancies involving more than two fetuses are quite rare unless ovulation-stimulating drugs have been used.
   a. **Triplets** are seen in 1 in 8100 pregnancies.
   b. **Quadruplets** are seen in 1 in 800,000 pregnancies.
2. Recently, new methods of treating infertility have resulted in an increase in multiple pregnancies.
   a. **Fertility drugs** are used to treat cases of ovulation incompetence due to hormonal imbalance. The drugs stimulate the development, maturation, and ovulation of multiple fertile ova in a single reproductive cycle.
   b. Multiple pregnancies can also occur when **in vitro fertilization (IVF)** is used, since multiple fertilized eggs are transferred into a mother (see Chapter 4, section IX).

STUDY QUESTIONS

Directions: Each question below contains five suggested answers. Choose the **one best** response to each question.

1. All of the following are features of placenta previa EXCEPT

   (A) it is a common complication, seen in 1 in 200 pregnancies
   (B) it is a type of ectopic pregnancy
   (C) the placenta forms across the cervical os
   (D) the gestational sac is inside the uterine cavity
   (E) delivery is more difficult than in normal pregnancy

2. All of the following are features of hydatidiform mole EXCEPT

   (A) it occurs in 1 in 2000 pregnancies in the United States
   (B) a fetus may be completely lacking
   (C) serum hCG levels are low
   (D) the uterus becomes filled with grape-like vesicles
   (E) edematous villi are present

3. All of the following structures are present in secondary chorionic villi EXCEPT

   (A) cytotrophoblast
   (B) syncytiotrophoblast
   (C) fetal connective tissue
   (D) mesoderm
   (E) fetal blood vessels

4. In the placenta at term, an oxygen molecule would need to cross several structures as it diffused from maternal blood to fetal blood. These structures include all of the following EXCEPT

   (A) syncytiotrophoblast
   (B) cytotrophoblast
   (C) basement membrane of trophoblast
   (D) fetal capillary endothelial basement membrane
   (E) fetal capillary endothelial cells

Directions: Each question below contains four suggested answers of which **one or more** is correct. Choose the answer

   A if **1, 2, and 3** are correct
   B if **1 and 3** are correct
   C if **2 and 4** are correct
   D if **4** is correct
   E if **1, 2, 3, and 4** are correct

5. The trophoblast forms which of the following structures?

   (1) Cytotrophoblast
   (2) Syncytiotrophoblast
   (3) Chorion
   (4) Intraembryonic mesoderm

6. True statements concerning the umbilical vein include which of the following?

   (1) It conveys oxygen-poor blood to the placenta
   (2) It contains smooth muscle in its wall
   (3) Its diameter is smaller than that of the umbilical arteries
   (4) It is surrounded by a hyaluronate-rich extracellular matrix

7. True statements concerning placental transport include which of the following?

(1) Sodium and potassium ions diffuse passively across the placenta
(2) Maternal immunoglobulin G (IgG) is transported across the placenta in functionally intact form
(3) Glucose is transported by a stereospecific carrier mechanism
(4) Conjugated bilirubin is transported across the placenta at a low rate

8. Twins can show which of the following characteristics?

(1) Dizygotic twins can have the same sex
(2) Monozygotic twins can be phenotypically different
(3) Dizygotic twins can share a placenta
(4) Dizygotic twins can share a single amniotic sac

9. The ultrastructure of the syncytiotrophoblast has which of the following characteristics?

(1) Its apical surface has many microvilli
(2) It has little rough endoplasmic reticulum
(3) It has many vesicles and vacuoles bounded by membranes
(4) It has little smooth endoplasmic reticulum

Directions: The groups of questions below consist of lettered choices followed by several numbered items. For each numbered item select the **one** lettered choice with which it is **most** closely associated. Each lettered choice may be used once, more than once, or not at all.

Questions 10–14

For each description below of a structure in the mature placenta, select the appropriate lettered area shown in the the accompanying diagram.

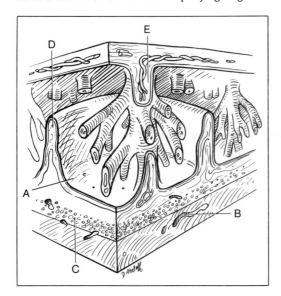

10. This structure joins the chorionic and decidual plates of the placenta and has branch villi on it

11. This structure conveys oxygenated blood to the intervillous space

12. This structure is a baffle which deflects blood from the intervillous space into vessels draining the intervillous space

13. This structure has columnar endothelial cells and injects blood into the intervillous space

14. This structure is filled with maternal blood and branch villi

Questions 15-19

For each description below of a structure in the conceptus, select the appropriate lettered component in the accompanying diagram.

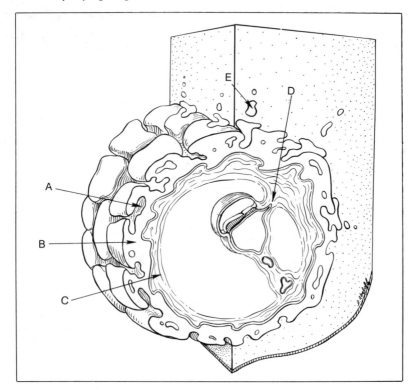

15. This structure becomes the umbilical cord

16. This structure is one of the invaginations in the surface of the syncytiotrophoblast known as lacunae

17. This cell layer produces the syncytiotrophoblast by proliferation and fusion

18. This layer becomes covered by microvilli and is bathed in maternal blood

19. This structure conveys maternal blood through the endometrium to the intervillous space

ANSWERS AND EXPLANATIONS

1. The answer is B. *(IX A 1, 2)* In placenta previa, the placenta forms across the cervical os, which is the canal that connects the lumen of the uterus with the vagina. Normally, the placenta forms in the upper, posterior portion of the uterus. Placenta previa is a common complication of pregnancy, occurring in 1 in 200 pregnancies. Normally, the placenta is delivered after the baby, but in placenta previa the outlet from the uterus is covered by the placenta, making the baby's exit more difficult. Placenta previa is not a type of ectopic pregnancy because the gestational sac and fetus are contained within the lumen of the uterus.

2. The answer is C. *(IX B 1)* Hydatidiform mole is an example of trophoblastic disease. It is seen in approximately 1 in 2000 pregnancies in the United States, but is more common in the Orient. In this disease, there may be no fetus at all or a dead and resorbed fetus. The placenta is abnormal, consisting of large numbers of abnormal edematous chorionic villi covered by syncytiotrophoblast. These villi secrete unusually high levels of chorionic gonadotropin (hCG), and a high titer of hCG in maternal serum is one of the ways that this disease is first detected. The mass of grape-like vesicles filling the uterus and the absence of a viable fetus can be diagnosed by ultrasonography.

3. The answer is E. *(III B 2)* During development of the placenta, the chorionic shell becomes covered with numerous villi. These first arise as simple projections, called primary villi, which consist of areas of cytotrophoblast covered by syncytiotrophoblast. As the extraembryonic mesoderm develops, tongues of fetal connective tissue push into the primary villi. Once fetal connective tissue is present, villi are called secondary villi. They become tertiary villi when fetal blood vessels appear in the fetal connective tissues. All types of villi have cytotrophoblast and syncytiotrophoblast, and therefore all contain mesoderm.

4. The answer is B. *(III F 1)* Early tertiary villi have a layer of cytotrophoblast and syncytiotrophoblast resting upon the trophoblastic basement membrane. Deep to this basement membrane are connective tissue and fetal blood vessels. These fetal blood vessels are typical continuous capillaries, consisting of endothelial cells surrounded by a basement membrane. In the term placenta, the cytotrophoblast has essentially proliferated itself out of existence, leaving only syncytiotrophoblast and trophoblastic basement membrane. In addition, the fetal capillaries have moved from the central core of tertiary villi toward the periphery of the villi. As they move, they displace some of the fetal connective tissue. Thus, at term, the placental tissue barrier between maternal and fetal blood is only a fraction of a micrometer thick.

5. The answer is A (1, 2, 3). *(II A)* In the blastocyst stage, the embryo consists of a trophoblast and an inner cell mass (embryoblast). The trophoblast forms most of the fetal membranes and placenta, including the cytotrophoblast and syncytiotrophoblast of the chorion. Much of the extraembryonic mesoderm in the placenta also comes from the cytotrophoblast. The intraembryonic mesoderm is derived from the epiblast during gastrulation.

6. The answer is C (2, 4). *(VIII A, B)* The umbilical cord has two umbilical arteries with relatively small diameters and a single umbilical vein with a relatively large diameter. Umbilical arteries convey oxygen-poor blood from the fetus to the placenta. The umbilical vein carries oxygen-rich blood from the placenta to the fetus. Both types of blood vessels have much smooth muscle in their walls and are surrounded by Wharton's jelly, a connective tissue consisting of fibroblasts and an extracellular matrix rich in hyaluronic acid.

7. The answer is E (all). *(VII B–E)* Most electrolytes diffuse freely across the placenta. There is evidence that calcium and phosphate ions are actively transported. Glucose and amino acids appear to cross the placenta by active transport. Maternal serum immunoglobulin G (IgG) is transported across the placenta by a mechanism involving specific receptors and endocytosis; the IgG molecules passively immunize the fetus. Unconjugated bilirubin diffuses freely across the placenta but conjugated bilirubin passes at a very slow rate. This serves as a mechanism for the elimination of unconjugated fetal bilirubin.

8. The answer is A (1, 2, 3). *(X B)* Dizygotic twins can be the same or different in sex, and they may share a single placenta due to secondary placental fusion during development. They will not share one amniotic cavity because they arise from separate ova and become two different developing systems. Monozygotic twins can share a single amniotic cavity. They can be phenotypically different if, for example, they received unequal blood supply from the placenta during development. They will, however, be genetically identical because they came from the same egg and sperm.

9. The answer is B (1, 3). *(IV B)* The syncytiotrophoblast has numerous apical microvilli for transporting substances across the placenta between the maternal and fetal circulations. The vesicles and vacuoles which impart a foamy character to the cytoplasm are bounded by membranes and are also involved in placental transport in both directions. The syncytiotrophoblast also has a rich supply of rough endoplasmic reticulum and a generous Golgi apparatus for synthesis and packaging of proteins such as chorionic gonadotropin, a glycoprotein hormone. Finally, it has abundant smooth endoplasmic reticulum, comprising intracellular membrane systems with enzymes for steroid biosynthesis.

10–14. The answers are: 10-E, 11-C, 12-D, 13-B, 14-A. *(VI A, B)* The diagram accompanying the questions shows the structure of the mature placenta. Anchoring villi *(E)* connect the chorionic plate on the fetal side of the placenta to the decidual plate *(C)* on the maternal side of the placenta. Anchoring villi have branch villi that project away from them into the intervillous space *(A)*. The intervillous space *(A)* receives maternal blood from the spiral arteries *(B)*, which are branches of the uterine arteries. The spiral arteries have columnar endothelial cells at the lumen just before they enter the intervillous space after penetrating the decidual plate. Thus, maternal blood is injected into the intervillous space under high pressure. The blood streams past the villi and then is deflected by decidual septa *(D)* toward the maternal veins draining the intervillous space. Oxygen-poor fetal blood enters the placenta via two umbilical arteries and oxygen-rich blood drains from the placenta via a single umbilical vein.

15–19. The answers are: 15-D, 16-A, 17-C, 18-B, 19-E. *(II A, B)* The cytotrophoblast *(C)* is a layer of proliferative cells lining the extraembryonic coelom. Cells of the cytotrophoblast fuse to form the syncytiotrophoblast *(B)*, a syncytial layer surrounding the cytotrophoblast. Lacunae *(A)* are deep invaginations in the surface of the syncytiotrophoblast, which is bathed in maternal blood coming from branches of the uterine arteries *(E)*. The connecting stalk *(D)*, which connects the embryo to the chorion, becomes the umbilical cord.

8
Development of Body Cavities, Mesenteries, and Diaphragm

I. INTRODUCTION

A. Basic anatomy
1. There are four separate cavities in the thorax and abdomen of the human body.
   a. One **pericardial cavity**, which surrounds the heart
   b. Two **pleural (thoracic) cavities**, which surround the lungs
   c. One **peritoneal cavity**, which surrounds the abdominal viscera
2. All of these cavities are lined by a simple squamous epithelium called **mesothelium**.
   a. The mesothelium secretes serous fluids into the cavities and provides a nonadhesive surface so that the organs within the cavities will not adhere to one another or to the body wall.
   b. The mesothelium has two **components**.
      (1) A **visceral layer** coats the organs projecting into the cavities
         (a) The visceral **pericardium** covers the heart.
         (b) The visceral **pleura** covers the lungs.
         (c) The visceral **peritoneum** covers visceral organs such as
            (i) The stomach and intestines
            (ii) The liver and spleen
            (iii) The upper portion of the bladder and uterus
      (2) A **parietal layer** coats the body wall of the cavity.
         (a) The parietal **pericardium** coats the inner surface of the pericardial cavity.
         (b) The parietal **pleura** coats the thoracic body wall.
         (c) The parietal **peritoneum** coats the abdominal body wall.
   c. The visceral and parietal layers are continuous with one another at their **reflections**, which are located at
      (1) The mediastinum of the heart
      (2) The mediastinum of the lungs
      (3) The attachment sites of abdominal organs to the body wall; for example, at the dorsal mesentery of the stomach
3. The four body cavities are **potential spaces** filled with a small amount of fluid. They can become real spaces, as when a knife penetrates the thoracic body wall, filling the pleural cavities with air (**pneumothorax**) or blood (**hemothorax**).

B. Overview of embryology
1. The four separate body cavities all arise from a single **intraembryonic coelom**, the space between the two components of the lateral plate mesoderm.
2. During development, there are two fundamental changes in the intraembryonic coelom.
   a. This single cavity is partitioned into four separate cavities.
   b. The communication between the intraembryonic and the extraembryonic coeloms is reduced and eventually obliterated.

II. EARLY DEVELOPMENT OF THE INTRAEMBRYONIC COELOM

A. Lateral plate mesoderm and formation of the intraembryonic coelom (see also Chapter 6, section II C 5).
1. The lateral portion of the intraembryonic mesoderm is at first a single sheet of cells.

2. Vacuoles form between cells, and these vacuoles begin to fuse and coalesce with one another, forming a cavity within the lateral plate mesoderm by about day 20 to 25.
   a. As a result, the lateral plate mesoderm is divided into a **somatic** and a **splanchnic mesoderm**.
   b. The cavity between these two mesodermal sheets is the **intraembryonic coelom** (Fig. 8-1).
3. The early intraembryonic coelom extends along the lateral flanks of the embryo and around the cranial end, forming a roughly horseshoe-shaped cavity.
4. At the lateral edges of the lateral plate mesoderm, the intraembryonic coelom opens directly into the extraembryonic coelom.

B. The early pericardial and peritoneal cavities

1. The cranial segment of the intraembryonic coelom represents the primordium of the **pericardial cavity**.
   a. This cavity forms just cranial to the developing heart.
   b. During flexion and growth of the forebrain and the amnionic head fold, the **pericardial cavity**, along with the **heart** and the **septum transversum**, a major precursor of the diaphragm, are all **rotated** about 180°, with an axis of rotation perpendicular to the long axis of the embryo.
2. On either side of the embryo the intraembryonic coelom forms a **coelomic duct**.
   a. These ducts are precursors of the **pericardioperitoneal canals**, which in turn are precursors of the **pleural cavities**.
   b. The coelomic ducts connect the pericardial and peritoneal cavity precursors. Figure 8-2 shows all of these cavities; note that they are in fact all connected to one another.

III. SEPARATION OF THE PERICARDIAL AND PLEURAL CAVITIES

A. Role of heart morphogenesis

1. During flexion, the rotation of the heart brings the originally cranial pericardial cavity and septum transversum ventrally and under the heart.
   a. The **septum transversum** is now a sheet of tissue crossing the body of the embryo transversally.
   b. It forms the caudal wall of the pericardial cavity.
2. The rotation of the heart also changes the shape of the pericardioperitoneal canals.

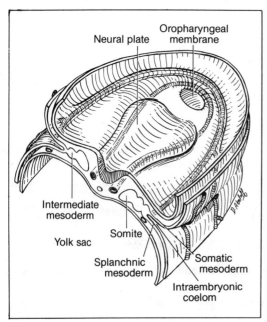

Figure 8-1. Pre-embryo in the bilaminar disk stage, showing the location of the intraembryonic coelom. As the intraembryonic coelom forms in lateral plate mesoderm, the layers of the somatic and splanchnic intraembryonic mesoderm lying lateral to the intermediate mesoderm appear. The intraembryonic coelom extends cranially around the oropharyngeal membrane and is in direct communication with the extraembryonic coelom.

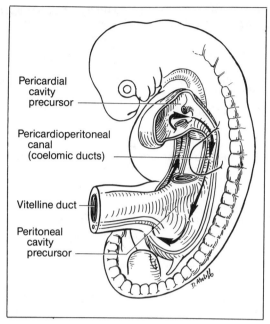

Figure 8-2. The intraembryonic coelom after flexion and growth of the amnionic folds and before the formation of the diaphragm. The intraembryonic coelom is still a single continuous space inside the embryo, as indicated by the *arrows*. An outline of a forelimb bud is shown as a landmark.

B. Role of lung bud morphogenesis (Fig. 8-3)

1. The **lung buds**, the precursors of the lungs, sprout laterally from the foregut.
    a. The lung buds grow laterally, toward the body walls, protruding into the enlarging pericardioperitoneal canals (see Fig. 8-3).
    b. As they grow, the lung buds carry with them a covering of splanchnic mesoderm and associated mesothelium.
2. At the same time, two folds of tissue, the **pleuropericardial membranes**, grow out from the body wall.
    a. The pleuropericardial membranes grow toward the midline, eventually fusing with one another (see Fig. 8-3).
    b. Ultimately, the fused pleuropericardial membrane becomes the **pericardium**.
3. The growing lung buds, the enlarging pericardioperitoneal canals, and the fusing pleuropericardial membranes all contribute to the partitioning and isolation of the pericardial and pleural cavities.

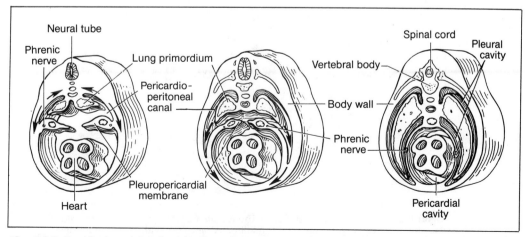

Figure 8-3. Partitioning of the pleural and pericardial cavities by growth of the lung buds and the pleuropericardial membranes. Note the movements of the phrenic nerve.

4. The caudal portions of the pericardioperitoneal canals persist for a time as the **pleuroperitoneal canals**. As the name suggests, the pleuroperitoneal canals connect the pleural and peritoneal cavities.

C. **Changes in the phrenic nerve**
1. The left and right phrenic nerves are initially widely separated from one another in the lateral portions of the pleuropericardial membranes.
2. As these membranes grow toward one another, the phrenic nerves are also brought together (see Fig. 8-3).
3. This morphogenetic event accounts for the presence of the phrenic nerves in the pericardium as they travel from their origin to the diaphragm (where they constitute the entire motor innervation of the diaphragm).

IV. MORPHOGENESIS OF THE DIAPHRAGM (Fig. 8-4)

A. **Components.** The diaphragm develops from four separate embryonic rudiments.
1. The **septum transversum** is the most important component of the diaphragm.
   a. **Growth of the septum transversum**
   (1) The septum transversum at first lies at the far cranial end of the embryo.

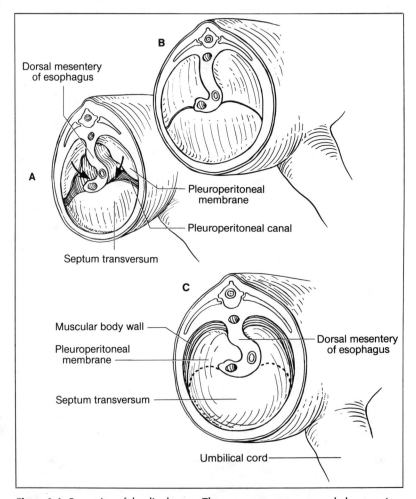

Figure 8-4. Formation of the diaphragm. The septum transversum and pleuroperitoneal membranes grow in toward the midline (A) and fuse with one another and with the dorsal mesentery of the esophagus (B) to form the bulk of the diaphragm. Ingrowth from the body wall (C) forms tissue on the periphery of the diaphragm.

- **(2)** It gains cells destined to differentiate into muscular tissue from the fusion of the third, fourth, and fifth cervical myotomes.
- **(3)** Next, it migrates caudally during flexion and comes to rest just cranial to the vitelline duct and caudal to the developing heart.
- **(4)** At this site, the septum transversum first forms a ventral mass of tissue which then extends dorsally and medially by growth toward the dorsal body wall.
- **(5)** As it grows, it leaves two dorsolateral gaps, which are the orifices of the **pleuroperitoneal canals**.

  b. The septum transversum forms two principal components of the definitive diaphragm:
  - **(1)** Most of the centrally placed skeletal muscle
  - **(2)** The central tendon

  c. The septum transversum also contributes to other important structures. It forms:
  - **(1)** Part of the fibrous pericardium
  - **(2)** The capsule of the liver
  - **(3)** The connective tissues and blood vessels in the liver

  2. The **pleuroperitoneal membranes** also make a major contribution to the development of the diaphragm (see Fig. 8-4).
  - **a.** The pleuroperitoneal membranes grow away from the dorsal body wall in a ventromedial direction.
  - **b.** Thus, they grow toward the septum transversum, which is expanding in the opposite direction.
  - **c.** The septum transversum fuses with the pleuroperitoneal membranes just ventral to the esophagus.

  3. The **dorsal mesentery of the esophagus**, the third embryonic structure which contributes to the diaphragm, fuses with the septum transversum and the pleuroperitoneal membranes, thereby closing off the pleuroperitoneal canals.

  4. Muscular ingrowth from the body wall, the fourth contribution, forms tissue on the periphery of the diaphragm after the formation of the pleuroperitoneal folds and membranes.

B. Innervation of the diaphragm

  1. The **phrenic nerve** supplies the motor innervation of the entire diaphragm and the sensory innervation of the central portion.

  2. The **seventh through twelfth thoracic nerves** provide the sensory innervation of the peripheral area of the diaphragm as a result of ingrowth from the body wall.

V. FORMATION OF THE MESENTERIES

A. General characteristics of mesenteries

  1. Functions of mesenteries
  - **a.** Mesenteries are structures that suspend visceral organs from the body wall.
  - **b.** Mesenteries also carry the following structures from the body wall to the suspended organ:
    - **(1)** Arteries
    - **(2)** Veins
    - **(3)** Lymphatic vessels
    - **(4)** Nerves

  2. Anatomic features of mesenteries
  - **a.** Mesenteries contain a generous supply of loose areolar connective tissue.
  - **b.** They are coated on both sides by a simple squamous **mesothelium**, which is part of the visceral peritoneal layer.

  3. Nomenclature. Mesenteries are named for the organ that they suspend. For example:
  - **a.** The **dorsal mesogastrium** suspends the stomach on the dorsal side of the body.
  - **b.** The **dorsal mesoduodenum** suspends the duodenum on the dorsal side of the body.
  - **c.** The **dorsal mesocolon** suspends the colon on the dorsal side of the body.

  4. Formation. Mesenteries are established as the visceral organs grow into the intraembryonic coelom and carry their mesothelial covering with them.
  - **a.** Some organs have both a dorsal and a ventral mesentery in both the embryo and the adult; for example, the stomach.

b. Some organs have both dorsal and ventral mesenteries in the embryo but only a dorsal mesentery in the adult; for example, the duodenum.
   c. Some organs have a dorsal mesentery transiently in the embryo but no mesenteries in the adult; for example, the heart.
   d. The lungs never form true mesenteries.

B. **Abdominal mesenteries**
   1. The **stomach** has both a dorsal and ventral mesogastrium (Fig. 8-5).
   2. The **spleen** arises in the dorsal mesogastrium (see Chapter 15, section V C), and this complicates the fate of the **dorsal mesogastrium** considerably.
      a. The dorsal mesogastrium forms a connection from the dorsal body wall to both the spleen and the stomach.
         (1) The mesentery connecting the spleen to the body wall becomes the **lienorenal ligament** in the adult.
         (2) The mesentery connecting the spleen to the stomach becomes the **gastrosplenic omentum** in the adult.
      b. The dorsal mesogastrium also grows tremendously after rotation of the stomach, to form the **greater omentum** (see Chapter 13, section II D 1).
   3. The **ventral mesogastrium** develops from the septum transversum. The liver diverticulum also grows into the septum transversum (see Chapter 13, section III A 1). This produces several adult **derivatives** of the ventral mesogastrium.
      a. The mesentery connecting the stomach to the liver later becomes the **lesser omentum**.
      b. The mesentery connecting the liver to the ventral body wall later becomes the **falciform ligament**. The falciform ligament carries the umbilical vein, which degenerates soon after birth, leaving a scarlike **ligamentum teres hepatis**.

VI. CONGENITAL ANOMALIES OF THE DIAPHRAGM

A. **Causes of developmental anomalies**
   1. The four embryonic rudiments that unite to form the diaphragm must fuse properly with one another.
   2. If they do not, a communication may remain between the pleural and peritoneal cavities.
      a. When this happens, peritoneal organs can herniate into the pleural cavities.
      b. This can cause secondary developmental anomalies in the lungs and perhaps the heart.

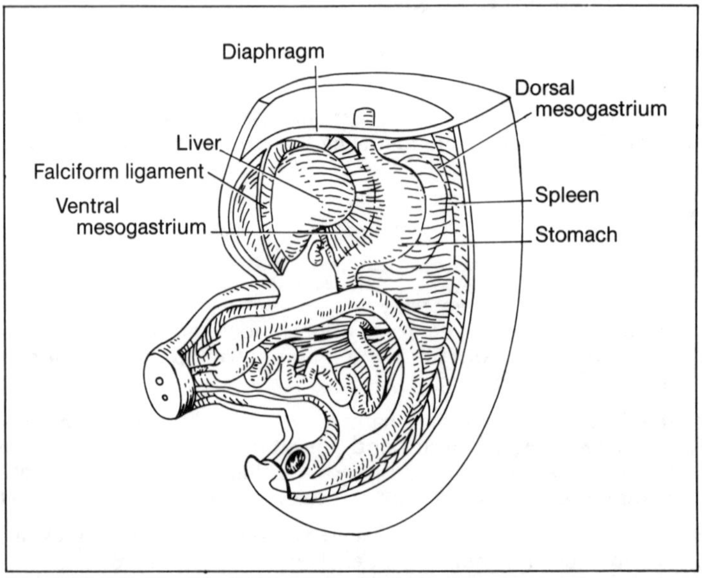

Figure 8-5. Relations of gastric mesenteries, spleen, and liver in the fetus.

B. Congenital diaphragmatic hernia. Large **dorsolateral hernias** (Fig. 8-6) represent 90% of all congenital diaphragmatic hernias; of these, 76% occur on the left side and 24% on the right.
1. This defect is caused by failure of the pleuroperitoneal folds to fuse with the septum transversum. The right pleuroperitoneal folds fuse before the left folds, and this may account for the higher incidence of defects on the left side.
   a. In this congenital anomaly, typically there is a large hole (**foramen of Bochdalek**) in the left dorsolateral diaphragm.
   b. As a result, loops of the small intestine can protrude into the left thoracic cavity (see Fig. 8-6), with several **consequences**:
      (1) Hypoplasia of the left lung
      (2) Displacement of the heart to the right
      (3) Associated anomalies in the development of the heart and great vessels, resulting from the displacement
2. Infants born with this congenital anomaly have the following **characteristics**:
   a. They appear nearly normal at birth, but close inspection reveals an enlarged thoracic cavity and a relatively small abdominal cavity.
   b. They become cyanotic and gasp for breath after feeding, because the bowel loops compress the lungs as they feed, making breathing difficult.
3. This defect can be corrected surgically if it is an isolated defect and if the amount of gut that has herniated is small enough to allow at least partial pulmonary development.
4. If the defect is severe and is associated with other anomalies, namely abnormal pulmonary and cardiac development, malrotation of the gut, cleft palate, and spina bifida, the child will probably die soon after birth.

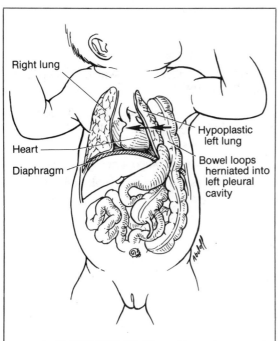

Figure 8-6. Congenital diaphragmatic hernia. Loops of bowel herniate into the pleural cavity because the pleuroperitoneal membrane does not fuse with the septum transversum during embryonic development of the diaphragm. Herniation is more common on the left side, as in the infant shown here.

STUDY QUESTIONS

Directions: Each question below contains five suggested answers. Choose the **one best** response to each question.

1. All of the following embryonic structures make substantial contributions to the adult diaphragm EXCEPT

(A) pleuroperitoneal membranes
(B) pleuropericardial membranes
(C) dorsal mesoesophagus
(D) septum transversum
(E) muscular ingrowth from the body wall

2. All of the following morphogenetic processes are involved in the separation of the pericardial and pleural cavities EXCEPT

(A) heart rotation
(B) lateral growth of lung buds
(C) medial growth of the pleuropericardial folds
(D) fusion of the pleuropericardial membranes
(E) medial growth of the pleuroperitoneal membranes

Directions: Each question below contains four suggested answers of which **one or more** is correct. Choose the answer

- A if **1, 2, and 3** are correct
- B if **1 and 3** are correct
- C if **2 and 4** are correct
- D if **4** is correct
- E if **1, 2, 3, and 4** are correct

3. True statements concerning congenital diaphragmatic hernia include which of the following?

(1) Most diaphragmatic hernias occur on the left side
(2) Diaphragmatic hernia is rarely complicated by pulmonary hypoplasia
(3) It is often associated with cardiac anomalies
(4) It is rarely fatal

4. True statements concerning the development of the intraembryonic coelom include which of the following?

(1) It originates by fusion of vesicles
(2) Its formation is linked to partitioning of the lateral plate mesoderm
(3) Initially, it is in broad communication with the extraembryonic coelom
(4) Its cranial component arises cranial to the developing heart

5. Mesothelium shows which of the following characteristics?

(1) It is a simple squamous epithelium lining the thoracic and abdominal cavities
(2) It is mesodermally derived
(3) Its visceral component covers organs
(4) It lines the intraembryonic coelom

Directions: The groups of questions below consist of lettered choices followed by several numbered items. For each numbered item select the **one** lettered choice with which it is **most** closely associated. Each lettered choice may be used once, more than once, or not at all.

Questions 6–10

Match each of the descriptions below with the type of mesentery that it best describes.

(A) Dorsal mesocardium
(B) Ventral mesocardium
(C) Dorsal mesogastrium
(D) Ventral mesogastrium
(E) Dorsal mesoduodenum

6. Never forms during development

7. Degenerates soon after its formation

8. Becomes the greater omentum

9. Becomes the falciform ligament

10. Becomes the gastrosplenic omentum

Questions 11–15

For each description of components of the developing intraembryonic coelom, select the appropriate lettered structure shown in the accompanying diagram.

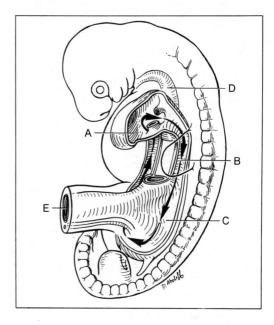

11. Pleuroperitoneal folds grow into this structure

12. This structure contains the developing heart

13. This structure receives the lungs as they grow away from the foregut

14. This structure receives peritoneal organs such as the stomach and spleen

15. This structure arose cranial to the developing head but becomes caudal to the head after head flexion is completed

ANSWERS AND EXPLANATIONS

1. The answer is B. *(IV A)* The pleuropericardial membranes form the fibrous pericardium. The pleuroperitoneal membranes form the dorsolateral portions of the diaphragm. The dorsal mesoesophagus forms a portion of the diaphragm around the esophagus. The septum transversum forms the central tendon and skeletal muscle of the diaphragm. The peripheral muscles of the adult diaphragm arise by ingrowth of the body wall.

2. The answer is E. *(III A, B)* Heart rotation causes a narrowing of the pericardioperitoneal canals. This in turn facilitates the medial growth of the pleuropericardial folds and membranes to close off these canals. The pleuropericardial membranes fuse with one another, creating the fibrous pericardium. The medial growth of the pleuroperitoneal membranes is an essential feature of the formation of the diaphragm, a structure which separates the pleural and peritoneal (not pericardial) cavities.

3. The answer is B (1, 3). *(VI B)* Large dorsolateral hernias of the diaphragm occur most often on the left side (76%) and result from failure of the left pleuroperitoneal fold to fuse with the septum transversum. There is a substantial hole in the diaphragm, called a foramen of Bochdalek. Often, loops of the bowel are herniated into the pleural cavity, resulting in pulmonary hypoplasia and abnormal development of the heart, which is displaced to the right. The gastrointestinal components in the pleural cavity often shown anomalous development as well. Consequently, patients with congenital diaphragmatic hernia also have associated malrotation of the gut. If the pulmonary hypoplasia is mild, and there are few other associated anomalies, the condition can be corrected surgically. If pulmonary hypoplasia is severe enough, and there are other associated anomalies (e.g., spina bifida), the child has a very great risk of dying soon after birth.

4. The answer is E (all). *(II A, B; III A)* The intraembryonic coelom forms by the fusion of vesicles that develop spontaneously in the lateral plate mesoderm. These vesicles coalesce into a single large cavity, the intraembryonic coelom, that is the precursor of the pericardial, pleural, and peritoneal cavities. Initially, the intraembryonic coelom extends along the lateral edges of the embryo and around the cranial end, so that the precursor of the pericardial cavity lies cranial to the developing heart and mouth. At its lateral edges, the intraembryonic coelom is in broad communication with the space around the embryo known as the extraembryonic coelom. As flexion occurs, the relative positions of portions of the intraembryonic coelom change. Also, the communication between the intraembryonic and extraembryonic coelom is first restricted and then obliterated.

5. The answer is E (all). *(I A; II A)* The intraembryonic coelom becomes lined by a simple squamous epithelium, called mesothelium, which is mesodermally derived. As visceral organs grow into the intraembryonic coelom, they carry a layer of mesothelial coating with them. This layer becomes the visceral layer of the appropriate mesothelium; for example, the visceral pleura covers the lungs.

6–10. The answers are: 6-B, 7-A, 8-C, 9-D, 10-D. *(V A, B)* The dorsal mesentery of the heart *(A)* forms transiently during embryonic development but then breaks down. No ventral mesocardium *(B)* ever develops. The dorsal mesogastrium *(C)* ultimately forms the greater omentum. It also serves as a location for the development of the spleen and becomes the gastrosplenic omentum. The ventral mesogastrium *(D)* attaches the stomach to the liver and body wall. Thus, it forms the lesser omentum (between the stomach and the liver) and the falciform ligament (between the liver and the body wall). The dorsal mesoduodenum *(E)* is the dorsal mesentery of the duodenum. It suspends the duodenum in the peritoneal cavity.

11–15. The answers are: 11-B, 12-A, 13-B, 14-C, 15-A. *(II A, B; III A, B)* The pericardial cavity *(A)* arises from the portion of the intraembryonic coelom that first forms cranial to the head. It moves ventral and caudal to the head during head flexion and is the cavity in which the heart develops. The pericardioperitoneal canals *(B)* connect the developing pericardial and peritoneal cavities. When the lung buds grow out from the foregut *(D)*, they grow into the pericardioperitoneal canals. The pleuroperitoneal folds (not shown in the diagram) also grow into the pericardioperitoneal canals *(B)* and make a contribution to the diaphragm. The midgut and hindgut form the various abdominal visceral organs that grow into the peritoneal cavity precursor *(C)*. The vitelline duct *(E)* connects the midgut to the yolk sac (not shown in the diagram).

9
Development of the Musculoskeletal System

I. INTRODUCTION

A. The vast bulk of the body is included in the musculoskeletal system. In spite of the huge size of the musculoskeletal system, its development is relatively simple and is amenable to a descriptive analysis based on variations on a few simple themes.

B. The composition of cartilage and bone
1. In the formation of cartilage and bone, mesodermally derived mesenchymal cells differentiate into **chondroblasts** and **osteoblasts**.
   a. The chondroblasts and osteoblasts secrete a different spectrum of extracellular macromolecules.
   b. The end result is the formation of connective tissues with very different physical properties and very different anatomic roles.
2. Cartilage and bone are specialized connective tissues. They share certain similarities with other connective tissues in that they are composed of cells, extracellular fibers, and extracellular amorphous ground substance.
3. The basic constituents of cartilage and bone are quite similar in some respects but are very different in other respects. For example:
   a. Both cartilage and bone contain **chondroitin sulfate** in the extracellular matrix, but they differ in the relative amounts of chondroitin sulfate.
   b. Both cartilage and bone contain **collagen** in the extracellular matrix, but the two collagens differ in molecular biology.
      (1) **Collagen** is composed of three polypeptide helices intertwined into one macromolecule.
      (2) There are several **varieties of polypeptide chains**, and they are combined in different ways in different kinds of collagen.
         (a) **Bone** contains **type I collagen**, which is composed of two $\alpha 1(I)$ chains and one $\alpha 2(I)$ chain. The $\alpha 1$ and $\alpha 2$ chains differ in their chromatographic behavior under certain conditions and amino acid sequence.
         (b) **Cartilage** predominantly contains **type II collagen**, which is composed of three $\alpha 1(II)$ chains.
         (c) **Other forms of collagen** have also been characterized by biochemists. Types III, IV, and V are major types of collagen; types VI through X are minor constituent collagens.
   c. The amorphous ground substance of bone is calcified under normal conditions, whereas the amorphous ground substance of cartilage is not.

II. EARLY EMBRYOLOGY OF THE MUSCULOSKELETAL SYSTEM

A. Subdivision of the intraembryonic mesoderm
1. Most of the musculoskeletal system develops from **intraembryonic mesoderm**, which forms from the epiblast during gastrulation.
2. Soon after it forms, the intraembryonic mesoderm becomes divided into three **components**:
   a. The **somites** are segmentally arranged, paired structures located just lateral to the notochord and spinal cord (Fig. 9-1). The somites run along the embryonic axis from the head to the tail (see Chapter 5, Fig. 5-6).
   b. **Intermediate mesoderm** forms lateral to the somites.
   c. **Lateral plate mesoderm** forms lateral to the intermediate mesoderm.

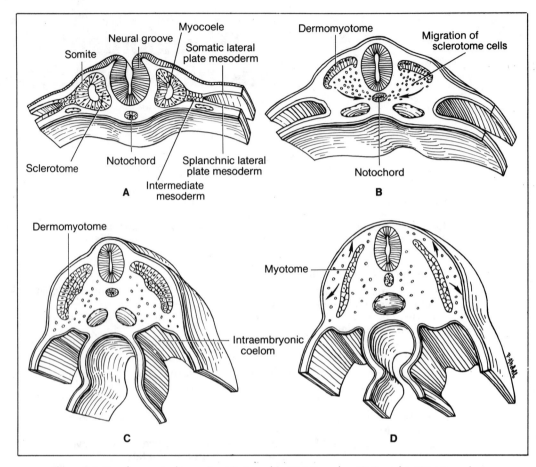

Figure 9-1. Development of a somite. (*A*) 4 weeks; (*B*) 3.5 weeks; (*C*) 4 weeks; (*D*) 4.5 weeks.

B. Fate of the mesoderm-derived tissues

1. **Intermediate mesoderm** makes a major contribution to the urogenital system.
2. With the formation of the intraembryonic coelom at about 3 weeks, the **lateral plate mesoderm** becomes divided into two components:
   a. **Somatic mesoderm**, which later contributes to the body wall musculature and the limbs
   b. **Splanchnic mesoderm**, which later contributes to the structure of various visceral organs, such as the trachea, lung, gastrointestinal tract, and pancreas
3. The **somites** become divided into two structures:
   a. The **sclerotomes**, which form vertebral bodies and associated connective tissue elements
   b. The **dermomyotomes**, which form dermal connective tissues and skeletal muscles
4. Much of the axial musculoskeletal system arises from the sclerotomes. The rest of the musculoskeletal system arises from limb bud mesenchyme and lateral plate somatic mesoderm.

III. CHONDROGENESIS AND OSTEOGENESIS (OSSIFICATION). Chondrogenesis is the process of cartilage formation, and **osteogenesis** is the process of bone formation.

A. Mechanism of cartilage formation

1. **Mesenchymal cell condensation and differentiation.** The formation of cartilage begins with the appearance of **centers of chondrification** (Fig. 9-2), which appear, for example, in parts of the axial skeleton and in limb buds.

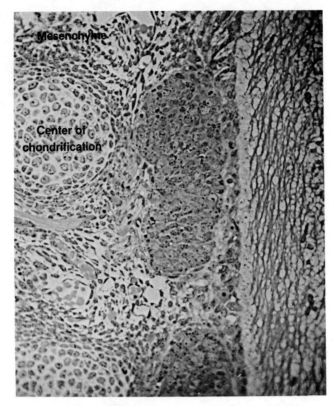

Figure 9-2. Centers of chondrification surrounded by undifferentiated mesenchymal cells. (Light micrograph)

    a. At first, these centers of chondrification represent little more than mesenchymal condensations.
    b. Soon, however, the **chondroblast** cells in the centers of chondrification secrete the extracellular matrix characteristic of cartilage.
    c. As chondroblasts become entrapped in the extracellular matrix that they secrete, they are now known as **chondrocytes**. As this entrapment occurs, **cartilage** begins to form.
  2. Later, the cartilage grows by two processes:
    a. Division of cells within the cartilage (**interstitial growth**), a process that is fundamental to the growth in length and width of bones
    b. The addition of newly differentiated cells onto the outer surface of the cartilage (**appositional growth**)

B. Mechanism of bone formation
  1. In the case of bone formation, the mesenchymal cells (Fig. 9-3) can differentiate spontaneously into **osteoblasts**.
    a. Osteoblasts then secrete a bone-specific extracellular organic matrix (**osteoid**), which later becomes calcified into bone.
    b. Osteoblasts become imprisoned in their own calcified secretion products and as they become surrounded by bone matrix, osteoblasts are converted into **osteocytes**.
  2. Thus **osteogenesis** occurs in one way, that is, by the secretion of bone organic matrix (osteoid) by osteoblasts, followed by the mineralization of this organic matrix. However, during embryonic development, the **bones themselves** are formed by two processes:
    a. Intramembranous ossification takes place without a pre-existing cartilaginous model. Bones are formed directly in undifferentiated mesenchymal fields in close association with blood vessels.
    b. Endochondral ossification takes place within the framework of a pre-existing cartilaginous model, which must be partially degraded before the bony tissue can form.

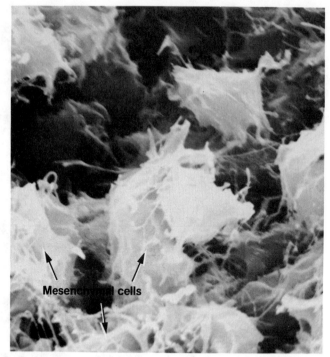

Figure 9-3. Human embryonic mesenchymal cells. (Scanning electron micrograph)

C. Intramembranous ossification

1. **Bones formed by intramembranous ossification** include:
   a. The flat bones of the skull (e.g., the frontal, parietal, upper part of the occipital, and squamous temporal)
   b. Other bones in the face (e.g., the maxilla, zygomatic arch, and mandible)
2. Bones formed by this process are commonly called **membrane bones**. They are sometimes called **dermal bones** because they arose during evolution as the result of ingression of hard dermal armor in primitive chordates.
3. **Steps in intramembranous bone formation**
   a. In this mode of bone formation, condensations of mesenchymal cells develop in close association with blood vessels. For unknown reasons, **osteoprogenitor cells** differentiate to **osteoblasts** and these cells begin to secrete **osteoid**.
   b. The osteoid becomes mineralized almost immediately after its secretion, and small spicules of bone begin to grow around many blood vessels (Fig. 9-4).
   c. These growing fragments of bone coalesce until they form large spongy networks of **trabeculae**, which contain many thin plates (lamellae) of bone and entrapped **osteocytes**.
   d. The trabeculae continue to thicken by the addition of many new layers of lamellae on the outer surface of the spicules and trabeculae.
   e. The osteoprogenitor cells on the outer surface of the growing bone continue to differentiate into osteoblasts, which in turn secrete more osteoid. When the bone reaches its final size, these osteoblasts revert to quiescent osteoprogenitor cells again.

D. Endochondral ossification

1. **Bones formed by endochondral ossification** include the long bones of the extremities and the bones forming the pelvis, vertebral column, and base of the skull.
2. These bones are sometimes called **cartilage bones** because of the **cartilaginous models** of the bones that appear in the embryo.
3. **Steps in endochondral bone formation.** Many of the separate steps occur simultaneously as the cartilage model grows and becomes converted into bone.
   a. **Formation of the cartilage model** (Fig. 9-5) begins the process of endochondral bone formation. The cartilage model serves as a scaffold for the developing bone.

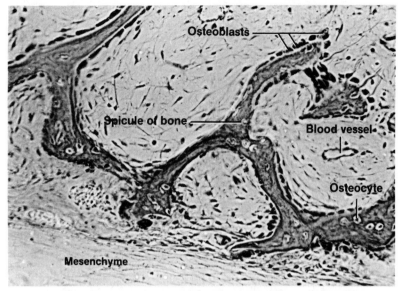

Figure 9-4. Intramembranous bone formation. (Light micrograph)

- (1) An area of cartilage has a dense, irregular connective tissue capsule around it called the **perichondrium**.
- (2) The inner layer of the perichondrium contains a layer of **chondroblasts**. These cells secrete **cartilage matrix** and entrap themselves in their own secretion product, thereby becoming **chondrocytes**.
- (3) As stated earlier, cartilage can grow by either interstitial growth or appositional growth. Bone, however, being rigid, cannot grow interstitially but can grow appositionally.
  - **b. Formation of the bony collar**
    - (1) In the diaphyseal region of the cartilage model the **perichondrium** differentiates into a layer of **osteoprogenitor cells**. These in turn differentiate into **osteoblasts** that secrete a layer of **osteoid** around the cartilage model.
    - (2) The layer of osteoid calcifies immediately, forming a bony collar.
  - **c. Degeneration of cartilage.** Meanwhile, in the center of the cartilage model, the cells of the cartilage hypertrophy and degenerate (Fig. 9-6), creating a cavity.
  - **d. Penetration by the vascular bud**
    - (1) Soon after the bony collar is formed, a **vascular bud**, aided by **osteoclasts** which have differentiated from surrounding mesenchymal cells, burrows a hole through the bony collar.
    - (2) The cavity in the cartilage, formed by the hypertrophy and degeneration of the cells of cartilage, is rapidly invaded by mesenchymally derived and growing blood vessels, hematopoietic stem cells, and osteoprogenitor cells.
    - (3) By this mechanism, a **marrow cavity** becomes established inside the growing bone (Fig. 9-7).
    - (4) Blood vessels proliferate toward both ends of the bone, enlarging the marrow cavity and stimulating further cartilage hypertrophy and degeneration.
    - (5) Meanwhile, the bony collar increases in thickness by appositional bone formation.
  - **e. Formation of the epiphyseal plate**
    - (1) The **cartilage** at the ends of the bones continues to proliferate, hypertrophy, and degenerate, leaving calcified cartilage at the ends of the bone. As this cartilage becomes transformed into bony spicules, **spongy bone** forms.
    - (2) The epiphyses are often invaded secondarily by new vascular buds, and the process repeats: progressive degeneration of cartilage, followed by ossification and the formation of more spongy bone.

- **E. Bone formation in later life**
  1. **Cartilage** persists at the **epiphyseal plate** (**growth plate**) in children with growing bones.
     a. During childhood and puberty, the cycle of proliferation, hypertrophy, degeneration,

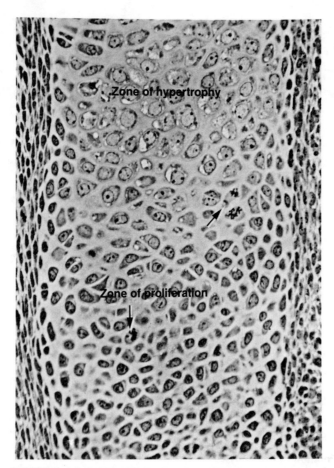

Figure 9-5. Early stages of endochondral ossification. (Light micrograph) *Below*, cartilage is growing in a zone of proliferation (*arrows* indicate mitotic figures). *Above*, cells have begun to undergo hypertrophy, which eventually will change to degeneration and the creation of a marrow cavity. At the periphery of the cartilage model there are many flattened cells in the perichondrium. Some of these will differentiate into osteoblasts to form a bony collar.

and calcification of cartilage continues at the epiphyseal plate, followed by the formation of more spongy or cancellous bone.
  b. Eventually, once the full adult stature has been reached, the epiphyseal plate stops growing and becomes completely ossified.
  c. Cartilage, however, persists throughout life on the articular surfaces of the bones.
 2. After closure of the epiphyseal plate, bone ceases to grow in length, but the bone is by no means static thereafter.
  a. Bones can continue to grow in diameter by appositional growth.
  b. In addition, the compact surface bone can be modified in adults by new bone formation.
  c. The spongy internal bone also can change in adults in response to changes in weight, age, and muscular loads placed on bones.
  d. Bones can also repair fractures by new bone formation.

IV. DEVELOPMENT OF THE AXIAL SKELETON

 A. Components. The **axial skeleton** consists of those skeletal elements that form **along the long axis** of the embryo:
  1. The vertebral column
  2. The attached ribs

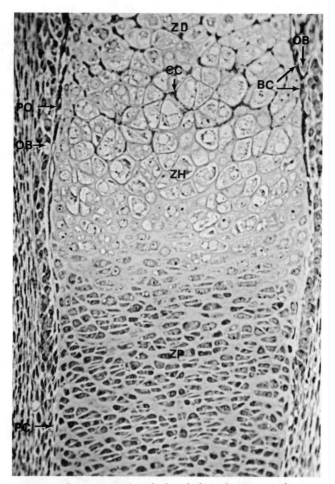

Figure 9-6. Intermediate stage of endochondral ossification. (Light micrograph) Zones of proliferation (*ZP*), hypertrophy (*ZH*), and degeneration (*ZD*) are all shown. A bony collar (*BC*) with a periosteum (*PO*) and osteoblasts (*OB*) is also visible. The cartilage is surrounded by a perichondrium (*PC*) in the zone of proliferation and is becoming calcified (*CC*) in the zone of degeneration.

   3. The sternum
   4. The skull

B. **Notochord, somites, and formation of vertebrae**
   1. The **notochord**, which develops during gastrulation, is the first embryonic component of the axial skeleton to form.
      a. The notochord extends only as far cranially as the prochordal plate.
      b. Therefore, the notochord represents the regions of the prospective vertebral column and base of the skull but not the skull region itself.
   2. Soon after the notochord forms (at about 3.5 weeks), the paired segmental **somites** begin to appear as blocks of tissue in the most medial part of the intraembryonic mesoderm (see Fig. 9-1). Cell division is intense in the somites.
      a. A cavity known as the **myocoele** forms in each somite.
      b. The cells in the ventromedial portion, or **sclerotome**, of the somite begin to migrate away from the myocoele and disperse themselves around the notochord and neural tube (Fig. 9-8).
   3. **Vertebral bodies** are derived from somite sclerotome.
      a. Each vertebral body has an **intersegmental origin**; that is, cells migrate both cranially and caudally from each somite to form a particular vertebral body.

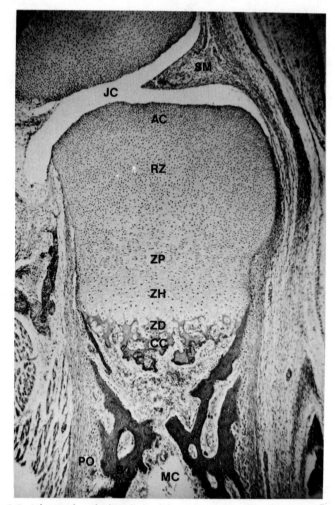

Figure 9-7. Advanced endochondral ossification. (Light micrograph) *SM*, synovial membrane; *JC*, joint cavity; *AC*, articular cartilage; *RZ*, resting zone; *ZP*, zone of proliferation; *ZH*, zone of hypertrophy; *ZD*, zone of degeneration; *CC*, calcified cartilage; *PO*, periosteum; *B*, bone; *MC*, marrow cavity.

  b. The migrating cells surround the notochord, which degenerates in the areas where the vertebral bodies form. The notochord persists, however, in the gaps between vertebral bodies.
 4. Immediately after the intersegmental vertebral bodies form, mesenchymal cells migrate dorsally and laterally away from the vertebral bodies.
  a. These cells form the rudiments of the **vertebral arches** that enclose the neural tube.
  b. These cells also produce the **costal processes**. In the thoracic vertebrae, these costal processes grow extensively, to give rise to the ribs.
 5. The vertebral processes and the motor nerves maintain a **segmented arrangement** throughout life. The sensory innervation of the skin also remains segmental, providing the **dermatomes** that are useful in neurologic evaluation of a patient.

C. Other somite derivatives

 1. The somites contribute to the muscles of the vertebral column that interconnect the ribs (intercostal muscles), as well as the flexors and extensors of the vertebral column.
 2. The **intervertebral disks** are also somite derivatives.
  a. The spaces between developing vertebral bodies quickly become densely packed

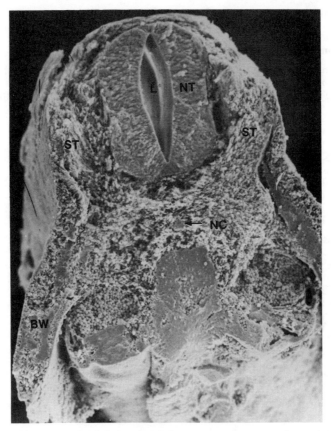

Figure 9-8. Beginning axial skeleton development in a human embryo of about 5 weeks. (Scanning electron micrograph) *L*, lumen of neural tube; *NT*, neural tube; *ST*, sclerotome; *NC*, notochord; *BW*, body wall.

with mesenchymal cells, which surround the notochord and differentiate into fibroblasts and chondrocytes.
   b. These cells subsequently form the fibrocartilage of the annulus fibrosus of the intervertebral disks.
   c. The **notochordal cells** also contribute to the intervertebral disks by forming the nucleus pulposus.

D. **Developmental variations in the vertebrae**
   1. The first cervical vertebra, the **atlas**, develops with an unusually large central foramen to accommodate the increased thickness of the spinal cord just after it exits through the foramen magnum at the base of the skull.
   2. The **thoracic vertebrae** have large costal processes that form the ribs.
   3. The **lumbar vertebrae**, which must support the weight of the vertebrae above them, form unusually large vertebral bodies.
   4. The **sacral vertebrae** have costal processes that fuse to form the sacrum.

E. **Formation of the sternum and clavicles**
   1. The **sternum** forms independently of the sclerotomes.
      a. **Sternal bars** arise as paired mesenchymal condensations just lateral to the ventral midline in the body wall. The paired cartilaginous bars fuse in a cranial to caudal sequence and then undergo ossification.
      b. The caudal tip persists in the adult as cartilage, the **xiphoid process**, which may be bifurcated due to incomplete fusion of the sternal bars.

2. The **clavicles** form partly by intramembranous ossification and partly by endochondral ossification.

F. **Development of the skull**
   1. The **neurocranium** is the portion of the skull that surrounds the brain and sense organs. It has two **components**.
      a. The **membranous neurocranium** forms by intramembranous ossification. Bones of the membranous neurocranium include:
         (1) The frontal bone
         (2) The parietal bones
         (3) The upper portion of the occipital bone
      b. The **cartilaginous neurocranium** forms by endochondral ossification. Bones of the cartilaginous neurocranium include:
         (1) The ethmoid bone
         (2) The sphenoid bone
         (3) The base of the occipital bone
         (4) The petrous portion of the temporal bone
   2. The **viscerocranium** completes the skull components. It develops from the **pharyngeal arches**. There are two **components** to the viscerocranium.
      a. The **membranous viscerocranium** forms by intramembranous ossification. Bones of the membranous viscerocranium all arise in the first pharyngeal arch and include:
         (1) The mandible
         (2) The maxilla and premaxilla
         (3) The zygomatic arch
         (4) The squamous portion of the temporal bone
         (5) The vomer
         (6) The palatine bones
      b. The **cartilaginous viscerocranium** forms by endochondral ossification. Bones of the cartilaginous viscerocranium and their sources include:
         (1) The middle ear ossicle (first and second pharyngeal arches)
         (2) The hyoid bone (second and third arches)
         (3) The laryngeal bones and cartilages (fourth to sixth arches)

V. DEVELOPMENT OF THE APPENDICULAR SKELETON

A. **Components.** The appendicular skeleton consists of the bones of the upper and lower limbs.

B. **Formation and development of the limb buds**
   1. The appendicular skeleton forms from mesenchymal elements within the limb buds.
      a. The limb buds (Fig. 9-9) consist of a mesenchymal core covered by ectoderm and capped by a distal **apical ectodermal ridge** (Fig. 9-10) that has special inductive capacity.
      b. The bones of the limbs are created by endochondral ossification, in the familiar mesenchyme → chondrogenesis → osteogenesis developmental sequence.
   2. Limb buds arise in somatic mesoderm at 4 weeks (see Fig. 9-9). The **forelimb buds** arise first, and the **hindlimb buds** soon follow. The forelimbs also develop more rapidly than the hindlimbs.
      a. By 5 weeks the forelimb buds have become slightly elongated, and soon after this they subdivide into components in which the precursors of the hand, forearm, and arm are visible. (The morphogenesis of a mouse forelimb is shown in Figure 9-11.)
      b. By the end of week 6, the hand has become partially subdivided into digits.
      c. By week 8, individual fingers and toes are clearly visible. These become demarcated by means of controlled **cell death** between digits.
   3. The bones of the limbs continue to grow rapidly after birth due to activity of the **epiphyseal plates**. The epiphyseal plates have a burst of activity at puberty and then ossify irreversibly, so that further increase in stature is not possible.

VI. DEVELOPMENT OF THE JOINTS

A. **Synarthroses** are joints with little mobility.
   1. The synarthroses have a relatively simple developmental history. They are formed from mesenchymal cells that arise between developing bones and that differentiate into connective tissue cells.

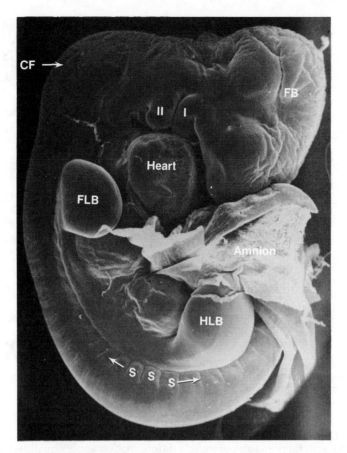

Figure 9-9. A human embryo at about 5 weeks. (Scanning electron micrograph) *FB*, forebrain; *CF*, cephalic flexure; *I* and *II*, first and second pharyngeal arches; *FLB*, forelimb bud; *HLB*, hindlimb bud; *SSS*, somites.

2. The **intervertebral disks** and the **symphysis pubis** are examples of a subclass of synarthroses known as **symphyses**. In symphyses, the cartilage at the ends of two opposed bones is united by a dense layer of fibrous connective tissue. The development of intervertebral disks is described above, in section IV C 2.

B. Diarthroses are joints with great mobility.
1. The highly mobile **diarthrodial (synovial) joints** occur most frequently between bones of the appendicular skeleton but may also be found between bones of the axial skeleton (e.g., the temporomandibular joint).
2. Diarthrodial joints have a somewhat more interesting developmental history than the synarthroses have.
    a. As cartilage models develop in the limb bud, the mesenchymal cells lying between the areas of cartilage begin to differentiate into the **joint capsule fibroblasts**.
    b. Spaces appear between the mesenchymal cells, and these spaces fuse with one another until a **joint cavity** forms.
    c. Meanwhile, the cartilage models are being ossified, except at the articular surfaces, where a thin sheet of **hyaline cartilage** persists until death in the healthy adult.
    d. The mesenchymally derived fibroblasts surrounding the joint differentiate into **synoviocytes**, while the surrounding mesenchymal cells differentiate into blood vessels, ligaments, and interrupted sheets of connective-tissue **synovial cells** that line the joint cavity.
    e. The **lining of the joint cavity** is not true epithelium because its component synovial cells do not form a continuous sheet, are not joined together by junctional complexes, and lack a distinct basement membrane.

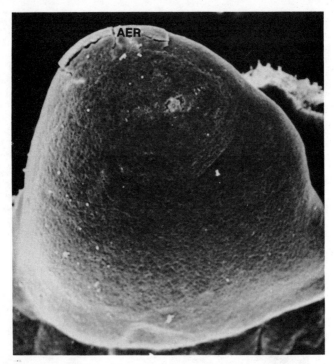

Figure 9-10. The apical ectodermal ridge (*AER*) on a human forelimb bud. (Scanning electron micrograph)

VII. MUSCLE DIFFERENTIATION. Although the formation of **skeletal muscle** is outlined here, many of the general principles of muscle differentiation apply equally well to **smooth and cardiac muscle**.

  A. Characteristics of myoblasts

  1. **Myoblasts**, the precursors of muscle cells, develop from mesenchymal cells.

  2. Myoblasts have a prominent nucleus and an enlarged nucleolus, many free ribosomes and polysomes in their cytoplasm, a few uniformly distributed globular mitochondria, and a sparse endoplasmic reticulum.

  3. In myoblasts, cell proliferation and protein synthesis are quite active, although most of the proteins synthesized are common to many cells.

  B. Myotube formation and myoblast differentiation

  1. Myoblasts aggregate and become committed to muscle cell differentiation. The individual cells then fuse with one another to form syncytial **myotubes**, multinucleated masses of primitive skeletal muscle (Fig. 9-12).

  2. As the myoblasts fuse into myotubes, a complex series of changes occur in the cytoarchitecture of the myoblast. It is important to realize that **cytodifferentiation of the myoblast** involves the accumulation of large quantities of tissue-specific proteins and a concomitant modification of the detailed fine structure of the cell.
      a. As the cell becomes committed to the muscle-specific differentiated state, the **proteins of the contractile apparatus** (actin, α-actinin, myosin, tropomyosin, and the troponin complex) accumulate in bulk and alter the cell structure.
      b. Filaments of actin and myosin assemble rapidly into **sarcomeres**, the fundamental contractile units of striated muscle. Most of the cytoplasm becomes filled with regular arrays of thick and thin filaments.
      c. With the formation of definitive sarcomeres, several **structural changes** take place:
          (1) The cell nuclei become pushed to the periphery of the cell.
          (2) The endoplasmic reticulum is transformed into the **sarcoplasmic reticulum**.

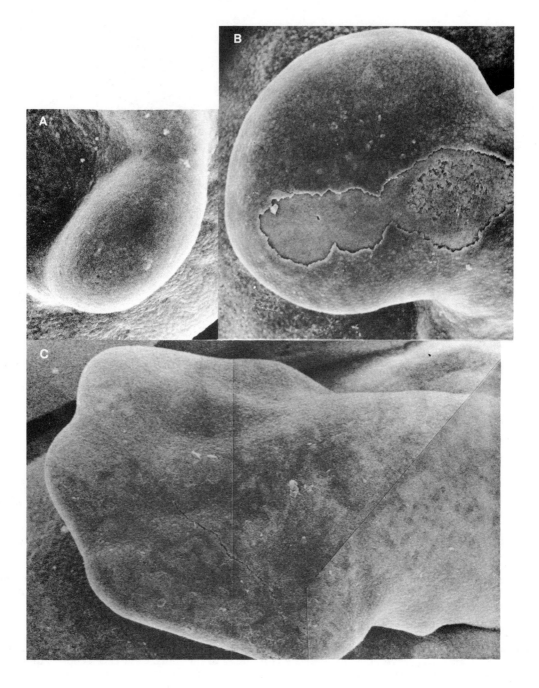

Figure 9-11. The forelimb buds of a mouse embryo. (Scanning electron micrograph) The stages of morphogenesis correspond approximately to human development at 27 days (A), 32 days (B), and 37 days (C).

        (3) Mitochondria become highly elongated and oriented parallel to the long axis of the sarcomeres.

VIII. CONGENITAL ABNORMALITIES OF THE MUSCULOSKELETAL SYSTEM

    A. Achondroplasia (chondrodystrophy) is a relatively common developmental abnormality of the skeletal system. The incidence is about 1 in 40,000 adults.

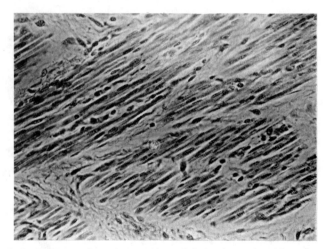

Figure 9-12. Human embryonic myotubes of skeletal muscle with sarcomeres visible. (Light micrograph)

1. **Bone formation**
   a. In achondroplasia, the development of bones formed by endochondral ossification is abnormal, while the development of bones formed by intramembranous ossification is essentially normal.
   b. Cell proliferation occurs in the epiphyseal plates, but at an apparently reduced rate.
2. **Physical features.** Achondroplastic dwarfs show the following characteristics:
   a. Short vertebral column
   b. Short limbs with thick diaphyses in long bones
   c. Sunken midfacial region
   d. Normal to superior mental capacity
3. **Etiology**
   a. **Genetic pattern.** Achondroplasia is usually caused by an autosomal dominant gene.
      (1) About 80% of cases arise as a spontaneous mutation in unafflicted families, while 20% of cases arise in a familial pattern.
      (2) In some cases, apparently normal parents have more than one achondroplastic child, suggesting a genetic pattern of recessive mutations, poor expressivity of a mutation, or gonadal mosaicism.
   b. **Role of growth hormone.** Growth hormone levels in achondroplastic persons are normal. Nevertheless, administration of growth hormone in childhood partially ameliorates this condition, suggesting that children may have partial growth hormone receptor deficiencies.
4. **Reproductive consequences**
   a. Achondroplastic persons are reproductively competent.
   b. An achondroplastic woman will always have a difficult vaginal delivery because of her small pelvis and the relatively large head of the fetus. Cesarean section is therefore indicated.

B. **Other limb defects.** A large number of developmental defects can alter the structure of the limb, leaving the rest of the musculoskeletal system more or less normal.

1. **Incidence**
   a. Except for achondroplasia, these limb defects are normally not common. In one study, for example, the total occurrence of twelve different kinds of limb defects was only 1 in 6438 people.
   b. In the late 1950s and early 1960s, a sudden striking increase in the frequency of formerly rare developmental limb defects was noticed in newborns. Epidemiologic studies quickly established a link between maternal **thalidomide** ingestion during pregnancy and these dramatic and unusual limb defects. When the treatment of pregnant women with thalidomide ceased, limb defects of the type seen in the

thalidomide embryopathy became much less common again. (See also Chapter 23, section V B 1.)
    c. Limb anomalies are also found in children with **Down syndrome**.
  2. **Types.** Several broad classes of limb defects have been identified.
    a. When limbs are completely absent, the condition is known as **amelia**.
    b. When there is a marked shortening of the limb with certain bones missing and others present and normal, the condition is known as **phocomelia**.
    c. **Digital abnormalities** are also seen (Fig. 9-13). These may involve fusion of digits (**syndactyly**) or duplication of digits (**polydactyly**). Digital anomalies arise spontaneously in most cases but can pass from parent to child under certain circumstances.

C. Skull defects

  1. In **achondroplastic dwarfs**, the developmental abnormalities that involve the cartilaginous neurocranium are largely cosmetic in nature and do not result in abnormal brain development.
  2. Other forms of developmental anomalies of the skull are considerably more serious. For example, **precocious fusion of sutures** in the membranous neurocranium (**craniosynostosis**) results in gross abnormalities in the shape of the skull and often causes attendant developmental defects in the brain.
    a. Premature closure of the **coronal sutures** (between the frontal and occipital bones) results in **acrocephaly**, in which the skull is abnormally tall.
    b. Premature closure of the **sagittal suture** results in **scaphocephaly**, in which excessive growth of the frontal and occipital portions results in a long and narrow skull.
    c. When several sutures fuse prematurely, the so-called **cloverleaf skull syndrome** (**kleeblattschädel anomaly**) results. The increased intracranial pressure results in extreme exophthalmia and is usually fatal or causes profound mental retardation.

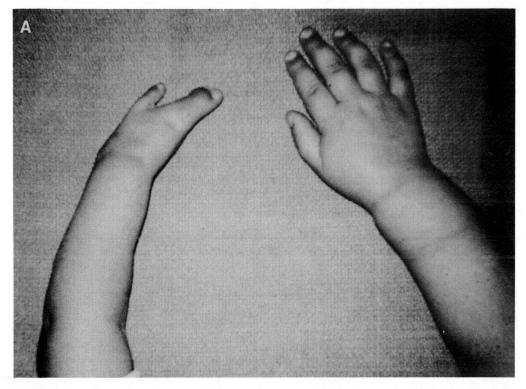

Figure 9-13. Examples of syndactyly (*A*, left hand) and a normal number of digits (*A*, right hand) and polydactyly (*B*) in the hand. (Courtesy of Mary H. McGrath, M.D., Division of Plastic and Reconstructive Surgery, George Washington University Medical Center, Washington, D.C.)

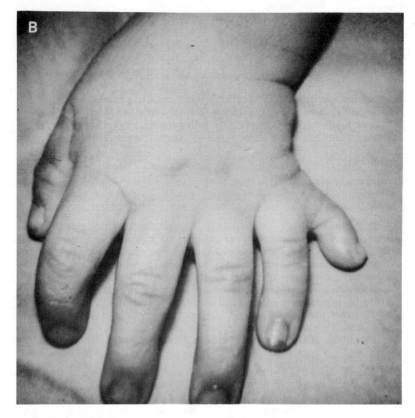

Figure 9–13. Continued.

STUDY QUESTIONS

Directions: Each question below contains four suggested answers of which **one or more** is correct. Choose the answer

- A if **1, 2, and 3** are correct
- B if **1 and 3** are correct
- C if **2 and 4** are correct
- D if **4** is correct
- E if **1, 2, 3, and 4** are correct

1. True statements concerning limb bud development include which of the following?

   (1) Limb bud mesenchyme forms skeletal muscle
   (2) Limb bones and the frontal bone of the skull form in a similar manner
   (3) The apical ectodermal ridge induces differentiation in limb bud mesenchyme
   (4) Digits arise in the hindlimb before the forelimb

2. Achondroplasia typically shows which of the following characteristics?

   (1) An autosomal recessive inheritance pattern
   (2) Excessive growth at the epiphyseal plate
   (3) Severe reduction in the volume of the skull vault
   (4) Normal mental capacity

3. Development of the intervertebral disks shows which of the following characteristics?

   (1) Sclerotome forms the annulus fibrosus
   (2) Notochord forms the nucleus pulposus
   (3) Intervertebral disks are arranged segmentally
   (4) Sclerotome mesenchymal cells do not form chondrocytes

4. True statements concerning muscle cell development include which of the following?

   (1) Soon after they appear in the cytoplasm, actin and myosin are arranged into sarcomeres
   (2) Myotubes form by large numbers of myoblast nuclear divisions without cytoplasmic division
   (3) Skeletal muscle tissue is a syncytium formed by myoblast fusion
   (4) The endoplasmic reticulum of myoblasts disappears after myotube formation

5. Cartilage and bone differ in which of the following ways?

   (1) Only cartilage contains substantial quantities of collagen
   (2) Only bone normally has a calcified matrix
   (3) Only cartilage can grow by an appositional mechanism
   (4) Only cartilage can grow by an interstitial mechanism

Directions: The groups of questions below consist of lettered choices followed by several **numbered** items. For each numbered item select the **one** lettered choice with which it is **most** closely associated. Each lettered choice may be used once, more than once, or not at all.

Questions 6–10

For each description of a region in a developing long bone of the limb, choose the appropriate lettered area shown in the accompanying micrograph.

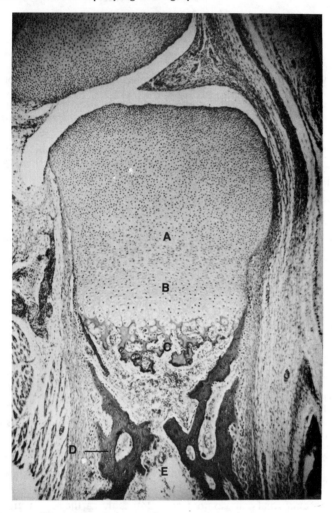

6. Part of the bony collar, later to become the metaphysis of the bone

7. Zone of cartilage calcification

8. Zone of chondrocyte proliferation

9. Marrow cavity, a site of hematopoiesis

10. Zone of chondrocyte hypertrophy

Questions 11–15

For each description of a bone of the skull below, choose the appropriate labelled area in the accompanying diagram.

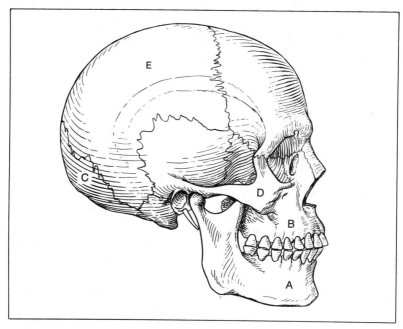

11. This bone is formed by intramembranous ossification and is part of the membranous viscerocranium; it contains no odontoblast derivatives

12. This bone is formed by endochondral ossification in its lower part and intramembranous ossification in its upper part

13. This bone is part of the membranous viscerocranium and is derived from the first maxillary component of the first pharyngeal arch; the lateral palatine processes form on its medial border

14. This bone is part of the membranous neurocranium and the anterior fontanelle forms on its anterior border

15. This bone forms by intramembranous ossification around Meckel's cartilage

ANSWERS AND EXPLANATIONS

1. The answer is B (1, 3). *(III C 1, D 1; V B 1 a, 2; VII A)* Limb bud mesenchyme is extensively involved in the formation of cartilage, bone, ligaments and tendons, joints, and skeletal muscles in the limb. The limb bones form by endochondral ossification. The frontal bone of the skull, by contrast, forms by intramembranous ossification. The apical ectodermal ridge induces differentiation of limb bud mesenchyme. The forelimb develops more rapidly than the hindlimb, and so the forelimb digits appear first, not the hindlimb digits.

2. The answer is D (4). *(VIII A)* Achondroplasia is caused by an autosomal dominant gene in most cases. It causes a generalized reduction in endochondral bone formation. There is an abnormal reduction in growth at the epiphyseal plate. Intramembranous bone formation is normal, and therefore the volume of the skull vault is normal. Mental function is not affected in persons with achondroplasia.

3. The answer is A (1, 2, 3). *(IV B 5, C)* The intervertebral disks have an annulus fibrosus derived from the sclerotome and a nucleus pulposus derived from the notochord. The intervertebral disks are segmentally arranged. The mesenchymal cells from the sclerotome differentiate into fibroblasts and chondrocytes.

4. The answer is B (1, 3). *(VII A, B)* Actin and myosin are synthesized in myoblasts and myocytes. Soon after their formation, actin and myosin become assembled into sarcomeres. Myotubes are formed by myoblast fusion rather than by nuclear division without cytoplasmic division. The endoplasmic reticulum of myoblasts and myocytes becomes arranged around sarcomeres, forming the sarcoplasmic reticulum.

5. The answer is C (2, 4). *[I B 3 ; III D 3 a (3)]* Cartilage and bone both contain substantial quantities of collagen and chondroitin sulfate, a proteoglycan. Both cartilage and bone can grow appositionally but only cartilage can grow interstitially. Only bone has an extensively calcified matrix.

6–10. The answers are: 6-D, 7-C, 8-A, 9-E, 10-B. *(III D)* The illustration shows endochondral bone formation occurring in an early embryonic digit, which is a long limb bone. In this developing cartilage model of a phalanx, the cartilage has a zone of chondrocyte proliferation (A), a zone of chondrocyte hypertrophy (B), and a zone of cartilage calcification (C). A newly ossified bony collar (D) will form the metaphysis in the labelled region and in the diaphysis further down the bone (not pictured). This bony material surrounds a marrow cavity (E) actively engaged in hematopoiesis.

11–15. The answers are: 11-D, 12-C, 13-B, 14-E, 15-A. *(Chapter 9 III C, D; IV F; Chapter 12 V A, B; Chapter 18 II C; III B)* The mandible (A) and maxilla (B) are both parts of the membranous viscerocranium, as is the zygomatic arch (D). The mandible forms around Meckel's cartilage. The maxilla has lateral palatine processes on its medial borders, and these form the secondary palate. Both the mandible and the maxilla have teeth with dentin (an odontoblast derivative) but the zygomatic arch does not. The parietal bone (E) is part of the membranous neurocranium and is on the posterior border of the anterior fontanelle. The lower part of the occipital bone (C) is part of the cartilaginous neurocranium and the upper part is part of the membranous neurocranium.

10
Development of the Heart and Major Blood Vessels

I. INTRODUCTION

A. General description of the cardiovascular system

1. The cardiovascular system is a collection of tubular channels designed to convey blood throughout the body, propelled by a four-chambered pump, the heart.
2. **Lining of the cardiovascular system.** The heart and vessels of the cardiovascular system are lined by a simple squamous epithelium known as **endothelium**. In most vessels, the endothelial cells are surrounded by muscular and connective tissue.
3. **Muscular tissue in the cardiovascular system**
   a. **Blood vessels** have **smooth muscle** in their walls.
   b. The **heart** has **cardiac muscle** in its walls.

B. Overview of cardiovascular development

1. **Early functional development of the cardiovascular system**
   a. The cardiovascular system is the first organ system to become functional in the embryo.
      (1) The **chorionic shell** that surrounds the embryo separates it from the maternal blood supply. At first, maternal–fetal exchange takes place by simple diffusion. The embryo has a rapid growth rate, however, that soon outstrips the exchange capacity met by diffusion.
      (2) The rapid development of the cardiovascular system supplements and then replaces diffusion as an exchange mechanism.
   b. By the beginning of the fourth week of development, the primitive heart and circulatory system (Fig. 10-1) have begun to move oxygen, nutrients, and wastes around the embryo and to the developing placenta via the connecting stalk.
2. **Later morphogenetic development of the cardiovascular system**
   a. **Relative size of the heart**
      (1) Initially, the chorionic shell and connecting stalk are more substantial than the embryo per se. Blood must be moved not only through the body of the growing embryo but also through the extraembryonic membranes.
      (2) As a result, the heart develops rapidly into a large organ out of proportion to the rest of the embryo.
      (3) After the fifth month of gestation, in the fetal period, the size of the body catches up with the heart, and the heart approaches the normal relative size found in the newborn.
   b. **Changes in heart structure**
      (1) **Morphogenesis**
         (a) When first formed (at about 3 weeks), the heart is a simple tubular organ without the four distinct chambers, septa, valves, and other components found in the adult heart.
         (b) By the end of the second month, the heart has undergone a morphogenesis from this chamberless tube to a morphology nearly like that found in the adult.
      (2) **Closure of the interatrial valve**
         (a) The fetus gets its oxygen from maternal blood, not from its own lungs. The fetal heart has a one-way valve that allows most oxygenated blood to bypass the pulmonary circulation.

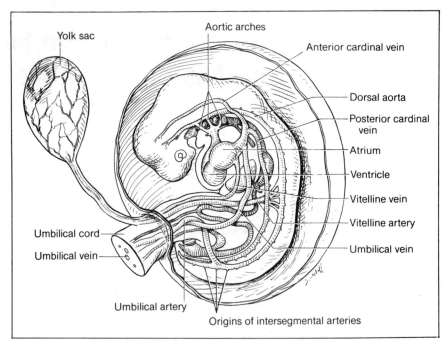

Figure 10-1. Primitive circulatory system in the human embryo.

       (b) As a result of the dramatic hemodynamic changes at birth, this one-way valve closes, permitting adequate blood flow to the pulmonary circulation.
    c. Changes in vascular symmetry
       (1) Initially, the great vessels form a symmetric network of arteries and veins.
       (2) By differential growth and asymmetric regression, the adult vascular patterns become grossly asymmetric.

II. EARLY EMBRYOLOGY OF THE CARDIOVASCULAR SYSTEM.
The formation of blood islands and the early development of the blood cells (hematopoiesis) are detailed in Chapter 6, section III. Thus, only a summary is presented here.

A. Blood islands. The development of the cardiovascular system begins with the formation of **blood islands (angiogenetic cell clusters)** in the intraembryonic and extraembryonic mesoderm.

1. Blood islands form as isolated cell clusters in several separate **locations**:
   a. The body of the embryo
   b. The connecting stalk
   c. The yolk sac
   d. The chorion

2. These groups of cells arise by the spontaneous differentiation of mesenchymal cells.

3. Mesenchymal cells at the periphery of the blood islands differentiate into endothelial cells which form vesicular sacs.
   a. At first, the sacs are isolated structures.
   b. The endothelial cells soon sprout branches, grow, and fuse with one another, forming larger vascular channels that constitute the precursors of the heart and blood vessels.

B. Early hematopoiesis. Mesenchymal cells in the blood islands also form the precursors of formed elements of the blood.

1. The mesenchymal cells differentiate into **primitive hemocytoblasts**, which later form **primitive erythrocytes** with nuclei.

2. This type of differentiation is particularly marked in the **yolk sac**, the first site of embryonic hematopoeisis.

C. The tubular heart and its origin

1. **Beginning as paired tubes**
   a. Formation of the heart begins at about 2.5 weeks, in a horseshoe-shaped region of blood islands at the most cranial portion of the embryo, the **cardiogenic area**.
   b. The angiogenetic cell clusters in the cardiogenic area form paired **endocardial heart tubes**, one on either side of the embryo, in a manner similar to the formation of other vascular channels.
2. **Relocation and fusion into a single tube**
   a. During flexion and growth of the amnionic folds, two important events occur:
      (1) First, head flexion rotates the cardiogenic area, with its paired developing heart tubes, and tucks it under the ventral surface of the embryo, caudal to the oropharyngeal membrane. [The septum transversum (precursor of the diaphragm) and the intraembryonic coelom (precursor of the pericardial cavity) also tuck under the body along with the developing heart tubes.]
      (2) Then, growth of the lateral folds of the amnion brings the paired tubes together in the ventral midline.
   b. The paired endocardial heart tubes now fuse with one another in a cranial to caudal sequence, forming a single **midline endocardial heart tube** (Fig. 10-2A).
      (1) Although a simple tubular structure, the heart tube has three **regions**; in cranial to caudal sequence, these are:
         (a) The **bulbus cordis**
         (b) The **ventricle**
         (c) The **atrium**
      (2) The heart tube has two large **bifurcations**, at its cranial and caudal poles.
3. **Surrounding tissues**
   a. After fusion, the endocardial heart tube grows into the pericardial cavity, carrying a layer of splanchnic mesoderm with it. Thus, the heart tube becomes surrounded by a layer called the **myoepicardial mantle**.
   b. An extracellular matrix known as the **cardiac jelly** for a time lies between the endocardial heart tube and the myoepicardial mantle.

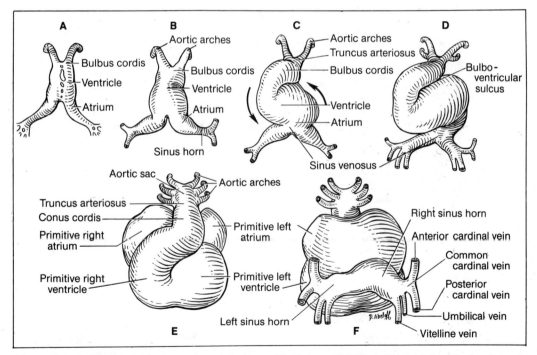

Figure 10-2. Early stages in the formation of the heart. (A) 21 days; (B) 22 days: The initially paired embryonic heart tubes fuse to form a single midline tube with three major subdivisions and a large bifurcation at either end. (C) 24 days; (D) 26 days: At the cranial and caudal poles, respectively, bilateral aortic arches and sinus horns form and develop branches. Simultaneously, growth of the heart within the confining pericardial cavity causes it to curve into an S-shaped heart loop. Arrows show the direction of the curving. (E) Ventral and (F) dorsal views (30–35 days), showing the external structures of the primitive heart and their relationships.

(1) The cardiac jelly is rich in collagen and several kinds of glycoproteins.
(2) It is thought to play an important role in early cardiac morphogenesis.

4. **Ultimate derivatives**
   a. As its name suggests, the **myoepicardial mantle** later differentiates to form:
      (1) **Myocardium**, after differentiation of striated cardiac muscle cells (**myocytes**)
      (2) **Epicardium**, after differentiation of the connective tissue cells characteristic of this layer
   b. The **endothelial cells** of the fused heart tubes later give rise to the definitive **endocardium**. This consists of:
      (1) The cardiac endothelium
      (2) The other connective tissue cells lying between the endothelial basement membrane and the myocardium

D. **Cardiac mesentery and the pericardial cavity**

   1. The primitive tubular heart is suspended in the pericardial cavity by a **dorsal mesocardium**. No ventral mesocardium ever forms.

   2. The dorsal mesocardium degenerates soon after its formation. The heart tube remains attached to the pericardial cavity at its cranial and caudal poles, and between these it is suspended freely in the pericardial cavity.

   3. A **mesothelium** later develops which covers both the pericardial cavity and the heart tube. This mesothelium forms:
      a. The **parietal pericardium**, which lines the pericardial cavity
      b. The **visceral pericardium**, which coats the heart

E. **The primitive great vessels** (see Fig. 10-2)

   1. The **cranial bifurcation** of the heart tube forms a pair of **aortic arches**.
      a. The aortic arches convey blood from the heart, through the pharyngeal arches, and up to the dorsal aortas (see Fig. 10-1), which run down both flanks of the embryo to end in the umbilical artery.
      b. The aortic arches later form a series of arches.

   2. The **caudal bifurcation** of the heart tube forms a **sinus venosus** with a left and right horn. Blood from the umbilical vein and other veins feeds into each sinus horn.

F. **Subdivisions of the primitive heart**

   1. Soon after the fusion of the endocardial heart tubes, by 3.5 weeks, subdivisions become evident (see Fig. 10-2).
      a. These arise largely as a result of differential growth of the heart tube.
      b. In a **caudal to cranial sequence** (the **direction in which blood flows** through the primitive heart), these structures include:
         (1) The left and right **horns of the sinus venosus**
         (2) The **sinus venosus**
         (3) The primitive **atrium**
         (4) The primitive **ventricle**
         (5) The **bulbus cordis**
         (6) The **truncus arteriosus**
         (7) The **aortic root**
         (8) The left and right **aortic arches**
      c. As the atrium separates from the ventricle, a single **atrioventricular canal** develops between them.

   2. The arrangement of heart structures at this stage is reminiscent of the arrangement found in mature fish and other primitive chordates.

G. **Establishment of the heart loop** (week 3.5)

   1. The heart is also growing rapidly in length within the pericardial cavity. Since it is fixed at both ends, the growth in length results in formation of the **heart loop**.
      a. Initially, this loop is U-shaped, with its convex side directed forward and to the right (Fig. 10-2C).
      b. As growth continues, ventricular growth predominates, so that the heart loop becomes S-shaped and a deep **bulboventricular sulcus** forms in the concave side of the loop (Fig. 10-2D).

2. The **primitive atrium**, originally attached to the septum transversum, now loses its attachment and moves dorsally and to the left as it becomes incorporated into the pericardial cavity.
3. Thus, the atrium is growing dorsally and to the left while the ventricle and bulbus cordis are growing ventrally and to the right (Figs. 10-2C–E).
4. Meanwhile, the future **heart chambers** become externally divided into primitive left and right atria and primitive left and right ventricles, although definitive septa do not yet form within.

III. ATRIAL SEPTATION AND CHANGES IN THE SINUS VENOSUS

A. Atrial septation

1. **Function of the interatrial septum**
   a. Once formed, the atrial septum functions as a **one-way valve**, allowing blood to pass from the right atrium to the left atrium.
      (1) The right atrium receives oxygenated blood from the umbilical vein by way of the inferior vena cava.
      (2) The left atrium sends this oxygenated blood to the fetal systemic circulation by way of the left ventricle.
   b. The valve closes at birth, ending the shunting of blood from right atrium to left atrium.

2. **Steps in atrial septation** (Fig. 10-3)
   a. **Formation of the septum primum** (weeks 5 to 6)
      (1) The **septum primum** is a curtain of tissue that arises in the cranial portion of the atrial roof near the midline.
      (2) It proceeds to grow downward toward the **endocardial cushions**, a pair of tissue mounds surrounding the atrioventricular canal.
      (3) As the septum primum grows toward the endocardial cushions, it leaves a hole on its inferior border called the **ostium primum**.
         (a) The ostium primum provides a passage between the right and left atria.
         (b) This passage becomes smaller and smaller as the septum primum grows and eventually becomes obliterated as the septum primum fuses with the endocardial cushions.

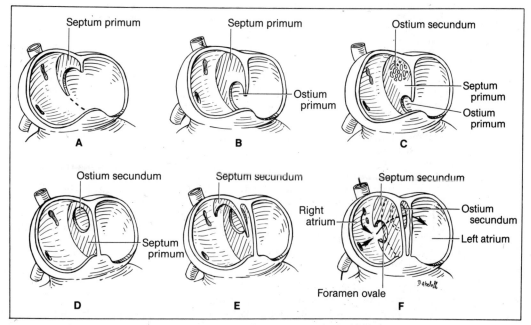

Figure 10-3. Atrial septation. (A–C) Events during week 5; (D–F) events during week 6. See text for description of the process. *Arrows* in (F) show the direction of blood flow across the fully developed septa, from the right atrium to the left atrium.

(4) Just before fusion of the septum primum, the **ostium secundum** appears in the septum primum. At first, the ostium secundum is a series of holes like those in Swiss cheese (Fig. 10-3C), but these soon coalesce to leave a single ostium secundum (Fig. 10-3D).
  b. **Formation of the septum secundum** (Figs. 10-3E–F)
     (1) The **septum secundum** is a second flap of tissue that forms to the right of the septum primum.
     (2) It also grows downward toward the endocardial cushions, but it never fuses with them. Instead, a persistent oval orifice, the **foramen ovale**, remains on its inferior border (see Fig. 10-3F).
3. **Mechanism of valve function**
  a. The septum primum and septum secundum together constitute the **interatrial septum**, which serves before birth as a one-way valve.
     (1) **Before birth**, the blood pressure in the right atrium is greater than in the left atrium because a large volume of blood is arriving from the placenta, reaching the right atrium via the umbilical vein and then the inferior vena cava.
     (2) After the blood enters the right atrium, the higher pressure pushes it through the foramen ovale, between the septum secundum and septum primum, and then through the ostium secundum into the left atrium (see Fig. 10-3F).
     (3) Blood does not flow in the reverse direction because interruption of the right-to-left pressure brings the septum primum and septum secundum together, effectively closing off the interatrial passage, since the foramen ovale and ostium secundum are not in a straight line.
  b. After birth, the one-way valve loses its functional value.
     (1) **After birth**, the pressure in the right atrium falls because the umbilical vein is closed off.
     (2) Simultaneously, the pressure in the left atrium increases because the pulmonary veins are now returning a large volume of blood from the lungs.
     (3) As a result of these pressure differentials, the one-way septal flap closes and prevents the shunting of blood from the left atrium to the right atrium.

4. **Fusion of the septa after birth**
  a. In the first few months after birth, the septum primum and septum secundum normally fuse with one another to form a single complete **interatrial septum**. The remnant of the foramen ovale is visible as the **fossa ovalis** in the right side of the interatrial septum.
  b. In about 20% of all adults, the septum primum and septum secundum fail to fuse and it is possible to pass a probe through the incomplete interatrial septum (**probe patency**). This anomaly usually goes undetected and has no clinical significance.

B. **Changes in the sinus venosus**
  1. In the primitive heart, the left and right horns of the sinus venosus are symmetric structures, each receiving blood from three major branches (see Fig. 10-2 and section VI A).
  2. Due to changes in the great veins (described in section VI), the left horn of the sinus venosus degenerates. Simultaneously, the right horn of the sinus venosus grows considerably and moves to the right side of the body.
  3. The following changes then occur by about 8 weeks:
     a. The **left sinus horn** becomes the coronary sinus.
     b. The **right sinus horn** becomes incorporated into the wall of the right atrium.
     c. The **sinoatrial orifice**, initially a transverse, round opening, shifts to the right and becomes elongated, vertical, and more oval. Because of the changes in the great veins, the sinoatrial orifice is now bordered by right and left **venous valves**.
        (1) The superior portions of these valves fuse to form a transient **septum spurium**.
        (2) The inferior part of the left venous valve and the septum spurium fuse with the growing **interatrial septum**.
     d. On the left side, **pulmonary veins** divide and become incorporated into the wall of the left atrium.
  4. **Fate of the sinoatrial structures**
     a. **Structures forming the definitive right atrium**
        (1) The **right horn of the sinus venosus** forms the **smooth portion** of the definitive right atrium (**sinus venarum**).
        (2) The original **primitive right atrium** forms the **rough trabeculated portion** of the definitive right atrium.

(3) The **dividing line** between these two portions of the definitive right atrium is the **crista terminalis**.
   b. **Structures forming the definitive left atrium**
      (1) The **pulmonary veins** form the **smooth portion** of the definitive left atrium.
      (2) The original **primitive left atrium** persists as the **trabeculated portion** of the definitive left atrium.
   c. The **left horn of the sinus venosus** persists as the **coronary sinus and associated vessels** draining the heart; for example, the oblique vein of the left atrium.
   d. The **right venous valve** persists only in its inferior portion, where it gives rise to the **valve of the inferior vena cava** and the **valve of the coronary sinus**.

IV. VENTRICULAR SEPTATION AND FORMATION OF CARDIAC VALVES (Figs. 10-4 and 10-5)

A. **The endocardial cushions**
   1. The endocardial cushions (see Fig. 10-4A) are two centers of mesenchymal cell proliferation distributed around the atrioventricular canal. There is experimental evidence from laboratory animals that the **neural crest** makes a contribution to endocardial cushion mesenchyme.
   2. The endocardial cushions begin to grow at about the same time that the septum primum begins to form (week 5).
   3. The septum primum fuses with the cranial margins of the endocardial cushions.
   4. Simultaneously, the two endocardial cushions grow toward one another to form a **septum intermedium**, which finally divides the common atrioventricular canal into **left and right atrioventricular canals**.

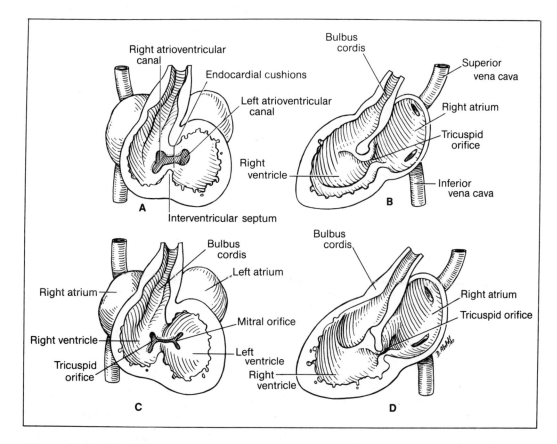

Figure 10-4. Ventricular septation at 35 days (A, B) and 40 days (C, D). See text for description of the process. (A) and (C) show the right and left ventricles; (B) and (D) show the right ventricle and right atrium.

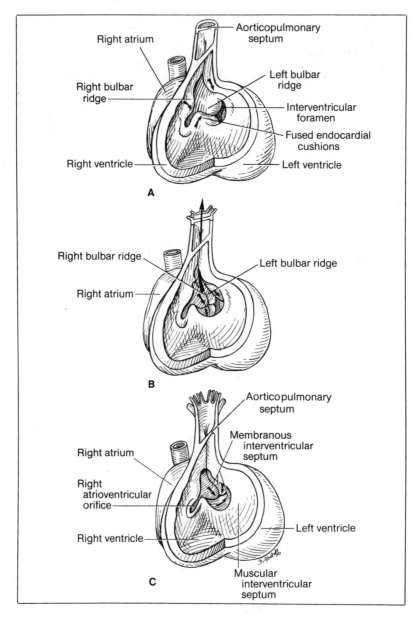

Figure 10-5. Partitioning of the ventricular outflow tract and formation of the interventricular septum at 5 weeks (A), 6 weeks (B), and 7 weeks (C), showing the role of the bulbar ridges and endocardial cushions. The wall of the right ventricle has been cut away to show the right ventricle and, beyond it, the right atrium and the left ventricle. *Arrows* show the directions of tissue growth.

B. Growth of the ventricular wall

1. While the septum intermedium is forming, a thick portion of the ventricular wall between the left and right ventricles starts to grow cranially toward the endocardial cushions.

2. As it grows cranially, this portion of the interventricular septum increasingly restricts the size of the interventricular orifice. However, there is still a **single ventricle** with a broad communication, the **interventricular foramen**, between its two halves.

C. Division of the ventricles and outflow tracts

1. The final formation of two ventricles and two ventricular outflow tracts requires the growth of the bulbar ridges and their fusion with the endocardial cushions.
   a. The left and right **bulbar ridges** are areas of thickened tissue that project into the bulbus cordis on either side near the atrioventricular canal (see Fig. 10-5).
   b. The caudal portions of the bulbar ridges and the cranial portions of the endocardial cushions proliferate in a spiralling pattern.
      (1) This forms the portion of the interventricular septum nearest the atrioventricular canals.
      (2) This **membranous interventricular septum** in the adult heart lacks cardiac muscle. Instead, it is composed of thick bands of dense connective tissue.
   c. The cranial portions of the bulbar ridges grow toward one another and fuse, forming a continuous septum.
2. In this way, the bulbar ridges make an important contribution to the **aorticopulmonary septum**, which divides the **bulbus cordis** and **truncus arteriosus** into two components:
   a. The **pulmonary trunk**, which becomes the outflow tract from the right ventricle to the lungs
   b. The **aortic trunk**, which becomes the outflow tract from the left ventricle to the systemic circulation

D. Formation of cardiac valves (weeks 6 to 7)

1. The cardiac valves form as a result of the proliferation of subendothelial connective tissue. Thus, in the adult, they consist of dense masses of connective tissue with an endothelial covering.
2. The **aortic and pulmonary valves** constitute the **semilunar valves**. These **half-moon-shaped** valves guard the aorta and pulmonary arteries.
   a. The semilunar valves are formed from the bulbar ridges in the bulbus cordis during the fusion of the bulbar ridges.
   b. The valves are later sculpted so that they become concave on one surface.
3. The **mitral and tricuspid valves** constitute the **atrioventricular valves**.
   a. These valves form by proliferation of subendothelial mesenchymal cells surrounding the atrioventricular canals. The endocardial cushions also make contributions to their formation.
   b. The **mitral valve**, between the left atrium and the left ventricle, forms only two cusps and thus resembles a bishop's **miter**.
   c. The **tricuspid valve**, between the right atrium and right ventricle, develops **three cusps**.
4. On the side of the valves facing the ventricles, some cell death occurs among myocardial cells, leaving finger-like projections of the myocardium (the **papillary muscles**) attached to flaps of the valves by narrow strands of connective tissue (the **chordae tendineae**).

V. DEVELOPMENT AND FATE OF THE AORTIC ARCHES (Fig 10-6)

A. General features of aortic arches

1. In the primitive heart before the interatrial and interventricular septa form, blood leaves the primitive ventricle, passes through the bulbus cordis and truncus arteriosus, and enters the **aortic sac** (see Fig. 10-2E).
2. The aortic sac communicates with a series of **aortic arches** (see Figs. 10-2 and 10-6).
   a. These pairs of arteries radiate bilaterally from the aortic sac and pass through the pharyngeal arches.
   b. Several aortic arches make important contributions to the great vessels that form as branches of the aorta in the adult.
3. After passing through the aortic arches, embryonic blood flows along the left and right **dorsal aortas** (see Fig. 10-1).
   a. These large vessels run along either side of the embryo.
   b. They join together caudal to the heart into a single **medial dorsal aorta**.
4. There are a number of important **branches from the dorsal aorta** (see also section V E):
   a. **Intersegmental arteries** supply the developing musculoskeletal somite derivatives and limbs.
   b. **Vitelline arteries** supply the yolk sac.
   c. **Umbilical arteries** supply the developing visceral organs and the placenta.

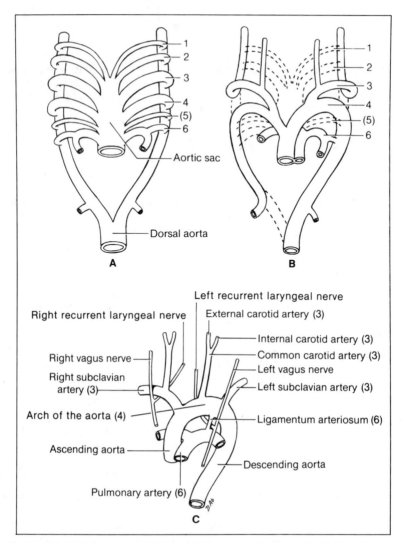

Figure 10-6. Development and fate of the aortic arches at 30 days' development (A), in the fetus (B), and in the adult (C). The fifth aortic arches are rudimentary or not present in humans. Note the dramatic changes in symmetry that take place during morphogenesis of the great vessels, due to differential growth and asymmetric regression of the aortic arches. Note also the resulting asymmetric route of the recurrent laryngeal nerve. Parenthetic numbers in (C) indicate the arches of origin.

B. Fate of the truncus arteriosus and aortic sac (Table 10-1)

1. The **truncus arteriosus** becomes incorporated into the proximal arch of the aorta and the roots of the pulmonary arteries.

2. The **aortic sac** becomes part of the arch of the aorta, specifically the segment between the portion derived from the truncus arteriosus and the portion derived from the fourth aortic arch. It also becomes part of the brachiocephalic artery.

C. Fate of the aortic arches (see Table 10-1 and Fig. 10-6). The aortic arches are initially arranged symmetrically along the left and right sides of the aortic sac. Some pairs of arches later regress completely, while the remainder become unevenly distributed as one member of a pair regresses while another grows more prominent.

  1. The first aortic arches

  a. The first aortic arches are small and transitory. They have formed and largely regressed by the end of the fourth week of development.

Table 10-1. Fate of Truncus Arteriosus, Aortic Sac, and Aortic Arches

Structure	Symmetry	Fate
Truncus arteriosus	Symmetric	Persists in adult; forms proximal root of pulmonary trunk on right and proximal root of aorta on left
Aortic sac	Asymmetric	Persists in adult: forms proximal part of arch of aorta and brachiocephalic artery on right
First aortic arches	Symmetric	Transient; persist as maxillary artery
Second aortic arches	Symmetric	Transient; persist as hyoid and stapedial arteries
Third aortic arches	Nearly symmetric	Persist in adult: form right and left common carotids and proximal part of internal carotid arteries
Fourth aortic arches	Asymmetric	Persist in adult: form proximal right subclavian artery on right, and arch of aorta, between common carotid and subclavian, on left
Fifth aortic arches	Symmetric	Transient or absent; form no adult vessels
Sixth aortic arches	Asymmetric	Form fetal ductus arteriosus on left. Proximal parts persist in adult: form right and left pulmonary arteries

    b. A small portion of each persists as the **maxillary artery** in adults and the rest degenerates.
 2. The second aortic arches
    a. The second aortic arches are also small and somewhat transitory embryonic structures, forming soon after the first aortic arches and degenerating almost as soon as they are formed.
    b. Small portions persist in the adult as two arteries:
       (1) The **hyoid artery**
       (2) The **stapedial artery**
 3. The third aortic arches
    a. The third aortic arches are important embryonic aortic arches.
    b. They persist on both sides of the body in the adult and make important contributions to the following structures:
       (1) The **common carotid arteries**
       (2) The proximal **internal carotid arteries** (the distal portions arise from the cranial dorsal aortas)
       (3) The **external carotid arteries**, which form as branches from the third aortic arches
 4. The fourth aortic arches
    a. The fourth aortic arches form large and persistent structures in the embryo and the adult.
    b. Their later development is asymmetric, because each member of the pair forms different structures.
       (1) As the heart is developing and the aorticopulmonary septum is forming to separate the outflow tracts for the left and right ventricles, the **aortic and pulmonary trunks** are forming toward the left side of the body (week 6).
       (2) Also, parts of the **dorsal aortas** degenerate.
          (a) On both sides of the body, the parts of the dorsal aortas between the third and fourth aortic arches degenerate.
          (b) On the right side, all of the dorsal aorta caudal to the seventh intersegmental artery breaks down and disappears.
       (3) On the **left side**, the **fourth aortic arch** forms the distal portion of the **arch of the aorta**. (The proximal portion is derived from the truncus arteriosus and the aortic sac.)
       (4) On the **right side**, the fourth aortic arch forms the proximal **right subclavian artery**. (The distal right subclavian artery arises from the dorsal aorta. The left subclavian artery comes from the seventh intersegmental artery.)
 5. The fifth aortic arches
    a. The fifth aortic arches are either absent or only rudimentary in humans.
    b. They have no adult derivatives.

6. The sixth aortic arches
   a. On the **right side**, the sixth arch forms the **right pulmonary artery**; the arch degenerates lateral to the lung buds.
   b. On the **left side**, the sixth arch forms the **left pulmonary artery**; the lateral portion of the arch persists as a fetal vessel, the **ductus arteriosus**. After birth, the ductus arteriosus degenerates and becomes the **ligamentum arteriosum**.

D. The recurrent laryngeal nerves and their relation to the sixth aortic arches
   1. Understanding the development of the sixth aortic arches also explains the course of the recurrent laryngeal nerves and their bilateral asymmetry.
   2. The **recurrent laryngeal nerve**, a branch of the **vagus nerve**, provides the nerve supply for the laryngeal derivatives of the sixth pharyngeal arch.
   3. Its anatomy is different on the right and left sides (see Fig. 10-6C).
      a. **On the right**, the recurrent laryngeal nerve ascends relative to the heart and passes under and behind the right subclavian artery, a derivative of the right fourth aortic arch. It takes this route because the distal portion of the right sixth aortic arch degenerates as the heart descends and the neck elongates during development.
      b. **On the left**, the recurrent laryngeal nerve passes under and behind the arch of the aorta, lateral to the ligamentum arteriosum. It takes this route for two reasons:
         (1) The distal portion of the sixth aortic arch on the left persists as the ductus arteriosus. This degenerates after birth, leaving the ligamentum arteriosum as a remnant.
         (2) Also, the fourth arch contributes to the arch of the aorta on the left side.

E. Derivatives of the dorsal aortas
   1. The left and right dorsal aortas form branches that supply the visceral organs, bones, and muscles developing in the body wall.
   2. There are three broad categories of these branches:
      a. **Intersegmental arteries** arise along the dorsal aortas between the somites (Figure 10-1 shows their sites of origin).
         (1) Branches of the intersegmental arteries supply various somitic derivatives such as ribs, intercostal muscles, and the spinal cord.
         (2) In the cervical and lumbar segments, intersegmental arteries supply the limbs.
      b. **Lateral splanchnic arteries** send branches from the dorsal aorta into derivatives of the intermediate mesoderm such as the kidneys and gonads.
      c. **Ventral splanchnic arteries** send branches from the dorsal aorta into the gut tube and its derivatives.
         (1) Initially, there are two major ventral splanchnic arteries:
            (a) The **vitelline arteries** supply the yolk sac.
            (b) The **umbilical arteries** supply the placenta and the developing visceral organs.
         (2) After the yolk sac degenerates, three new large vessels form:
            (a) The **celiac arteries** supply the foregut derivatives such as the stomach.
            (b) The **superior mesenteric arteries** supply the midgut derivatives such as the duodenum and ileum.
            (c) The **inferior mesenteric arteries** supply the hindgut derivatives such as the descending colon and rectum.

VI. DEVELOPMENT OF THE VEINS

A. Early venous system.
In the primitive heart, three major vessels empty into the sinus venosus and the atria (see Figs. 10-1 and 10-2F):
   1. The **vitelline veins**, which drain the yolk sac
   2. The **umbilical veins**, which drain the placenta
   3. The **common cardinal veins**, which drain the body of the embryo, and which themselves receive branches:
      a. The **anterior cardinal veins**, which drain the body cranial to the heart
      b. The **posterior cardinal veins**, which drain the body caudal to the heart

B. Fate of the anterior cardinal veins
   1. In the eighth week of development, an oblique vessel forms, which shunts blood from the left to the right anterior cardinal veins.

2. The caudal portion of the left anterior cardinal vein later degenerates, and the oblique shunt then becomes the **left brachiocephalic vein**.
3. The right anterior cardinal and common cardinal veins become the **superior vena cava**.

C. Fate of the posterior cardinal veins

1. With the development of the definitive metanephric kidney, the posterior cardinal veins degenerate in most places.
2. The persisting portions form:
   a. The **common iliac veins**
   b. The **root of the azygos vein**
3. As the posterior cardinal veins disappear, they are supplanted by two large, but temporary, venous systems:
   a. The **subcardinal veins**, which later form:
      (1) The left **renal vein**
      (2) The **gonadal veins**
      (3) The **suprarenal veins**
      (4) The **inferior vena cava** between the renal veins and the liver
   b. The **supracardinal veins**, which later form:
      (1) The **azygos vein**
      (2) The **hemiazygos vein**
      (3) The **lower inferior vena cava**

D. Fate of the vitelline and umbilical veins (Fig. 10-7). These blood vessels have a complex and informative developmental history. Understanding this history will clarify the hemodynamic changes that take place in other parts of the circulatory system.

1. The **vitelline veins** pass over the developing gut tube and through the septum transversum, and then enter the sinus horns.
   a. The vitelline veins make an important contribution to the **blood vessels of the liver** and to the **inferior vena cava**.
   b. As the liver diverticulum grows from the gut tube into the septum transversum, and the midgut undergoes rotation, the vitelline veins are converted into a network of liver sinusoids, hepatic veins, and portal veins.
   c. The **left vitelline vein** degenerates cranial and caudal to the liver but persists within the liver as the hepatic sinusoidal system and the hepatic portal system.
   d. The **right vitelline vein** persists as the short segment of the posthepatic inferior vena cava.
2. The **umbilical veins** run lateral to the vitelline veins as paired structures passing through the septum transversum to the sinus horns.
   a. The development of the liver cords in the septum transversum causes the umbilical veins to differentiate into **hepatic sinusoids**.
   b. As a result of degeneration of the left sinus venosus and degeneration of parts of the umbilical veins, blood begins to flow from left to right through the liver by way of a new vessel, the **ductus venosus**. The ductus venosus results from the coalescence of many sinusoids.
   c. Subsequently, most of the right umbilical vein degenerates.
   d. The **left umbilical vein** also degenerates cranial to its entry into the septum transversum, but the caudal portion of the left umbilical vein persists in fetal life as a single umbilical vein to drain the placenta.
   e. The **ductus venosus** also persists until the placental blood flow is interrupted at birth.

VII. FETAL CIRCULATION AND CHANGES AT BIRTH. There are striking hemodynamic differences between fetus and newborn.

A. The fetal circulation (Fig. 10-8)

1. The fetus receives oxygenated blood from the placenta.
   a. The **umbilical vein** carries the oxygenated blood from the placenta through the ductus venosus and into the inferior vena cava.
   b. The **inferior vena cava** transports blood from the liver, lower extremities, and kidneys. The inferior vena cava passes through the liver.

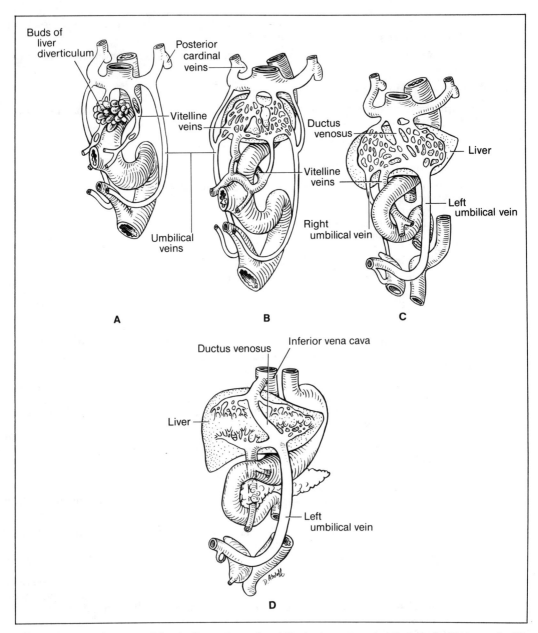

Figure 10-7. Development of the vitelline veins and umbilical veins at 4 weeks (*A*), 5 weeks (*B*), 2 months (*C*), and 3 months (*D*). The vitelline and umbilical veins differentiate into a sinusoidal network of small vessels throughout the liver. The right vitelline vein contributes to the inferior vena cava. The ductus venosus forms from the coalescence of many sinusoids. During fetal life, the ductus venosus carries blood through the liver from left to right between the left umbilical vein and the inferior vena cava.

    2. The **ductus venosus** joins the inferior vena cava, which subsequently empties into the right atrium.
    3. The **superior vena cava** also empties into the right atrium. It drains oxygen-poor blood from the cranial portions of the body, including the head and upper extremities.
    4. There is mixing of oxygen-rich and oxygen-poor blood in the inferior vena cava and the right atrium.
        a. After mixing in the **right atrium**, some of this blood passes into the **left atrium**. It is deflected by the free margin of the septum secundum (the **crista dividens**) so that it passes through the **foramen ovale** into the left atrium.

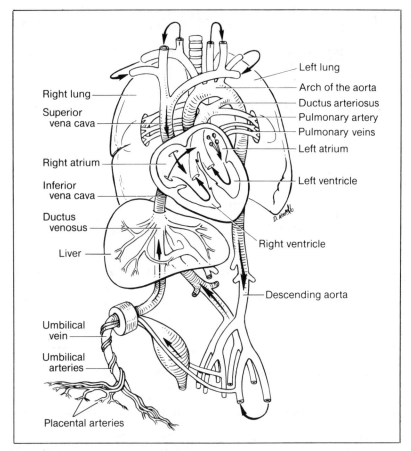

Figure 10-8. Fetal circulatory pattern prior to birth. *Arrows* indicate the direction of blood flow.

    b. From the left atrium, this mixed blood enters the **left ventricle** and then the **aorta**.
5. The fetal lungs are not inflated, and consequently pulmonary perfusion is minimal.
   a. **Oxygen-poor blood** leaves the **right atrium** and enters the **right ventricle**.
   b. From the right ventricle, this oxygen-poor blood is pumped into the **pulmonary arteries**. However, the blood bypasses the lungs because of the ductus arteriosus and enters the systemic circulation.

B. **Circulatory changes in the newborn**
   1. At birth, profound **hemodynamic changes** result from two major events:
      a. The connection to the placenta is severed by clamping of the umbilical cord.
      b. The lungs become inflated, assuming their normal extrauterine respiratory function.
   2. **Clamping of the umbilical cord** has several effects.
      a. Blood flow from the **placenta** via the umbilical vein suddenly ceases, and the umbilical vein closes.
      b. The **ductus venosus** also closes off. This causes increased blood flow through the liver sinusoids.
   3. **Inflation of the lungs** has multiple consequences also.
      a. Peripheral vascular resistance in the lungs suddenly decreases, causing a sudden **increase in pulmonary perfusion**.
      b. The inflated lungs release **bradykinin**, a vasoactive polypeptide (i.e., one that affects the caliber of blood vessels). The bradykinin specifically stimulates smooth muscle contraction in the **ductus arteriosus**, narrowing the lumen of this pulmonary shunt.
      c. With the ductus arteriosus no longer patent, **oxygen-rich blood** now pours back from the lungs through the **pulmonary veins**.

(1) This causes a sudden increase in pressure in the left atrium.
(2) In addition, there is a decrease in blood pressure in the right atrium because umbilical vein blood no longer drains into it via the inferior vena cava.
(3) This **pressure differential** pushes the septum primum against the septum secundum, **closing the foramen ovale**.

C. Fate of fetal circulatory structures

1. The **umbilical vein** eventually degenerates, leaving behind a streak of connective tissue called the **ligamentum teres hepatis**.
2. The **ductus venosus** ultimately degenerates into a connective tissue band known as the **ligamentum venosum**.
3. The **ductus arteriosus** also undergoes degeneration, leaving behind the **ligamentum arteriosum**.
4. With the clamping and cutting of the umbilical cord, the paired **umbilical arteries** degenerate near their attachment to the umbilicus, leaving the **medial umbilical ligaments**. Branches of the umbilical arteries persist as the **blood supply to the urinary bladder**.

VIII. COMMON CONGENITAL ANOMALIES OF THE CARDIOVASCULAR SYSTEM

A. Etiology

1. Considering the complexity of the cardiovascular system, it is probably not surprising that a high frequency of congenital anomalies occur during the formation of this system.
2. The cause is usually unknown in an individual case, but several **etiologic factors** are known to be associated with congenital cardiovascular defects.
   a. **Disorders of chromosomal number.** Congenital heart defects are seen in infants with trisomy 21, 18, or 13. Trisomy syndromes are pleiotropic; that is, they affect more than one organ system (see Chapter 23, section II B).
   b. **Familial disorders.** Heart defects show an increased frequency in some families, suggesting a genetic etiology.
   c. **Teratogenic viral infections. Rubella** infections during the first trimester of pregnancy are known to be teratogenic, causing various congenital anomalies including heart defects.

B. Common congenital heart defects

1. **Atrial septal defects** (persistent patency of the interatrial septum)
   a. Atrial septal defects are the most common and least severe cardiac defects.
      (1) **Probe patency of the foramen ovale** is present in 20% of all adults. It causes no symptoms, since the atrial septum can function as a one-way valve even if a probe patency is present.
      (2) More extensive atrial septal defects are seen in 1 of 13,500 live births. Most are seen near the foramen ovale.
   b. Atrial septal defects cause a **left-to-right shunting** of blood, with increased flow across the tricuspid and pulmonary valves.
   c. Children with atrial septal defects usually have normal stature but may weigh less than normal and may have heart murmurs.

2. **Ventricular septal defects** (persistent patency of the interventricular septum)
   a. Ventricular septal defects are rare as isolated defects but are common in association with other defects, as in the tetralogy of Fallot.
      (1) All ventricular septal defects taken together occur in 1 in 500 live births but are considerably less common at autopsy, suggesting that some are corrected on their own during life.
      (2) Ventricular septal defects are common in **trisomy syndromes**. They occur in 74% of children with trisomy 18 and in 47% with trisomy 21.
   b. Fully 90% involve the membranous portion of the septum; the rest are in the muscular portion.
   c. In ventricular septal defects, high-pressure blood is **shunted from the left to the right ventricle** and into the pulmonary arteries.
   d. Children with ventricular septal defects have heart murmurs. Symptoms are minor if the defect is minor, but large defects can cause severe disability.

3. **Tetralogy of Fallot**
   a. The tetralogy of Fallot (Fig. 10-9) combines **four anomalies**:
      (1) Ventricular septal defect
      (2) Pulmonary artery stenosis
      (3) Overriding aorta (displaced so that its outlet lies partly over the left ventricle and partly over the right ventricle)
      (4) Right ventricular hypertrophy
   b. It probably represents a defect in the development of the **bulbus cordis**.
   c. Tetralogy of Fallot occurs in 1 in 8500 live births.
   d. In children with tetralogy of Fallot, symptoms include:
      (1) Cyanosis, due to poor perfusion of the lungs
      (2) Exhaustion or even fainting after mild exertion
      (3) Stunted growth and delayed puberty
      (4) Clubbing of the distal portions of fingers and toes
   e. Surgery can improve the blood flow to the lungs, ameliorating the symptoms.
4. **Tricuspid atresia** (absence or severe narrowing of the tricuspid valve)
   a. Tricuspid atresia occurs in 1 in 5000 live births.
   b. It usually causes a small (hypoplastic) right ventricle and an enlarged (hypertrophic) left ventricle.
   c. In tricuspid atresia, **blood enters the left atrium from the right atrium** through an atrial septal defect. The septum remains open because of the persistent high pressure in the right atrium, due in part to the smallness of the right ventricle.
   d. Children with tricuspid atresia are cyanotic at birth and have a very short life span unless the defect is corrected surgically.
5. **Patent ductus arteriosus** (failure of the ductus arteriosus to close)
   a. Patent ductus arteriosus occurs in 1 in 3500 live births.
   b. It causes the **shunting** of high-pressure, oxygen-rich blood **back into the pulmonary artery**.
   c. Children with patent ductus arteriosus have heart murmurs and may develop congestive heart failure unless the ductus arteriosus is closed surgically.
   d. Premature infants are often given **prostaglandin synthetase inhibitors** such as indomethacin to promote closure of the ductus arteriosus.

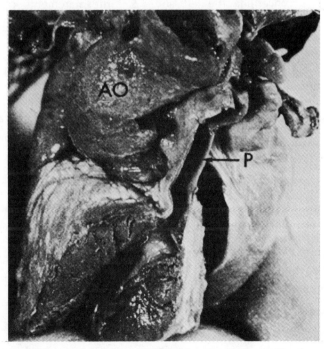

Figure 10-9. The heart of a newborn who died from tetralogy of Fallot. The stenosis of the pulmonary artery (P) leads to right ventricular hypertrophy. In this specimen, the aorta (AO) is also grossly enlarged. (Reprinted with permission from Warkany J: *Congenital Malformations*. Chicago, Year Book, 1971, p 497.)

STUDY QUESTIONS

Directions: Each question below contains five suggested answers. Choose the **one best** response to each question.

1. At birth, when the lungs become inflated, they release bradykinin, a vasoactive peptide that stimulates smooth muscle contraction. Which blood vessel, among those listed below, is most sensitive to bradykinin?

(A) Inferior vena cava
(B) Superior vena cava
(C) Internal iliac artery
(D) Ductus arteriosus
(E) Umbilical vein

2. All of the following contribute to the formation of the interventricular septum EXCEPT

(A) muscular growth of the ventricular walls
(B) septum secundum
(C) left bulbar ridge
(D) right bulbar ridge
(E) endocardial cushions

Directions: Each question below contains four suggested answers of which **one or more** is correct. Choose the answer

A if **1, 2, and 3** are correct
B if **1 and 3** are correct
C if **2 and 4** are correct
D if **4** is correct
E if **1, 2, 3, and 4** are correct

3. True statements concerning the left and right sinus horns include which of the following?

(1) The ductus venosus is directly connected to the left sinus horn
(2) The coronary sinus is a derivative of the right sinus horn
(3) The right atrium has a trabeculated portion derived from the right sinus horn
(4) Most of the left sinus horn degenerates

4. True statements concerning the interatrial septum include which of the following?

(1) The ostium secundum is a hole in the septum primum
(2) The foramen ovale is located at the inferior border of the septum primum
(3) The septum primum has an incomplete inferior border at the ostium primum before the ostium secundum forms completely
(4) The septum secundum closes the interatrial septum during fetal life

5. True statements concerning congenital cardiovascular defects include which of the following?

(1) Cardiovascular defects are often accompanied by other congenital anomalies
(2) Chromosomal anomalies can result in cardiovascular defects
(3) Atrial septal defects can be asymptomatic
(4) Right ventricular hypertrophy is part of the tetralogy of Fallot

Directions: The groups of questions below consist of lettered choices followed by several numbered items. For each numbered item select the **one** lettered choice with which it is **most** closely associated. Each lettered choice may be used once, more than once, or not at all.

Questions 6–10

For each description below of a structure in the developing cardiovascular system, choose the structure that it best describes.

(A) Umbilical vein
(B) Ductus venosus
(C) Ductus arteriosus
(D) Foramen ovale
(E) Left atrium

6. Found at the inferior border of the septum secundum

7. Receives oxygen-rich blood and passes it through the liver prior to birth

8. Receives oxygen-rich blood after birth, due to inflation of the lungs

9. Derived from the left sixth aortic arch; normally closes soon after birth

10. Originally a paired vessel that empties into the sinus venosus

Questions 11–15

For each description below of the fate of an aortic arch, choose the appropriate aortic arch, as shown in the accompanying diagram.

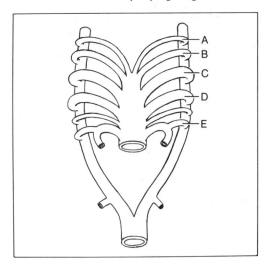

11. Forms the pulmonary artery and the ductus arteriosus

12. Forms the common carotid artery

13. Forms part of the arch of the aorta

14. Forms the maxillary artery

15. Forms the hyoid artery

ANSWERS AND EXPLANATIONS

1. The answer is D. *(VII B 3)* The ductus arteriosus is a derivative of the left sixth aortic arch. Prior to birth, it serves as a shunt to bypass the pulmonary arteries and carry blood directly from the right ventricle into the aorta. Soon after birth, when the lungs become inflated, blood begins to flow to the lungs by way of the pulmonary arteries. The inflated lungs release bradykinin, which stimulates smooth muscle contraction in the ductus arteriosus. As the ductus arteriosus closes down, all of the right ventricular output now flows to the lungs.

2. The answer is B. *(IV A, B, C).* The septum secundum forms part of the interatrial septum, not the interventricular septum. The formation of the interventricular septum is a complex process. The muscular portion of the definitive interventricular septum is formed by growth of muscular tissue from the apex of the heart toward the atrioventricular canal. The membranous portion of the definitive interventricular septum is formed by a fusion of the endocardial cushions and the left and right bulbar ridges.

3. The answer is D (4). *(III B)* The primitive heart has a left and a right horn of the sinus venosus. Each sinus horn receives three major blood vessels: the common cardinal vein, the vitelline vein, and the umbilical vein. The left sinus horn undergoes substantial degeneration but persists as the coronary sinus and the oblique vein of the heart. The right sinus horn persists and becomes incorporated into the wall of the right atrium, giving rise to the smooth portion of the definitive right atrium. The trabeculated portion of the definitive right atrium is derived from the primitive embryonic right atrium.

4. The answer is B (1 and 3). *(III A)* The interatrial septum is formed by the septum primum and the septum secundum. The ostium primum is a hole at the inferior border of the septum primum. As the ostium primum closes, an ostium secundum forms in the septum primum. The foramen ovale is a hole at the inferior border of the septum secundum. Prior to birth, the two flaps of the atrial septum, with their eccentric openings, form a one-way valve that allows the shunting of blood from the right atrium to the left atrium. At birth, closure of the umbilical vein and ductus venosus causes the blood pressure to decrease in the right atrium. Simultaneously, the blood pressure increases in the left atrium because inflation of the lungs causes a sudden increase in the return of pulmonary blood through the pulmonary veins. This pressure differential closes the one-way valve, completing the process of atrial septation.

5. The answer is E (all). *(VIII A, B)* Congenital anomalies of the heart rarely occur in total isolation, without other congenital anomalies. In patients with trisomies 21, 18, or 13, for example, cardiovascular defects are associated with mental retardation and with numerous physical malformations. Atrial septal defects are the most common congenital anomalies of the heart and if mild they can be completely asymptomatic, as in probe patency of the foramen ovale. In these cases, even though the foramen ovale remains open, the anatomic one-way valve of the interatrial septum functions normally because blood pressure is higher in the left atrium than in the right atrium. The tetralogy of Fallot comprises four cardiac defects: a ventricular septal defect, pulmonary artery stenosis, a displaced (overriding) aorta, and right ventricular hypertrophy.

6–10. The answers are: 6-D, 7-B, 8-E, 9-C, 10-A. *(II E 2; III A 2 b; V C 6 b; VI D 2; VII B 3)* The umbilical veins (A) begin as a pair of blood vessels that empty into the sinus venosus and then largely degenerate. The caudal portion of the left umbilical vein remains, forming a single umbilical vein which carries oxygen-rich blood from the placenta to the ductus venosus (B), in the liver. The blood then passes into the inferior vena cava and from there to the right atrium. Much of this oxygen-rich blood then flows from the right atrium to the left atrium (E) through the foramen ovale (D). This blood then enters the left ventricle, and is pumped out into the systemic circulation. Blood leaving the right ventricle shunts past the pulmonary circulation by way of the ductus arteriosus (C), and it then enters the systemic circulation via the aorta. After birth, when blood flow from the placenta ceases, the umbilical vein and ductus venosus close off. This decreases the pressure in the right atrium. Meanwhile, the lungs are inflating and the ductus arteriosus closes, and pulmonary circulation increases suddenly. This causes a sudden increase in pressure in the left atrium, which closes the one-way valve in the interatrial septum, establishing an adult circulatory pattern.

11–15. The answers are: 11-E, 12-C, 13-D, 14-A, 15-B. *(V C; Table 10-1)* The first and second aortic arches are largely embryonic arches, and most of their embryonic components degenerate soon after they are formed. However, remnants of the first arch (A) persist as the maxillary artery, and parts of the second arch (B) persist as the stapedial and hyoid arteries. The third arch (C) persists to form the right and left common carotid arteries, the proximal right and left internal carotid arteries, and, by outgrowths, the external carotid arteries. The fourth arch (D) forms the arch of the aorta on the left side and the proximal subclavian artery on the right side. The fifth arch is rudimentary or may not form at all in human embryos and has no adult derivatives. The sixth arch (E) forms the pulmonary arteries on both sides and the ductus arteriosus on the left side; the ductus arteriosus degenerates after birth.

11
Development of the Nervous System

I. OVERVIEW OF ORGANOGENESIS OF THE NEURAXIS (CENTRAL NERVOUS SYSTEM; CNS)

A. Beginnings of the nervous system. Neurulation and the formation of the neural crest are described in Chapter 5. To summarize:

1. The **neural plate** is induced by the notochord and paraxial mesoderm after gastrulation.
   a. The neural plate soon thickens and invaginates, forming first a neural groove and neural folds, and then a **neural tube**.
   b. With closure of the neuropores at either end of the neural tube, the neuraxis becomes a fluid-filled tube that is sealed at either end.
2. Before the dorsal edges of the neural folds fuse to form a complete neural tube, certain neuroepithelial cells emigrate from the neural groove to establish a widely dispersed population of pluripotent **neural crest cells**.

B. Formation of the spinal cord and brain

1. Soon after its initial formation, the **caudal** portion of the neural tube begins a relatively slow growth to form the **spinal cord**. The lumen remains small and becomes the **central canal** of the spinal cord.
2. The **cranial** portion of the neural tube grows very rapidly to form the **brain**. The lumen expands rapidly to form the **brain ventricles**.
3. Three **primary brain vesicles** soon become evident:
   a. **The prosencephalon (forebrain)**
      (1) The cranial portion of the prosencephalon soon becomes hugely dilated into two lateral **telencephalic vesicles**. These later develop into the **cerebral hemispheres**.
      (2) The caudal portion of the prosencephalon forms the **diencephalon**. This later contributes to the **optic vesicle** and **optic stalk**, which finally form the **retina** and **optic nerve**, respectively.
   b. **The mesencephalon (midbrain).** The mesencephalon undergoes only minor changes in later development.
   c. **The rhombencephalon (hindbrain)**
      (1) The cranial portion of the rhombencephalon later becomes the **metencephalon**.
         (a) The metencephalon is attached to the mesencephalon.
         (b) It gives rise to the **cerebellum** and the **pons**.
      (2) The caudal portion of the rhombencephalon later becomes the **myelencephalon**.
         (a) The myelencephalon is continuous with the spinal cord.
         (b) It gives rise to the **medulla oblongata**.
4. The **lumen** of the neural tube remains to form the fluid-filled **ventricular system** of the brain and the **central canal** of the spinal cord.

C. Derivatives of the neural crest. The neural crest cells give rise to a wide variety of structures, not all of them components of the nervous system. **Neural derivatives** of the neural crest cells include:

1. **Sympathetic ganglia** of the autonomic nervous system
2. **Dorsal (sensory) ganglia** of the peripheral nervous system
3. **Supporting cells** of the nervous system, including:

168 Human Developmental Anatomy

      a. Schwann cells, which wrap nerve axons in myelin
      b. Some meningeal cells

II. PRINCIPLES OF CELL AND TISSUE FORMATION (CYTOGENESIS AND HISTOGENESIS) IN THE NERVOUS SYSTEM. The vast bulk of the nervous system is derived from the ectoderm; the microglia arise from the mesoderm via monocytes.

  A. Structure of neuroepithelium. The neural tube is composed of a pseudostratified epithelium, called the **neuroepithelium** (Fig. 11-1).

    1. The neuroepithelium has two **limiting membranes**:
      a. An **external limiting membrane** is merely the basement membrane of the neuroepithelium.
      b. An **internal limiting membrane**, at the lumen of the neural tube, is a place where epithelial cells are joined together by junctional complexes typical of the apical portion of many epithelial cells.

    2. The **pseudostratified appearance** of the neuroepithelium is due to the fact that it consists of cells of many different heights with their nuclei in different portions of the neuroepithelium (see Fig. 11-1).

  B. Formation and development of neuroblasts and glioblasts. Cell division is particularly important in the differential growth of the nervous system. The entire nervous system, except for the meninges, ganglia, and microglia, develops as a result of astronomic numbers of cell divisions of the germinal cells in the neuroepithelium of the neural tube.

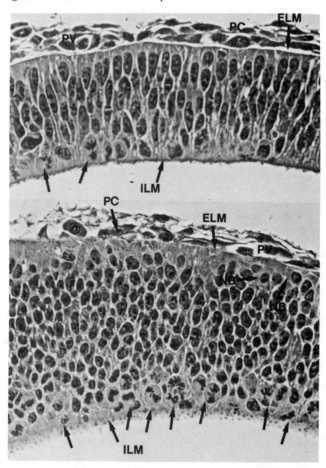

Figure 11-1. The neuroepithelium. (Light micrograph) *Top*, soon after closure of the neural tube; *bottom*, later, after there have been several rounds of cell divisions (*arrows*) and the establishment of neuroblasts (*NB*). *ELM*, external limiting membrane; *ILM*, internal limiting membrane; *PC*, pial cell; *PV*, pial vessel.

1. **Interkinetic nuclear migration and the mitotic cell cycle**
   a. As a general principle, cells have a tendency to lose their attachments to neighboring cells and to become rounder when they undergo mitosis.
   b. This phenomenon occurs in the pseudostratified neuroepithelium, in a process known as **interkinetic nuclear migration** (Fig. 11-2).
      (1) The pseudostratified neuroepithelium contains tall columnar cells that stretch all the way from the internal limiting membrane to the external limiting membrane.
      (2) As these cells begin to synthesize DNA in preparation for a mitotic event (the S phase of the mitotic cell cycle), the cells begin to grow shorter and rounder as they temporarily lose their attachments to the external limiting membrane.
      (3) The cells continue to shorten during the G_2 (gap 2) phase of the cell cycle, and they become completely rounded during the M (mitosis) phase.
      (4) In the G_1 (gap 1) phase that follows mitosis, the cells elongate again, and their nuclei begin to migrate away from the internal limiting membrane and back toward the external limiting membrane at the peripheral portion of the neural tube (see Fig. 11-2).
      (5) After the cells become elongated again, a new S phase begins and the cycle repeats itself over and over.

2. **Fate of mitotic daughter cells: origin of neuroblasts and glioblasts**
   a. In the early neuroepithelium, both daughter cells of the mitotic event continue on as discrete elements of the pseudostratified neuroepithelium. Soon after the closure of the neural tube, however, some of the daughter cells have very different fates.
      (1) One of the two daughter cells creates a **stem cell** population that continues to go through many more mitotic cycles and interkinetic nuclear migrations.
      (2) The other daughter cell begins to differentiate into either **neuroblasts**, which are cells destined to become mature **neurons**, or **glioblasts**, cells destined to become mature **glial cells**.
   b. Once the neuroblasts and glioblasts have been produced, they may either undergo subsequent cell divisions to produce more neuroblasts or glioblasts, or they may differentiate directly into neurons and glial cells.

3. **Neuroblast differentiation: principles of neuron formation**
   a. Characteristics of neurons
      (1) Neurons are the **functional cellular elements** of the nervous system. They generate impulses, conduct the impulses from one place to another, and send them across synaptic connections to neighboring neurons.

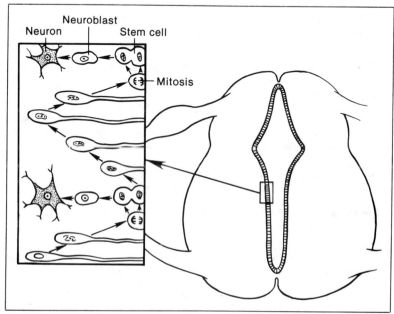

Figure 11-2. Interkinetic nuclear migration, followed by neuroblast differentiation into neurons.

(2) Neurons vary widely in **structure**, but each neuron has a **cell body** (which contains the nucleus) and one or more **processes**, typically an **axon** and one or more **dendrites**.
  (a) The **dendrite** is the receiving end of the neuron. It conducts impulses toward the cell body. Dendrites are typically short and have many branches.
  (b) The **axon** is the transmitting end of the neuron. It conducts impulses away from the cell body. Axons are typically longer than dendrites and have fewer branches.

b. **Principles of neuronal differentiation.** There is a fantastic variety in the neuronal family (see Chapter 1, Fig. 1-3). Nevertheless, the differentiation of a motor neuron in the spinal cord will serve to illustrate the major principles of neuronal differentiation.
  (1) The motor neurons in the spinal cord develop from neuroblasts that have very few processes. The **neuroblasts**, once formed, migrate away from the lumen of the spinal cord, and as they do so they begin to form a small number of **processes**.
    (a) Some of these processes develop into a **dendritic group** of moderately long processes that receive inputs from other cells via synapses.
    (b) One **axonal process** becomes extremely elongated and may grow extensively in the marginal layer (see section II C 2) if it is destined to carry impulses parallel to the long axis of the spinal cord, or it may grow a process that begins to project through the marginal layer out of the central nervous system into the peripheral nervous system.
  (2) Motor neurons eventually will contact developing **muscle fibers** and form **motor end plates** with them.

c. Some neuroblasts form motor neurons, while others form small interneurons, or large pyramidal neurons of the cerebral cortex, or Purkinje cells of the cerebellum, or another of the many types of neurons. These diverse cell types differ in the size and shape of their cell bodies, extent of dendritic arborization, and length of axons (see Chapter 1, Fig. 1-3), and in many functional criteria as well.

4. **Glioblast differentiation**
  a. The **glia**, or **neuroglia**, are the **supporting tissue** of the nervous system. Glial cells differ in location and function, as well as in morphology; some of their functions are not as well understood as those of neurons.
  b. **Glioblasts** of the primitive neuroepithelium differentiate into either **oligodendroblasts** or **astroblasts**, and these in turn differentiate into **oligodendroglia (oligodendrocytes)** or **astroglia (astrocytes)**, respectively.
    (1) **Oligodendrocytes** are responsible for the synthesis of **myelin** in the central nervous system. This function in the peripheral nervous system is subserved by **Schwann cells**, which are neural crest derivatives.
    (2) **Astrocytes** are thought to have **support functions** for neurons, but these are poorly understood. Astrocytes are widely distributed throughout both the white and the gray matter in the central nervous system. They are also prominent in two boundary locations:
      (a) The **glia limitans** is a layer which forms as astrocytes and their end processes are added at the basement membrane (external limiting membrane) of the neuroepithelium.
      (b) Astrocytes also form **around blood vessels** in large numbers, although their function there is not well understood. The earlier notion that astrocytes form the so-called blood–brain barrier has been disproved by recent tracer experiments.

5. There are two **other groups of glial cells** in the central nervous system.
  a. The **microglia** are known to be a component of the **mononuclear phagocyte system** and as such are derived from the **bone marrow** stem cells (mesodermal derivatives) just as monocytes and macrophages are.
  b. **Ependymal cells**, which line the central canal and brain ventricles, are also considered to be glial cells.

C. **Formation of mantle, marginal, and ependymal layers**
  1. **The mantle layer** is a densely packed zone of cell **nuclei**.
    a. Once the neuroblasts and glioblasts have formed in the germinal layer near the lumen of the neural tube, they migrate outward from this zone toward the external limiting membrane.
    b. The entire wall of the neural tube increases in thickness as many layers of nuclei become piled on top of the original layer (Fig. 11-3).

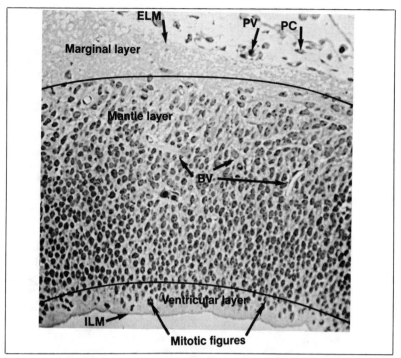

Figure 11-3. The wall of the neural tube after myelin accumulation has begun to thicken the marginal layer. (Light micrograph) Note the numerous mitotic figures near the lumen of the neural tube, at the ventricular layer. *BV*, blood vessels; *ELM*, external limiting membrane; *ILM*, internal limiting membrane; *PC*, pial cells; *PV*, pial vessels.

  c. The mantle layer becomes the **gray matter** of the central nervous system.
 2. **The marginal layer** is a zone composed mostly of **axons** and **dendrites**.
    a. As the neurons differentiate and sprout axons and as the glioblasts differentiate into glial cells, a layer of nonmyelinated and myelinated nerve cell processes develops external to the inner mantle layer, between the mantle layer and the external limiting membrane (see Fig. 11-3).
    b. This **marginal layer** is devoid of the cell bodies of large neurons and consists primarily of cell processes, although the cell bodies of glial elements are also common here.
    c. The marginal layer becomes the **white matter** of the central nervous system.
 3. The **ependymal layer** develops from the original germinal layer.
    a. Eventually, no new neuroblasts or glioblasts are "born" from the neuroepithelium.
    b. The quiescent epithelial layer at the lumen of the central nervous system, now called the **ependymal layer**, consists of ependymal cells, a kind of glial cell.

D. **Formation of alar and basal laminae**
 1. As the neuroepithelium proliferates, forming the mantle and marginal layers, the proliferation thickens the wall of the neural tube.
    a. The **central lumen** of the tube also changes shape, elongating in the dorsal-ventral axis and becoming roughly diamond-shaped (Fig. 11-4).
    b. The dorsomedial and ventromedial parts of the neural tube remain thin, to form a **dorsal roof plate** and a **ventral floor plate**, respectively.
 2. The thick lateral walls on either side of the neural tube are each divided into a **dorsal alar plate** and a **ventral basal plate** (see Fig. 11-5) by a recess known as the **sulcus limitans**.
    a. The **sulcus limitans** thus serves to divide the developing central nervous system into two functionally important components.
       (1) The **dorsal regions (alar laminae)** will be **afferent** and will have **sensory** functions.
       (2) The **ventral regions (basal laminae)** will be **efferent** and will have **motor** functions.
    b. The sulcus limitans extends from the caudal end of the neural tube to the junction between the midbrain and the forebrain.

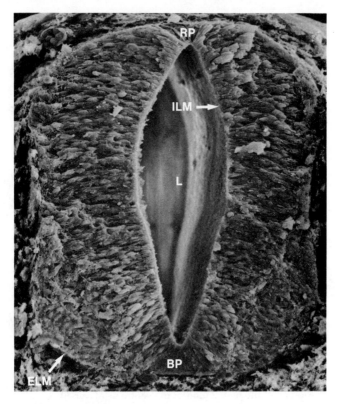

Figure 11-4. The human neural tube soon after closure. (Scanning electron micrograph) *ELM*, external limiting membrane; *ILM*, internal limiting membrane; *L*, neural tube lumen; *RP*, roof plate; *BP*, basal plate.

      (1) Because of this, the midbrain and the hindbrain derivatives have an arrangement of alar and basal laminae very like the arrangement found in the spinal cord.
      (2) The forebrain is thought to have only alar laminae.

E. **Formation of meninges and intermeningeal spaces**
  1. The **meninges** form chiefly from **neural crest cells**.
      a. Neural crest cells develop into a loose mesenchyme-like network surrounding the entire neural tube.
      b. This meshwork soon becomes differentiated into an inner **endomeninx** and an outer **ectomeninx**.
          (1) The **ectomeninx** later develops into the tough outer **dura mater**.
          (2) The **endomeninx** develops into the inner **leptomeninges**; that is, the **pia mater** and the **arachnoid membrane**.
  2. During the formation of the endomeninx, intercellular spaces form.
      a. These coalesce into a **subarachnoid space** between the pia mater and arachnoid. The subarachnoid space eventually becomes filled with cerebrospinal fluid.
      b. A **subdural space** also forms, between the arachnoid and the dura mater.

F. **Myelination of axons**
  1. **Myelin** is a substance that surrounds many axons in both the peripheral and central nervous systems. It is composed of numerous concentrically arranged layers of the membranes of the myelinating cells that surround the neuronal axon.
  2. **Myelination in the peripheral nervous system**
      a. In the peripheral nervous system, myelin is derived from the cell membranes of **Schwann cells**.
          (1) The point of reflection of the Schwann cell membrane around the axon is known as the **mesaxon**.

- (2) The Schwann cell begins to elongate and then rotates around the axon and the mesaxon, forming layers much like a jelly roll, with the Schwann cell cytoplasm representing the cake of the jelly roll and the mesaxon representing the jelly.
- (3) As the Schwann cell rotates (or the mesaxon elongates; it is not clear which actually occurs), a new apposed double layer of Schwann cell membrane from the mesaxon is laid down with each revolution of the Schwann cell.
- (4) In many instances, there are hundreds of lamellae of myelin forming a thick **myelin sheath** around the axon.
  - b. A typical long axon in the peripheral nervous system is myelinated by a large number of different Schwann cells, arranged end to end. Between each Schwann cell, there is a bit of naked axon at a location known as the **node of Ranvier**, which represents a gap where one Schwann cell ends and the next begins.
- 3. **Myelination in the central nervous system**
  - a. In the central nervous system, myelin is derived from the cell membranes of **oligodendroglia**.
    - (1) Oligodendroglial cells have several cell processes, each of which invests and myelinates a different neuronal axon.
    - (2) The oligodendroglial cell also forms multiple lamellae of its own cell membrane around each axon.
      - (a) However, it can not do so by a rotation of the entire cell, because one oligodendrocyte myelinates more than one axon.
      - (b) Instead, the oligodendroglial cell (and probably the Schwann cell as well) is thought to form the myelin sheath by growth of the mesaxon, which sends the mesaxon tip spiralling around the neuronal axon.
    - (3) The glial cells produce myelin first near the cell body of the neuron and then more or less sequentially along the length of the axon away from the cell body.
  - b. Myelination begins in the central nervous system of the human fetus during the fourth month of development and is not complete until several years after birth. Different portions of the nervous system become myelinated at different times of gestation. As a general rule, however, there is a good correlation between the functional development of a system and the completion of its myelination.
- 4. **Function of myelin.** Myelin is an **insulating substance** on the axon. It prevents ionic efflux from the axoplasm where it is present.
  - a. In myelinated fibers, ionic efflux is restricted to the **nodes of Ranvier**, and conduction velocity is greater due to **saltatory conduction**; that is, the action potential jumps from node to node, thus increasing conduction velocity.
  - b. There is a clear relationship between **conduction velocity** of a nerve fiber and the myelination of it. Unmyelinated fibers have a slow conduction velocity and myelinated fibers have a higher conduction velocity.

III. DEVELOPMENT OF THE SPINAL CORD

- A. **Early events**
  1. The spinal cord develops in the neural tube caudal to the **cervical flexure** of the brain (see Fig. 11-7).
     - a. Soon after the neural folds fuse to form a neural tube, some neural crest cells have migrated out into the tissues of the embryo and have become widely dispersed.
     - b. Other **neural crest cells** form segmentally arranged precursors of **dorsal root ganglia**.
  2. The **neural tube** now consists of a neuroepithelium and is surrounded by a basement membrane, the external limiting membrane.
  3. As described in section II B, the neuroepithelium produces many neuroblasts and glioblasts by mitotic cell divisions. This proliferation thickens the wall of the neural tube and distorts the lumen, or **central canal**, which elongates in the dorsal–ventral axis and becomes roughly diamond-shaped (see Fig. 11-4).

- B. **Formation of mantle and marginal layers**
  1. Proliferation results in establishment of a **mantle layer** with many cell nuclei.
  2. Production of large numbers of cell processes which become myelinated results in the establishment of a **marginal layer** with very few cell nuclei in it.

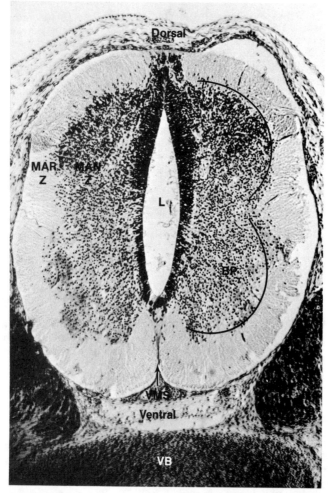

Figure 11-5. The developing spinal cord. (Light micrograph) *AP*, alar plate; *BP*, basal plate; *L*, lumen; *MAN Z*, mantle zone; *MAR Z*, marginal zone; *VB*, vertebral body; *VMS*, ventral median fissure (sulcus). The *semicircular lines* drawn on the right represent the approximate boundary between the gray matter and the white matter.

C. Formation of alar and basal plates (Fig. 11-5)

1. The dorsomedial and ventromedial parts of the neural tube remain thin to form a **roof plate** and a **floor plate**, respectively.
2. The lateral walls of the neural tube are thick and are divided into a **dorsal alar plate** and a **ventral basal plate** by the **sulcus limitans**.
   a. The **alar plate** contains many neuroblasts that will differentiate into **afferent neurons**.
      (1) These neurons receive sensory input from the peripheral nervous system via **dorsal root ganglia**. The dorsal root ganglia contain neural crest–derived neurons that send one process centrally and another peripherally.
      (2) Thus, the alar plate produces **sensory neurons** and eventually gives rise to the **dorsal (sensory) horns** of the grey matter in the spinal cord.
   b. The **basal plate** grows more rapidly than the alar plate and forms a large mass of neuroblasts that will differentiate into **efferent neurons**.
      (1) These neurons send axons out of the central nervous system to peripheral muscles.
      (2) Thus, the basal plate produces **motor neurons** and gives rise to the **ventral (motor) horns** of the grey matter in the spinal cord.
3. An **intermediate plate**, which straddles the sulcus limitans, forms neurons for the **autonomic nervous system** and gives rise to the **intermediate horn** of the spinal cord.
4. As the alar and basal plates grow, the wall of the spinal cord thickens, the spinal canal becomes smaller, and **dorsal and ventral median septa** become recognizable.

5. Also, the relatively more rapid growth in the basal plate results in an overgrowth of the floor plate to form a deep indentation of the ventral spinal cord, the so-called **ventral median fissure (ventral median sulcus)**.

D. Formation of the meninges
1. As described in section II E, the spinal cord develops an inner endomeninx and an outer ectomeninx from a loose mesenchyme-like network formed by the neural crest cells.
2. The **ectomeninx** later develops into the tough outer dura mater while the **endomeninx** develops into the inner **pia-arachnoid**.
3. During the formation of the endomeninx, intercellular spaces develop into the fluid-filled **subarachnoid space** between the pia mater and the arachnoid, and the **subdural space** between the arachnoid and the dura mater.

E. The caudal spinal cord
1. When the neural tube first forms, it extends all along the length of the embryonic axis. Later, the **motor nerve roots** leave the cord at their segmental level of origin and project laterally through the intervertebral foramina and nearly perpendicular to the long axis of the spinal cord.
2. With the elongation of the fetus, the **caudal portion of the spinal cord** undergoes some changes.
    a. Few if any neurons differentiate in the caudal cord. Instead, a **filum terminale** forms. This strand of connective tissue connects the caudal termination of the spinal cord (the **conus medullaris**) to the bones of the vertebral column.
    b. Simultaneously, the growth rate of the vertebral column outstrips growth of the spinal cord, so that the conus medullaris lies at progressively more cranial spinal segments.
        (1) At 24 weeks of development, the spinal cord terminates at sacral spinal segment S1.
        (2) In a newborn it ends at lumbar spinal segment L3.
        (3) In an adult the spinal cord usually ends at L1 but may be as low as L3.
    c. The **subarachnoid space** extends well below the conus medullaris. Consequently, **lumbar puncture** between lumbar vertebrae L4 and L5 allows the physician to sample cerebrospinal fluid with reduced risk of damaging the spinal cord.
    d. The nerve roots that extend caudally from the conus medullaris are gathered into a group known as the **cauda equina**.

IV. DEVELOPMENT OF DORSAL ROOT GANGLIA, SPINAL NERVES, AND SYMPATHETIC GANGLIA. Neural crest cells play an important role in the formation of the dorsal root ganglia and the sympathetic ganglia.

A. Dorsal root ganglia and spinal nerves
1. As neural crest cells migrate out of the neuroepithelium, some of them become segmentally arranged as paired structures on the dorsolateral aspect of the neural tube.
    a. These paired structures, which form the **dorsal root ganglia**, initially are loose aggregations of neuroblasts.
    b. The neuroblasts soon develop into **pseudounipolar neurons** as a result of fusion of the dendrite and axon of the neuron near the cell body.
2. **Connections between dorsal root ganglia, spinal cord, and peripheral structures** (Fig. 11-6)
    a. The pseudounipolar neurons send their axons and dendrites out from the dorsal root ganglia.
        (1) An **axon** from the dorsal root ganglion grows into the dorsal portion of the spinal cord. Here, the axon either synapses with another neuron in the spinal cord or it projects all the way up to the brain.
        (2) A **dendrite** from the dorsal root ganglion grows away from the spinal cord and comes to provide sensory innervation for peripheral structures such as the skin and muscle spindles.
    b. Bundles of dendrites and bundles of axons become gathered together.
        (1) The axon bundles eventually contribute to the **dorsal roots**.
        (2) The dendrite bundles become the **spinal nerves**.
    c. In this manner, the **alar laminae** of the spinal cord, which give rise to the **dorsal horns**, form neurons which receive synapses from large numbers of **afferent, sensory inputs**.

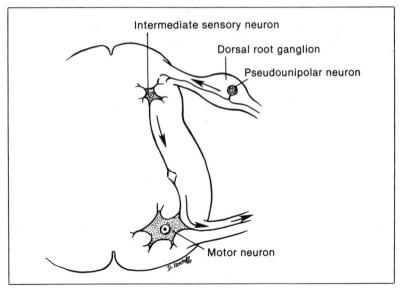

Figure 11-6. Connections between neurons of a dorsal root ganglion, the spinal cord, and a ventral root. *Arrows* show the direction of a nerve impulse traveling along this route.

    d. In contrast, the **basal laminae** of the spinal cord, which give rise to the **ventral horns**, form neurons which project axons into the peripheral portions of the body to innervate various muscles; that is, the ventral horn neurons generate **efferent, motor impulses**.

B. Sympathetic ganglia

1. Neural crest cells also form a complex sympathetic chain of ganglia.
2. Neurons differentiate in these ganglia and send out long processes that innervate peripheral structures such as blood vessels or the smooth muscle cells in visceral organs.
3. In addition, neurons differentiate in the **intermediate horns of the spinal column** and send out processes that synapse with the cell bodies of sympathetic neurons located in the sympathetic ganglia.

V. EARLY DEVELOPMENT OF THE BRAIN (Fig 11-7)

A. The three primary brain vesicles.
Soon after the neural tube forms, it begins to grow rapidly in the portion cranial to the fourth somite so that the walls become thickened conspicuously and the three primary brain vesicles form (see Fig. 11-7): the **prosencephalon (forebrain)**, the **mesencephalon (midbrain)**, and the **rhombencephalon (hindbrain)**.

B. Formation of the first two flexures.
As the brain grows rapidly, two flexures form:

1. The **cranial flexure** is known as the **midbrain flexure**.
2. The **caudal flexure** is known as the **cervical flexure**.

C. Subdivision of the prosencephalon.
The prosencephalon rapidly becomes subdivided into a **telencephalon** and a **diencephalon**.

1. This event is marked by the rapid lateral expansion of the walls of the forebrain to form the precursors of the **cerebral hemispheres**.
2. The walls of the diencephalon also become modified extensively by the formation of the **optic vesicles** (see Chapter 20, section II A).

D. Formation of the third flexure and subdivision of the rhombencephalon (see Fig. 11-7)

1. The **hindbrain** now begins to grow rapidly to produce a **third flexure**, the **pontine flexure**.

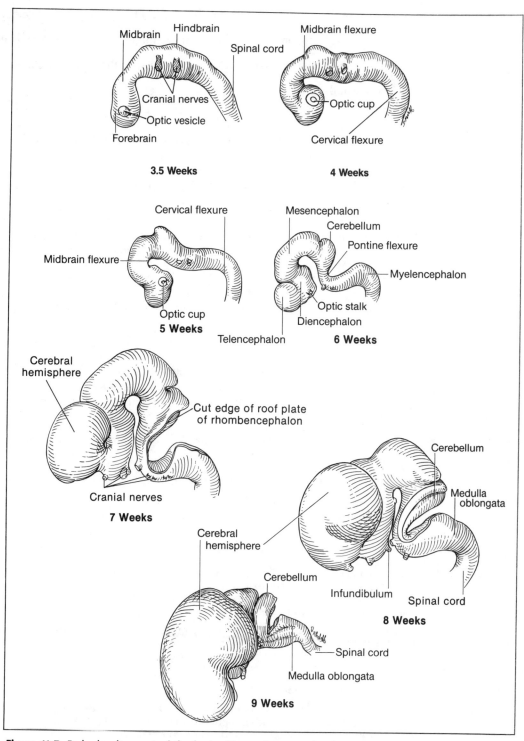

Figure 11-7. Early development of the brain. First to form are the three primary vesicles [prosencephalon (forebrain), mesencephalon (midbrain), and rhombencephalon (hindbrain)]. The midbrain and cervical flexures appear shortly thereafter, followed by establishment of the pontine flexure. Later, the cerebral hemispheres develop from the telencephalon; the mesencephalon remains relatively unchanged; and the rhombencephalon subdivides into the metencephalon, which forms the pons and cerebellum cranial to the pontine flexure, and the myelencephalon, which becomes the medulla oblongata caudal to the pontine flexure.

2. With the formation of the pontine flexure, the rhombencephalon now has two components:
   a. The cranial component, the **metencephalon**, will eventually give rise to the **cerebellum** and the **pons**.
   b. The caudal component, the **myelencephalon**, will give rise to the **medulla oblongata**.

E. Alar and basal laminae in the brain
   1. With the rapid growth of the cranial portion of the neural tube, the originally similar cranial and caudal portions become quite different.
   2. Nevertheless, a **sulcus limitans** extends all the way to the junction between the forebrain and the midbrain.
   3. Because of this, the midbrain and the hindbrain derivatives have an arrangement of **alar and basal laminae** that is closely related to the arrangement found in the spinal cord.

VI. DEVELOPMENT OF THE PROSENCEPHALON

A. **Cytogenesis and histogenesis in the cerebral hemispheres.** The histogenesis of the cerebral cortex follows much the same basic principles as for the development of the rest of the neural tube, but with an interesting variation on the general theme of interkinetic nuclear migration, namely the addition of new layers of neurons superficial to the white matter.
   1. As discussed in section II, the neural tube is made up of **pseudostratified neuroepithelium** (see Fig. 11-1), and nuclear divisions of cells in the neuroepithelium occur at the ependymal layer.
      a. Daughter cells from these mitotic divisions can differentiate now into **neuroblasts** (and later into neurons) as well as a host of **glioblasts** (and later glial cells).
      b. By repeated divisions and the formation of neurons and processes, the cerebrum thickens rapidly to form a **mantle layer** and a **marginal layer** (Fig. 11-8).
   2. In the early cerebral cortex, the neuroepithelial cells extend all the way from the ependymal layer to the external limiting membrane. These cells undergo nuclear division at the ependymal layer, but they undergo cytoplasmic division elsewhere.
      a. Following nuclear division, the daughter nucleus and a mass of cytoplasm migrates away from the ependymal surface to a subpial position toward the external limiting membrane.
      b. **Cytoplasmic division** is accomplished only after this migration has taken place, so that it occurs just below the external limiting membrane rather than at the ependymal surface.
      c. Once cytoplasmic division occurs, a new neuroblast is formed, and this cell then differentiates, sprouting dendrites and an axon to become a **neuron** of the cerebral cortex.
   3. This process occurs in successive waves, with newly formed neurons being layered over older neurons.
      a. The neurons formed in the earlier wave of nuclear migration later contribute to the deeper layers of the cerebral cortex (layers V and VI).
      b. The neurons formed in the later waves of nuclear migration later contribute to the more superficial layers of the cerebral cortex (layers II, III, and IV).
   4. The formation of a large number of neurons in the more superficial portions of the cerebral cortex also explains how a layer of gray matter comes to lie outside the white matter in the cerebral cortex. This relationship is the reverse of the arrangement in the spinal cord, where the white matter is external to the gray matter.

B. Development of the telencephalon
   1. The telencephalon grows first as two large dilations, which represent the precursors of the cerebral hemispheres. These dilations later grow cranially, caudally, dorsally, and ventrally, eventually to engulf the diencephalon nearly completely.
   2. Two **lateral ventricles** form as cavities inside each of the cerebral hemispheres (Fig. 11-9).
      a. Each lateral ventricle communicates with the third and fourth ventricles by means of an **interventricular foramen** (the **foramen of Monro**).
      b. The lateral ventricles are distorted extensively by the growth of the cerebral hemispheres so that they eventually become almost C-shaped.
      c. The dorsomedial wall of the developing telencephalon becomes very thin and gives rise to the **choroid plexus** (see Fig. 11-9).

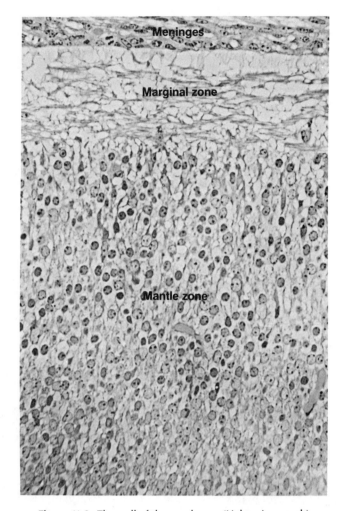

Figure 11-8. The wall of the cerebrum. (Light micrograph)

      (1) The choroid plexus is found in both lateral ventricles and the third ventricle.
      (2) The **cerebrospinal fluid** is a secretion product of the choroid plexus in all ventricles.
  3. Continued localized proliferation of neuroblasts in the floor of each cerebral hemisphere results in the formation of the **corpus striatum**.
     a. The corpus striatum curls around inferiorly and distorts the lateral ventricle as it does so.
     b. In addition, the **lateral ventricles** grow in a posterior direction.
     c. These changes finally result in the formation of **inferior and posterior horns** of the lateral ventricles.
     d. Nerve fiber tracts also divide the corpus striatum into a **lentiform nucleus** and a **caudate nucleus**.
  4. The walls of the telencephalon now undergo a fantastically complex series of growth and differentiation events to form the **cerebral cortex**. The histogenesis of the cerebral cortex proceeds as described above, in section VI A.

C. Formation of the cerebral hemispheres and other telencephalic structures (Fig. 11-10)
  1. The cerebral hemispheres first appear during the fifth week. During the second month, the basal portions of the cerebral hemispheres grow in size and consequently project into the lateral ventricles and the floor of the interventricular foramen.
     a. This region of active growth is known as the **corpus striatum**.

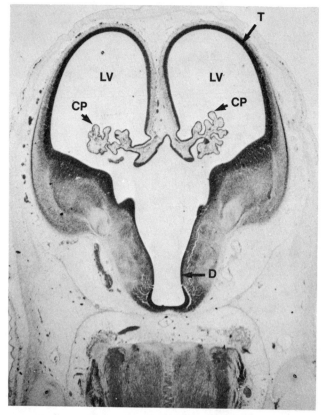

Figure 11-9. Coronal section of the telencephalon *(T)* and the diencephalon *(D)*, showing the lateral ventricles *(LV)* and the choroid plexus *(CP)*.

    b. The roof plate in this region is particularly thin and invaginates to form the **choroid fissure**, a precursor of the **choroid plexus** of the lateral ventricles and the third ventricle.

  2. Another bilateral zone of proliferative activity appears just dorsal to the choroid fissure and this eventually becomes the **hippocampus**. As it grows, the hippocampus bulges laterally into the lateral ventricles.

  3. Meanwhile, the medial wall of each cerebral hemisphere fuses with the lateral wall of the diencephalon, bringing the **caudate nucleus** of the telencephalon into contact with the **thalamus** of the diencephalon.

  4. The **frontal, temporal, and occipital lobes** of the cerebral cortex now arise by differential growth, and these lobes eventually overgrow the **insula**, which represents cortical tissue overlying the relatively more slowly growing corpus striatum.

D. Development of the diencephalon. The development of the diencephalon is considerably less complicated than the development of the telencephalon.

  1. Three swellings form in the lateral walls of the third ventricle. These swellings are the precursors of the **epithalamus, thalamus,** and **hypothalamus**.
    a. The precursor of the thalamus grows rapidly, and as it does so, it reduces the lumen of the third ventricle to a small slit.
    b. The thalamic masses most often become fused together.
    c. The epithalamus and hypothalamus do not grow as extensively as the thalamus.

  2. The **pineal gland (epiphysis cerebri)** develops as a diverticulum of the roof of the diencephalon near the epithalamus.

  3. The hypothalamic nuclei and pituitary gland
    a. The hypothalamus contains several areas where neuroblasts proliferate extensively, giving rise to the **supraoptic and paraventricular nuclei** and the **mammillary bodies**.

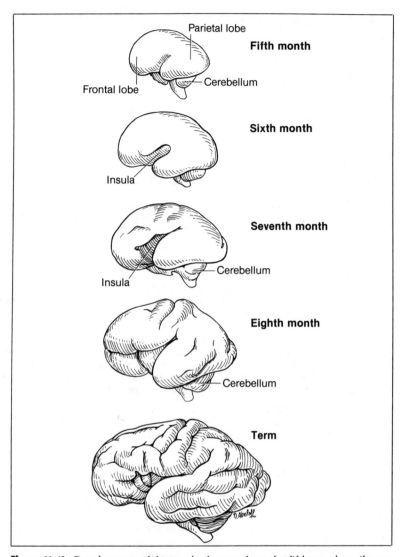

Figure 11-10. Development of the cerebral cortex from the fifth month until term.

    b. The **pituitary gland (hypophysis cerebri)** is formed in part by an evagination of the floor of the diencephalon which arises near the hypothalamic nuclei.
        (1) This evagination, called the **infundibulum**, is responsible for forming the **neurohypophysis**.
        (2) The **adenohypophysis** forms from **Rathke's pouch**, an evagination of the roof of the oral cavity (see Chapter 19, section II B).
    c. The hypothalamic nuclei are very important in the regulation of **endocrine function**, for some of their neurons have axons that terminate near blood vessels which transport **releasing hormones** from the neurohypophysis to the adenohypophysis.

VII. DEVELOPMENT OF THE MESENCEPHALON. The development of the mesencephalon is relatively simple when compared to the development of the prosencephalon or the rhombencephalon.

    A. The midbrain ventricle
        1. The midbrain ventricle is at first quite large compared to the relatively thin walls of the midbrain vesicle.

2. As the midbrain grows, however, the midbrain ventricle becomes reduced until it eventually forms the narrow **aqueduct of Sylvius**, which joins the third ventricle to the fourth ventricle.
3. The mesencephalon has a definite **sulcus limitans** and clearly demarcated alar and basal laminae.

B. **Alar and basal laminae**
   1. **Development of the alar laminae.** The alar (dorsal) laminae of the mesencephalon develop into the **tectum**.
      a. At first, the alar laminae are two broad hillocks that are separated by a superficial midline groove.
      b. Later, a second groove forms perpendicular to the first groove, and the **superior and inferior colliculi** are formed anteriorly and posteriorly, respectively.
         (1) The **superior colliculus** is involved in processing visual inputs.
         (2) The **inferior colliculus** is involved in auditory reflexes.
      c. Several waves of proliferative activity in the alar laminae result in the formation of markedly stratified colliculi.
   2. **Development of the basal laminae**
      a. The basal (ventral) laminae of the mesencephalon form the **tegmentum** dorsally and the **crura cerebri** ventrally.
         (1) The **tegmentum** is a region of the brain which forms from the basal lamina and the floor plate of the mesencephalon. It forms the **nuclei** for the **oculomotor nerve** (cranial nerve III) and the **trochlear nerve** (cranial nerve IV).
         (2) The most ventral portion of the mesencephalon becomes considerably enlarged by the formation of the **crura cerebri**. These structures represent large numbers of nerve fibers connecting the cerebral cortex to lower centers, such as the **corticospinal tracts** of the tectal nuclei and the **corticopontine tracts**.
      b. The basal laminae of the mesencephalon also give rise to the **Edinger-Westphal nucleus**, which innervates the sphincter muscles of the pupil of the eye.
   3. There is some controversy regarding the origin of the **red nucleus** and the **substantia nigra**. These structures may be derived from the nearby basal laminae, or they may arise from migration of cells from the more distant alar laminae into the ventral portion of the mesencephalon.

VIII. **DEVELOPMENT OF THE RHOMBENCEPHALON**

A. **General features of rhombencephalic development**
   1. The most caudal of the three primary brain vesicles, the rhombencephalon, or hindbrain, becomes subdivided into a cranial **metencephalon** and a caudal **myelencephalon**.
      a. The **metencephalon** forms the **pons** and the **cerebellum**.
      b. The **myelencephalon** forms the **medulla oblongata**.
   2. The metencephalon has a clearly demarcated sulcus limitans and therefore well defined alar and basal laminae. However, its **roof plate** becomes considerably expanded.
      a. This expansion causes the walls of the hindbrain to become separated from one another, much like the pages in a book with the binding of the book placed ventrally (Fig. 11-11).
      b. Thus, the **alar laminae** are widely spaced and lie dorsolateral to the closely spaced and ventromedial **basal laminae**.
      c. This arrangement helps one to understand some of the functional arrangement of brain nuclei.
   3. The development of the myelencephalon into the medulla oblongata is relatively straightforward.

B. **Development of alar laminae of the myelencephalon to form the medulla oblongata**
   1. The alar laminae of the myelencephalon release some cells that migrate cranially and ventrally to form the **olivary nucleus**.
   2. The alar laminae next become differentiated into three **afferent (sensory) nuclei**.
      a. The most dorsolateral of these nuclei, the **somatic afferent nuclei**, receive sensory input from the ear (via the **vestibulocochlear nerve**) and head (via the **trigeminal nerve**).

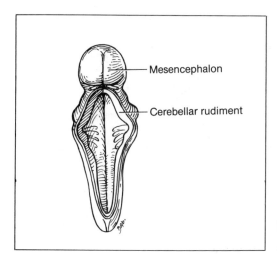

Figure 11-11. Dorsal view of the early rhombencephalon (1 month), with the roof of the fourth ventricle removed to show the cerebellar rudiment.

     b. Intermediate **special visceral afferent nuclei** receive nerve fibers from the taste buds on the tongue and from other nerve endings in the oral cavity and pharynx.
     c. The most ventromedial of these nuclei, the **general visceral afferent nuclei**, contribute mainly to the sensory component of the dorsal nucleus of the vagus nerve.

C. Development of the basal laminae of the myelencephalon to form the medulla oblongata. The basal laminae of the myelencephalon also form three different nuclei, in this case **efferent (motor) nuclei.**

    1. The most dorsolateral of these nuclei, the **general visceral efferent nuclei**, form nearest the sulcus limitans. These nuclei contain the cell bodies of motor neurons that supply the involuntary muscles in the gastrointestinal tract, the respiratory tract (which, after all, arises as a diverticulum of the gastrointestinal tract), and the heart.
    2. **Special visceral efferent nuclei** form as well. These contain motor neurons for cranial nerves IX (glossopharyngeal), X (vagus), and XI (accessory).
    3. The most ventromedial nuclei to form are called the **somatic efferent nuclei.** These contribute to cranial nerve XII (hypoglossal), which supplies the motor innervation for the muscles of the tongue.

D. The rhombic lip–cerebellum

    1. The arrangement of alar and basal laminae in the **metencephalon** is distorted to a certain extent due to the fact that the dorsal part of the metencephalic alar laminae forms **the rhombic lip.**
    2. The cranial portion of the rhombic lip becomes extensively thickened to form the **cerebellar rudiment.**
    3. The rhombic lip is V-shaped at first, with the point of the V pointing in a cranial direction, but it soon becomes compressed in a cranial–caudal axis by the pontine flexure, so that it forms a **cerebellar plate.**
    4. Later, the cerebellar plate gains a central **vermis** and two **lateral hemispheres.** A transverse fissure then forms and separates a **nodule** from the vermis and a **flocculus** from the hemispheres (Fig. 11-12). Other fissures also form, producing other structures in the vermis and lateral hemispheres.

E. Histogenesis of the cerebellum (Fig. 11-13)

    1. The histogenesis of the cerebellar cortex differs significantly from the development of the rest of the neural tube.
    2. As in the rest of the neural tube, the cerebellum arises from a pseudostratified neuroepithelium, in this case the neuroepithelium of the rhombic lip.
    3. Cell proliferation is also quite active in the neuroepithelium near the fourth ventricle.
    4. In addition, however, an entire population of proliferative neuroepithelial cells migrates

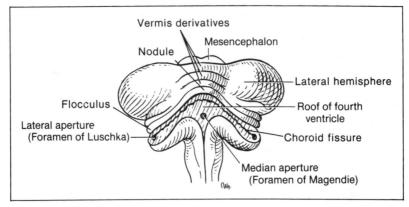

Figure 11-12. Dorsal view of the later rhombencephalon (5 months), showing the apertures in the roof of the fourth ventricle and formation of the extraventricular cerebellum.

away from the ventricular mantle layer and through the deep part of the marginal layer, to the superficial portion of the marginal layer.
   a. This superficial layer of cells is the **external granular layer**.
   b. These displaced neuroepithelial cells begin to proliferate extensively, so that the marginal layer expands more quickly than the mantle layer, resulting in the formation of marked **folds** on the surface of the cerebellar cortex, the so-called **folia**.

5. While the surface of the cerebellum is becoming folded due to differential cell proliferation, an **internal granular layer** is established. The cells of the internal granular layer arise from division of neuroepithelial cells in the mantle layer, followed by migration of neuroblasts into the deep portion of the marginal layer.

6. **Cell types produced in the various layers**
   a. The neuroblasts of the **internal granular layer** differentiate into two types of neurons, the **Purkinje cells** and **Golgi neurons.**
   b. Other neuroepithelial cells in the mantle layer proliferate to form the **dentate nucleus** and other cerebellar nuclei.
   c. At the same time, the **external granular layer** produces some cells that differentiate into neurons and glia. These migrate toward the internal granular layer and become associated with Purkinje cells.

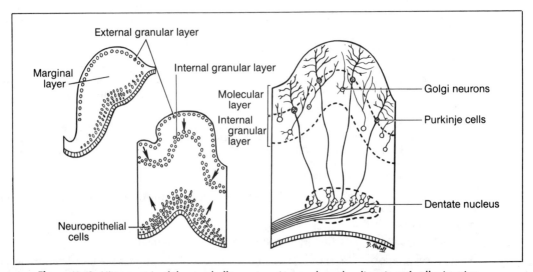

Figure 11-13. Histogenesis of the cerebellar cortex. *Arrows* show the direction of cell migration.

F. **Development of the pons**
 1. The pons carries nerve fibers that connect the spinal cord to the cerebellum and the cerebrum.
 2. The alar plates of the caudal metencephalon and cranial myelencephalon give rise to populations of migrating neurons that migrate ventral to the basal plates and establish **pontine nuclei**.
 3. The basal plates of the metencephalon show extensive expansion of their marginal layers as they produce large numbers of fiber tracts connecting the spinal cord with the cerebellum and cerebrum.

G. **Development of the roof plate of the rhombencephalon.** The roof plate of the rhombencephalon lies over the fourth ventricle and has an unusual developmental history.
 1. The rhombencephalic roof plate becomes extremely attenuated early in its development.
 2. In addition, it becomes deeply invaginated by a **choroid fissure** which later develops into the **choroid plexus** of the fourth ventricle. The choroid plexus, as in all ventricles, is the site of production of cerebrospinal fluid.
 3. The roof of the fourth ventricle forms an **ependymal diverticulum** which bulges away from the ventricle and eventually ruptures to form a single **median aperture** (the **foramen of Magendie**).
 4. Later, two **lateral apertures (foramina of Luschka)** also form by a similar mechanism.
 5. These apertures (see Fig. 11-12) represent holes in the wall of the neural tube derivatives which form a continuous sheet of epithelium elsewhere in the brain and spinal cord.
 6. These holes represent an outflow tract for the **cerebrospinal fluid** from the source of its production at the choroid plexus into the **subarachnoid space**.
 7. In essence, these apertures represent a breach in the neuroepithelial surface so that the luminal surfaces and the external surfaces are continuous with one another. Both surfaces are also bathed constantly in cerebrospinal fluid.

IX. **CONGENITAL ABNORMALITIES OF THE NERVOUS SYSTEM.** As one might imagine from a system with such a complex developmental history, there are a host of congenital defects that have profound effects on the structure and function of the nervous system.

A. **Neural tube defects.** Neural tube defects are by far the most common group of congenital anomalies of the nervous system. Because they result from a failure of neural tube closure during neurulation, they are discussed in Chapter 5.

B. **Hydrocephalus.** In addition to failures of neural tube closure, the developing brain can be altered by conditions that **restrict the outflow of cerebrospinal fluid** from the brain. In such cases, the condition known as **hydrocephalus** develops.
 1. **Causes of hydrocephalus**
    a. Hydrocephalus is caused by the congenital accumulation of cerebrospinal fluid, resulting in expansion of the brain ventricles.
    b. It may also result from a blockage of the median or lateral apertures in the roof of the fourth ventricle.
 2. **Consequences**
    a. The accumulation of fluid in the ventricles of the brain causes them to expand abnormally. The eventual consequences may be:
       (1) A marked increase in the diameter of the skull
       (2) Thinning of the membranous neurocranium, with or without improper closure of the sutures
    b. Hydrocephalic children often exhibit mental retardation to a variable extent.
 3. Recent studies in nonhuman primates suggest that congenital hydrocephalus can be corrected by placing shunts in fetuses in utero, prior to irreversible brain damage. Such techniques offer great promise for application to human subjects in the future.

C. Plasticity and mental retardation
 1. Some parts of the developing brain show a striking **plasticity**, in that gross morphologic defects can be compensated for by some poorly understood mechanism.

- a. For example, there are instances in the medical literature of patients entirely **lacking a cerebellum.** Nevertheless, the patients exhibit only mild lack of coordination.
- b. Similarly, **defects in the corpus callosum** have been reported with only modest clinical symptoms.

2. Many congenital syndromes have **mental retardation** as one of the components, but are not associated with obvious structural abnormalities in the brain. For example, children with **Down syndrome** invariably show mental retardation, but there is no clear-cut anatomic abnormality in their brains.

STUDY QUESTIONS

Directions: Each question below contains four suggested answers of which **one or more** is correct. Choose the answer

- A if **1, 2, and 3** are correct
- B if **1 and 3** are correct
- C if **2 and 4** are correct
- D if **4** is correct
- E if **1, 2, 3, and 4** are correct

1. True statements about the proliferating neuroepithelium include which of the following?

   (1) The internal limiting membrane is a basement membrane at the lumen of the neural tube
   (2) The external limiting membrane is a basement membrane at the periphery of the neural tube
   (3) The neuroepithelium is a stratified epithelium at first
   (4) Interkinetic nuclear migration is responsible for the pseudostratified character of the epithelium

2. The glia limitans has which of the following characteristics?

   (1) Neuronal cells are part of it
   (2) Glial cells have their foot processes on the external limiting membrane
   (3) The glia limitans has no astrocytes
   (4) The glia limitans forms the outer boundary of the nervous system

3. Characteristics of neuroblasts include which of the following?

   (1) They form neurons
   (2) They form glial cells
   (3) They form Purkinje cells in the cerebellum
   (4) They are postmitotic cells

4. Glioblasts form which of the following cell types?

   (1) Astrocytes
   (2) Oligodendroglial cells
   (3) Myelinating cells in the central nervous system
   (4) Microglia

5. True statements about myelination include which of the following?

   (1) Neural crest derivatives myelinate cell processes in the peripheral nervous system
   (2) Oligodendroglial cells myelinate cell processes in the central nervous system
   (3) The mesaxon grows to form multiple layers of membrane
   (4) Myelination is completed by birth

6. Which of the following would be alar plate or alar lamina derivatives?

   (1) Spinal cord sensory neurons
   (2) Spinal cord motor neurons
   (3) Mesencephalic tectal nuclei
   (4) Dorsal root ganglia

7. Which of the following would be basal plate or basal lamina derivatives

   (1) Mesencephalic tegmental nuclei
   (2) Motor neurons in the spinal cord
   (3) Rhombencephalic general visceral efferent nuclei
   (4) Rhombencephalic special visceral afferent nuclei

Directions: The groups of questions below consist of lettered choices followed by several numbered items. For each numbered item select the **one** lettered choice with which it is **most** closely associated. Each lettered choice may be used once, more than once, or not at all.

Questions 8–12

For each description below of the development of an adult brain structure, select the appropriate lettered structure shown in the accompanying drawing of an adult brain.

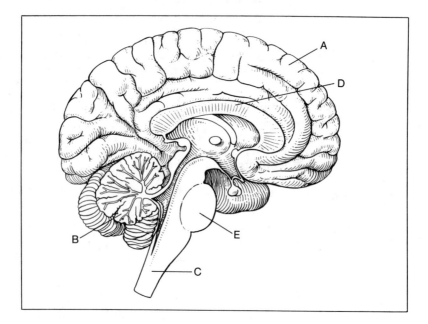

8. This structure develops from the myelencephalon of the rhombencephalon

9. This structure develops from the telencephalon of the prosencephalon

10. This structure develops from the rhombic lip

11. This structure develops from the metencephalon of the rhombencephalon but not from the rhombic lip

12. This structure contains Purkinje cells, Golgi neurons, and cortical gray matter

Questions 13–17

For each description below of a structure in the developing spinal cord, select the appropriate lettered portion of the developing spinal cord shown in the accompanying photomicrograph.

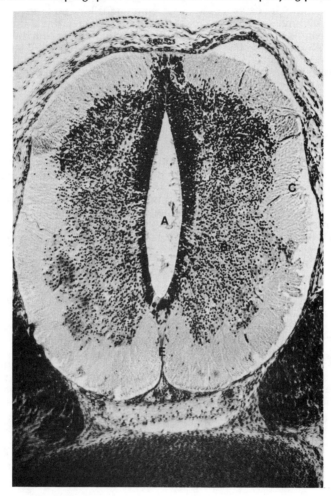

13. This structure is formed by rapid growth of motor neurons in the basal plate

14. This structure was once continuous with the amniotic cavity but now communicates with the brain ventricles

15. This structure contains neuroblasts that will differentiate into neurons which synapse with neural crest–derived neurons in the dorsal root ganglia

16. This structure contains many neuronal cell bodies and relatively little myelin

17. This structure contains relatively few neuronal cell bodies and many myelinated axons and dendrites

ANSWERS AND EXPLANATIONS

1. The answer is C (2, 4). *(II A, B)* The internal limiting membrane is located at the lumen of the neural tube, but it is not really a membrane. Instead, it consists of tight apical junctions between neuroepithelial cells. The external limiting membrane is located at the periphery of the neural tube and is the basement membrane for the neuroepithelium. The neuroepithelium is a pseudostratified epithelium, and this characteristic is due to interkinetic nuclear migration. The neuroepithelium is never truly stratified.

2. The answer is C (2, 4). *(II B 4)* The glia limitans forms at the external limiting membrane as astrocyte foot processes become pushed up against the external limiting membrane from within the neuroepithelium. Astrocytes (a kind of glial cell) are definitely part of the glia limitans. It does indeed form the outer boundary of the nervous system.

3. The answer is B (1, 3). *(II B 2, 3)* Neuroblasts form many different types of neurons in the nervous system, including the cerebellar Purkinje cells. Glioblasts form glial cells. The neuroblasts are capable of extensive mitotic divisions. For example, in the cerebral and cerebellar cortex, an entire population of neuroblasts divides extensively to form the peripheral gray matter of the brain.

4. The answer is A (1, 2, 3). *(II B 4)* Glioblasts form several different kinds of glial cells, including astrocytes and oligodendroglial cells. The latter cells are responsible for myelination in the central nervous system. The microglia are part of the mononuclear phagocyte system and arise from monocytes, a form of white blood cell, rather than from the neuroepithelium, the source of all glioblasts.

5. The answer is A (1, 2, 3). *(II F 2, 3)* Myelination is performed by Schwann cells (which are neural crest derivatives) in the peripheral nervous system, and by oligodendroglial cells (glioblast derivatives) in the central nervous system. The mesaxons of the myelinating cells grow extensively in a spiral fashion around processes (axons and dendrites) to be myelinated. Myelination occurs extensively both before and after birth. Myelination serves to isolate nerve processes from one another so that impulses are conducted in a separated manner.

6. The answer is B (1, 3). *(II D 2 a; III C 2; VII B 1)* The alar plate and alar laminae are dorsal structures in the neural tube. They contain the cell bodies of developing sensory neurons in the spinal cord and developing neurons that form the tectal nuclei in the mesencephalon. The motor neurons develop in the basal plates. The neurons in dorsal root ganglia are neural crest derivatives.

7. The answer is A (1, 2, 3). *(II D 2 a; VII B 2)* The basal plate and basal laminae are ventral structures in the neural tube. They contain the cell bodies of developing motor neurons in the spinal cord and developing neurons that form the tegmental nuclei in the mesencephalon. They also form general visceral efferent nuclei in the rhombencephalon. The special visceral afferent nuclei in the rhombencephalon form from the alar laminae.

8–12. The answers are: 8-C, 9-A, 10-B, 11-E, 12-B. *(V A, C, D)* The cerebrum (A) is formed by the telencephalic hemispheres, which are in turn derived from the prosencephalon (forebrain). The cerebellum (B) forms in the rhombic lip of the metencephalon, which is in turn derived from the rhombencephalon (hindbrain). The cerebellum has cortical gray matter like the cerebrum but contains Purkinje cells (neurons) and Golgi neurons peculiar to the cerebellum. The medulla oblongata (C) forms from the myelencephalon, which in turn develops from the caudal portion of the rhombencephalon. The origin of the corpus callosum (D) is not described by any of the questions. The corpus callosum is the most important commissure of the brain. It connects the non-olfactory areas of the cerebral hemispheres. It forms as a small bundle of nerve fibers in the medial portion of the telencephalon (lamina terminalis) and expands over the diencephalon. The pons (E) forms from the metencephalon of the rhombencephalon.

13–17. The answers are: 13-E, 14-A, 15-D, 16-B, 17-C. *(III A, B, C)* The central canal of the spinal cord (A) faces onto the amniotic cavity when the neural plate is still flat. It becomes the lumen of the neural tube, and is a continuous cavity from the ventricles of the brain to the central canal of the spinal cord. This cavity contains cerebrospinal fluid. The mantle layer (B) contains many neuroblasts but little myelin. The marginal layer (C) contains few neurons and many myelinated processes. The alar plate (D) lies dorsally and contains neuroblasts that differentiate into sensory neurons which in turn synapse with the pseudounipolar neurons formed in the dorsal root ganglia (neural crest derivatives). The ventral median fissure (E) is a deep recess that appears in the neural tube as a result of the relatively greater growth in the flanking basal plates. These basal plates (unlabelled) contain neuroblasts that differentiate into large motor neurons.

12
Development of the Integument and Teeth

I. INTRODUCTION: General features of the skin and its appendages

A. Functions of the skin
1. The entire outer surface of the body, except for the cornea, is covered by skin.
2. This complex covering layer is essential to life. It serves as:
   a. A barrier against infection
   b. A hydrophobic layer to prevent loss of vital tissue fluids
   c. A mechanism to alter the core body temperature, performing this function in two ways:
      (1) By regulating blood flow through the capillary beds serving the skin
      (2) By producing sweat, an evaporating fluid that can cool the body

B. Histology of the skin and its appendages
1. The skin is made up of a stratified squamous keratinized epithelium known as the **epidermis** and a dense irregular connective tissue known as the **dermis**.
   a. The **epidermis** is derived from the ectoderm.
   b. The **dermis** is derived from the mesoderm of the dermatomes.
2. The **epidermis** is made up of a number of **layers**.
   a. Proceeding from the innermost layer outward, the layers are:
      (1) Stratum basale (stratum germinativum)
      (2) Stratum spinosum
      (3) Stratum granulosum
      (4) Stratum lucidum (present only in very thick areas, such as the sole of the foot)
      (5) Stratum corneum
   b. The stratification represents different **stages of keratinization**, with cells becoming more and more keratinized as they progress to the outermost layers of the epidermis.
3. The skin produces acellular **protective appendages**, the **hair** and **nails**, in several locations.
   a. These structures are formed entirely from the epidermis.
   b. However, formation is under the inductive influence of the dermis closely associated with hair follicles or nail beds.
   c. The development of the skin's appendages is also partially under hormonal control.
4. **Skin color**, with its variations in different ethnic and racial groups, is due to the action of the **melanocyte**, a neural crest derivative and therefore ectodermal in origin.
5. On the surface of the body, the skin is constantly subjected to abrasion. The basal layer of cells in the skin proliferates constantly and then differentiates into **keratinized cells** which eventually dry out and desquamate from the surface.
6. **Glands** in the skin come in several varieties.
   a. The **eccrine** and **apocrine sweat glands** produce perspiration for cooling and specialized secretions, respectively.
   b. The **sebaceous glands** produce sebum for lubricating and conditioning the skin.
7. The **mammary glands** are highly modified sweat glands and they develop as appendages of the skin.
8. **Teeth** develop in the oral cavity from oral ectoderm, neural crest cells, and associated mesenchyme.

II. EMBRYOLOGY OF THE SKIN

A. Development of the skin

1. **Epidermis.** The epidermis of the skin is derived from the **ectoderm**.
   a. In the 5-week fetus, the skin is a simple cuboidal epithelium.
   b. By 7 weeks, the ectodermal component of the skin is two layers thick (Fig. 12-1).
      (1) The single squamous layer on top is known as the **periderm**, or **epitrichium** (Fig. 12-2).
      (2) Beneath the periderm is a basal layer of cuboidal cells.
   c. By 4 months, an intermediate layer, three to five cell layers in thickness, has been interposed between the cuboidal basal cells and the periderm (Figs. 12-3 and 12-4).
   d. After 4 months, the epidermis continues to increase in thickness, until at birth it has the essential histologic characteristics of adult skin.

2. **Dermis**
   a. The dermis develops from **mesenchymal cells** derived from the somite by way of the **dermatome**. This mesenchymal domain is known as the **corium** (see Fig. 12-1).
   b. A basement membrane separates the corium from the basal layer of the epidermis (see Fig. 12-4).
   c. As the epidermis thickens, the corium also thickens into a dense, irregular connective tissue domain by mesenchymal cell proliferation.
   d. **Dermal papillae** arise during the fourth month by differential growth in the epidermis, and become increasingly complex in their foldings. The dermal papillae serve to anchor the epidermis firmly to the dermis.
   e. Most of the increase in the thickness of the skin is due to an increase in the thickness of the dermis.

3. At birth, the epidermis and dermis have the essential histologic features of adult skin, although newborn skin is not yet as thick as adult skin (Fig. 12-5).

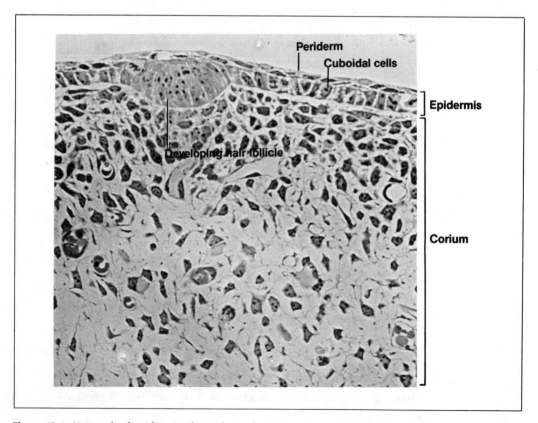

Figure 12-1. Human fetal epidermis when it has only two layers, an outer periderm and an inner basal layer. Note the condensation of mesenchymal cells in the corium, a precursor of the dermis.

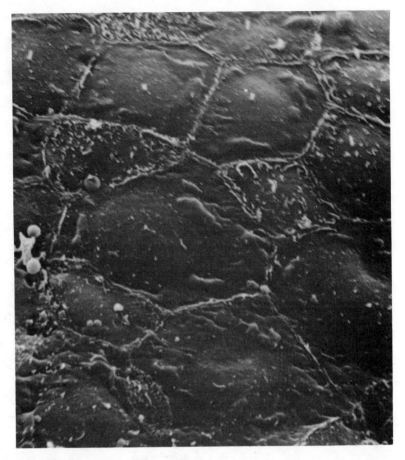

Figure 12-2. Squamous cells of the periderm, viewed from the external surface (apical surface) of the epidermis. (Scanning electron micrograph)

B. Neural crest contributions

1. The neural crest produces a migratory population of cells called **melanoblasts**. During the fourth month, **melanocytes** invade the epidermal component of the skin.
2. Melanocytes produce **melanin granules** and pass them into cells in the stratum basale.

III. KERATINIZATION

A. General features of keratinization

1. Keratinization begins in late fetal life and continues throughout adult life.
   a. Keratinization is the process whereby the living, dividing cells in the stratum basale are converted into the dried, keratin-filled dead cells of the stratum corneum.
   b. These dead, dried cells filled with hydrophobic proteins serve two major **functions.**
      (1) They limit water loss from the body.
      (2) They restrict the entry of noxious substances and microorganisms into the body.
   c. Although stratified squamous epithelium is present wherever body surfaces are subjected to abrasion (skin, oral cavity, esophagus, vagina), only the skin is also keratinized.
2. Keratinization is a particularly evident example of **terminal cellular differentiation**.
   a. This growth process is characterized by the continuous proliferation of an undifferentiated stem cell population, resulting in large numbers of cells that undergo terminal differentiation but can no longer divide (see Chapter 1, section III B 5). In the case of keratinization,
      (1) The stem cell population consists of the dividing cells in the stratum basale.

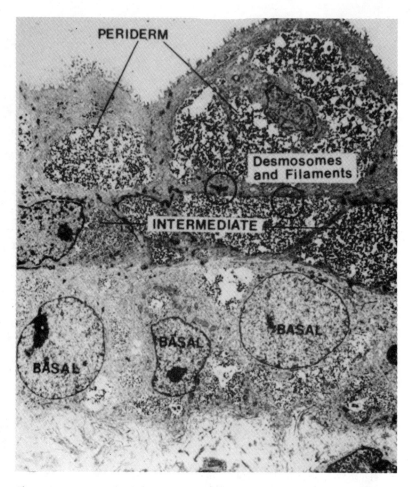

Figure 12-3. Human fetal skin after the establishment of an intermediate layer between the basal layer and the periderm. (Transmission electron micrograph). (Reprinted with permission of the National Foundation from Holbrook KA, Smith LT: Ultrastructural aspects of human skin during the embryonic, fetal, premature, neonatal, and adult periods of life. In *Morphogenesis and Malformation of the Skin*, edited by Blandau RF. New York, Alan R. Liss, 1981, p 21.)

      (2) The terminally differentiated cells are the dead cells of the stratum corneum.
   b. The death of a cell in the epidermis is more rapid, but no less inevitable, than the death of a highly differentiated red cell in the blood or pyramidal neuron in the cerebrum. All three cells have become highly differentiated and have also lost the ability to proliferate, thus ensuring that they will have a shortened life span.
   c. In contrast, the cells in the stratum basale of the epidermis, along with spermatogonia, hematogenous cell lines, and cells lining the crypts in the intestines do not differentiate but remain proliferative throughout the life of the organism.

B. The process of keratinization

  1. Keratinization has three **stages**.
    a. First, of course, the cells that will become committed to the "fatal" differentiation step must be produced. This is accomplished by repeated mitotic divisions of proliferative cells in the stratum basale.
    b. Second, cells in the stratum basale and stratum spinosum must become committed to the production of certain proteins characteristic of keratinized cells.
    c. Third, these proteins must be produced in large quantity. In fact, they accumulate within the cells to such an extent that they dominate the cell and lead to the exclusion of all other organelles.

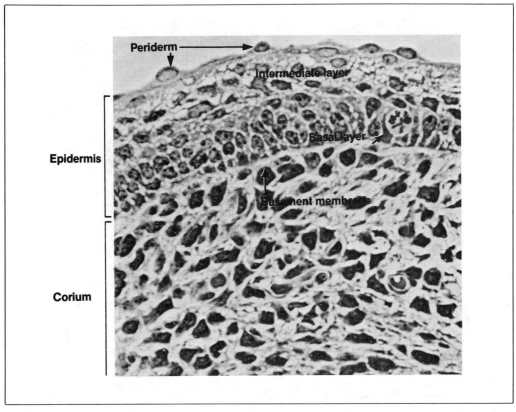

Figure 12-4. Full thickness of human fetal skin after the establishment of an intermediate layer. (Histologic section)

2. The **stratifications** in the epidermis are merely different stages in the process of keratinization.
   a. The completely proliferative, unkeratinized cells lie near the basement membrane.
   b. The nonproliferative, completely keratinized cells make up the outermost layers of the epidermis.
   c. Between these two extremes, intermediate stages in the accumulation of keratin are evident.
3. While keratin is accumulating within cells, lamellated **granules** also accumulate.
   a. These granules are composed of lipids and proteins.
   b. The bipolar lipids derived from the lamellated granules are expelled from cells during keratinization.
4. The end result of keratin accumulation and expulsion of the bipolar lipids is the death of the cell and the erection of a substantial **hydrophobic barrier**, preventing passage of water into or out of the body.

C. **Characteristics of keratin and other proteins of the stratum corneum.** Because of extensive **crosslinking**, the proteins of the stratum corneum are very resistant to dissolution.
   1. **Keratin** is a very stable, highly insoluble protein because it contains some sulfur with crosslinking by disulfide bridges. Keratin can be dissolved by strong acid but otherwise it remains insoluble.
   2. The **proteins derived from keratohyalin granules** are also extensively crosslinked, via disulfide bonds, both to their own kind and to the other proteins of the keratin.

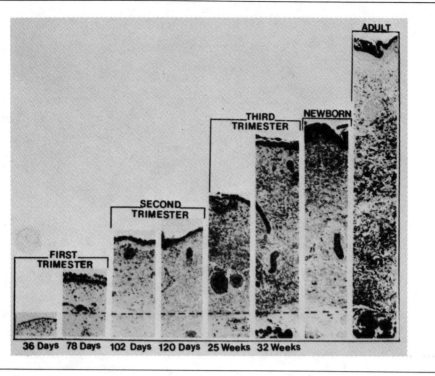

Figure 12-5. Changes in the thickness of human skin at different stages of development. (Reprinted with permission of the National Foundation from Holbrook KA, Smith LT: Ultrastructural aspects of human skin during the embryonic, fetal, premature, neonatal, and adult periods of life. In *Morphogenesis and Malformation of the Skin*, edited by Blandau RF. New York, Alan R. Liss, 1981, p 11.)

IV. DEVELOPMENT OF APPENDAGES OF THE SKIN

A. Role of inductive interaction

1. The epidermal appendages include:
   a. Eccrine and apocrine sweat glands
   b. Sebaceous glands
   c. Hairs
   d. Fingernails and toenails
2. These appendages of the skin are all derived from the **ectoderm**. Their formation, however, is controlled at least partially by the inductive influence of the underlying **mesoderm**.
   a. The appendages form first as **epidermal invaginations**. Mesenchymal cells become condensed around these surface invaginations (Fig. 12-6).
   b. This association between mesodermal cells and the ectodermal invaginations is important in inducing the differentiation of specific types of appendages.
      (1) Experimental studies with animals show that the **ability** to form appendages is an innate property of the **epidermis**, but the **specific kind of appendage** formed is dictated by the underlying **mesenchymal inducer**; that is, the local dermal cells.
      (2) In these studies, microsurgical techniques are used to separate embryonic epidermis and dermis and then recombine them in different ways. For example, recombinations in birds give the following results:
         (a) If wing epidermis is combined with belly mesenchyme and the combination is transplanted into the wing, then belly-type feathers will form in the wing region.
         (b) If belly epidermis is combined with wing mesenchyme and the combination is transplanted into the belly, then wing-type feathers will form in the belly region.

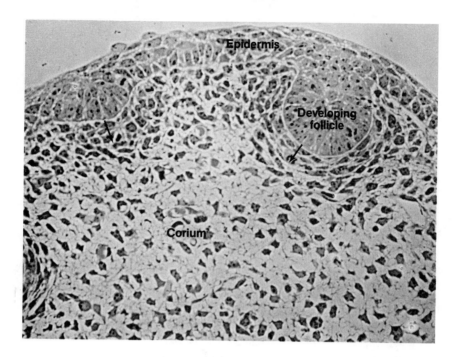

Figure 12-6. Early development of hair buds in human fetal skin. Note the mesenchymal condensations around the developing hair follicles (*arrows*). (Light micrograph)

3. The development of the skin's appendages is also partially under **hormonal control**. For example, the amount and pattern of hair on the body which contribute to secondary sexual differences are clearly under the control of estrogen and androgen levels.

B. Development of hair follicles and hair
1. Hair follicles begin to develop in the skin early in the third month.
    a. The follicles develop first as localized regions of epidermal proliferation and invagination, called **hair buds**, which grow down into a region of mesenchymal condensation (see Figs. 12-1 and 12-6).
        (1) At first, the hair bud is cylindrical, but the distal tip soon becomes bulbous as it is deeply invaginated by a mesodermally derived **hair papilla** (Figs. 12-7 and 12-8). The hair papilla probably has an inductive influence on the epidermal cells, promoting hair formation.
        (2) Some of the mesenchymal cells in the hair papilla now differentiate into **blood vessels**.
    b. As the hair bud elongates, cells in the wall of the developing hair follicle send out secondary buds of proliferating cells which differentiate into **sebaceous glands** (see Fig. 12-7).
    c. Other mesenchymal cells differentiate into small slips of smooth muscle called the **arrector pili muscle** (see Figs. 12-7 and 12-8).
2. The **hair** itself is composed of keratin secreted by epidermal cells.
    a. Hairs become visible on the surface of the body after the fifth month.
        (1) The first fine hairs to form are known as the **lanugo**.
        (2) At about the time of birth, lanugo hairs are replaced by the larger **vellus** hairs.
    b. At **puberty**, coarse hairs appear on the body.
        (1) These grow in the axilla, the pubic region, and other areas such as the legs, chest, face, and stomach.
        (2) The amount and distribution of **secondary body hairs** is under the control of sex hormones and is one of the important secondary sexual characteristics.

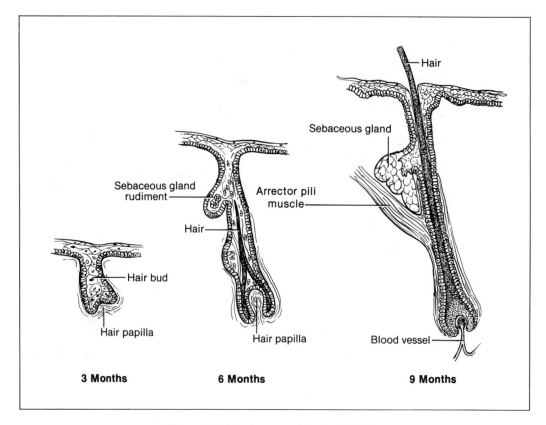

Figure 12-7. Development of the hair follicle.

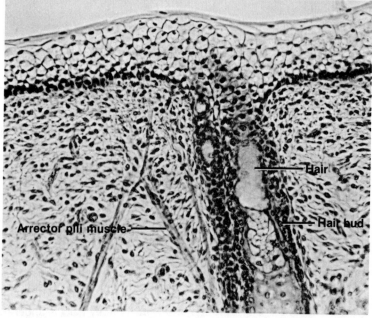

Figure 12-8. A developing hair follicle in human fetal skin. (Light micrograph)

C. Development of sebaceous glands

1. During the fifth month, peripheral cells in the hair follicle begin a localized proliferation to form a sebaceous gland (see Fig. 12-7).
2. As the cell nest grows away from the axis of the hair shaft, the central cells in the nest undergo a differentiation into cells laden with lipid droplets.
3. Next, these lipid-rich cells degenerate, spilling their **sebum** into the hair follicle.
   a. The sebum mixes with desquamated epidermal cells to make up the **vernix caseosa**.
   b. This protective material is a whitish, cheesy substance which coats the embryo, protecting the skin as the embryo develops in the fluid-filled environment of the amniotic cavity.

D. Development of sweat glands

1. Eccrine sweat glands develop as downgrowths of epithelial cords of cells in much the same way as the hair follicles develop.
2. However, the eccrine glands do not become associated with a mesenchymal papilla. Instead, they become canalized by a lumen and become extensively coiled as they continue to grow downward away from the epidermal surface.

V. DEVELOPMENT OF TEETH (Fig. 12-9)

A. The process of tooth formation

1. **The dental lamina**
   a. In a 7-week fetus, it is possible to observe a thickening in the oral epithelium covering both the developing mandible and the developing maxilla.
   b. This thickening, the **dental lamina**, sends out localized proliferations which penetrate the underlying mesenchyme and (by 2 to 4 months) give rise to cup-shaped **enamel organs**.

2. **Enamel organs and dental papillae** (see Fig. 12-9)
   a. A separate enamel organ forms for each of the primary teeth.
      (1) The enamel organ grows larger and becomes deeply invaginated.
      (2) Within the deep invagination, a mesenchymal condensation, the **dental papilla**, forms.

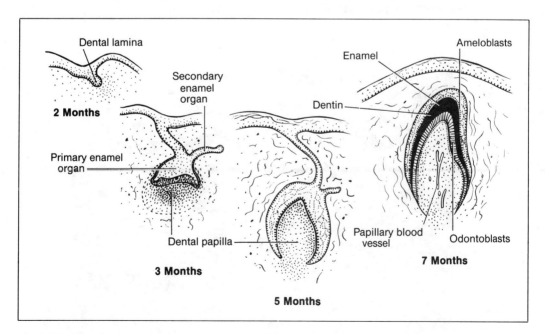

Figure 12-9. Development of a tooth. The secondary enamel organ has been omitted from the 7-months tooth for simplicity.

(3) The dental papilla consists of a dense collection of stellate cells that will eventually form most of the tooth proper, including the pulp cavity, dentin, and blood supply for the tooth.
  b. Tooth formation involves an **epithelial–mesenchymal interaction** between the ectodermally derived enamel organ and the mesenchymally derived dental papilla: The enamel organ is induced to form a tooth by the dental papilla.
  c. The specific **morphology** of the tooth in terms of shape and number of cusps is controlled by the dental papilla.

3. **Formation of dentin and enamel.** On one surface of the enamel organ, a layer of ectodermally derived **ameloblasts** form **enamel** and mesenchymally derived **odontoblasts** form **dentin** (Figs. 12-9 and 12-10), beginning at about 7 months. The mesenchyme which forms odontoblasts receives a contribution from the **neural crest**.
  a. Initially, **odontoblasts** secrete a collagenous extracellular matrix known as **predentin**. This becomes calcified extracellularly to result in **dentin**, a hard bone-like material.
  b. The formation of dentin seems to induce **ameloblasts** to produce a **crown** consisting of a second calcified extracellular matrix, the **enamel**.
    (1) The crown forms first on the **cusps** of the developing tooth.
    (2) It then grows toward the area where the **roots** of the tooth will form.

4. **Formation of tooth roots and cementum**
  a. The **roots** are next formed by odontoblast secretion of predentin. The roots of teeth lack enamel. Roots begin to form at about 7 months and continue to grow after birth.
  b. The formation of the root seems to induce certain mesenchymal cells to differentiate into **cementoblasts**.
    (1) These cells then secrete a third calcified extracellular matrix, the **cementum**.
    (2) This material aids in fixing the teeth in their bony sockets in the maxilla and mandible.

B. **Odontoblasts, predentin, and dentin**

1. **Odontoblasts** differentiate from neural crest–derived mesenchymal cells of the dental papilla immediately adjacent to the basement membrane of the enamel organ.
  a. They become extremely elongated and form an epithelioid layer adjacent to the enamel organ.
  b. As they lay down predentin and dentin, they recede centripetally, resulting in a progressive decrease in the size of the dental papilla.
  c. As odontoblasts lay down an ever thickening layer of dentin, they leave behind **odontoblast processes (Tomes fibers)** similar to the processes of osteocytes. These pro-

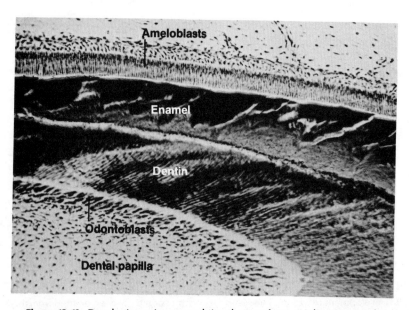

Figure 12-10. Developing primary tooth in a human fetus. (Light micrograph)

cesses become surrounded by dentin and are contained in **dentinal tubules** that are much like the canaliculi in bone.
2. **Predentin** is a mixture of collagen, glycoproteins, and several kinds of proteoglycans.
3. Following its secretion from the odontoblasts, predentin becomes calcified into dentin by the accumulation of **hydroxyapatite**.
4. **Dentin** is a good deal like bone in many respects but it is denser and harder than bone.

C. **Deciduous and permanent teeth**
1. As the enamel organs grow, the **primary (deciduous) teeth** erupt into the oral cavity for use by the child in mastication. The eruption of primary teeth may begin prior to birth and continues through early childhood.
2. The enamel organs for the primary teeth also form a branch, the **secondary enamel organ** (see Fig. 12-9), which gives rise in turn to the **secondary (permanent) teeth** of the adult.
   a. The secondary enamel organs grow during childhood, forming the secondary teeth in the same manner as described above.
   b. Eventually, the growing secondary teeth force the shedding of the deciduous teeth, thereby inducing a raid on parental wallets to appease the tooth fairy.
3. Deciduous teeth are shed in different parts of the mouth at different times, leaving the child for a time with a serviceable set of mixed primary and secondary teeth that are able to prepare food properly for digestion.

VI. DEVELOPMENT OF THE MAMMARY GLANDS

A. **Early development**
1. The first evidence of the formation of the mammary glands is seen at about the sixth week of development, when a ridge-like ectodermal thickening, the **mammary ridge**, appears.
2. The mammary ridge originally extends along the ventral body wall from the base of the forelimb buds all the way to the future inguinal region at the level of the hindlimb buds.
3. In most locations the mammary ridge regresses, but over the pectoral muscles it begins to proliferate, forming an epithelial cord of cells which grows downward into the surrounding mesenchyme of the skin.

B. **Histogenesis during embryonic life**
1. The downgrowth of epithelial tissue continues to proliferate and bifurcate during the second trimester until about 20 major branches form.
2. The branches develop a lumen and represent the precursors of the major **lactiferous ducts** draining the mammary gland into the nipple.
3. The ducts now contain several types of cells:
   a. **Columnar cells** with an apical–basal polarization
   b. Undifferentiated **basal stem cells**
   c. **Myoepithelial cells**
      (1) Myoepithelial cells are isolated smooth muscle–like cells that are interspersed between the secretory elements of a gland and the basement membrane of the glandular epithelium.
      (2) When the cells contract, they aid in expressing secretion products from the gland.
      (3) Myoepithelial cells are intraepithelial cells and are derived from surface ectodermal invaginations, rather than from mesenchyme as one might suppose from the fact that they are similar to smooth muscle cells.
4. During the third trimester, the ducts continue to elongate and branch, until eventually they begin to penetrate the subcutaneous connective tissue.

C. **Histogenesis after birth**
1. Due to hormonal influences, presumably related to the physiology of the birth process, there is a final burst of glandular proliferation in the **newborn**. In some cases, there is a transient secretory activity and fluid production (**"witch's milk"**) in the newborn's mammary gland.
2. During **childhood**, the mammary tissue grows along with the rest of the body. With the **approach of puberty** in female children, the mammary glands undergo increased growth.

3. During **puberty**, the ducts of the mammary glands proliferate extensively. Once the breast has reached its adult size, the breast ducts and glands undergo cyclic proliferation and regression so that the absolute amount of glandular tissue remains essentially constant.
4. If **pregnancy** occurs, the ducts proliferate extensively and the glandular alveoli increase in number to a marked degree in preparation for lactation.
5. The growth and function of the mammary glands are under **hormonal control** from a number of different sources. Although the entire story is far from complete, three broad generalizations can be made.
   a. First, the **pituitary gland** of the female has a strong influence on the development and secretory activity of the mammary gland.
      (1) **Prolactin** and **adrenocorticotropic hormone (ACTH)** are released from the adenohypophysis during pregnancy.
      (2) These hormones stimulate functional development of the mammary glands.
   b. Second, the **ovary** produces estrogen and progesterone, and these have an important role in the development of the mammary glands.
      (1) **Estrogen** is thought to stimulate ductal growth.
      (2) Estrogen in combination with **progesterone** stimulates development of the secretory alveoli of the glands.
   c. Third, during pregnancy the **placenta** augments the ovarian production of steroid hormones, and it also secretes human placental lactogen (see Chapter 19, section VII).
      (1) **Progesterone** has a stimulatory effect on alveolar proliferation, but it has an inhibitory effect on lactation. Perhaps the abrupt decrease in maternal progesterone levels following parturition is related to the onset of lactation.
      (2) **Human placental lactogen** is very similar to growth hormone. It plays a role in the mobilization of lipids to form free fatty acids and probably also has a nonspecific stimulatory effect on the mammary glands.

VII. CONGENITAL ABNORMALITIES

A. Diseases involving the skin

1. **Congenital ectodermal dysplasia** is a rare hereditary disease in which the development of all ectodermal structures except the neural plate is altered to a variable extent. Mild ectodermal dysplasia can cause only scanty hair and distorted fingernails, but more severe forms also affect the sweat and sebaceous glands and the teeth.
2. Rarely, the skin may be abnormally **hyperkeratinized**, leading to dry and scaly skin, as in the condition known as congenital **ichthyosis**.
3. The skin is also markedly altered in **albinism**, a condition caused by lack of **tyrosinase**, an enzyme involved in melanin synthesis. True albinos lack pigmentation in the skin and hair; even the retina lacks pigmentation.
4. **Ehlers-Danlos syndrome** is a complex of diseases. Several varieties are caused by autosomal dominant mutations.
   a. In Ehlers-Danlos syndrome, dermal collagen fibers are large and irregular in shape.
   b. The skin is thin and shows hyperextensibility.

B. Congenital anomalies in mammary glands and teeth

1. Mammary glands
   a. **Supernumerary nipples (polythelia)** or **mammary glands (polymastia)** are usually found along the mammary ridge on the ventral body wall.
   b. In rare cases, polymastia may occur in other sites, or the mammary glands may be entirely absent (**amastia**).
2. Teeth
   a. There may be minor numerical abnormalities in either the primary or the secondary teeth.
   b. The teeth may show minor abnormalities in the shape of the crown or the root or both.
   c. The formation of enamel on all teeth may also be abnormal, resulting in poorly calcified, brittle enamel (**amelogenesis imperfecta**).

STUDY QUESTIONS

Directions: Each question below contains five suggested answers. Choose the **one best** response to each question.

1. Which of the following statements concerning the developing skin is correct?

   (A) It has an epithelium derived from sclerotome mesenchyme
   (B) It has melanoblasts derived from sclerotome mesenchyme
   (C) It has a basal layer that is proliferative
   (D) It forms hair follicles from the corium
   (E) It forms vellus hairs before lanugo hairs

2. Which of the following statements concerning hair follicles is correct?

   (A) They form by mesenchymal proliferation
   (B) They form by epithelial invagination and are induced by underlying mesenchymal condensations
   (C) They are rarely associated with sebaceous glands
   (D) They form lanugo hairs after birth
   (E) They contribute to the vernix caseosa

3. Keratinization shows which of the following characteristics?

   (A) It involves extensive proliferation but little cell differentiation
   (B) It involves only proliferation of cells in the stratum basale
   (C) It is an example of terminal cell differentiation leading to cell death
   (D) It involves only cell division in the stratum corneum
   (F) It involves formation of keratohyalin granules in the stratum basale

4. Which of the following statements concerning developing teeth is correct?

   (A) The dental lamina forms by mesenchymal proliferation
   (B) Primary teeth lack cementum
   (C) The enamel organ is a neural crest derivative
   (D) Secondary teeth arise from enamel organs after the primordia of primary teeth have formed
   (E) The odontoblasts are enamel organ derivatives that secrete dentin

5. The developing mammary glands show which of the following characteristics?

   (A) They have ductal epithelium derived from mesenchyme
   (B) Multiple hormones control their development
   (C) They have lactiferous sinuses derived from mesenchyme
   (D) They can differentiate to a lactogenic state without estrogen
   (E) They have mesodermally derived myoepithelial cells

Directions: The groups of questions below consist of lettered choices followed by several numbered items. For each numbered item select the **one** lettered choice with which it is **most** closely associated. Each lettered choice may be used once, more than once, or not at all.

Questions 6-10

For each description below of a congenital anomaly of the skin, select the anomaly being described.

(A) Congenital ectodermal dysplasia

(B) Congenital ichthyosis

(C) Albinism

(D) Ehlers-Danlos syndrome

(E) Amastia

6. The dermis is abnormally thin and hyperextensible

7. There is generalized abnormal development of skin, hair, sebaceous glands, and nails

8. The enzyme tyrosinase is congenitally lacking

9. Formation of the mammary glands is defective

10. Keratinization is excessive

ANSWERS AND EXPLANATIONS

1. The answer is C. *(IB; II A1, B 1; IV A, B 2 a)* The stratum basale of the skin is highly proliferative. In fact, it produces all of the other epithelial layers of the skin by mitotic divisions and later differentiation. The sclerotomes are somite derivatives, and thus mesodermal. The epithelium of the skin, the epidermis, is derived from ectoderm. Melanoblasts are neural crest derivatives. Hair follicles form as epidermal invaginations, while the papilla of the hair forms from mesenchymal condensations in the corium. The lanugo hairs form before the vellus hairs.

2. The answer is B. *(IV A, B, C)* The epidermal appendages of the skin all form as epidermal invaginations under the inductive influence of the underlying mesenchyme. Only the papilla of a hair follicle forms from mesenchymal cells. Hair follicles are invariably associated with sebaceous glands. Lanugo hairs form before birth. Hair follicles per se do not contribute to the vernix caseosa, which is a mixture of sloughed dead cells and sebaceous gland secretions.

3. The answer is C. *(III B)* Keratinization involves both cell proliferation (which occurs exclusively in the stratum basale, not in the stratum corneum) and terminal differentiation. In many instances, there is a mutual antagonism between proliferation and differentiation. Thus, highly proliferative cells are not usually highly differentiated. Similarly, highly differentiated cells are not often highly proliferative. The keratohyalin granules are formed in the stratum granulosum, not in the stratum basale.

4. The answer is D. *(V A, 1, 3, 4, C)* The dental lamina is an ectodermal invagination. Primary teeth are anchored to the upper and lower jaw by a layer of cementum. The enamel organ is an ectodermal derivative. The neural crest contributes to the formation of teeth by way of the dentin-secreting odontoblasts. Primary teeth form from an enamel organ that also sends out a branch, the secondary enamel organ, leading to the formation of secondary teeth after the primordia of primary teeth have formed.

5. The answer is B. *(VI B, C 1, 4)* The mammary glands require at least estrogen, progesterone, prolactin, and human placental lactogen for complete development from the embryonic state, through female pubertal development, to full lactogenic differentiation during pregnancy and birth. The ductal, sinusoidal, and secretory alveolar epithelial cells and also the myoepithelial cells are all ectodermal derivatives. Only the connective tissue, fat, and blood vessels in mammary glands are mesodermal derivatives. Estrogen and progesterone are important for the extensive pubertal development of mammary glands in the female.

6–10. The answers are: 6-D, 7-A, 8-C, 9-E, 10-B. *(VII A, B)* Congenital ectodermal dysplasia *(A)* in its severe form affects the development of all non-neural ectodermal derivatives, including the skin, sweat glands, sebaceous glands, hair follicles, and nails. Congenital ichthyosis *(B)* is a disease of excessive keratinization. Albinism *(C)* is an anomaly in which no melanin is formed because of a lack of the enzyme tyrosinase, which is required for melanin synthesis. The Ehlers-Danlos syndrome *(D)* is a complex of several different clinical entities, some of which are caused by autosomal dominant mutations. In this syndrome, the skin is thin and shows hyperextensibility.

13
Development of the Digestive System

I. INTRODUCTION

A. Components of the digestive system (Fig. 13-1)

1. The adult digestive system includes the oral cavity and salivary glands (see Chapter 18), pharynx, esophagus, stomach, small intestines, large intestines, rectum, and anus.
2. The liver, pancreas, and gallbladder are also parts of the digestive system.

B. Early embryology of the digestive system

1. As discussed in Chapter 6, section IV D, the **primitive gut** forms during body flexion when part of the **yolk sac** is incorporated into the embryo. The primitive gut tube remains connected medially to the yolk sac by the **vitelline duct**.
   a. The yolk sac lining is derived from **endoderm**.
   b. Consequently, all of the **epithelial linings** of the digestive system, except for the anterior portion of the mouth and the lower portion of the anal canal, are endodermally derived.
2. The **splanchnic mesoderm** comes to lie over the endodermally derived luminal linings of the digestive system and eventually gives rise to the connective, vascular, and muscular tissues surrounding the gut tube.
3. The intrinsic **enteric nervous system** is a part of the autonomic nervous system. Its neurons are **neural crest** derivatives.
4. The cranial and caudal ends of the gut tube at first are covered over by a thin membrane.
   a. The **stomodeum**, at the cranial entrance to the gut tube, is covered by the **oropharyngeal membrane**.
   b. The **proctodeum**, at the caudal exit of the gut tube, is covered by the **cloacal membrane**.
   c. Both of these thin sheets of tissue are regions where ectodermally and endodermally derived epithelial tissues are closely apposed to one another, without any intervening layer of mesodermally derived mesenchyme.
5. The primitive gut tube is divided into three **subdivisions** (Fig. 13-2):
   a. The **foregut** extends from the **stomodeum** to the **anterior intestinal portal**, the point where the foregut joins the midgut.
   b. The **midgut** extends from the anterior intestinal portal to the posterior intestinal portal.
   c. The **hindgut** extends from the **posterior intestinal portal** to the **proctodeum**.
6. The **liver**, **biliary apparatus**, and **pancreas**, as well as the entire **respiratory system**, arise as diverticula from the foregut; consequently, they have large numbers of glandular epithelial cells derived from endoderm as well as connective tissue and muscular tissue derived from adjacent splanchnic mesoderm.
7. Along its entire length, the gut tube is suspended from the dorsal body wall by a **dorsal mesentery**. Along part of its length, it is attached to the ventral body wall by a **ventral mesentery**.

208 Human Developmental Anatomy

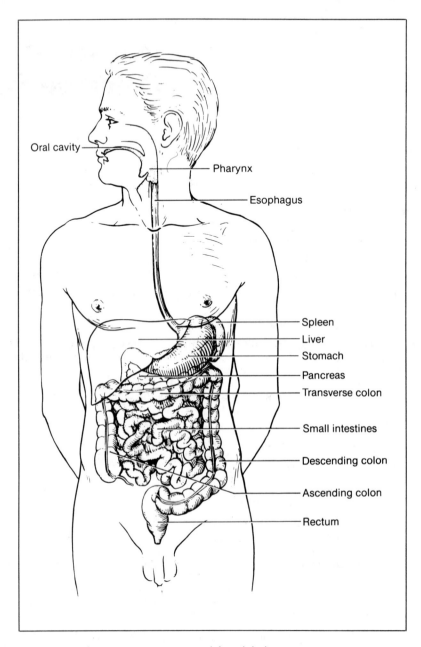

Figure 13-1. Components of the adult digestive system.

II. DEVELOPMENT OF THE FOREGUT

A. Foregut derivatives and blood supply

1. The foregut gives rise to the epithelial linings of:
   a. The pharynx
   b. The trachea, bronchi, and other airways in the lungs
   c. The esophagus
   d. The stomach
   e. The duodenum proximal to the biliary tract
   f. The liver, pancreas, biliary tract, and gallbladder
2. Foregut derivatives are supplied with blood from the **celiac artery**.

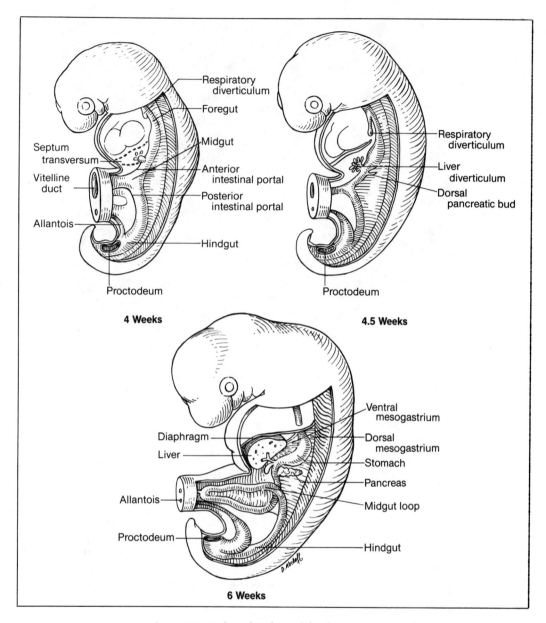

Figure 13-2. Early embryology of the digestive system.

B. Development of the esophagus. Figure 13-3 shows the histologic details of a section of the esophagus in a first-trimester human embryo.

1. At first, the esophagus is relatively short. By 7 weeks, the body elongates in a cranial direction. The esophagus becomes elongated as well, reaching its approximate length relative to the rest of the body.

2. The esophagus is initially lined by an endodermally derived epithelium that nearly obliterates the lumen of this organ. Later in development the esophagus is recanalized by cell death.

3. **Muscles and nerve supply**
   a. The **skeletal muscle** of the proximal portion of the esophagus is derived from pharyngeal arch mesenchyme, while the **smooth muscle** of the remainder of the esophageal wall is derived locally from splanchnic mesoderm.

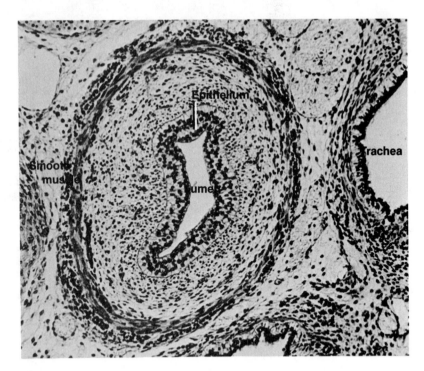

Figure 13-3. The developing esophagus in a first-trimester human embryo. (Light micrograph)

      b. The **vagus nerve**, which supplies the caudal pharyngeal arches, also supplies the motor innervation for the esophagus.

C. Development of the stomach. The stomach has a somewhat more complicated developmental history.

  1. The stomach first forms (week 4) as a fusiform dilation of the foregut, suspended from the body wall by a dorsal mesogastrium and a ventral mesogastrium (see Fig. 13-2).

  2. A branch of the dorsal aorta, the **celiac artery**, reaches the stomach via the dorsal mesogastrium and sends branches over the surface of the stomach, creating the afferent blood supply for the stomach.

  3. The dorsal portion of the stomach grows more rapidly than the rest of the stomach as the entire organ becomes expanded in a dorsoventral direction, leading to the formation of the greater curvature of the stomach.

  4. Rotation of the stomach (Fig. 13-4)
      a. As the stomach grows larger, it rotates 90° **about its longitudinal axis** in a counter-clockwise fashion, moving the ventral border to the left. Thus the original left side becomes shifted ventrally and the original right side becomes shifted dorsally.
      b. The stomach also undergoes a rotation **in the frontal plane** so that the cranial portion (the future cardia) is shifted to the left and inferiorly while the caudal portion (the future pylorus) is shifted to the right and superiorly.
      c. This rotation accounts for the fact that the stomach in the adult lies nearly in a transverse plane, with the long axis of the stomach lying perpendicular to the long axis of the body.

D. Development of gastric mesenteries (Fig. 13-5) [see also Chapter 8, section V]. The rotation of the stomach alters the relations of the mesenteries of the stomach (**mesogastrium**).

  1. Dorsal gastric mesentery
      a. The dorsal mesogastrium is carried from the median plane to the left by the rotation of the stomach.

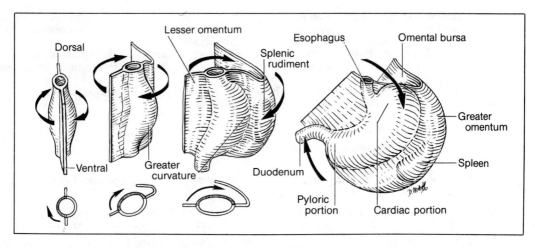

Figure 13-4. Rotation of the stomach.

   b. The dorsal mesogastrium also grows rapidly to create a blind-ending **omental bursa (lesser peritoneal sac)**, which opens into the rest of the peritoneal cavity by way of the **epiploic foramen**.
   c. While the stomach is rotating in the frontal plane, the dorsal mesogastrium extends tremendously as a double-layered flap of mesentery, the **greater omentum**, which comes to lie over the intestines (see Fig. 13-5).
      (1) At first, there is a small gap between the apposed layers of the greater omentum, resulting in a large inferior recess of the omental bursa.
      (2) Later, the two layers of the greater omentum fuse, obliterating most of the inferior recess and leaving a single flap of mesentery.
   d. As the stomach rotates, the **epiploic foramen** becomes constricted to a narrow opening situated near the upper margin of the superior portion of the duodenum (see Fig. 13-5).
   e. The **spleen** forms in the dorsal mesogastrium.
      (1) It becomes attached to the posterior body wall by a remnant of the dorsal mesogastrium known as the **lienorenal ligament**.
      (2) The spleen is also attached to the stomach by another remnant of the dorsal mesogastrium, the **gastrolienal ligament**.

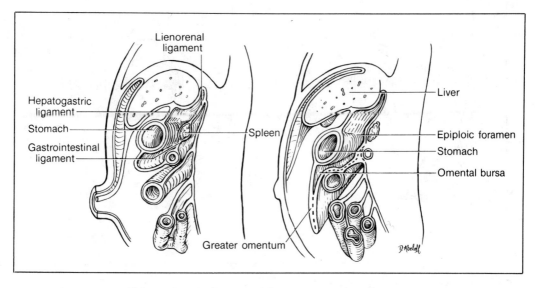

Figure 13-5. Development of the gastrointestinal mesenteries.

2. The ventral gastric mesentery

a. The ventral mesogastrium attaches the ventral border of the lower esophagus, stomach, and proximal duodenum to the ventral body wall.
b. It forms the **hepatogastric ligament (lesser omentum)** and the **falciform ligament**, which attach the stomach to the liver and the liver to the ventral body wall, respectively.
c. The liver undergoes an extensive growth into the ventral mesentery of the stomach and the septum transversum (see section III A).

E. Development of the proximal duodenum

1. The duodenum develops from the caudal portion of the foregut and the cranial portion of the midgut.
2. The entrance of the **bile duct** into the duodenum is located just proximal to the junction between the foregut and the midgut.
3. The duodenum grows in length to form a short loop. As the stomach rotates, the loop of the duodenum also rotates to the right, but it remains in a retroperitoneal location.
4. Early in development, the duodenal epithelium grows rapidly for a time, obliterating the lumen of the gut tube. Later, the duodenal lumen is recreated by secondary canalization due to cell death.

III. DEVELOPMENT OF THE LIVER, BILIARY APPARATUS, AND PANCREAS

A. Embryology of the liver and biliary apparatus

1. **The liver diverticulum.** The liver and biliary apparatus first form as the **liver diverticulum**, a ventral bud from the caudal portion of the foregut.
   a. Initially, the liver diverticulum is a simple evagination of the wall of the foregut which grows into the **septum transversum** and the **ventral mesogastrium** (Figs. 13-2 and 13-6).
      (1) Both of these structures are mesenchymally derived.
      (2) Thus, the growth of the liver diverticulum into these structures explains why most of the liver is surrounded by a connective tissue capsule (**Glisson's capsule**) and covered by a mesothelium.

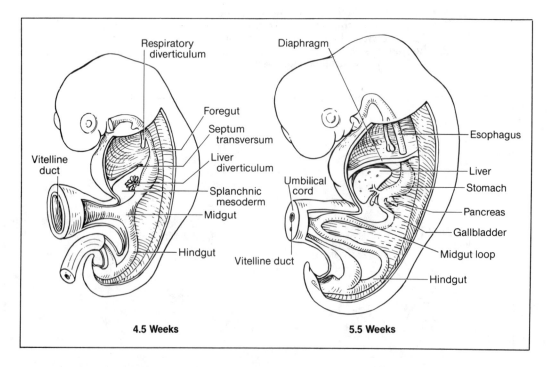

Figure 13-6. Development of the liver, pancreas, and gallbladder.

b. During weeks 4 to 5, the liver diverticulum begins to branch extensively. These branches give rise to:
  (1) Interconnected cords of hepatic parenchymal cells
  (2) The **biliary apparatus** within the liver (see section III A 4)
  (3) The epithelial lining of the extrahepatic portion of the biliary apparatus, including the **hepatic duct** and the **gallbladder**

2. Supporting tissues
  a. The connective tissue of the liver is derived from septum transversum mesenchyme.
  b. Vascular elements arise from vitelline and umbilical blood vessels as well as septum transversum mesenchyme. The vascular elements include:
  (1) Blood vessels
  (2) Hematopoietic cells
  (3) Hepatic sinusoidal endothelial cells (Fig. 13-7)
  (4) Phagocytic Kupffer cells
  c. Connective tissue and smooth muscle in the **hepatic ducts** and **gallbladder** arise from the splanchnic mesoderm surrounding appropriate branches of the liver diverticulum.

3. The liver as hematopoietic organ
  a. During its early development, the liver occupies a large portion of the peritoneal cavity (Fig. 13-8). It grows much more rapidly than the other nearby derivatives of the gut tube. This is due in part to the fact that the liver is a major hematopoietic organ after the sixth week of development.

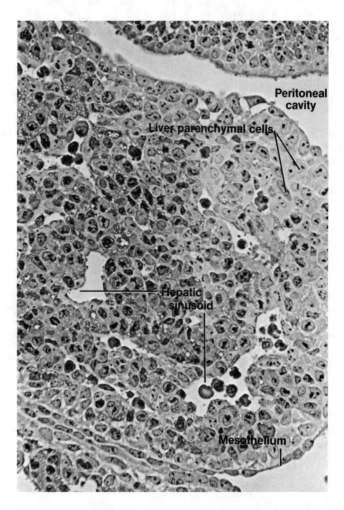

Figure 13-7. The developing liver in a mammalian embryo. (Light micrograph)

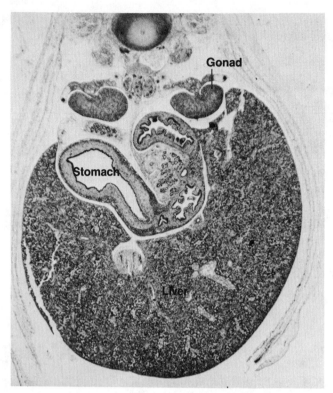

Figure 13-8. Light micrograph showing the liver occupying most of the peritoneal cavity.

    b. Cells lining the hepatic sinusoids are actively involved in erythropoiesis. Their activity is most intense during the first and second trimesters, gradually subsiding at term.

  4. Embryology of the biliary apparatus
    a. Distal branches of the liver diverticulum form the **intrahepatic biliary apparatus** and the **hepatic duct**.
    b. A small intermediate branch gives rise to the **gallbladder** and the **cystic duct** (Fig. 13-9).
    c. The most proximal portion of the liver diverticulum becomes the **bile duct** draining the liver and gallbladder into the duodenum.

B. Embryology of the pancreas
  1. The pancreas develops from two separate foregut diverticula, the **dorsal** and the **ventral pancreatic buds** (see Fig. 13-9).
    a. The **ventral pancreatic bud** forms as an evagination of the proximal liver diverticulum.
    b. The **dorsal pancreatic bud** forms as an evagination of the foregut in the proximal portion of the duodenum, opposite to the liver diverticulum and ventral pancreatic bud.

  2. The rotation of the duodenum to the right carries the ventral pancreatic bud dorsally, where it fuses with the dorsal pancreatic bud.

  3. The **ventral pancreatic bud** forms:
    a. The main pancreatic duct
    b. The uncinate process
    c. The inferior portion of the head of the pancreas

  4. The **dorsal pancreatic bud** forms:
    a. The accessory pancreatic duct
    b. The remainder of the pancreas not formed by the ventral bud

  5. The main and accessory ducts usually fuse to form a single **pancreatic duct**.
    a. About 10% of all humans retain two separate pancreatic ducts, reflecting the dual embryonic origin.
    b. This minor anatomic variation is seldom clinically significant.

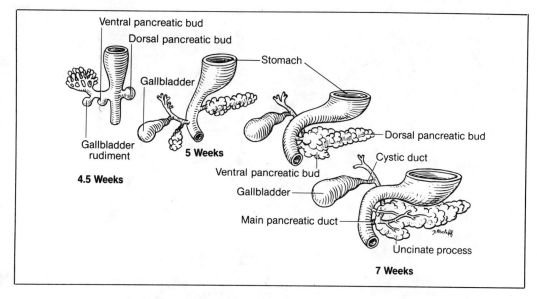

Figure 13-9. Development of the pancreatic buds and gallbladder.

6. Pancreatic development involves an **endodermal–mesodermal inductive interaction**.
    a. The **pancreatic acinar cells**, the alpha and beta cells of the **islets of Langerhans** (see Chapter 19, section V), and the epithelial cells lining the intra- and extrapancreatic ducts are **endodermally derived**.
    b. They are supported by connective tissue and smooth muscle that is derived from the **splanchnic mesodermal anlage** that surrounds the growing pancreatic buds. These mesenchymal cells induce:
        (1) Branching in the distal tips of the pancreatic buds
        (2) Differentiation of the secretory pancreatic acinar cells

IV. DEVELOPMENT OF THE MIDGUT

A. Midgut derivatives

1. The midgut extends from the anterior intestinal portal to the posterior intestinal portal.
2. The midgut forms:
    a. The small intestines distal to the opening of the bile duct
    b. The cecum and appendix
    c. The ascending colon
    d. The proximal part (right one-half to two-thirds) of the transverse colon

B. Midgut mesentery and blood supply

1. The midgut is suspended from the dorsal wall by a short **dorsal mesentery** which carries the **superior mesenteric (midgut) artery**, a branch of the dorsal aorta.
2. All of the midgut derivatives are supplied by the superior mesenteric artery.

C. Physiologic herniation and rotation of midgut loops

1. Herniation
    a. The midgut begins to grow extensively during the sixth week to form a U-shaped midgut loop.
    b. Because the liver is a relatively large organ at this time, it bulges prominently into the abdominal cavity, nearly filling the abdomen and occupying space that might otherwise be occupied by the midgut.
    c. As a consequence, the growing midgut loop herniates into the umbilical cord (Fig. 13-10).
        (1) In histologic sections, the midgut loop appears to project through the body wall.
        (2) In fact, it projects into the **extraembryonic coelom** and it is surrounded by components of the **umbilical cord** (Fig. 13-11).

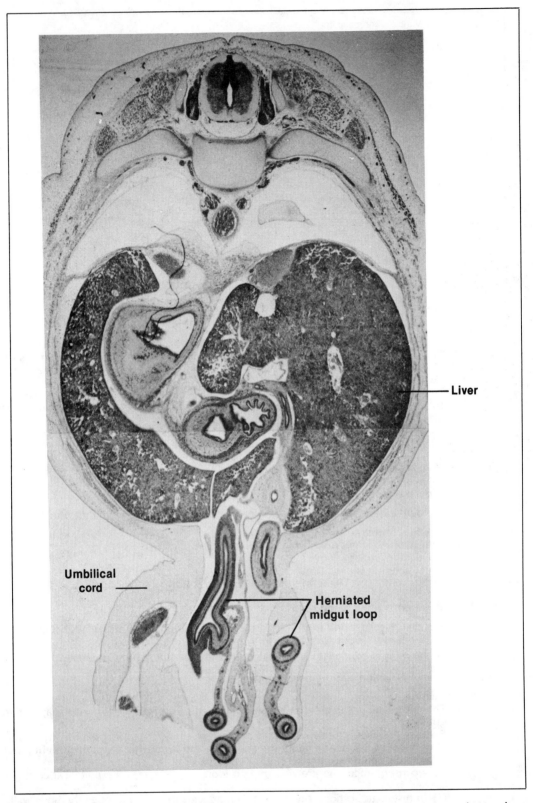

Figure 13-10. Physiologic herniation of the midgut loop into the umbilical cord. (Light micrograph) Note how the size of the liver leaves little room for the growing midgut within the peritoneal cavity.

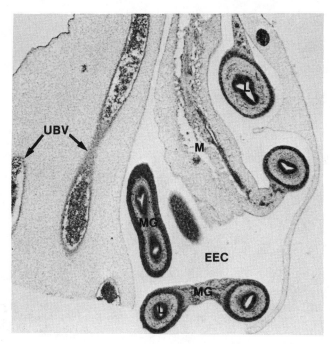

Figure 13-11. Physiologic herniation of the midgut loop into the umbilical cord. (Light micrograph) *EEC,* Extraembryonic coelom; *L,* lumen of midgut; *M,* mesentery; *MG,* midgut loop; *UBV,* umbilical blood vessel.

2. **Rotation of midgut loops**
   a. The midgut is connected to the yolk sac by a narrow **vitelline duct** at the level of the main branch of the superior mesenteric artery.
   b. The midgut loop has a **cranial limb** and a **caudal limb** (Fig. 13-12). The division point between the two limbs is at the site of attachment of the vitelline duct.
   c. The cranial limb grows much more rapidly than the caudal limb, and while the midgut is herniated into the umbilical cord, it undergoes a 90° rotation in a counterclockwise fashion as viewed from the ventral aspect of the embryo (see Fig. 13-12).
      (1) The rotation occurs in the frontal plane of the embryo.
      (2) The vitelline duct and the superior mesenteric artery provide an axis of rotation of the midgut loop as it rotates.
3. **Reduction of the midgut herniation and further rotation**
   a. The abdominal cavity expands as the body grows, and the liver and kidneys become relatively less massive.
   b. Consequently, during the tenth week, the midgut loop is drawn back into the abdominal cavity.
   c. This reduction of the umbilical herniation of the midgut loop is accompanied by a further 180° counterclockwise rotation. The rotation is around the same axes and in the same plane as the initial rotation.
   d. The two rotations add up to a **total rotation** of about 270°. This total rotation, plus a subsequent descent of the cecum and appendix into the right iliac fossa, result in the following **relationships** (see Fig. 13-12):
      (1) The cecum and appendix come to lie in an inferior position on the right side.
      (2) The ascending colon and the proximal portion of the transverse colon project anteriorly and to the left, while resting ventral to the cranial portion of the midgut loop.
4. **Attachments of the midgut loop**
   a. As the midgut loop is drawn back into the abdominal cavity and rotated, it also becomes attached in some portions to the posterior body wall by a dissolution of the mesenteries.
   b. Eventually, the ascending and descending colon become fixed to the posterior body wall and the transverse colon becomes fused to the greater omentum.

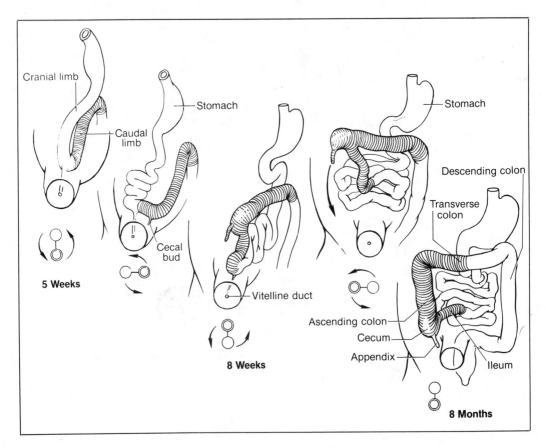

Figure 13-12. Rotation of the midgut loop.

    c. The proximal portion of the duodenum also becomes fixed to the posterior body wall.
    d. The jejunum and the ileum remain suspended in the abdominal cavity by a dorsal mesentery.

D. Development of the appendix
1. The **vermiform appendix** forms from the **cecal bud**, which arises in the caudal portion of the midgut loop.
2. The cecal bud first appears in the sixth week as a small evagination of the midgut loop opposite the mesentery.
3. The appendix forms at the apex of this diverticulum and becomes displaced into the right iliac fossa during the growth, rotation, and descent of the cecum.
4. **Anatomic variants of the appendix**
      a. The position of the appendix is of considerable clinical significance in the diagnosis of **appendicitis**, an infection requiring prompt surgical intervention.
         (1) The appendix may lie behind the cecum (**retrocecal appendix**) or behind the colon (**retrocolic appendix**) or even over the brim of the pelvis (**pelvic appendix**).
         (2) In most people (64%) the appendix is located retrocecally.
      b. There is often considerable variation in the length and mesenteric attachments of the appendix.

V. DEVELOPMENT OF THE HINDGUT

A. Hindgut derivatives and blood supply
1. The hindgut extends from the posterior intestinal portal to the proctodeum. A large caudal **cloaca** forms as an expansion of the hindgut at its most caudal extent.

2. The hindgut forms:
   a. The distal portion (left one-half to one-third) of the transverse colon
   b. The descending colon
   c. The rectum and upper portion of the anal canal
   d. The lining of the urinary bladder (see Chapter 16 section IV C)
3. The **blood supply** for the hindgut derivatives comes from the **inferior mesenteric artery**, a branch of the dorsal aorta.
4. The boundary between the midgut portion and the hindgut portion of the transverse colon can be inspected, because it is defined by the respective distributions of tributaries from the superior and inferior mesenteric arteries.

B. **The allantois.** The allantois is a blind-ending diverticulum that projects into the umbilical cord away from the cloaca.
   1. In human embryos, it has little functional significance, but in some mammals it is a major excretory organ of the fetus and becomes elaborately developed and vascularized.
   2. The allantois gives rise to the **urachus**, a degenerate cord-like band of fibrotic connective tissue which attaches the bladder to the umbilicus.

C. **The cloaca**
   1. The **cellular origins** of the cloaca are the same as in other portions of the developing gut tube.
      a. The luminal epithelial cells of the cloaca are derived from endoderm.
      b. The mural connective tissues and muscular tissues are derived from splanchnic mesoderm or the mesenchymal cells of the urorectal septum.
   2. **Subdivisions**
      a. The growth of the **urorectal septum** divides the cloaca into a posterior **rectum** and **anal canal** and an anterior **urogenital sinus**.
      b. The urorectal septum fuses with the cloacal membrane, partitioning the cloaca and the cloacal membrane.
         (1) The **cloaca** is divided into a **rectum** and **anal canal** and a **urogenital sinus**.
         (2) The **cloacal membrane** is divided into a posterior **anal membrane** (covering the anal canal) and an anterior **urogenital membrane** (covering the urogenital sinus).

D. **Hindgut mesenteries**
   1. Initially, the hindgut derivatives are suspended from the dorsal body wall by a **dorsal mesentery**.
   2. Eventually, the dorsal mesentery dissolves and the organs become fixed to the posterior body wall.

E. **The anal canal**
   1. The **proctodeum** becomes somewhat invaginated after the formation of the anal membrane.
   2. Consequently, the anal canal has a mixed origin.
      a. The **proximal (upper) two-thirds** are hindgut derivatives and are thus lined by an endodermally derived epithelium.
      b. The **distal (lower) one-third** is a proctodeal derivative and is thus lined by an ectodermally derived epithelium.
      c. In the adult, the approximate **boundary** between these two primordia lies at the level of the **anal valves** (the **pectinate line**).

VI. CONGENITAL MALFORMATIONS OF THE GASTROINTESTINAL TRACT

A. **Stenotic disorders**
   1. **Esophageal and duodenal stenosis**
      a. As mentioned earlier, the esophagus and duodenum have a rapidly growing epithelial lining that obliterates the lumen for a time and is only **secondarily canalized** later in development.
         (1) If this canalization is faulty for some reason, then the lumen of the tube fails to form and the passage of food is obstructed.

- **(a)** If the lumen completely **fails to form**, then the child would be afflicted with **esophageal** or **duodenal atresia**.
- **(b)** If the lumen forms but is **constricted**, then **esophageal** or **duodenal stenosis** would result.
- (2) In both conditions, there might be a reduction in resorption of amniotic fluid and a consequent increase in the volume of amniotic fluid (**polyhydramnios**).
- (3) In cases of polyhydramnios **without bile** in the amniotic fluid, one might suspect foregut atresia.
  - **b.** **Duodenal stenosis** can also be caused by the formation of an **annular pancreas**, in which pancreatic tissue surrounds the duodenum. This in turn is caused by abnormal rotation and fusion of the two pancreatic buds.
    - (1) With annular pancreas, the stenosis is usually found proximal to the site of origin of the pancreatic buds (i.e., in the proximal midgut).
    - (2) Therefore, the amniotic fluid might be expected to contain bile.
    - (3) Thus, in cases of polyhydramnios **with bile** in the amniotic fluid, one might suspect duodenal stenosis due to annular pancreas.
  - **2. Pyloric stenosis** is a quite common congenital anomaly, affecting 1 in 150 males and 1 in 750 females.
    - **a.** This condition is apparently due to a poorly understood multifactorial mechanism of genetic transmission.
    - **b.** Children with pyloric stenosis have an unusually thick band of smooth muscle around the pylorus which severely restricts the entrance to the small intestine.
      - (1) Children so afflicted are asymptomatic at birth but soon after birth they begin projectile vomiting.
      - (2) The vomit is not bile-stained.
    - **c.** Pyloric stenosis can be corrected surgically.

- **B. Meckel's diverticulum**
  1. **Meckel's diverticulum** is the most common congenital abnormality of the gastrointestinal tract. It occurs in about 3% of all live births, with males outnumbering females 3 to 1.
  2. This curious anatomic variant arises when a small portion of the **vitelline duct** persists as a diverticulum from the gut tube. The anomaly is most often located in the ileum.
  3. Meckel's diverticulum is usually asymptomatic but may present clinical complications when it becomes inflamed or ulcerated.
  4. In many cases, the diverticulum contains **ectopic tissue**.
     - **a.** Often, the ectopic patch is gastric mucosa and thus may become ulcerated.
     - **b.** Ectopic pancreatic acinar tissue can also be found in a Meckel's diverticulum.

- **C. Abnormalities of gut rotation.** The complex herniation and rotation of the midgut loop can result in several related congenital anomalies.
  1. **Omphalocele** results when the physiologic herniation and reduction of the midgut loop fail to occur normally.
     - **a.** In omphalocele, loops of midgut project into the umbilical cord to a variable extent.
       - (1) The newborn baby will exhibit loops of small intestine on the ventral surface of the body.
       - (2) These loops will be covered by a thin layer of umbilical cord and amnion.
     - **b.** Omphalocele is one of several lesions that can be suspected when elevated amniotic fluid α-fetoprotein levels are detected during amniocentesis. The omphalocele can then be diagnosed by sonography (Fig. 13-13).
     - **c.** Omphalocele can be corrected surgically if it is an isolated defect and is not overly extensive.
  2. In **gastroschisis**, the midgut loop herniation is associated with a large defect in the anterior body wall, and the visceral organs are not covered by a thin sac but are bathed directly in amniotic fluid.
  3. **Failure of rotation of the midgut loop** may occur to a variable degree so that the colon may reside on the left rather than the right side.
     - **a.** If uncomplicated by **volvulus** (strangulation by twisting), malrotation will not be associated with symptoms.
     - **b.** Often, however, malrotation is associated with **volvulus** or with **peritoneal bands**. Either

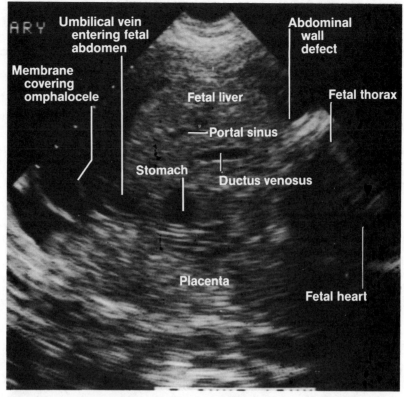

Figure 13-13. Sonogram of an example of omphalocele. (Courtesy of Teresita L. Angtuaco, M.D., Assistant Professor, Department of Obstetrics and Gynecology, University of Arkansas for Medical Sciences, Little Rock.)

of these can cause obstruction of the gut tube. They can also compromise the blood supply, followed by gangrenous degeneration of tissues.
    c. Malrotation can accompany omphalocele or gastroschisis.
D. **Congenital anomalies of the hindgut.** These vary considerably, both in nature and in extent.
    1. **Abnormalities in the caudal portion of the anal canal**
        a. These range from the less severe cases of **imperforate anus** to the more severe forms of **rectal atresia** with or without **rectovaginal** or **rectourethral fistula**.
        b. Such malformations are due to abnormalities in the formation of the urorectal septum or rectum, or to abnormalities in the breakdown of the anal membrane.
        c. Many of these anatomic problems can be corrected by plastic surgery.
    2. **Congenital aganglionic megacolon (Hirschsprung's disease)**
        a. Sometimes portions of the colon do not receive **neural crest cells** which differentiate into the **myenteric plexus**.
        b. In this case, peristalsis does not occur in the portion lacking the neural crest cell derivatives.
        c. As a result, the portion proximal to the aganglionic segment will become congenitally distended.

STUDY QUESTIONS

Directions: Each question below contains five suggested answers. Choose the **one best** response to each question.

1. All of the following are true statements about liver development EXCEPT

   (A) the liver parenchymal cells are derived from the liver diverticulum
   (B) hepatic duct epithelial cells are derived from splanchnic mesoderm
   (C) the hepatic sinusoidal endothelium is derived from vitelline and umbilical vessels
   (D) rapid growth of the liver fills much of the peritoneal cavity during early gastrointestinal development
   (E) the liver succeeds the yolk sac as a hematopoietic organ

2. The development of the stomach shows all of the following characteristics EXCEPT

   (A) the greater curvature of the stomach is attached to the dorsal mesogastrium
   (B) the first rotation of the stomach brings its dorsal side to the right
   (C) the second rotation of the stomach carries the pyloric stomach to the right side
   (D) the omental bursa is partially obliterated by fusion of flaps of the greater omentum
   (E) chief and parietal cells in gastric glands are endodermal derivatives

3. The ventral pancreatic bud of the developing pancreas shows all of the following characteristics EXCEPT

   (A) it forms as a branch from the liver diverticulum
   (B) it fuses with the dorsal pancreatic bud
   (C) it forms most of the body of the pancreas
   (D) it forms the main pancreatic duct
   (E) it forms pancreatic acinar cells

Directions: Each question below contains four suggested answers of which **one or more** is correct. Choose the answer

   A if **1, 2, and 3** are correct
   B if **1 and 3** are correct
   C if **2 and 4** are correct
   D if **4** is correct
   E if **1, 2, 3, and 4** are correct

4. Foregut derivatives include which of the following?

   (1) The esophagus
   (2) The stomach
   (3) The proximal duodenum
   (4) The ileum

5. Midgut derivatives include which of the following?

   (1) The distal duodenum
   (2) The appendix
   (3) The jejunum
   (4) The descending colon

6. Which of the following cells are endodermal derivatives?

   (1) Pancreatic acinar cells
   (2) Alpha and beta cells in the islets of Langerhans
   (3) Liver parenchymal cells
   (4) Cells lining the lumen of the gallbladder

7. True statements concerning the development of the midgut include which of the following?

   (1) The initial 90° rotation occurs in a clockwise fashion
   (2) The final 180° rotation occurs as the loop is withdrawn into the peritoneal cavity
   (3) The ascending colon keeps its dorsal mesentery and does not become fixed to the body wall
   (4) Physiologic herniation occurs as a result of the large size of the liver

Directions: The groups of questions below consist of lettered choices followed by several numbered items. For each numbered item select the **one** lettered choice with which it is **most** closely associated. Each lettered choice may be used once, more than once, or not at all.

Questions 8–11

For each characteristic of a congenital anomaly of the gastrointestinal tract given below, select the diagnosis that is most appropriate.

(A) Omphalocele
(B) Hirschsprung's disease
(C) Both
(D) Neither

8. Detectable by sonography

9. Due to a lack of neural crest cell derivatives

10. Associated with oligohydramnios

11. Associated with increased levels of amniotic fluid α-fetoprotein

Questions 12–16

For each description of a structure in the developing gastrointestinal tract given below, select the appropriate lettered component shown in the accompanying diagram.

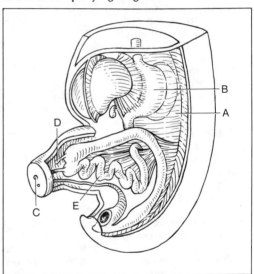

12. This structure is a foregut derivative

13. This structure serves as part of the axis of rotation of the midgut loop

14. This dorsal mesentery becomes the greater omentum

15. This structure descends into the right iliac fossa and becomes the vermiform appendix

16. This structure is a midgut derivative

ANSWERS AND EXPLANATIONS

1. The answer is B. *(III A 1, 2, 3)* The liver diverticulum forms hepatic parenchymal cells and the lining of the intrahepatic ducts and biliary apparatus. Hepatic blood vessels and the endothelial cells lining hepatic sinusoids come from septum transversum mesenchyme, vitelline blood vessels, and umbilical blood vessels. The liver is a hematopoietic organ after the yolk sac serves this function, but before the bone marrow takes over. This accounts for the relatively large size of the liver and the small remaining volume in the peritoneal cavity, leading to physiologic herniation of the midgut loop.

2. The answer is B. *(II C, D)* The first stomach rotation brings the dorsal side of the stomach to the left, while the second rotation brings the pyloric stomach up and to the right. The greater omentum forms from an extensive growth of the dorsal mesogastrium along the greater curvature of the stomach, followed by a partial collapse of the omental bursa due to fusion of the flaps of mesentery. All of the epithelial cells lining the gastrointestinal tract are endodermally derived.

3. The answer is C. *(III B)* The ventral pancreatic bud forms as a branch of the liver diverticulum. It rotates toward and fuses with the dorsal pancreatic bud. It forms the uncinate process and the main pancreatic duct. Both pancreatic acinar cells and islet tissue differentiate from each pancreatic bud.

4. The answer is A (1, 2, 3). *(II A)* The foregut extends from the stomodeum to the anterior intestinal portal. The foregut forms everything from the esophagus to the proximal duodenum. The midgut extends from the anterior intestinal portal to the posterior intestinal portal. The midgut gives rise to the remainder of the duodenum, the jejunum and ileum, the ascending colon, and the proximal half of the transverse colon.

5. The answer is A (1, 2, 3). *(IV A)* The midgut extends from the anterior intestinal portal to the posterior intestinal portal. The midgut loop undergoes a 270° counterclockwise rotation during development. The midgut forms the distal duodenum and the rest of the small intestines. It also forms the ascending colon, appendix, and proximal half of the transverse colon.

6. The answer is E (all). *(I B 1; III A 1, B 6)* The endoderm forms the liver diverticulum and pancreatic buds. These structures, in turn, form all of the epithelial parenchymal cells of the liver and pancreas and also the alpha and beta cells of the islets of Langerhans in the pancreas. Finally, the linings of the pancreatic ducts are endodermal derivatives, as are the cells lining the gallbladder.

7. The answer is C (2, 4). *(IV C)* Both the initial and final rotations of the midgut loop are counterclockwise. The final 180° rotation occurs as the herniated gut loops are drawn back into the peritoneal cavity. Herniation occurs because the large size of the liver fills the peritoneal cavity, leaving no room for the rapidly growing midgut loop. The transverse colon keeps its dorsal mesentery and stays mobile, while the ascending and descending colon both become fixed by losing their mesenteries.

8–11. The answers are: 8-C, 9-B, 10-D, 11-A. *(VI C 1, D 2)* Omphalocele is a congenital abnormality in the withdrawal of the midgut loop from the umbilical herniation. Omphalocele is visible on sonograms and is associated with increased levels of α-fetoprotein in the amniotic fluid. Hirschsprung's disease (congenital megacolon) is characterized by abnormal distension of the colon due to a failure of the formation of the neurons of the myenteric plexus. These neurons are neural crest cell derivatives. Congenital megacolon can also be detected on sonograms. Neither of these diseases is associated with oligohydramnios (decreased volume of amniotic fluid). Blockage of the gastrointestinal tract can result in polyhydramnios if the fetus is unable to swallow amniotic fluid.

12–16 The answers are: 12-B, 13-C, 14-A, 15-D, 16-E. *(II C 1, D 1; IV C 2, D 1)* The dorsal mesogastrium *(A)* forms the greater omentum on the greater curvature of the stomach *(B)*, a foregut derivative. The vitelline duct *(C)* connects the lumen of the gastrointestinal tract with the yolk sac. The vitelline duct, along with the superior mesenteric artery, serves as the axis of rotation of the midgut loop. The cecal bud *(D)* is located on the midgut loop *(E)*. The cecal bud forms the appendix and descends into the right iliac fossa after rotation has been completed.

14
Development of the Respiratory System

I. INTRODUCTION. The development of the nose and mouth are covered in Chapter 18, and the respiratory aspects of these organs are discussed in this chapter.

A. Components of the respiratory system
1. The respiratory system is composed of a **conducting airway** and an **epithelium** specialized for **gas exchange**.
   a. The **conducting airway** consists of:
      (1) The nasal cavities
      (2) The nasopharynx
      (3) The larynx
      (4) The trachea
      (5) The bronchi
      (6) The bronchioles
      (7) The respiratory bronchioles and alveolar ducts
   b. The **epithelium for gas exchange** lines the alveoli, providing the **respiratory surface** of the lungs.
   c. An overview of the gross anatomy of the lower portion of the respiratory system is shown in Figure 14-1.

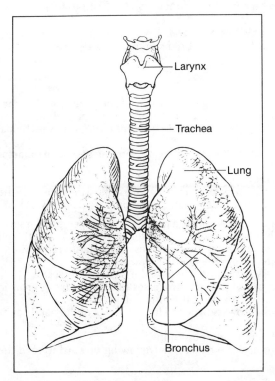

Figure 14-1. Gross anatomy of the lower portion of the adult respiratory system.

2. The airway has various **supportive structures**:
   a. Cartilage and smooth muscle, to prevent its collapse and to regulate the diameter of its lumen
   b. Glands, to keep it moistened
   c. Cilia, to propel inspired debris toward the gut
   d. A blood supply
   e. Innervation

3. **Other structures** also lie in the respiratory system.
   a. The **larynx** contains the vocal cords and thus plays a key role in phonation.
   b. The **organ of olfaction** is also located in the respiratory system. The nasal cavity is equipped with a highly modified **olfactory epithelium** (see Chapter 18, section III F 1).

B. Functions of the respiratory system

1. The **epithelium** of the respiratory portion of the lungs is a thin layer of cells lining the alveoli. It is specialized to function in two ways, by virtue of two **types of cells**.
   a. **Type I cells** facilitate **gas exchange** between the blood and air.
      (1) These cells are extremely attenuated.
      (2) Oxygen and carbon dioxide cross the thin epithelial barrier in the alveoli with ease.
   b. **Type II cells** are specialized for secreting **surfactant**, a mixture of lipid, protein, and polysaccharide.
      (1) The surfactant spreads over the vast surface area of the alveoli, reducing the surface tension of the fluid covering the alveolar surface.
      (2) Surfactant thereby reduces the surface tension forces that tend to collapse the inflated lungs.

2. Air that enters the respiratory system through the nasal cavity is warmed, moistened, and often cleared of significant amounts of water-soluble air pollutants. These varied functions are all accomplished by the **respiratory mucosa** of the nasal cavity.
   a. The nasal cavity is built in such a way that the entering air flows over the nasal mucosa with considerable turbulence.
   b. The nasal mucosa has a pseudostratified ciliated columnar epithelium covering the nasal turbinates.

3. **Phonation** and **olfaction**, which both involve the passage of air (and, in the case of olfaction, air-borne chemicals), could also be considered functions of the respiratory system.

II. DEVELOPMENT OF THE UPPER RESPIRATORY SYSTEM. Development of the nasal and oral cavities is described in Chapter 18. Therefore, only a brief summary is given here.

A. Formation of the nasal and oral cavities

1. **Beginnings of the nasal cavities**
   a. The **nasal placodes** are ectodermal thickenings that appear during week 4 on either side of the face just above the maxillary processes of the first pharyngeal arch.
   b. **Nasal swellings** develop around the nasal placodes by proliferation of mesenchymal cells.
   c. The placodes invaginate into the proliferating mesenchyme, forming two **nasal (olfactory) pits**.
   d. The nasal pits then deepen by further growth to form **nasal sacs**.
   e. Mesenchymal cells between the nasal sacs form a medial mass of tissue known as the **primary palate**, and the nasal sacs grow caudally around the primary palate (week 6).

2. **Development of the palate and nasal cavities.** While the nasal sacs are developing, important changes take place in the **maxillary processes** (see Chapter 18, sections II and III and Fig. 18-4). Through these changes, left and right nasal cavities are formed cranially, and the nasal and oral cavities are separated from one another by the **palate**.
   a. First, the medial tips of the maxillary processes fuse with the nasal processes.
   b. Second, two shelves of tissue, the **lateral palatine processes** (**palatal shelves**), grow in from the maxillary processes along either side of the tongue (Fig. 14-2).
   c. In addition, a primitive **nasal septum** grows downward from the roof of the nasal cavity (see Fig. 14-2).
   d. The **primary palate** also expands laterally and posteriorly.
   e. The **tongue** now moves downward and the palatal shelves swing upward toward the nasal septum.

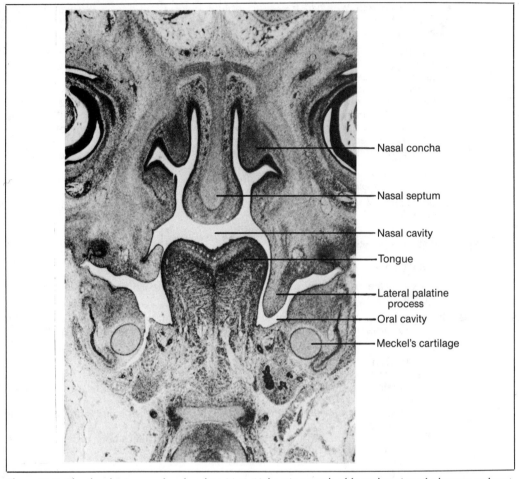

Figure 14-2. The developing nasal and oral cavities. (Light micrograph of frontal section of a human embryo)

    f. The palatal shelves then fuse with one another, with the primary palate, and with the nasal septum (weeks 8 to 9).
3. While the palate is forming, three shelf-like structures begin to form the future superior, medial, and inferior **nasal conchae** in the lateral walls of each nasal cavity.
4. For a brief time, a **bucconasal membrane** separates the nasal and oral cavities. The bucconasal membrane later breaks down and the **posterior nares** form, completing the communication between the surface of the face, the **anterior nares** (the nasal cavity), and the **nasopharynx** (the oral cavity posterior to the developing palate).

B. **Histodifferentiation in the nasal cavities**
  1. **Ectodermal and endodermal derivations**
     a. For a time, the **stomodeum** (the precursor of the oral cavity) is covered over by a **buccopharyngeal (oropharyngeal) membrane**. When this breaks down, the gut tube is connected to the amniotic cavity.
     b. Therefore, the oral and nasal cavities are both lined by an epithelium derived from ectoderm anteriorly and from endoderm posteriorly.
        (1) All epithelial structures and derivatives arising **anterior to the oropharyngeal membrane**, including the tooth-forming enamel organ, perhaps some salivary glands, and the linings of the nasal and oral cavities, are all **ectodermal derivatives**.
        (2) All epithelial structures and derivatives arising **posterior to the oropharyngeal membrane** are **endodermal (foregut) derivatives**.

228 *Human Developmental Anatomy*

   c. **Rathke's pouch**, which forms the adenohypophysis (see Chapter 19, section II B), arises as an ectodermal evagination of the roof of the mouth just anterior to the oropharyngeal membrane.
2. **Respiratory and olfactory epitheliums**
   a. The **nasal cavities** become lined in most places by a typical pseudostratified ciliated columnar epithelium with goblet cells (**respiratory epithelium**).
   b. However, high in the nasal cavities the respiratory epithelium elaborates into two patches of **olfactory epithelium** (see Chapter 18, section III F 1).
      (1) The olfactory epithelium is pseudostratified, columnar, and ciliated like the typical respiratory epithelium, but it lacks goblet cells and the cilia are immobile and highly elongated.
      (2) The **olfactory cilia** contain chemoreceptors that respond to chemical substances in the air.
      (3) The ciliated cells are bipolar neurons with axons that project directly into the olfactory bulb of the brain.
   c. **Bowman's glands**, which secrete a serous fluid onto the surface of the olfactory epithelium, form as invaginations from the developing olfactory epithelium.

III. MORPHOGENESIS OF THE TRACHEA, BRONCHI, AND LUNGS

A. **Development of the respiratory diverticulum and lung buds** (Fig. 14-3)
   1. At 3 weeks, the **respiratory diverticulum (tracheobronchial groove)** forms as a ventral epithelial evagination of the foregut.
   2. The groove begins to elongate in a caudal direction and soon becomes separated from the foregut proper by formation of an **esophagotracheal (tracheo-esophageal) septum**.
   3. By 4 weeks, this separation is nearly completed, and the respiratory diverticulum is beginning to branch into a left and right **lung bud**.
      a. The **branching of the lung buds** progresses rapidly.
      b. Three main branches form in the right lung bud and two main branches form in the left lung bud.
         (1) These first branches that form in the lung buds correspond to the **lobar bronchi** that are part of the adult lungs.
         (2) Eventually, in the adult, there are three main lobes and lobar bronchi in the right lung but only two of each in the left lung.

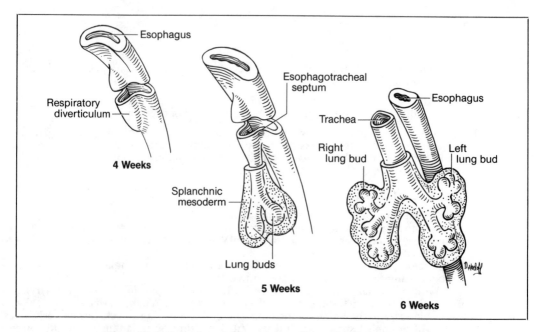

Figure 14-3. Formation of the respiratory diverticulum and lung buds.

4. The lung buds continue to grow caudally and laterally and continue to branch (Fig. 14-4). After forming the lobar bronchi, the respiratory diverticulum undergoes about 20 generations of dichotomous branching.

B. Splanchnic mesoderm

1. As the lung buds grow caudally and laterally, they grow into a second primordium which is a mass of splanchnic mesoderm (Fig. 14-5).
2. As the lung buds branch and extend, they carry this mass of mesodermal tissue along with them.

C. Derivatives of the respiratory diverticulum and the splanchnic mesoderm

1. The lung buds and the associated splanchnic mesoderm undergo a **reciprocal inductive interaction** that is essential for normal pulmonary development.
2. These two primordia contribute to the formation of the definitive respiratory system.
   a. The **epithelium** lining the entire respiratory system posterior to the stomodeum develops from the **respiratory diverticulum** and is therefore of **endodermal origin**.
   b. The **splanchnic mesoderm** forms the connective tissue, cartilage, smooth muscle cells, and blood vessels surrounding the epithelium.
   c. For example, in the **trachea**, the **derivations** are as follows:
      (1) The **respiratory diverticulum** forms:
         (a) The respiratory epithelium of the trachea
         (b) The mucosal and submucosal tracheal glandular elements connected to the lumen of the trachea
      (2) The **splanchnic mesoderm** forms:
         (a) The connective tissue of the tracheal lamina propria
         (b) The tracheal cartilage rings and smooth (trachealis) muscles in the dorsal portion of the trachea
         (c) The blood vessels and lymphatics of the trachea
   d. In the more **distal portions** of the respiratory system, the **derivations** are as follows:
      (1) The **respiratory diverticulum** forms the type I and type II epithelial cells lining the alveolar airways.

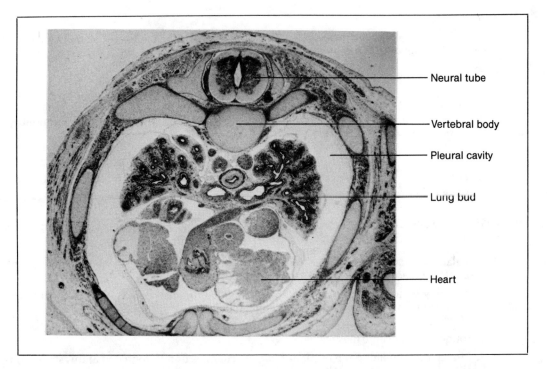

Figure 14-4. The developing lung buds of a human embryo. (Light micrograph; low power)

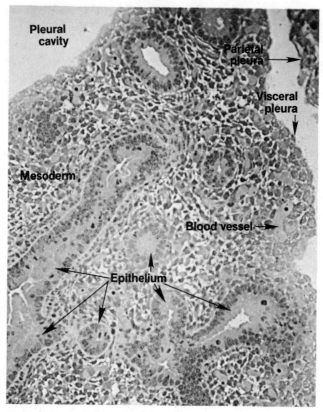

Figure 14-5. A developing lung bud in a mammalian embryo. Note the splanchnic mesoderm surrounding the epithelial lung bud branches. (Light micrograph; high power)

   (2) The **splanchnic mesoderm** forms the mural connective tissue, blood vessels, and lymphatics in the pulmonary alveoli.

   D. Formation of the pleural cavities and pleura
   1. The lateral growth of the lungs causes a progressive obliteration of the **pericardioperitoneal canals**, the immediate precursors of the **pleural cavities** (see Chapter 8, section III).
      a. In the primitive condition, the pericardioperitoneal canals are part of the **intraembryonic coelom**.
      b. They are lined with the same **mesothelium** that lines the pericardial cavity and the peritoneal cavity.
   2. The developing lungs become coated with a **visceral pleura** which is reflected upon a **parietal pleura** at the mediastinum.

IV. **HISTOGENESIS OF THE LUNGS.** During their histologic development, the **lungs** pass through three **developmental stages** (Fig. 14-6).

   A. **The glandular stage** (Fig. 14-7; see also Figs. 14-4 and 14-5) extends from the branching of the respiratory diverticulum to the fourth month of development.
   1. The growth and branching of the respiratory diverticulum occurs incessantly until the embryonic lungs take on a **glandular appearance**.
   2. It is during the glandular stage that the lung buds proliferate and branch into the surrounding splanchnic mesenchyme.
   3. The epithelium lining the respiratory diverticulum is undifferentiated at this stage, consisting of unremarkable columnar cells.

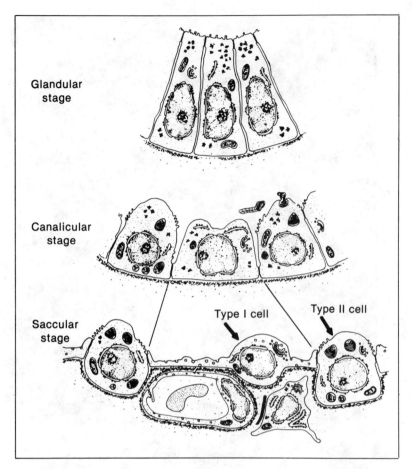

Figure 14-6. The three stages of pulmonary development. In the glandular stage (week 4 to month 4), the respiratory epithelium is undifferentiated. In the canalicular stage (month 4 to month 6), the epithelium becomes cuboidal and the parenchyma becomes highly vascularized. In the saccular stage (month 6 to term), blood vessels proliferate and the alveolar epithelium thins and gradually differentiates into type I (squamous) cells and type II (surfactant-secreting) cells. (Adapted from Burri PH, Weibel ER: Ultrastructure and morphometry of the developing lung. In *Development of the Lung*. Edited by Hodson WA. New York, Marcel Dekker, 1977, p 230.)

B. The canalicular stage (Fig. 14-8) occurs between the fourth and sixth months of fetal life. During this stage, the airways become lined by a **cuboidal epithelium** and the parenchyma of the lungs becomes highly **vascularized**.

C. The saccular stage (Fig. 14-9) extends from the end of the canalicular stage until term.

1. During the saccular stage, the **epithelium** that lines the many branches of the lung bud descendants becomes thinner and thinner, while the **blood vessels** proliferate and become more intimately associated with this alveolar epithelium.

2. Between the sixth and seventh month, the **alveolar epithelium** begins to differentiate into the two types of **alveolar cells**:
   a. **Squamous type I cells** (Fig. 14-10)
   b. **Surfactant-secreting type II cells (great alveolar cells)**
      (1) Type II cells possess numerous intracellular **inclusion bodies (multilamellar bodies)**, which represent a storage form of the pulmonary **surfactant** synthesized in type II cells.

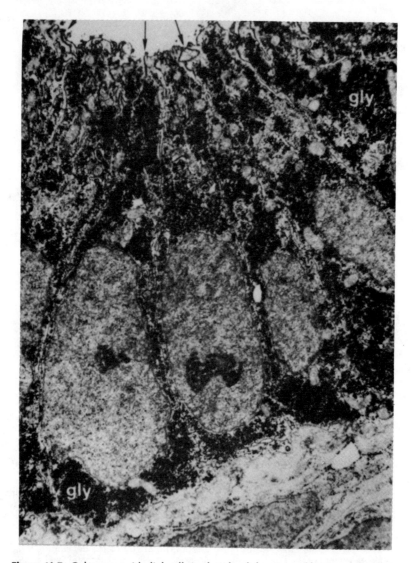

Figure 14-7. Columnar epithelial cells in the glandular stage of human pulmonary development. (Electron micrograph) *Arrows* indicate the apical tight junctions that join these epithelial cells together. *gly*, glycogen. (Reprinted with permission from Burri PH, Weibel ER: Ultrastructure and morphometry of the developing lung. In *Development of the Lung*. Edited by Hodson WA. New York, Marcel Dekker, 1977, p 220.)

        (a) Pulmonary surfactant is made up of phospholipoprotein complexes.
        (b) Phosphatidylcholine (**lecithin**) is the most abundant phospholipid in surfactant.
    (2) The phospholipoprotein complexes are secreted from the type II cells onto the apical surface of the alveolar epithelial lining.
    (3) Here the complexes form a thin but continuous film of phospholipid and protein that reduces the surface tension at the interface between the fluid-filled alveolus and the alveolar epithelium.
  3. Once adequate numbers of type II cells have formed, a fetus is viable in the extrauterine environment.
    a. Until enough type II cells form, premature infants are at high risk of developing respiratory distress syndrome (see section V A).
    b. These infants have great difficulty inflating their lungs, due to the lack of surfactant.
  4. The secretion of surfactant is also a clinically useful indication of fetal lung maturity (see section V B).

V. RESPIRATORY DISTRESS SYNDROME AND ASSESSMENT OF FETAL MATURITY

A. Respiratory distress syndrome (RDS; hyaline membrane disease)

1. Each year, a large number of infants are born prematurely; that is, before the normal 38-week term of normal pregnancy.
2. Many of these infants are at risk of developing **respiratory distress syndrome (RDS)**, the leading cause of mortality and morbidity among premature infants.
   a. In this affliction, functional immaturity of the lungs causes inadequate secretion of surfactant from type II alveolar cells. (The alveolar surfaces also become coated with a clear **hyaline membrane** of vascular transudates—the reason for the alternative name for this disorder.)
   b. The lack of surfactant results in **atelectasis** (incomplete expansion of the lungs), which in turn leads to respiratory distress.
   c. Research pediatricians noticed that the lungs of children who died from RDS contained significantly less surface-active material (surfactant) than lungs of age-matched children who died from other causes unrelated to pulmonary function.
3. The state of differentiation of type II cells in the alveolar epithelium is thus of particular significance to the development of RDS.

B. Assessment of fetal maturity

1. **Clinical usefulness**
   a. An elective cesarean-section delivery of the preterm fetus is indicated on clinical grounds in certain maternal conditions.
   b. Pregnant patients suffering from diabetes mellitus, hypertension, sickle-cell disease, and Rh isoimmunization all are at considerable risk for an intrauterine fetal demise.
   c. For these women, a determination of the maturity of fetal pulmonary function can guide the obstetrician in making a judgment as to the appropriate time to deliver the baby.

2. **Method of assessment: the lecithin/sphingomyelin (L/S) ratio**
   a. The **L/S ratio**, measured in amniotic fluid samples taken by amniocentesis, can be used as a guide to fetal pulmonary maturity, and thus as a reasonably sensitive predictor of the possibility of development of RDS in the fetus.
      (1) Before birth, the fetal lungs are filled with amniotic fluid, and lecithin secreted from type II pneumocytes enters the amniotic fluid. The amniotic fluid also contains other phospholipids, among them sphingomyelin.

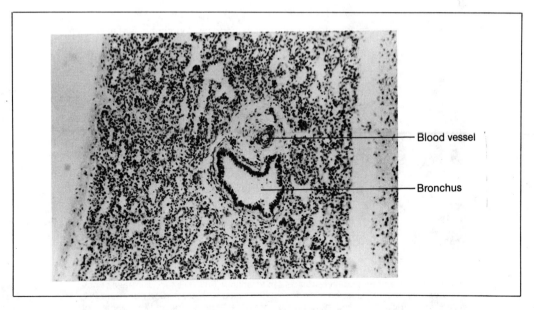

Figure 14-8. The canalicular stage of human pulmonary development. (Light micrograph)

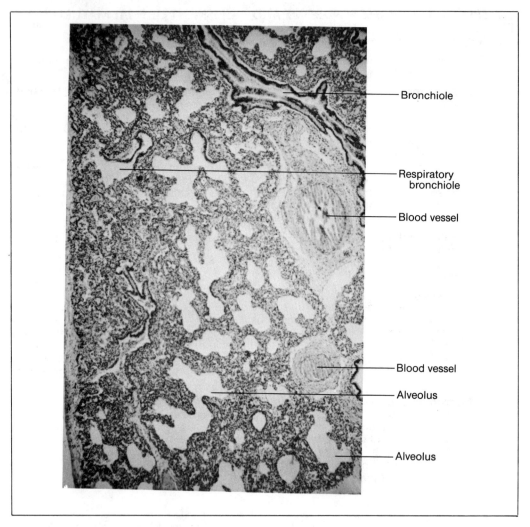

Figure 14-9. The saccular stage of human pulmonary development. (Light micrograph)

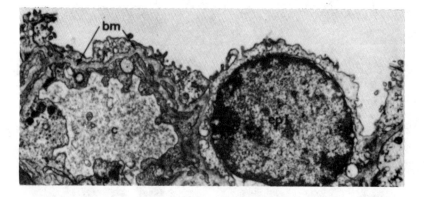

Figure 14-10. A type I squamous alveolar epithelial cell (*cpl*) resting on basement membrane (*bm*) and immediately adjacent to a capillary (*c*) in the saccular stage of pulmonary development. (Electron micrograph) (Reprinted with permission from Burri PH, Weibel ER: Ultrastructure and morphometry of the developing lung. In *Development of the Lung*. Edited by Hodson WA. New York, Marcel Dekker, 1977, p 226.)

       (2) The amount of **lecithin** in amniotic fluid increases dramatically as the type II pneumocytes secrete **surfactant**. By contrast, the content of **sphingomyelin** in the amniotic fluid remains relatively invariant throughout gestation.
          (a) Both lecithin and sphingomyelin appear in amniotic fluid at about 24 weeks of development.
          (b) For a time, both levels rise slowly.
          (c) Suddenly, at 35 weeks, the lecithin levels rise rapidly, so that by term lecithin accounts for about 75% of the phospholipid in amniotic fluid.
  b. In common practice, once the L/S ratio is greater than a certain value (established by each laboratory because of technical differences), the obstetrician can then be confident that an unborn child will be at acceptably low risk for developing RDS.

STUDY QUESTIONS

Directions: Each question below contains five suggested answers. Choose the **one best** response to each question.

1. Cells derived from the respiratory diverticulum, an endodermal diverticulum of the foregut, include all of the following EXCEPT

   (A) chondrocytes
   (B) tracheal goblet cells
   (C) ciliated tracheal epithelial cells
   (D) type I alveolar epithelial cells
   (E) type II alveolar epithelial cells

2. A child is born prematurely after 30 weeks of development. It would be likely to show all of the following clinical findings EXCEPT

   (A) apnea
   (B) hyaline membranes on alveolar epithelium
   (C) cyanosis
   (D) a high lecithin/sphingomyelin (L/S) ratio
   (E) reduced chance of survival

Directions: Each question below contains four suggested answers of which **one or more** is correct. Choose the answer

   A if **1, 2, and 3** are correct
   B if **1 and 3** are correct
   C if **2 and 4** are correct
   D if **4** is correct
   E if **1, 2, 3, and 4** are correct

3. Type II cells in the developing lungs show which of the following characteristics?

   (1) They differentiate from cells in the respiratory diverticulum
   (2) Their differentiation causes the lecithin/sphingomyelin (L/S) ratio to fall
   (3) They secrete lecithin into the amniotic fluid
   (4) They become functionally differentiated during the twentieth week of development

4. Respiratory distress syndrome (RDS) shows which of the following characteristics?

   (1) It is an uncommon cause of death in premature infants
   (2) Lung lavages from infants with RDS would be deficient in surfactant
   (3) It is less common in 28-week fetuses than in 37-week fetuses
   (4) It is often caused by lack of type II cell differentiation

5. True statements concerning stages of lung histodifferentiation include which of the following?

   (1) Bronchioles are established during the glandular stage
   (2) Bronchi are established during the saccular stage
   (3) Type II cells form during the canalicular stage
   (4) Alveolar ducts are established during the saccular stage

Directions: The groups of questions below consist of lettered choices followed by several numbered items. For each numbered item select the **one** lettered choice with which it is **most** closely associated. Each lettered choice may be used once, more than once, or not at all.

Questions 6–9

Listed below are structures that form during the development of the lungs. For each structure formed, select the embryonic rudiment that forms it.

(A) Respiratory diverticulum
(B) Splanchnic mesoderm
(C) Both
(D) Neither

(6) Epithelial cells lining blood vessels
(7) Structures making up the alveolar walls
(8) Surfactant-secreting cells in the distal lung
(9) Tracheal smooth muscles and bronchial cartilages

Questions 10–14

For each of the following descriptions of structures in the developing nasal cavities, select the appropriate lettered component shown in the accompanying micrograph.

10. This portion of the maxilla forms most of the hard palate

11. When this structure is depressed, the lateral palatine processes become elevated

12. This structure fuses with the primary and secondary palate to form the nasal septum

13. This structure is the precursor of the nasal cavity (at this stage, it is in direct communication with the oral cavity)

14. This structure forms the soft palate

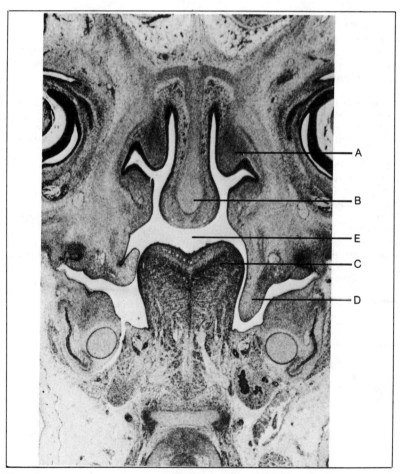

Questions 10–14

ANSWERS AND EXPLANATIONS

1. The answer is A. *(Chapter 9 II B 2; III A 1; Chapter 14 III C 2)* Chondrocytes are cartilage cells. They are present in the respiratory system in the cartilages found, for example, in the trachea and in bronchi. Chondrocytes are derived from splanchnic mesoderm. All of the other cell types in the question are epithelial cells lining the airways of the lungs. Goblet cells and ciliated cells are in the tracheal airways. Type I and type II cells are in the alveoli. All of the cells lining the airways and respiratory surfaces of the lungs are derived from the endodermal respiratory diverticulum.

2. The answer is D. *(V A, B)* The normal duration of intrauterine development is 38 weeks. A 30-week premature infant would have an increased chance of having respiratory distress syndrome (RDS), the leading cause of death among premature infants. Infants with RDS often exhibit apnea (difficulty in breathing), cyanosis (bluish cast to the skin), and a membranous hyaline transudate on the alveolar epithelium. RDS is caused by a significant immaturity of the lungs, with inadequate numbers of surfactant-secreting type II alveolar epithelial cells. After 35 weeks, the type II cells are numerous enough to produce adequate amounts of surfactant (lecithin), so that the lecithin/sphingomyelin (L/S) ratio of the amniotic fluid rapidly increases. Thereafter, the risk of RDS decreases significantly.

3. The answer is B (1, 3). *(IV C 2; V B)* Type II cells develop from the respiratory diverticulum. When they mature, beginning around the twenty-fifth week, they secrete surfactant into the amniotic fluid. Surfactant contains lecithin, and when type II cells differentiate, the amount of lecithin in the amniotic fluid increases, causing the lecithin/sphingomyelin (L/S) ratio to rise slowly. Once there is adequate surfactant production, at about the thirty-fifth week, the L/S ratio shows a sudden increase. As a result, the risk of developing respiratory distress syndrome decreases rapidly.

4. The answer is C (2, 4). *(V A, B)* Respiratory distress syndrome is the leading cause of death among premature infants. It is most often caused by delivery prior to the time when type II alveolar cell differentiation has led to the production of large amounts of surfactant. It decreases in frequency and severity with increasing fetal age. This decrease in frequency and severity is due primarily to the production of surfactant by type II cells.

5. The answer is D (4). *(IV A, B, C)* The first period of lung histogenesis is the glandular stage. During this stage, branches of the respiratory diverticulum form the bronchi. During the second, or canalicular, stage, the bronchioles are formed. During the final stage, the saccular stage, the alveolar ducts and alveoli differentiate. Type II cells do not form until the saccular stage.

6-9. The answers are 6-B, 7-C, 8-A, 9-B. *(III C)* The respiratory diverticulum is a branch of the foregut. It is lined by endodermally derived cells. It gives rise to the entire epithelial lining of the lumen of the respiratory system, including the lining of the conducting airways and the lining of the surfaces specialized for respiratory gas exchange. The splanchnic mesoderm forms connective tissue elements, blood vessels (including their linings), cartilage, and smooth muscle in the respiratory system.

10-14. The answers are 10-D, 11-C, 12-B, 13-E, 14-D. *(II A 2)* The photomicrograph accompanying the questions is a frontal section through the developing nasal cavities. The nasal conchae (A) are shelves that develop in the upper portion of the nasal cavity (E). The nasal septum (B) divides the nasal cavity into left and right sides after it has fused with the lateral palatine processes (D), the precursors of most of the hard palate (posterior to the incisive foramen) and all of the soft palate. The tongue (C), initially high (as in the micrograph), moves downward, allowing the lateral palatine processes to swing upward. The lateral palatine processes then fuse with one another, with the primary palate, and with the nasal septum, forming the complete palate.

15
Development of the Immune System

I. INTRODUCTION

  A. The immune system provides the body with the ability to mount a defense against foreign organisms and antigenic substances. Perhaps because of this widespread function, the immune system is a complex system, both structurally and functionally, and it has a complex developmental history.

  B. **Components of the immune system** (Fig. 15-1)

   1. The immune system is is widely dispersed throughout the body.
   2. It is composed of organs, cellular elements, and soluble (humoral) elements.
      a. **Organs of the immune system**
         (1) The organs of the immune system consist of:
             (a) Lymph nodes
             (b) The spleen
             (c) The thymus
             (d) Tonsils
             (e) Gut-associated lymphoid tissue (GALT)
             (f) Various lymphatic vessels
             (g) Bone marrow
         (2) Except for the spleen, the lymphoid organs are rather straightforward histologically, yet they are a good deal more complex than would appear at first glance.
      b. **The cellular elements of the lymphoid system** are the lymphocytes and macrophages. The **lymphocytes** are a diverse group of cells in the circulating blood and tissue spaces.
         (1) The lymphocytes are similar in appearance and appear to be morphologically simple.
         (2) This simple, similar morphology is highly deceptive, however, because lymphocytes are functionally heterogeneous and complex.
         (3) The complexities of lymphocytes involve both their developmental differentiation and their interaction in the immune response.
      c. **The humoral elements of the lymphoid system** are the **antibodies**, or **immunoglobulins**, that are chiefly found circulating in the blood.

II. MOLECULAR BIOLOGY OF IMMUNOGLOBULINS

  A. **Nature of immunoglobulins**

   1. **Immunoglobulins are a series of closely related glycoproteins.**
      a. They are called **immunoglobulins** because they are found in the **globulin fraction** of blood serum.
         (1) The immunoglobulins in serum are dissolved and circulate in high concentrations.
         (2) The circulating **antibodies** in human serum are immunoglobulins.
      b. Some immunoglobulins are associated with the **surface of cells** of the immune system.
   2. **Five broad classes** of immunoglobulins are known:
      a. Immunoglobulin G (IgG), the most prevalent in serum
      b. Immunoglobulin M (IgM)
      c. Immunoglobulin A (IgA)
      d. Immunoglobulin D (IgD)
      e. Immunoglobulin E (IgE)

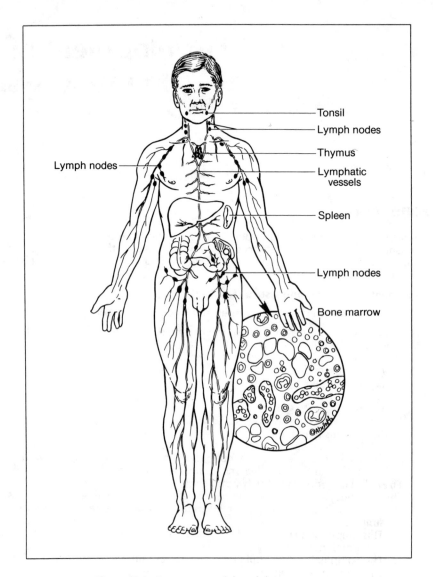

Figure 15-1. Components of the adult immune system.

3. Immunoglobulin molecules can aggregate with one another and can also bind to cells and to antigens that enter the body.
   a. The resulting **antigen-antibody complexes** then set off intricate responses in the organism that eventually result in the elimination of the antigen-antibody complexes from the body.
   b. One important response stimulated by antigen-antibody complexes is activation of the **complement cascade**.
      (1) While traditionally not considered a part of the immune system, the complement system is an important element in antigen-antibody reactions.
      (2) The complement system consists of a complex interlocking cascade of serum proteins.
         (a) These proteins exist in the serum as inactive **precursors**. Activation of the first protein in the complement series (for example, through binding by an antigen-antibody complex) sets off the activation of the second protein, which in turn activates the third, and so on through the entire cascade.
         (b) Once fully activated, the complement cascade can result in the lysis and destruction of many different kinds of microorganisms and cells.

B. Basic immunoglobulin structure

1. The molecular structure of IgG (Fig. 15-2) is representative of the basic structure of all immunoglobulin molecules.
   a. Like other immunoglobulins, IgG is composed of four **polypeptide chains** linked to one another into a macromolecular complex by **disulfide (-S-S-) bonds**.
      (1) Two of the polypeptides are large and **heavy (H chains)** and two are small and **light (L chains)**.
      (2) They are assembled as shown diagrammatically in Figure 15-2.
   b. An area at each outer end of the light and heavy chains of the immunoglobulin molecule is referred to as the **variable region**. (These are the areas marked V_L and V_H in Figure 15-2.)
      (1) This variable region contains the **antigen-binding site**.
      (2) Variations in the amino acid sequences in this region are thought to be the basis for the **antigenic specificity** shown by different IgG subtypes.

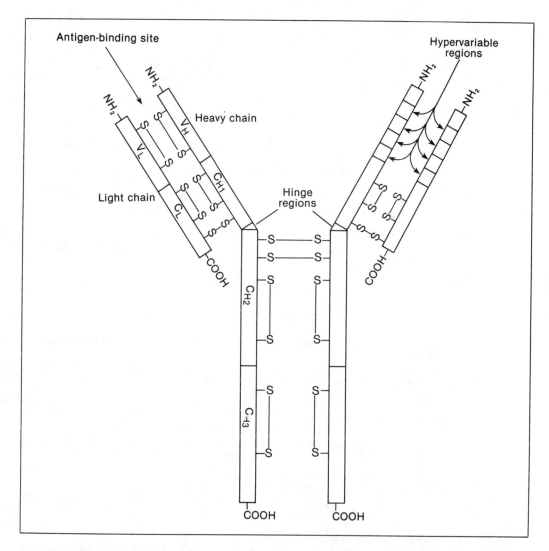

Figure 15-2. The human immunoglobulin G molecule. Right and left sides of the molecule are symmetric; components are identified on one side only for simplicity. S–S, disulfide bonds; V_H and V_L, variable regions on the heavy and light chains, respectively; C_H and C_L, constant regions on the heavy and light chains, respectively; COOH, carboxyl terminal; NH_2, amino terminal. (Adapted from Halkerston IDK: *NMS Biochemistry*, 2nd ed. Media, Pa., Harwal/Wiley, 1988, p 140.)

c. Both heavy and light chains also have **constant regions**; in heavy chains, this is divided into three homologous subregions. (These are the areas marked C_L and C_{H1}, C_{H2}, and C_{H3} in Figure 15-2.) The amino acid sequences in the constant regions are nearly identical within each immunoglobulin class.
2. All of the immunoglobulins can occur in the body as **monomers**, the structure shown in Figure 15-2. IgA and IgM also occur as **polymers**.
   a. **IgA** can occur as a **dimer** (two joined monomers).
   b. **IgM** occurs in the blood as a **pentamer** (five joined monomers).
   c. Polymeric immunoglobulins have an additional type of chain, the **joining (J) chain** (see Fig. 15-3).

C. **Properties of the five immunoglobulin types**
1. **IgG**
   a. IgG is a monomer with a molecular weight of 150,000 daltons (150 kDa).
   b. IgG is the most common immunoglobulin in the serum and the major antibody type appearing in response to an antigen.
   c. IgG is especially important in fetal development, because it is the only immunoglobulin to cross the placenta.
      (1) The fetus receives a good deal of IgG from the mother by active **transport across the placenta**.
      (2) This has both beneficial and potentially harmful aspects.
         (a) Maternal IgG **protects the fetus** against harmful antigens, an effect that persists for several months after birth.
         (b) IgG is the immunoglobulin that **reacts with Rh antigen**, causing erythroblastosis fetalis (see section VIII).

2. **IgM**
   a. IgM is a pentamer; that is, an aggregate of five IgG-like units. The IgM pentamer has a molecular weight of about 900 kDa.
   b. In contrast to IgG, IgM is not transported across the placenta, perhaps because of its large molecular weight.
   c. Unlike the antigen-binding sites of IgG, those of IgM do not have a high affinity for antigens, but the IgM pentamers are particularly potent as activators of the complement system.
   d. **IgM monomers** are constituents on the surface of B lymphocytes, the precursors of immunoglobulin-secreting cells. Thus, IgM may play a role in stimulating immunoglobulin production.

3. **IgA**
   a. IgA in the blood serum is a **monomer**. The IgA monomer is similar to the IgG monomer but it has a slightly higher molecular weight.
   b. IgA **dimers** are found in **secretions**—tears, sweat, saliva, breast milk, colostrum, and mucus.
      (1) IgA dimers have a **J (joining) polypeptide** and a glycoprotein **secretory component** (Fig. 15-3).
      (2) **Secretory IgA**, the dimeric form, is thought to reduce local damage to the body from antigens entering via the gastrointestinal, respiratory, and urogenital tracts, for example.
      (3) They may bind to enteric bacteria, preventing bacterial adhesion to enteric epithelial cells.
      (4) Secretory IgA is important from a developmental perspective, in that it is found in high concentrations in **colostrum** (a kind of breast milk, produced transiently after childbirth as lactation begins), and in **breast milk** itself (see section VI B 1).

4. **IgE and IgD** are present in only trace amounts.
   a. **IgE** is a monomer with a molecular weight of 190 kDa.
      (1) IgE is involved in histamine release from mast cells and basophils, and thus is important in immediate hypersensitivity (allergic) reactions such as asthma and hay fever.
      (2) IgE may play a protective role in parasitic infections.
   b. **IgD** is a monomer with a molecular weight of 180 kDa. Its biologic role is still poorly understood.
      (1) IgD monomers, like IgM monomers, are found on the surface of B lymphocytes, and thus may play a role in stimulating immunoglobulin production.
      (2) IgD may represent an immunoglobulin found predominantly on fetal and malignant cells.

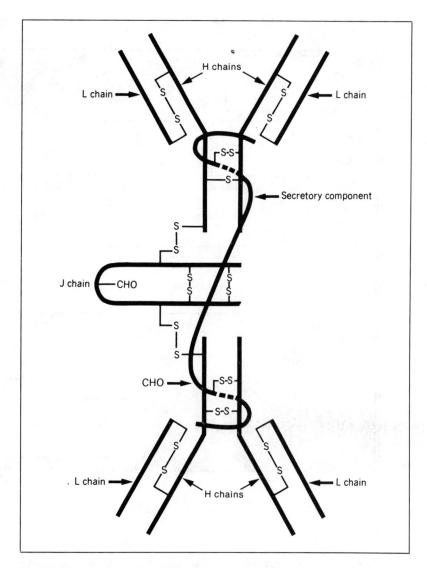

Figure 15-3. The human dimeric secretory IgA molecule, showing the postulated arrangement of IgA monomers, secretory component, and the J chain. -S-S-, disulfide bridges; CHO, carbohydrate. (Adapted from Klein J: *Immunology.* New York, Wiley, 1982, p 193.)

III. **HEMATOPOIESIS.** It is not possible to study the ontogeny of the immune system without considering hematopoiesis, as it relates so closely to the development of the rest of the immune system.

  A. **The periods of hematopoiesis during human development** (Fig. 15-4)
    1. **The yolk sac**
      a. Blood cell formation begins in **blood islands** in the yolk sac during the third week of development (see Chapter 6, section III A).
        (1) In the yolk sac, mesodermally derived cells differentiate into **hematopoietic stem cells**.
        (2) At first, in the yolk sac, these stem cells differentiate further only into **primitive erythroblasts** and **primitive erythrocytes**.
      b. Later, stem cells migrate from the yolk sac into the **liver**.

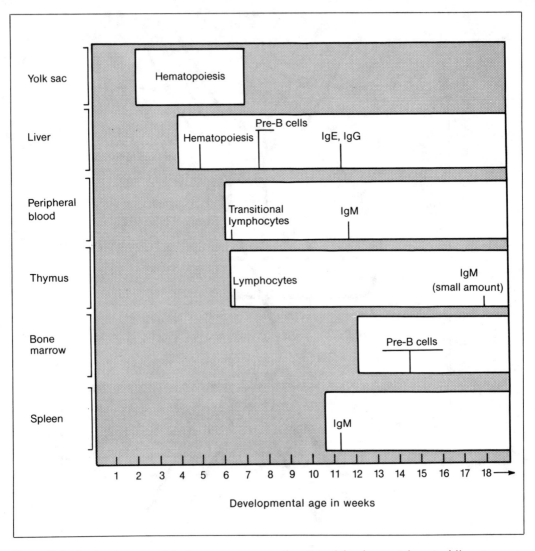

Figure 15-4. The development of the immune system as a function of developmental age in different organs. (Adapted from Klein J: *Immunology.* New York, Wiley, 1982, p 312.)

2. **The liver and spleen**
   a. From about the sixth week on, until bone marrow takes over hematopoietic function, the liver and, to a lesser extent, the spleen serve as the major source of blood cells (Fig. 15-5).
   b. In the liver and spleen, the stem cells differentiate into all the blood cell types: erythrocytes, megakaryocytes, monocytes, lymphocytes, and the cells of the granulocytic series.
3. **The bone marrow**
   a. During the period of hepatic blood cell formation, cartilage and bones are forming. As the bones take shape, **central cavities** are formed and are invaded by **hematopoietic stem cells**.
   b. **Bone marrow** differentiates in this way during osteogenesis and subsequently replaces the liver and spleen as the major hematopoietic site.
   c. The bone marrow is the site of hematopoiesis in later fetal life and in the child and adult.

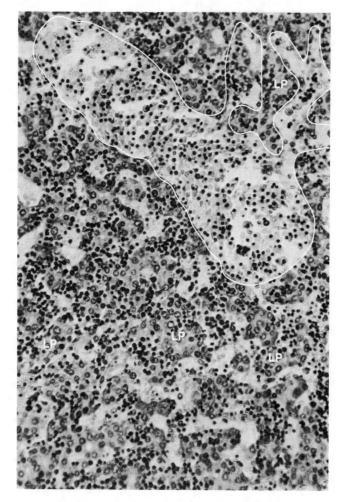

Figure 15-5. Hematopoietic area in the human liver (*outlined*), surrounded by numerous liver parenchymal cells (*LP*). (Light micrograph)

B. Origin of hematopoietic stem cells
1. There is some controversy surrounding the actual origin of stem cells.
   a. Some believe that all stem cells originate in the yolk sac and that these yolk sac–derived stem cells subsequently populate other hematopoietic organs.
   b. Others feel that stem cells arise de novo in various other intraembryonic sites as well as in the yolk sac.
2. Recent experiments using chick–quail chimeric embryos favor the latter interpretation.
   a. The nuclei of chick and quail embryonic cells are morphologically distinct from one another.
   b. It is possible by transplantation to attach chick embryos to quail yolk sacs (or vice versa), and such chimeras can be used to test cell lineages.
   c. When the transplants were performed, it was clear that some stem cells were derived from embryonic cells rather than yolk sac cells, supporting the notion that liver and bone marrow stem cells may arise in situ.
3. Because there may be differences between birds and mammals, the question of stem cell origins is not fully answered at the present time. However, with advances in mammalian (and human?) embryo culture techniques, it will be possible to approach these intellectual challenges experimentally.

IV. LYMPHOCYTE DIFFERENTIATION (Fig. 15-6)

A. Characteristics of B cells and T cells

1. **Lymphocytes** are the key cellular elements of the immune system. They are essential for mounting immune responses against cellular and soluble antigens.
2. There are two **subpopulations** of lymphocytes, **T cells** and **B cells**. In the peripheral adult circulation, T cells comprise about 65% of the total lymphocytes and B cells comprise about 35%.
   a. **T (thymus-dependent) cells**
      (1) T cells are named from the fact that they require "processing" by the **thymus** in order to differentiate into T cells.
      (2) T cells are responsible for the **cell-mediated immune response**, so called because the cells themselves take part in the immune response.
         (a) T cells combat fungal and viral infections.
         (b) T cells, along with macrophages, are involved in B cell differentiation into antibody-secreting plasma cells.

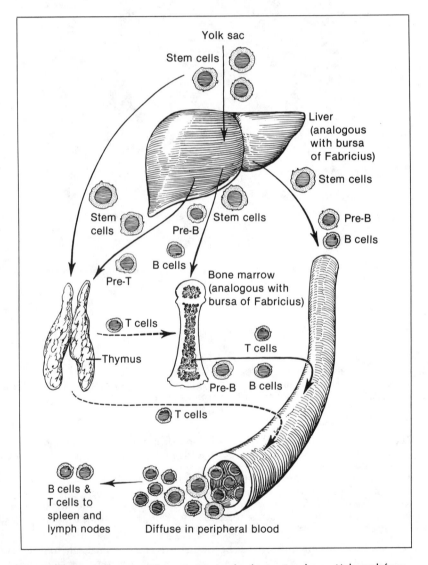

Figure 15-6. Lymphocyte differentiation in the human embryo. (Adapted from Klein J: *Immunology*. New York, Wiley, 1982, p 632.)

(c) They are also involved in graft rejection and destruction of tumor cells.
b. **B (bursa-dependent) cells**
    (1) B cells are so named because their differentiation from stem cells is presumed to require processing by an organ analogous to the **bursa of Fabricius** in birds (see section IV C 2).
    (2) B cells are responsible for **humoral immunity**, so called because **humoral (soluble) elements**—the **immunoglobulins (antibodies)**—take part in the immune response, rather than the B cells themselves.
    (3) B cells **differentiate** further into **plasma cells** after appropriate stimulation. This differentiation process involves the help of T cells and macrophages (Fig. 15-7).

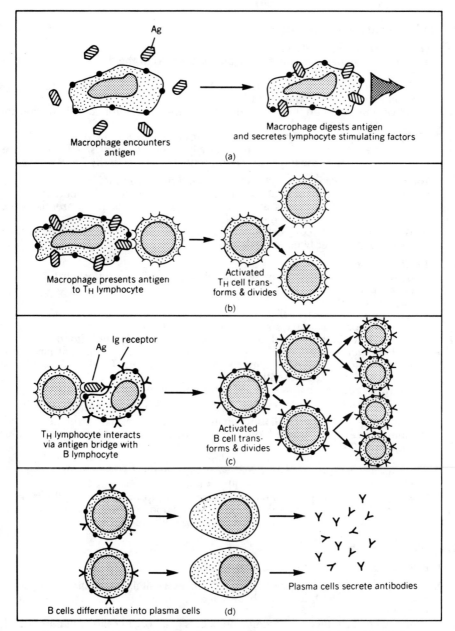

Figure 15-7. The salient features of B cell differentiation. T_H, T helper cell. (Adapted from Klein J: *Immunology.* New York, Wiley, 1982, p 513.)

(4) The **plasma cells** secrete large quantities of **specific antibodies** which circulate in the blood and bind to foreign antigens.
3. T cells and B cells are not strikingly different from one another morphologically unless specific immunohistochemical tests are performed to differentiate them.
4. Nevertheless, they are **functionally very different** from one another and they have very different developmental histories.
5. Both T and B cells are found in the lymph nodes, spleen, thymus, and bone marrow as well as in the peripheral blood.
   a. The distribution and relative abundance of T and B lymphocytes varies tremendously in these organs and in the peripheral blood.
   b. For example, T cells outnumber B cells in the peripheral blood and thymus, but B cells predominate in the bone marrow.

B. **T cell differentiation**
   1. **The process of T cell differentiation**
      a. T cells originate from **undifferentiated stem cells** in the liver, spleen, and bone marrow.
      b. These stem cells produce **lymphoblasts** which migrate from sites of stem cell populations to the **thymus** gland.
         (1) Undifferentiated stem cells enter the thymic cortex from the circulation and begin to divide rapidly.
         (2) The cells then migrate from the thymic cortex toward the thymic medulla. As they migrate, they become morphologically recognizable as **small lymphocytes**. They have also become functionally differentiated as **T cells** (by 7 to 9 weeks).
   2. The **thymic medulla** is clearly the **site** of T cell differentiation.
      a. However, the **mechanism of differentiation** is not clearly understood. It is thought that thymic protein hormones attach to the cell surface of undifferentiated cells and induce their differentiation to T cells.
      b. The thymus influences T cell differentiation even after T cells have left the thymus and have seeded other lymphoid organs.
   3. **T cell subclasses**
      a. Following thymic processing, several subclasses of T cells differentiate:
         (1) Helper T cells
         (2) Suppressor T cells
         (3) Cytotoxic (killer) T cells
      b. The functional subclasses arise as a result of further T cell differentiation, but the factors controlling this further differentiation are poorly understood.
         (1) However, experimental studies on mouse T cell development have shown that there are cell surface antigens expressed on pre-T cells that are replaced or masked during differentiation.
         (2) These antigens may be related to the later differentiation of subclasses, since each subclass, once formed, can be identified by its particular cell surface markers.
   4. Experimental studies on **T cell function** in human embryos have been performed.
      a. Human T cells will respond to stimulation by certain plant lectins such as **phytohemagglutinin (PHA)**.
         (1) Soluble PHA will stimulate a proliferative response in T cells, and PHA stimulation has been used as a criterion of T cell differentiation.
         (2) Fetal T cells are responsive to PHA stimulation as early as 10 weeks.
      b. Also, in several experimental series a relationship has been noted between thymic responsiveness to PHA stimulation, demarcation of cortical and medullary thymic zones, and increased T cell counts in peripheral blood.

C. **B cell differentiation**
   1. B cells also originate from **bone marrow stem cells**.
   2. There is presumed to be an organ that influences B cell differentiation, comparable to the thymus for T cells, but no such B-cell–differentiating organ has been identified in mammals.
      a. In the **chicken**, B cell differentiation occurs in an organ called the **bursa of Fabricius**.
         (1) The bursa of Fabricius is a derivative of the caudal hindgut.
         (2) Like the thymus, the bursa of Fabricius develops as a diverticulum from the gut tube.

(3) Also like the thymus, the bursa of Fabricius is seeded by undifferentiated lymphocyte stem cells which come from the yolk sac and liver.

    b. Extensive searches for the bursa equivalent in mammals have been unsuccessful. Experiments have ruled out the appendix, Peyer's patches, and other gut-associated lymphoid tissue.
    c. Most investigators feel that the **bone marrow**, the **liver**, or **both**, is the probable bursa equivalent in mammals.
3. B cells are characterized by possessing large numbers of surface immunoglobulins, and the appearance of IgM on the cell surface is a hallmark of B cell differentiation.
    a. IgM-bearing B cells are found in the human fetal liver at about 9 weeks, and a few days later IgG-bearing B cells are also detectable.
    b. By about 12 weeks, IgA-bearing cells are found, and differentiated B cells bearing IgM, IgG, and IgA on their cell surfaces are found in the liver, peripheral blood, spleen, and bone marrow.
4. **After birth**, antigenic challenge causes B cells to undergo further differentiation into **plasma cells**, which then produce circulating immunoglobulins (see Fig. 15-7). However, the **fetus** normally does not encounter such antigens, and therefore **plasma cells** (and their secreted circulating immunoglobulins) are not present in the normal fetus.

V. EMBRYOLOGY OF LYMPHATIC VESSELS AND MAJOR LYMPHATIC ORGANS

A. **Lymphatic vessels**
   1. **Mode of formation**
      a. Lymphatic vessels are thought to form either by evagination of the walls of the developing blood vessels or by confluence of perivenous mesenchymal tissue spaces.
      b. It is clear that lymphatic vessels form in intimate association with the developing venous system (see Fig. 15-12, *left*).
   2. **Stages of formation**
      a. **Four major lymphatic vessels** form first. They are completely formed by around 9 weeks. These vessels are:
         (1) Paired **jugular lymph sacs** (in the neck)
         (2) Paired **ilioinguinal lymph sacs** (in the pelvis)
         (3) Unpaired **retroperitoneal sacs** (in the posterior abdominal wall)
         (4) The **cisterna chyli**, which runs from the ilioinguinal to the jugular sacs
      b. The remaining lymphatics of the body probably develop as branches of these major sacs.
      c. **Lymphatic valves** appear in some locations by the end of the second month.
      d. By the beginning of the fifth month, the fetus is equipped with large numbers of lymphatic vessels with functional valves.

B. **Lymph nodes** (Fig. 15-8)
   1. Lymph nodes arise as lymphocytes aggregate around the major lymphatic sacs.
      a. These lymphocytes have differentiated from **hemocytoblasts (stem cells)** in the liver and bone marrow and have migrated to the lymph nodes.
      b. T lymphocytes arrive at lymph nodes after processing in the thymus.
      c. Small aggregates of lymphocytes are seen around lymphatic sacs as early as the seventh week, but these clusters remain small and indistinct until about the tenth week.
   2. The complete histologic differentiation of lymph nodes normally does not occur until after birth, and lymph nodes normally are not functional in mounting an immune response until after birth.
      a. Normally, **germinal centers** appear in lymph nodes as a result of the **antigenic challenges** presented to the newborn. These germinal centers are morphologic expressions of plasma cell differentiation.
      b. **Plasma cells**, the immunoglobulin-secreting B cell derivatives, are not present in the normal fetus.
         (1) In fetuses aborted as a result of intrauterine rubella, toxoplasma, or *Treponema pallidum* (syphilis) infections, plasma cells are present and germinal centers can be observed in lymph nodes.
         (2) This suggests that the fetus is **immunocompetent** but does not express this ability unless there is an intrauterine infection.

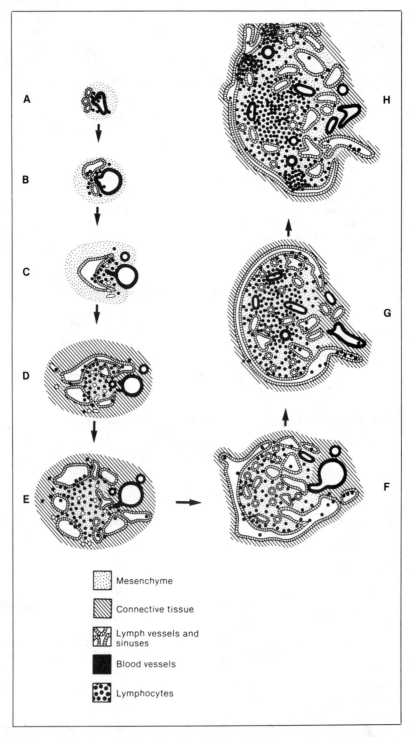

Figure 15-8. Steps in the development of a lymph node. (A) Lymph vessels and blood vessels form in mesenchyme. (B) Lymphocytes from lymphatic vessels and blood vessels invade the mesenchyme. (C–H) Lymph vessels and blood vessels proliferate; more lymphocytes enter lymph nodes; mesenchyme forms a capsule around the organ; lymphatic vessels penetrate the capsule. (Reprinted with permission from Klein J: *Immunology*. New York, Wiley, 1982, p. 632.)

C. The spleen

1. The spleen appears at about 5 weeks.
   a. It begins as a condensation of mesenchymal cells in the **dorsal mesogastrium** (the mesentery that suspends the stomach from the dorsal body wall).
   b. As the condensation grows, it projects into the peritoneal cavity.
   c. This is how the spleen comes to be encapsulated in mesothelium.
2. At about the ninth week of development, just as the embryo has entered the fetal period, mesenchymal cells arrange themselves into anastomosing networks of trabeculae.
   a. The trabecular masses also enclose other mesenchymally derived cells, which remain free in the spaces between trabeculae.
   b. These free cells differentiate into lymphoblasts, erythroblasts, myeloblasts (granulocyte precursors), and megakaryocytes.
3. **Hematopoiesis** is intense in the spleen during the fourth and fifth intrauterine months. Later, **myelopoiesis** decreases in significance but **erythropoiesis** continues in the spleen.

D. The thymus has a complex embryologic history.

1. The thymus, along with the parathyroid glands, arises from the third and fourth pharyngeal pouches.
   a. The third and fourth pharyngeal pouches rapidly grow ventromedially and caudally, and fuse in the ventral midline inferior to the developing thyroid gland, at a point near the arch of the aorta.
   b. As these pouches grow downward they carry the parathyroid rudiments with them.
   c. Eventually, however, the parathyroids separate from the thymic rudiments.
2. The endodermal derivatives of the third and fourth pharyngeal pouches give rise to the reticular epithelial cells of the thymus.
   a. These epithelial cells are known to secrete a polypeptide hormone known as **thymosin**.
   b. Thymosin is required for the differentiation of lymphoblasts into mature **T cells**.
3. Mesenchymally derived blood vessels grow into the endodermally derived thymic rudiments.
   a. In the process, the gland is divided up into a series of lobules which persist into adult life.
   b. Each lobule has a cortex and a medulla (Fig. 15-9).
4. As the blood vessels grow into the gland, they also carry in circulating lymphocytes, which come to be intimately associated with the epithelial elements of the gland.
5. In the thymus, certain lymphoblasts are programmed to differentiate into **T cells**.

E. The tonsils and gut-associated lymphoid tissue (GALT)

1. The **tonsils** are lymphoid organs in the vicinity of the oral cavity and pharynx.
   a. The **palatine tonsils** are the largest tonsils.
      (1) They arise from the paired second pharyngeal pouches.
      (2) These paired evaginations give rise to the stratified squamous epithelium lining the palatine tonsillar crypts.
      (3) Soon after their formation, the tonsillar crypts become invaded by masses of B and T lymphocytes which travel to the crypts from the bone marrow and the thymus respectively.
   b. The **pharyngeal tonsils** form from a single median evagination of the dorsal wall of the nasopharynx.
      (1) The pharyngeal tonsils are usually lined by pseudostratified epithelium but may also have small patches of stratified squamous epithelium as well.
      (2) Here too, once the tonsillar crypt is formed, B and T lymphocytes invade it.
      (3) In childhood, the pharyngeal tonsils may become substantially enlarged due to chronic infection, forming the **adenoid tonsils**.
2. **Gut-associated lymphoid tissue (GALT)** is a diffuse collection of lymph nodules and nodes found all along the gastrointestinal tract. Although it has not been closely studied embryologically, GALT probably forms in much the same manner as other lymph nodes.

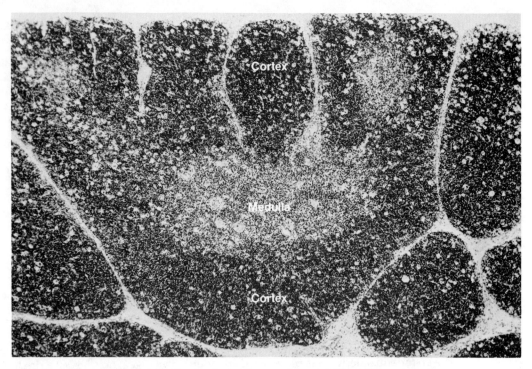

Figure 15-9. The developing human thymus. (Light micrograph)

VI. MATERNAL IMMUNOLOGIC AIDS FOR THE FETUS AND NEWBORN

A. Passive fetal immunization

1. Prior to birth, the normal **fetus** does not mount an immune response to environmental antigens, merely because the fetus is not normally exposed to these antigens in utero.

2. Usually, the **newborn** deals with the onslaught of new antigens by **passive immunization**—that is, by utilizing maternally produced IgG that has been transported across the placenta.

3. As the maternally derived IgG molecules are catabolized in the newborn, the child's own immune system matures and the child can begin to produce its own IgG.

B. Immunologic function of breast milk

1. **Colostrum** and **breast milk** contain additional immunologic aids for the newborn in the form of a substantial concentration of **IgG** and a very high concentration of **secretory IgA (sIgA)**. These immunoglobulins help protect the infant from gastrointestinal infections.
    a. **Structure of secretory IgA** (see Fig. 15-3)
        (1) Secretory IgA is a **dimer** of two molecules much like a single IgG molecule.
        (2) It also has a **J (joining) polypeptide chain** and a **secretory component (SC)**.
            (a) The **J chain** links the IgA monomers into a dimer.
            (b) The **secretory component** covers the protease-sensitive sites of IgA and thus protects the molecules from digestion in the gastrointestinal tract after they are ingested by the suckling infant.
    b. **Transport of secretory IgA**
        (1) Apparently, IgA-producing plasma cells enter the breast and release the dimeric IgA into the vicinity of glandular secretory cells.
            (a) The secretory component of the sIgA may be a membrane receptor for dimeric IgA on local cells.
            (b) Some authors feel that IgA dimers are released from plasma cells and bind to secretory components in the surface of the glandular cells, thus forming complete sIgA.

(2) Next, the sIgA complex is endocytosed, transported through the epithelial cells, and secreted into the breast milk with the secretory component attached to the IgA dimer to make complete sIgA.

(3) Some IgA of sIgA is made locally by plasma cells in the mammary gland, and some is synthesized in other sites and removed from serum to enter the milk. Amazingly enough, even IgA-secreting plasma cells make their way into colostrum.

2. Breast milk also contains lymphocytes, in addition to immunoglobulins.

3. Human breast milk is also rich in lysozyme, lactoperoxidase, lactoferrin, and other antibacterial and opsonizing factors.

VII. IMMUNOLOGIC ASPECTS OF FETAL-MATERNAL INTERACTION.
A complex problem has intrigued and baffled students of maternal–fetal interaction for many years: Why does the mother fail to recognize the foreign antigenic nature of the conceptus developing within the uterus?

A. Differences in maternal and fetal immunologic makeup

1. Usually, the developing fetus and the maternal host are immunologically different from one another.
2. This is due, at least in part, to the fact that **histocompatibility antigens** (see section VII B) are genetically determined.
   a. The fetus has a set of chromosomes partially derived from its father and partially derived from its mother.
   b. Therefore, except in extremely rare cases of consanguinity or chance, the paternal contribution to the fetal histocompatibility antigens ensures that there will be substantial differences between fetus and mother.

B. Histocompatibility antigens

1. Differences between individuals are partially determined by certain **cell surface antigens** which are widely expressed on many different tissues.
2. These so-called **histocompatibility antigens** are controlled by a series of closely linked genes.
3. Histocompatibility antigens are present on the surface of many different cells in the body, including the cells of the immune system, enabling the host to recognize and reject a foreign antigenic material.
4. When **T cells** with one set of histocompatibility antigens confront cells with a different set of histocompatibility antigens, a **rejection reaction** occurs.

C. The nature of the problem

1. Humans have a thoroughly developed capacity to reject grafts of foreign tissue.
   a. Even when tissues are closely matched for histocompatibility antigens, there is still a strong tendency for the body to respond to minor differences in tissue types.
   b. Successful organ transplants require extensive treatment with potent immunosuppressive drugs.
2. The mother clearly has the ability to mount an immunologic response to foreign antigens.
   a. In animal studies, graft rejection is fully developed if fragments of fetal tissue are placed in extrauterine sites.
   b. Pregnant women also have the ability to mount T-cell–mediated responses to viral and fungal infections.
3. Why then is it possible for a developing conceptus to survive in the uterus in spite of the fact that the fetus and mother are different in their histocompatibility antigens?
4. The answer to this perplexing question is far from settled, but certain features are emerging from the experimental literature.

D. Immunosuppressive mechanisms

1. The **interface** between the developing conceptus and the maternal immune system resides at the **syncytiotrophoblastic layer** of the placenta.
   a. There is usually a thick layer of fibrinoid material at the maternal–fetal interface, and

this may prevent maternal T cells from invading the immediate vicinity of the syncytiotrophoblast.
- (1) This cell layer is derived solely from the developing conceptus with no maternal components.
- (2) It appears to be fundamentally different from other tissues of the conceptus.
  - (a) Experimental studies using antibodies to histocompatibility antigens clearly show that these antigens are not fully expressed on the surface of the syncytiotrophoblast, in spite of the fact that the connective tissue cells of chorionic villi and the endothelial cells lining the placental blood vessels do express histocompatibility antigens.
  - (b) This **lack of antigenic expression** is poorly understood at present. It may be due to a lack of antigenic content, or it may be the result of **masking** caused by substances derived from the maternal circulating system.
  - (c) **Blood group substances**, in addition to histocompatibility antigens, are also poorly expressed on the syncytiotrophoblast, suggesting that there is a fundamental difference between the cell surface of the maternal–fetal interface and elsewhere in the developing system.
- b. **Maternal suppressor T cells** have been found near the placenta and they may cause a local modulation of maternal T cell function.

2. **Steroids** have a well-known immunosuppressive quality. The developing **placenta** is a source of tremendous quantities of **steroidal hormones**.
   - a. The placental steroids, principally **estrogen** and **progesterone**, can reach very high concentrations at the maternal–fetal interface and as a result of these high concentrations, may have a potent immunosuppressive effect.
   - b. The steroids in the maternal circulation derived from the developing placenta are not a substantial proportion of the total maternal steroid load. Thus, the mother still can mount an immune response to foreign antigens.

3. **Other complexities** exist that are also poorly understood.
   - a. For example, it is now clearly established that **fetal blood cells** enter the maternal circulation, perhaps to signal the maternal immune system not to reject the fetal antigens expressed in the fetal components of the placenta.
   - b. Recently, a maternal urinary glycoprotein, called **uromodulin**, has been discovered.
     - (1) Uromodulin has an inhibitory effect on in vitro assays for T cell and monocyte function.
     - (2) Uromodulin may play some role in specific immunosuppression which allows the mother to recognize foreign non-placental cellular antigens and reject them, while maintaining, at the same time, an immunosuppressed state with respect to distinct placental antigens.

VIII. Rh ISOIMMUNIZATION

A. Etiology

1. As described above, there are antigenic differences between the fetus and the mother. In most instances, there is no clinical manifestation of these differences, due to poorly understood immunosuppressive mechanisms.
2. This is not the case, however, when one considers the **Rh antigen**.
   - a. The Rh antigen is a cell surface antigen on red blood cells (RBCs).
   - b. In **mothers** who lack this antigen, and thus are **Rh-negative**, there is a potential for **Rh incompatibility** when the **father** of the fetus is **Rh-positive**.
     - (1) If the fetus inherits the Rh-positive trait from the father, the **fetus will be Rh-positive**, and thus there will be striking antigenic differences between the fetal and maternal RBCs.
     - (2) Due to the intimate nature of the connection between the fetal and maternal blood supply of the human hemochorial placenta, there is a good chance that Rh-positive fetal RBCs will enter the maternal circulation and result in the production of **maternal immunoglobulins** directed **against the fetal RBCs**.
     - (3) These antibodies are transported across the placenta and will attach to fetal RBCs, leading to their destruction in the fetal liver and spleen. The consequence is fetal **hemolytic anemia**.

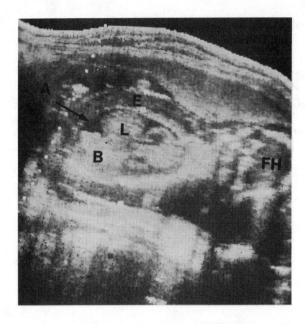

Figure 15-10. Sonogram of cutaneous edema (*E*) in a hydropic fetus with ascites (*A*) near the liver (*L*) and bowel (*B*). The fetal head (*FH*) is also shown. (Reprinted with permission of the Massachusetts Medical Society from Chervenak FA et al: Fetal cystic hygroma. *N Engl J Med* 309:822–825, 1983.)

B. Characteristics of Rh isoimmunization

1. In severe cases of Rh isoimmunization, the fetus suffers from **erythroblastosis fetalis**.
   a. The excessive destruction of fetal RBCs results in the formation of large amounts of fetal **bilirubin**, a hemoglobin breakdown product, which the fetus can not process and eliminate.
   b. Erythroblastosis fetalis is marked clinically by an enlarged liver and spleen, fetal edema (**hydrops fetalis**) [Fig. 15-10], severe jaundice, and potentially lethal sequelae resulting from the jaundice, such as brain damage.

2. The severity of the erythroblastosis fetalis will be lowest in first pregnancies where there is Rh incompatibility and will become progressively more severe with subsequent pregnancies.

3. In many instances, the Rh incompatibility will threaten a premature termination of the pregnancy if untreated.

C. Treatment of Rh isoimmunization

1. In recent years, several medical advances have improved the obstetrician's ability to treat Rh incompatibility.
   a. The severity of the disease can be assessed in the fetus by measuring the amount of **bilirubin in the amniotic fluid**, which is obtained by amniocentesis.
   b. **Intrauterine blood transfusion** will often have a transient effect on the fetus, relieving some of the symptoms of the hemolytic anemia.
      (1) Several intrauterine blood transfusions can be performed, allowing the fetus to mature sufficiently so that it can survive in the extrauterine environment after premature delivery by cesarean section.
      (2) The intrauterine blood transfusions are done through the wall of the uterus by injecting a needle into the fetal peritoneal cavity and transfusing whole blood into the fetus. A large number of the transfused cells make their way from the fetal peritoneal cavity into the fetal circulation, apparently by resorption via lymphatics around the diaphragm.

2. At the present time, correct obstetric practice requires that all **Rh-negative mothers** be treated with **Rh immune globulin (RhoGAM™)** after the birth of an Rh-positive child.

RhoGAM reduces the concentration of maternal serum anti-Rh antibody. This treatment reduces the risk to subsequent fetuses of developing erythroblastosis fetalis due to Rh-isoimmunization.

IX. IMMUNODEFICIENCY DISORDERS AND CYSTIC HYGROMA

A. Immunodeficiency disorders. In recent years, a number of immunodeficiency diseases have been characterized. The examples that are considered here were chosen because they reveal fundamental aspects of the development of the immune system.

1. **Congenital X-linked hypogammaglobulinemia: a B cell disorder**
   a. This disease is characterized by gross reductions in the amount of serum immunoglobulins in male children.
   b. Affected infants begin to develop recurrent infections soon after birth, as maternally derived IgG is catabolized.
   c. Patients with this disease have lymphocytes, but laboratory tests soon show that these are almost exclusively T cells with few B cells or even none at all.
      (1) Affected infants may have abnormally low levels of circulating IgG and extremely low levels of IgM.
         (a) Histologic examinations quickly reveal a severely reduced number of B cells and few if any plasma cells.
         (b) The lack of plasma cells accounts for the hypogammaglobulinemia, since plasma cells are derived from B cells and are responsible for antibody synthesis.
      (2) Other laboratory tests suggest that T cell function is normal but that B cell differentiation is suppressed or absent.
   d. **Genetic studies** of this disease suggest that there is a single gene defect causing the disease.
      (1) The condition is not a mutation of the structural genes for immunoglobulins, since the low levels that are produced are apparently normal in their structure.
      (2) Perhaps some inducer of B cell function, analogous to thymosin, is altered by the mutation.

2. **DiGeorge syndrome: a T cell disorder** (see also Chapter 18, section VI C)
   a. DiGeorge syndrome represents a failure of the development of the thymus and parathyroids. Presumably, the third and fourth pharyngeal pouches fail to develop, resulting in **thymic and parathyroid agenesis**.
   b. In addition, cardiovascular and craniofacial anomalies (Fig. 15-11) are present in this disease.
   c. These athymic patients reveal the importance of the **thymus** in promoting **T cell differentiation**.
      (1) Upon laboratory examination, these patients show normal or near-normal numbers of peripheral lymphocytes but a severely reduced proportion of them are T cells.

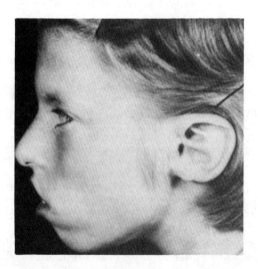

Figure 15-11. DiGeorge syndrome. Note the shape of the mouth, due to the shortened philtrum; the low-set, notched pinna; and the shortened jaw. The eyes are also widely spaced. (Reprinted with permission from Klein J: *Immunology*. New York, Wiley, 1982, p 86.)

(2) Because of the T cell deficiency, patients with this affliction are highly susceptible to opportunistic yeast and fungal infections such as *Pneumocystis carinii* infections.
   d. If the cardiovascular anomalies can be managed and the hypocalcemia (due to the lack of parathyroid glands) can be controlled by administration of calcium, patients can live after birth.
   e. Some relief has been given to these patients by thymic grafts or by thymosin treatment.
   f. Some research workers feel that DiGeorge syndrome is caused by defective neural crest cell migration into the pharyngeal arches and the endocardial cushions of the heart.

B. **Cystic hygroma**
   1. Fetal cystic hygromas are congenital anomalies involving abnormal development of the lymphatic vessels.
      a. When no connection forms between the lymphatic vessels and the adjacent veins, a closed lymphatic vessel forms and becomes distended by the accumulation of lymphatic fluid.
      b. This results in the formation of a large, fluid-filled cyst.
   2. Cystic hygromas occur most frequently in the cervical region (Fig. 15-12), probably due to the complexity of the jugular lymph sacs and their relationship to the internal jugular vein.
   3. Cystic hygromas are readily detectable by sonography (Fig. 15-13), and they often can be larger than the head.
   4. Curiously enough, cystic hygromas are often seen in fetuses with the 45, X karyotype characteristic of **Turner syndrome**. When a cystic hygroma is detected by sonography, amniocentesis should be performed to allow a cytogenetic analysis of the fetal karyotype.

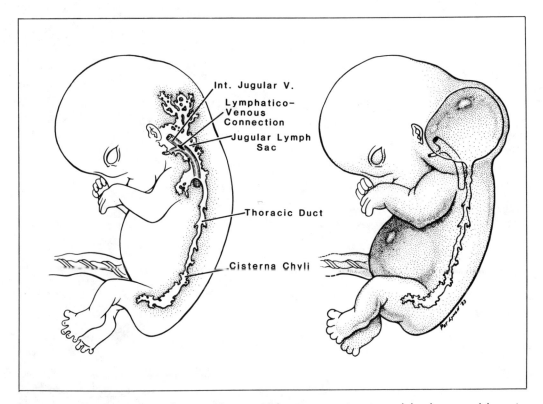

Figure 15-12. Cystic hygroma in the cervical region (*right*). For comparison, normal development of the major lymphatic vessels is shown at *left*. (Reprinted with permission of the Massachusetts Medical Society from Chervenak FA et al: Fetal cystic hygroma. *N Engl J Med* 309:822–825, 1983.)

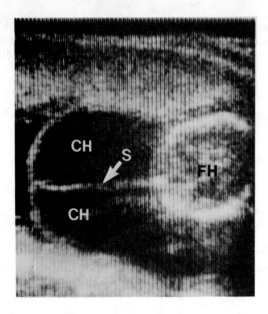

Figure 15-13. Sonogram of cystic hygroma (CH) with a septum (S) near the fetal head (FH). The placenta (P) is also shown. (Reprinted with permission of the Massachusetts Medical Society from Chervenak FA et al: Fetal cystic hygroma. N Engl J Med 309:822–825, 1983.)

STUDY QUESTIONS

Directions: Each question below contains five suggested answers. Choose the **one best** response to each question.

1. All of the following characteristics or symptoms are found in children with congenital X-linked hypogammaglobulinemia EXCEPT

   (A) absence of normal numbers of B cells
   (B) normal titer of IgG
   (C) substantial numbers of T cells
   (D) few if any plasma cells
   (E) recurrent infections

2. All of the following statements concerning passive fetal immunization are true EXCEPT

   (A) maternal IgG is transported across the placenta
   (B) maternal antibodies to fetal antigens are transported across the placenta
   (C) maternal IgM is transported across the placenta
   (D) maternal IgG is catabolized after birth
   (E) fetal IgG is synthesized after birth once the fetus has become exposed to environmental antigens

Directions: Each question below contains four suggested answers of which **one or more** is correct. Choose the answer

   A   if **1, 2, and 3** are correct
   B   if **1 and 3** are correct
   C   if **2 and 4** are correct
   D   if **4** is correct
   E   if **1, 2, 3, and 4** are correct

3. The thymus contains which of the following kinds of cells?

   (1) Pre-B cells programmed to differentiate in the bursa equivalent
   (2) Mesodermally derived cells
   (3) Ectodermally derived cells
   (4) Endodermally derived cells

4. True statements about the embryology of the spleen include which of the following?

   (1) It is attached to the kidneys by a mesenteric remnant called the lienorenal ligament
   (2) It contains endodermally derived cells
   (3) Its sinusoidal cells are derived from mesenchymal cells in the dorsal mesogastrium
   (4) It serves no hematopoietic function during development

5. True statements about the embryology of the tonsils include which of the following?

   (1) The palatine tonsils are derived from the first pharyngeal pouch
   (2) The pharyngeal tonsils have an ectodermally derived epithelium
   (3) The pharyngeal tonsils arise as an invagination of the oropharynx
   (4) The palatine tonsils have an endodermally derived epithelium

6. Breast milk shows which of the following characteristics?

   (1) It contains monomeric secretory IgA and a J polypeptide
   (2) It contains dimeric secretory IgA and a secretory component
   (3) It lacks IgG and lymphocytes
   (4) It protects the fetus from enteric infections

SUMMARY OF DIRECTIONS				
A	B	C	D	E
1, 2, 3 only	1, 3 only	2, 4 only	4 only	All are correct

7. Characteristics of Rh isoimmunization include which of the following?

(1) It is more severe in second than in first pregnancies
(2) It is observed in Rh-negative mothers
(3) It results in hemolytic anemia in the fetus
(4) Amniocentesis is of little value in evaluating severity of the disease

8. Patients with DiGeorge syndrome show which of the following characteristics?

(1) An increased incidence of *Pneumocystis* infections and viral infections
(2) A lack of functional B cells
(3) An increased incidence of malignant diseases
(4) Reduced levels of IgG in their blood

Directions: The groups of questions below consist of lettered choices followed by several numbered items. For each numbered item select the **one** lettered choice with which it is **most** closely associated. Each lettered choice may be used once, more than once, or not at all.

Questions 9–13

For each of the following characteristics of lymphocytes, select the type of lymphocyte that it describes.

(A) B cells
(B) T cells
(C) Both
(D) Neither

9. Derive from lymphoblasts arising in the liver and bone marrow

10. Require a specialized microenvironment of the thymus for differentiating from lymphoblasts

11. Derive from lymphoblasts arising before primitive erythrocytes

12. Are functionally deficient in a disease associated with craniofacial and cardiovascular anomalies

13. Are deficient in X-linked hypogammaglobulinemia

Questions 14–16

For each of the following characteristics of a lymphatic organ, select the organ which it best describes.

(A) Spleen
(B) Thymus
(C) Both
(D) Neither

14. Contains epithelial cells derived from the third and fourth pharyngeal pouches

15. Develops in the dorsal mesogastrium

16. Contains cells programmed in the thymus and the bursa equivalent

ANSWERS AND EXPLANATIONS

1. The answer is B. *(IX A 1)* Congenital X-linked hypogammaglobulinemia is a disease found in male children. It is characterized by recurrent infections and gross reductions in serum IgG. Laboratory tests show that these children have some lymphocytes, but these are mostly T cells, whereas B cells and plasma cells are lacking. A small amount of apparently normal IgG is synthesized in these patients, suggesting that the structural gene for IgG is intact but that some regulatory gene controlling B cell differentiation is abnormal.

2. The answer is C. *(II C 1, 2; VI A)* Under normal circumstances, the fetus develops in a sterile environment. Thus, the fetus is not normally exposed to bacterial antigens in utero. At birth, however, the newborn infant is immediately exposed to bacteria in the environment. During pregnancy, maternal antibodies to bacterial antigens, especially low-molecular-weight IgG molecules, are transported transplacentally, in a functionally intact state, into the fetal circulation. At birth, the placental input of maternal antibodies ceases, but the infant still has maternally derived antibodies. Since these are slowly catabolized, the infant remains protected. The fetal plasma cells, now exposed to environmental antigens, begin to synthesize new antibodies which replace the diminishing maternal antibodies, thus ensuring continuous protection of the newborn infant.

3. The answer is C (2, 4). *(V D)* The thymic reticular epithelium is formed by an invagination from the second pharyngeal pouch and contains endodermally, not ectodermally, derived cells. The blood vessels, connective tissue, and both B and T lymphocytes are mesodermally derived. Pre-T cells, not pre-B cells, are found in the thymus, the site of T cell differentiation.

4. The answer is B (1, 3). *(V C)* The lienorenal ligament is a remnant of the dorsal mesogastrium. The spleen has a hematopoietic function along with the liver during fetal development. There are no endodermally derived cells in the spleen. All splenic sinusoidal cells are derived from mesenchymal cells in the dorsal mesogastrium.

5. The answer is D (4). *(V E)* The palatine tonsils have an epithelium derived from the second pharyngeal pouch. The first pouch forms the auditory tube. Both the palatine and pharyngeal tonsils have endodermally derived epithelium. The pharyngeal tonsils form from an endodermal invagination of the nasopharynx.

6. The answer is C (2, 4). *(II C 3 b; VI B)* Breast milk contains dimeric secretory IgA. It also has a J (joining) polypeptide, which joins the two monomeric subunits, and a secretory component, which protects the molecule from enteric proteolysis. IgA molecules protect infants against enteric infections. Breast milk also contains IgG and lymphocytes.

7. The answer is A (1, 2, 3). *(VII A; VIII A, B)* Rh isoimmunization occurs in Rh-negative mothers carrying Rh-positive fetuses. It is usually more severe with each pregnancy after the first. It results in destruction of fetal erythrocytes (hemolytic anemia) and can be detected by measurement of bilirubin levels in amniotic fluid sampled by means of amniocentesis.

8. The answer is B (1, 3). *(IX A 2)* DiGeorge syndrome is due to a congenital lack of the thymus. Consequently, T cell function is abnormal, leading to opportunistic infections by *Pneumocystis* and viruses, and to an increased risk of developing a malignancy. B cell function is essentially normal and, as a result, normal levels of IgG are present. Cardiovascular and craniofacial anomalies are also associated with this disease.

9–13. The answers are: 9-C, 10-B, 11-D, 12-B, 13-A. *(III A; IV A 2, B 1, C 1; IX A)* Both B cells and T cells are derived from lymphoblasts arising in the liver and bone marrow. T cells are programmed to differentiate in the thymus and are lacking in patients with DiGeorge syndrome. All lymphoblasts, whether destined to become B cells or T cells, arise after the formation of primitive erythrocytes in the yolk sac. B cells are deficient in patients with X-linked hypogammaglobulinemia.

14–16. The answers are: 14-B, 15-A, 16-C. *(V C, D)* The thymus contains reticular epithelial cells derived from the third and fourth pharyngeal pouches. Both the spleen and the thymus contain T cells and B cells. Pre-T cells are programmed to differentiate into T cells in the thymus. Pre-B cells are programmed to differentiate into B cells in an unidentified site known as the bursal equivalent because the bursa of Fabricius serves this function in birds. The spleen develops in the dorsal mesogastrium.

16
Development of the Urinary System

I. INTRODUCTION

A. General description of the urinary system

1. **Components and function of the urinary system**
   a. The urinary system is composed of the kidneys, the ureters, the urinary bladder, and the urethra.
   b. The kidneys produce urine, which is a blood filtrate, and regulate its volume and composition, thereby maintaining the proper volume and composition of the body's fluids.
   c. The rest of the urinary system is specialized for the transport of urine out of the body or the storage of urine for periodic elimination from the body.

2. **Gross anatomy of the kidney** (Fig. 16-1)
   a. The two **kidneys** are located retroperitoneally, on either side of the vertebral column.
   b. They are concave medially, and in the concavity is a **hilus** where the ureter exits and the blood vessels, lymphatics, and nerves enter.
   c. The parenchyma of the kidney surrounds a cavity called the **renal sinus**, which holds the **renal pelvis** and **calyces**.
      (1) The **renal pelvis** is the expanded upper end of the ureter. Into it feed two or three **major calyces**.
      (2) Several **minor calyces** feed in turn into each major calyx.
   d. When a kidney is hemisected, the **parenchyma** is seen to contain a lighter inner **medulla** and a darker outer **cortex**.
      (1) The **medulla** is made up of a number of **renal pyramids**.
         (a) The bases of the pyramids abut on the cortex, and the apices of the pyramids (the **papillae**) end in the minor calyces.

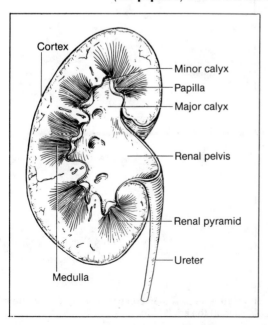

Figure 16-1. Major components of an adult human kidney, seen in hemisection.

264 Human Developmental Anatomy

        (b) The tip of each papilla is perforated by many **papillary ducts** emptying into the minor calyces.
        (c) Each pyramid contains **uriniferous tubules** and **blood vessels**.
    (2) The **cortex** contains the **glomeruli** and portions of the **tubules**.
3. **Anatomy of the nephron and collecting tubules** (Fig. 16-2)
    a. The functional units of the kidney are the **uriniferous tubules**. These are composed of the **nephron** for producing urine and the **collecting tubules** for concentrating and transporting urine.
        (1) The **nephrons** develop from the **metanephric blastema**, a mass of mesenchyme at the caudal end of the urogenital ridge.
        (2) The **collecting ducts** develop from the **ureteric bud**, a diverticulum of the **mesonephric duct**.
    b. The **nephron** is the most complex element of the uriniferous tubule, both structurally and functionally.
        (1) The renal corpuscle
            (a) The most proximal portion of the nephron is a cuplike structure called **Bowman's capsule**. Within this capsule is a **glomerulus** (cluster) of capillaries. Together, the glomerulus and Bowman's capsule comprise a **renal corpuscle**.
            (b) Filtrate from the plasma exudes through fenestrations in the glomerular capillaries into Bowman's capsule.
                (i) The parietal layer of Bowman's capsule is a simple squamous epithelium, while the visceral portion is composed of extremely complicated and highly modified epithelial cells called **podocytes**.
                (ii) The basement membrane lying between the podocytes and the fenestrated glomerular capillaries is extremely thick and serves as one of the sites of retention of blood proteins.
            (c) The renal corpuscle has a **vascular pole** where the blood vessels enter and leave the glomerulus, and a **urinary pole** where the parietal epithelium of Bowman's capsule is continuous with the proximal tubule.
        (2) The proximal and distal tubules and Henle's loop (see Fig. 16-2)
            (a) The proximal part of the proximal tubule is convoluted, as is the distal portion of the distal tubule.
            (b) Between the convoluted portions of the proximal and distal tubules lies the **loop of Henle**.

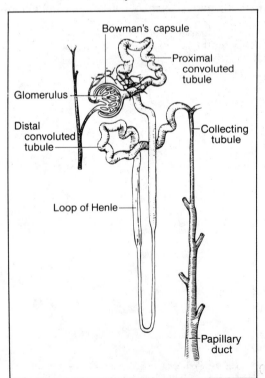

Figure 16-2. Major components of the uriniferous unit in the adult kidney.

- (c) The proximal tubule is convoluted as it leaves Bowman's capsule and has a straight portion in the loop of Henle which passes into the thin segment of the loop of Henle.
  - (i) The thin segment has a squamous epithelium.
  - (ii) The epithelium of the thin segment is directly continuous with the epithelium of the **distal tubule**.
- (d) The volume and composition of the urine are regulated by a complex transporting of fluid, ions, and other substances across the elongated surfaces and convolutions of the tubules of the nephron.
- c. **The collecting tubules (collecting ducts)**
  - (1) The collecting tubule receives urine from the distal tubule and passes it on to the papillary duct.
  - (2) In the collecting tubules, the cells grow in height as the diameter of the collecting tubules increases.
- d. **Papillary ducts** are lined by a simple columnar epithelium.

B. Overview of development of the urinary system

1. During fetal life, **three separate pairs of nephric structures** arise successively.
   - a. These embryonic nephric structures develop from intermediate mesoderm.
   - b. They form in a cranial to caudal sequence. The cranial nephric structures degenerate soon after their formation, being quickly replaced by the development of more caudal nephric structures.
   - c. The **pronephros**, the first to form, does not become active in urine production and undergoes a complete regression soon after its formation.
   - d. The **mesonephros**, the second kidney to form, probably functions in human fetal urine production. The body of the mesonephros undergoes degenerative changes, but parts of the **mesonephric duct** (which drains the mesonephros) persist to form the entire excurrent drainage system of the male gonad (see Chapter 17, section III).
   - e. The **metanephros**, the third and definitive nephric structure, forms from two different rudiments which together contribute to the complete adult kidneys and the ureters.
2. The urinary bladder and the urethra both develop from the **urogenital sinus**, which is a derivative of the embryonic hindgut.

II. DEVELOPMENT OF THE PRONEPHROS AND MESONEPHROS

A. The pronephros

1. The pronephros is a transient structure that arises in the intermediate mesoderm associated with cervical and cranial somites.
2. Pronephric structures may be either solid cords of tissue or small vesicles. They are first visible at the beginning of the fourth week and begin to regress almost as soon as they form.
3. By the beginning of the fifth week, pronephric regression is complete.
4. The pronephros forms in a cranial to caudal sequence. It also degenerates in a similar sequence.
   - a. The cranial vesicles degenerate first, followed by the caudal vesicles.
   - b. As a result of the sequential degenerative activity, the position of the mass of pronephric tissue shifts caudally.
5. Based on morphologic observations, it is certain that the pronephros does not function in urine production.
   - a. Pronephric glomeruli have not been observed.
   - b. Pronephric vesicles are not connected to the pronephric duct.

B. The mesonephros

1. Before the pronephros has undergone complete degeneration, a mesonephros begins to form (Fig. 16-3).
2. The mesonephros (Figs. 16-4 and 16-5) arises in the **nephrogenic cord**, a component of the intermediate mesoderm.
   - a. While the nephrogenic cord is elongating by growth in a caudal direction, it undergoes differentiation into **mesonephric vesicles**.
   - b. The mesonephric vesicles arise along the nephrogenic cord from the first thoracic segment all the way to the third lumbar segment.

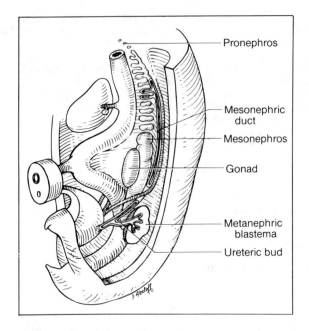

Figure 16-3. The urinary system in the 6-week human embryo.

3. Soon after they arise, the mesonephric vesicles increase in number by bifurcation or subdivision and begin to undergo elongation into pear-shaped and S-shaped vesicles.
4. The mesonephric vesicles develop into rudimentary **nephrons**.
   a. The S-shaped vesicles make communication with the mesonephric duct.
   b. Branches from the dorsal aorta grow toward the S-shaped mesonephric vesicles.
   c. Meanwhile, the S-shaped bodies are forming primitive **Bowman's capsules**, and blood vessels begin to form **capillary tufts (glomeruli)** that indent the developing Bowman's capsule and connect up with branches from the dorsal aorta (see Figs. 16-4 and 16-5).
   d. The remainder of the S-shaped loop often becomes more **convoluted** and develops in close association with the efferent arterioles which carry blood from the glomerulus to the posterior cardinal vein.
5. The mesonephros undergoes a cranial to caudal degenerative sequence.
   a. In the fifth week, cranial structures are regressing while caudal structures are still differentiating.
   b. By the eighth week, many parts of the mesonephros have degenerated.
6. Not all parts of the mesonephros degenerate completely, as is the case for the pronephros.
   a. Around the sixth week, the mesonephros forms a large ovoid mass (Fig. 16-6) just lateral to the midline.
      (1) This mass, along with the developing gonad, makes a major contribution to the **urogenital ridge**.
         (a) The urogenital ridge is a dynamic structure.
         (b) It is difficult to portray in diagrams, because the pronephric component has formed and disappeared by the time the mesonephric and metanephric components are clearly delineated.
      (2) The **mesonephric duct** runs along the lateral border of the urogenital ridge and drains the nephrons into the **urogenital sinus** (see Fig. 16-6). The urogenital sinus, a hindgut derivative, later becomes the urinary bladder and the urethra.
   b. The **mesonephric tubules** near the gonad persist in the male as the efferent ductules of the testis and other, minor structures.
   c. The **mesonephric duct** gives rise to the duct of the epididymis, the ductus (vas) deferens, the seminal vesicles, and the ejaculatory duct in the male. It also forms minor cystic structures in the female. (See Chapter 17, section III.)
   d. A branch of the mesonephric duct, the **ureteric bud** (see Fig. 16-3), contributes the urine-collecting elements of the definitive kidney (see sections III A 2 and IV A).
7. It is not known with certainty if the human mesonephros produces urine, but morphologic studies on human embryos, coupled with structural and functional observations on

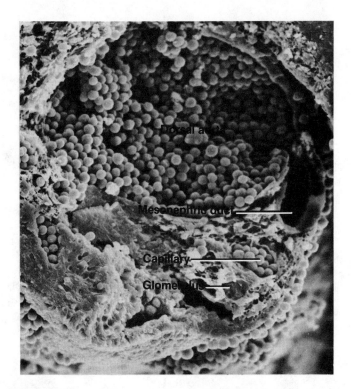

Figure 16-4. Mesonephric kidney in the 6-week human embryo. (Scanning electron micrograph)

laboratory animals, give strong evidence to support the notion that the human mesonephros produces hypotonic urine.

III. DEVELOPMENT OF THE METANEPHROS

A. Morphogenesis of the metanephros

1. The metanephric kidney, the last nephric organ to develop, is the **definitive kidney**. It is functional with respect to urine production in both the fetus and the adult.

2. The metanephros arises from two separate rudiments, the **metanephric blastema** and the **ureteric bud** (see Fig. 16-3).
   a. The **metanephric blastema** arises in the caudal portion of the nephrogenic cord. The metanephric blastema gives rise to the **excretory components** of the metanephros. These include:
   (1) Bowman's capsule
   (2) The proximal convoluted tubule
   (3) The loop of Henle
   (4) The distal convoluted tubule
   b. The **ureteric bud** is a branch from the mesonephric duct. It contributes the definitive **urine-collecting elements**.
   (1) Within the kidney these include:
      (a) The collecting tubules within the kidney
      (b) The papillary ducts
      (c) The major and minor calyces
   (2) The ureters also come from the ureteric bud.

B. Histogenesis of the metanephros

1. **Formation of the collecting system from the ureteric bud**
   a. The ureteric bud begins as a diverticulum of the mesonephric duct.
   b. The bud grows dorsally and becomes distended at its cranial extremity, forming an **ampulla**.

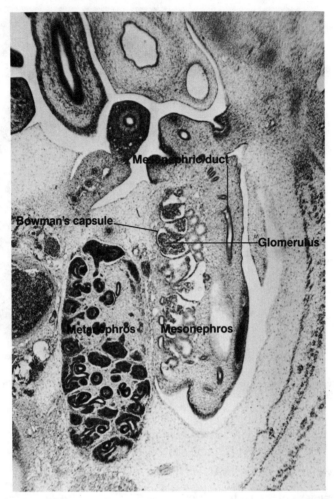

Figure 16-5. The human embryonic mesonephros and metanephros at 8 weeks' development. (Light micrograph)

(1) The ampulla comes in contact with the metanephric blastema in the caudal portion of the nephrogenic cord.
(2) The ampullary portion of the ureteric bud next begins to undergo a series of bifurcations.
  (a) These are at first symmetric but later occur most often at the cranial and caudal extremities of the kidney.
  (b) The result is a fanning out of the collecting system to form a diverging system of major and minor **calyces** and medullary **collecting ducts**.

2. **Formation of nephrons from the metanephric blastema** (Fig. 16-7)
  a. The dilated portions of the ureteric bud become surrounded by dense caps of mesenchymal cells (Fig. 16-8).
    (1) These caps are local condensations of cells of the metanephric blastema.
    (2) The condensations are **induced** by the branches of the ureteric bud to differentiate into vesicles and then into **S-shaped tubules** in a manner similar to that seen in the formation of the mesonephric nephrons.
  b. As nephrons are induced, the branches of the ureteric bud continue to grow centripetally and as they do so, they induce new generations of nephrons.
  c. While new nephrons are forming, the older ones continue to mature. Their maturation involves an increase in the convolutions in the **proximal and distal convoluted tubules** and also an increase in the length of the **loop of Henle** (see Fig. 16-8).

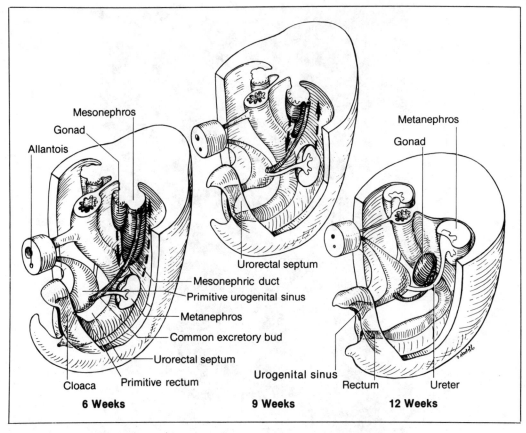

Figure 16-6. Relations between mesonephros, gonad, and metanephros during their formation and relative movements. Note that the kidney ascends and the gonad descends (*arrows*).

C. **Ascent of the metanephros** (see Fig. 16-6)

1. The metanephros originates at the level of the upper sacral segment. It also receives its blood supply from sacral branches of the dorsal aorta.
2. During the sixth to eighth weeks of development, the metanephros undergoes an ascent from a pelvic position to a lumbar position. This ascent is partly apparent, resulting from the rapid elongation of the sacral segments, but it is also partly due to an actual ascent of the organ.

D. **Blood supply of the metanephros**

1. The ascent of the metanephros is accompanied by changes in the blood supply. As it ascends, the metanephros takes branches from the dorsal aorta at progressively higher levels until the definitive blood supply, the **renal arteries**, arise at the level of the second lumbar segment.
2. The kidneys are sometimes supplied by **supernumerary renal arteries**, which are usually located caudal to the main renal arteries.
   a. These supernumerary blood vessels are remnants of branches of the dorsal aorta formed during ascent of the kidneys.
   b. They are end arteries. Therefore, damage to these blood vessels will result in damage to the renal parenchyma that they supply.

IV. DEVELOPMENT OF THE URINARY BLADDER

A. **The ureters.** The ureters are formed from the proximal portion of the ureteric bud. The transitional epithelium lining the ureters is a mesodermal derivative, as is the smooth muscle in the wall of the ureters.

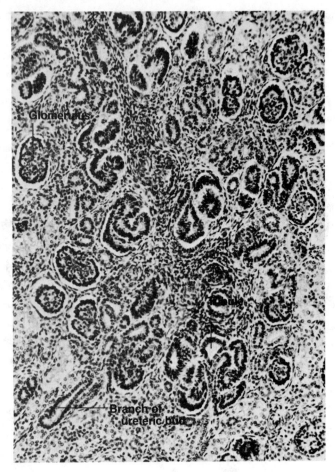

Figure 16-7. Early stage of formation of metanephric nephrons in the definitive human embryonic kidney in a 12-week fetus. (Light micrograph)

B. Division of the cloaca

1. The urinary bladder is derived from the **cloaca**, a slightly distended portion of the caudal hindgut (see Fig. 16-6).

2. The cloaca is divided into a dorsal (posterior) **primitive rectum** and a ventral (anterior) **primitive urogenital sinus** by the growth of the urorectal septum toward the proctodeum or cloacal membrane, a double epithelial layer covering the cloaca (see Fig. 16-6).

C. The urogenital sinus.
The primitive urogenital sinus becomes elongated in a cranial–caudal direction in the portion cranial to its junction with the ureter, and flattened in its portion caudal to the ureteric junction.

1. **The vesicourethral canal**
   a. The cranial portion of the urogenital sinus, now the **vesicourethral canal**, gives rise to the **urinary bladder** and part of the **urethra**.
      (1) The mucosa of the urinary bladder is largely derived from the vesicourethral canal.
      (2) The smooth muscle is derived from splanchnic mesoderm surrounding the vesicourethral canal.
   b. The **urethral portion** of the vesicourethral canal differs in the male and the female.
      (1) In the male, it forms the part of the urethra between the common urethral orifice and the ejaculatory ducts.
      (2) In the female, it forms most of the adult urethra.
   c. The most cranial portion of the vesicourethral canal communicates directly with the **allantois**, a blind-ending hindgut diverticulum that projects into the umbilical cord

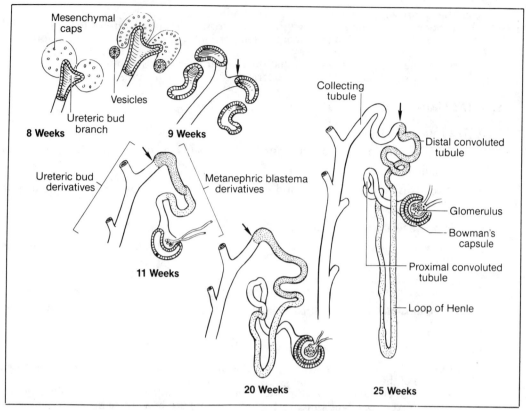

Figure 16-8. Development of metanephric nephrons. The *arrows* indicate the approximate boundary between ureteric bud derivatives (proximal) and metanephric blastema derivatives (distal). The dates shown in the figure are approximate because nephrons do not all mature simultaneously. Thus at 25 weeks some nephrons are more mature, as shown, while others may still be at the 9-week stage.

(see Fig. 16-6). Later in development, the allantois degenerates, leaving a fibrotic cord known as the **urachus** which runs from the bladder to the umbilicus.

2. **The caudal urogenital sinus**
   a. The caudal part of the urogenital sinus forms the **urethra**.
   b. The caudal urogenital sinus is covered over by a **urogenital membrane** which persists in the female as the **hymen**.

D. **The mesonephric duct**

1. As stated earlier in this chapter, the ureteric bud forms as a branch from the mesonephric duct (see sections III A and B).

2. The portion of the mesonephric duct between the ureteric bud and the vesicourethral canal is known as the **common excretory bud**. The common excretory bud apparently becomes incorporated into the wall of the developing bladder, and the sites where the ureters enter the bladder (the ureteric orifices) exhibit an apparent cranial migration.

3. In the male, the mesonephric ducts persist as the left and right **ductus (vas) deferens**.
   a. These ducts migrate caudally with respect to the ureteric orifices. This may be due to differential growth of the tissue lying between the ureteric orifices and the orifices of the left and right ductus deferens.
   b. As the testis descends and the kidneys ascend, each ductus deferens loops over and behind the ureters.

E. **The trigone**

1. The **trigone** is the roughly triangular segment of the bladder between the ureteric and the urethral orifices. It has a muscular layer that fuses neatly into the ureteric musculature.

2. The embryology of this region is poorly understood.
   a. Some embryologists believe that the mucosa and musculature of the trigone of the bladder comes from the incorporated portions of the ureters and is therefore strictly mesodermal in origin.
   b. An alternative theory holds that the mesodermally derived mucosa of the bladder is overgrown secondarily by endodermally derived epithelium.

V. FETAL URINE PRODUCTION

A. The nature of fetal urine
1. Fetal urine is hypotonic to fetal plasma with respect to sodium and chloride concentration.
2. It is slightly acidic (pH 6.0).
3. It contains very little protein and glucose, but has more urea and creatinine than fetal plasma.

B. Role of the fetal nephric structures
1. The **mesonephric kidneys** probably function for a brief time in the production of fetal urine.
2. By the end of the fourth month, the fetal mesonephros completes its degeneration and its function in urine production is assumed by the metanephros.
3. The human **fetal metanephros** is clearly involved in the production and excretion of large volumes of fetal urine.

C. Regulation of amniotic fluid volume
1. One of the main functions for the fetal urinary system is in the maintenance of the volume of the amniotic fluid.
   a. Urine is eliminated from the fetal urinary bladder into the amniotic cavity around the ninth week of development, at which time the urethral orifice becomes patent.
   b. From that time onward, the fetus contributes to amniotic fluid production by urine secretion, and also removes amniotic fluid by swallowing it.
2. Fetal swallowing and absorption of amniotic fluid normally amounts to as much as one-half liter per day.
   a. Small volumes of amniotic fluid (**oligohydramnios**) may be indicative of **renal agenesis** or an **obstruction of the urethra**.
   b. Large volumes of amniotic fluid (**polyhydramnios**) may be indicative of an **anencephalic fetus** unable to swallow or of **esophageal atresia**.

D. Fetal waste elimination
1. The elimination of fetal nitrogenous wastes occurs by diffusion across the placenta into the maternal blood. The maternal kidneys then serve to eliminate both maternal and fetal nitrogenous wastes.
2. Fetal waste elimination, therefore, occurs primarily by **maternal urination**.
3. **Urea** can cross the placenta with ease.
   a. Some fetal urea is eliminated immediately via the placenta after direct diffusion from the amniotic fluid.
   b. The remainder is first carried in the fetal blood, after absorption from the gastrointestinal tract, before proceeding to the placenta and the maternal blood for elimination in the maternal urine.

VI. CONGENITAL ANOMALIES OF THE URINARY SYSTEM

A. Anomalies involving the kidney
1. **Renal agenesis**
   a. Renal agenesis may be due to a failure of formation of the ureteric bud or to failure of a suitable inductive interaction between the ureteric bud and the metanephric blastema.
   b. Renal agenesis may be bilateral or unilateral.
      (1) **Bilateral renal agenesis** is relatively rare, occurring in about 1 in 4000 deliveries. It is

fatal and would be associated with oligohydramnios, since there could be no fetal urine to contribute to the amniotic fluid.

(2) **Unilateral renal agenesis** is much more common, although incidence statistics are hard to establish because the condition is often asymptomatic and compatible with a healthy life.

2. **Congenital cystic disease of the kidneys**
   a. Congenital cystic disease of the kidneys represents several different entities grouped under one name.
   b. Even though the pathogenesis of the different forms is very different, the several separate clinical entities all involve **multiple renal cysts**.
      (1) In one form, there is marked proliferation of collecting tubules, so that the kidneys become grossly enlarged.
         (a) In this type, cyst formation is not restricted to the kidneys but may also be seen in the hepatic bile ducts, lungs, and pancreas.
         (b) This condition is rapidly fatal and is seen only rarely in newborns. However, it shows a strong genetic component, and the occurrence in siblings is markedly elevated.
      (2) In another type, a large number of cystic elements of variable size are scattered throughout both kidneys, intermingled with normal tissue.
         (a) In these infants, the greater the amount of abnormal tissue, the greater the chances of death soon after birth.
         (b) This type may be due to abnormal subdivisions of the ureteric bud or to an improper union between ureteric bud branches and the nephric vesicles that the ureteric bud induces in the metanephric blastema.
      (3) **Ureteric obstruction** can also lead to cystic renal disease.

3. **Anomalies of anatomic location**
   a. Large amounts of renal tissue may arise in abnormal locations associated with abnormal ascent of the kidney.
   b. The so-called **pelvic kidneys** are a notable example of an **ectopic kidney**.
   c. A **horseshoe kidney** (Fig. 16-9) forms if the two separate metanephroi become fused at their caudal poles.
      (1) As the kidneys attempt to ascend, their fused caudal poles hook around the inferior mesenteric artery (hindgut artery), leading to an arrest of ascent.
      (2) This is a relatively common anomaly, seen in 1 in 400 people. It may be asymptomatic in childhood, but in later life people with horseshoe kidney are more likely to have infections of the kidney and kidney stones.

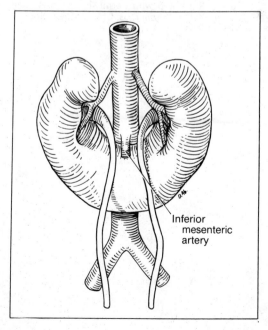

Figure 16-9. Horseshoe kidney anomaly. Note that the normal ascent of the kidneys is restricted by the inferior mesenteric artery, which supplies the hindgut.

B. Anomalies of the ureter and bladder

1. Partial or complete **ureteric duplication** is quite common, occurring in about 1 in 150 necroscopies. It may be asymptomatic or may cause recurrent kidney infections or kidney stones.
2. **Bladder exstrophy** (Fig. 16-10) is due to a ventral body wall defect in which the bladder is everted and opens onto the surface of the body.
3. In some cases, the **allantois** fails to degenerate correctly. This may have several consequences.
   a. The bladder may be connected to the umbilicus by a **fistula**.
   b. Isolated **cystic structures** may be found in the body wall anywhere along the path of normal urachal degeneration.

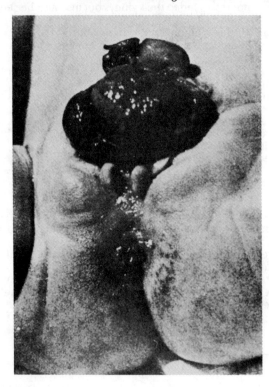

Figure 16-10. Bladder exstrophy in a human newborn infant. (Reprinted with permission from Warkany J: *Congenital Malformations.* Chicago, Year Book, 1971, p 1075.)

STUDY QUESTIONS

Directions: Each question below contains five suggested answers. Choose the **one best** response to each question.

1. All of the following statements concerning the development of the urinary bladder are correct EXCEPT

    (A) the urinary bladder is derived from a subcomponent of the cloaca
    (B) part of its epithelium is derived from the vesicourethral canal
    (C) its smooth muscle is derived from splanchnic mesoderm
    (D) part of its epithelial lining is ectodermally derived
    (E) most of its epithelial lining is endodermally derived

2. Renal agenesis can be associated with all of the following causes or clinical features EXCEPT

    (A) abnormal allantoic regression
    (B) failure of inductive interaction between the ureteric bud and the metanephric blastema
    (C) an absence of symptoms
    (D) oligohydramnios
    (E) death soon after birth

Directions: Each question below contains four suggested answers of which **one or more** is correct. Choose the answer

A	if **1, 2, and 3** are correct
B	if **1 and 3** are correct
C	if **2 and 4** are correct
D	if **4** is correct
E	if **1, 2, 3, and 4** are correct

3. The mesonephros shows which of the following characteristics?

    (1) It produces hypotonic urine
    (2) It contains functional nephrons
    (3) Most of it degenerates while the metanephros is forming
    (4) Its duct degenerates completely

4. True statements about the metanephros include which of the following?

    (1) It becomes functional before complete mesonephric degeneration
    (2) The ureteric bud forms Bowman's capsule
    (3) The metanephric blastema forms the distal convoluted tubule
    (4) The metanephric blastema forms papillary ducts

5. The urogenital sinus shows which of the following characteristics?

    (1) It has a mesodermally derived epithelium outside the trigone
    (2) It has an endodermally derived epithelium inside the trigone
    (3) It is a midgut diverticulum
    (4) It has a diverticulum, the allantois, projecting from it into the umbilical cord

6. True statements about fetal urine production include which of the following?

    (1) In renal agenesis, oligohydramnios would be present
    (2) In an anencephalic fetus, polyhydramnios would be present
    (3) Fetuses urinate into the amniotic fluid
    (4) Fetal urine is hypotonic prior to birth

Directions: The group of questions below consists of lettered choices followed by several numbered items. For each numbered item select the **one** lettered choice with which it is **most** closely associated. Each lettered choice may be used once, more than once, or not at all.

Questions 7–12

For each description of a component of the developing urinary system, choose the appropriate lettered structure shown in the accompanying diagram.

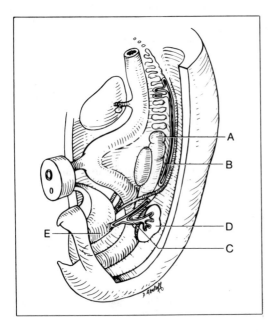

7. This structure drains the mesonephros and makes an important contribution to the excurrent ducts of the male reproductive system

8. This structure is involved in fetal urine production but its nephrons degenerate before birth

9. This structure is the precursor of the definitive urinary bladder

10. This structure develops into metanephric nephrons

11. This structure develops into the papillary ducts and lining of the renal sinus

12. This structure forms the ureters

ANSWERS AND EXPLANATIONS

1. The answer is D. *(IV B, C, E)* The urinary bladder develops from the vesicourethral canal, which in turn derives from the urogenital sinus, a portion of the cloaca. The cloaca is a diverticulum of the hindgut and is therefore lined by an endodermally derived epithelium. The cloaca becomes divided by the urorectal septum into the urogenital sinus and the rectum. The urogenital sinus forms much of the urinary bladder and all of the urethra. In addition, the proximal roots of the ureteric buds become incorporated into the wall of the urogenital sinus. Some authors feel that the mesodermally derived ureteric buds make a transient contribution to the epithelial lining in the trigone of the urinary bladder. Later, this mesodermally derived epithelial lining is replaced by endodermally derived epithelium from the urogenital sinus. The smooth muscle of the bladder is derived from splanchnic mesoderm surrounding the urogenital sinus.

2. The answer is A. *(VI A 1)* Normally, a reciprocal inductive interaction between the ureteric bud and the metanephric blastema leads to the development of the definitive adult kidney. Failure in this inductive system leads to renal agenesis. Failure of allantoic degeneration leads to urinary bladder fistula or to cysts in the umbilical region.

Renal agenesis can be unilateral or bilateral. Unilateral renal agenesis is often asymptomatic and is compatible with a normal life due to compensatory hypertrophy of the single normal kidney. Bilateral renal agenesis is associated with oligohydramnios (decreased volume of amniotic fluid) because of an absence of fetal urine production. A newborn infant with complete renal agenesis can be born normally at term because of the maternal elimination of fetal nitrogenous wastes by way of the placenta, but the infant will die soon after birth.

3. The answer is A (1, 2, 3). *(II B; V A, B)* The mesonephros becomes functional during fetal life and secretes a dilute, hypotonic urine due to the fact that it contains functional nephrons. It degenerates for the most part while the metanephros is forming, but parts of its duct persist in the adult as, for example, the vas deferens in males and the ureteric bud, which forms the ureters.

4. The answer is B (1, 3). *(III A, B)* The metanephros becomes functional in urine production before the complete degeneration of the mesonephric nephrons. The ureteric bud forms the ureters, the lining of the renal pelvis, the lining of the calyces, and the papillary ducts. The metanephric blastema forms Bowman's capsule, the convoluted tubules, and the loop of Henle.

5. The answer is D (4). *(IV C, E)* The urogenital sinus is a diverticulum of the hindgut which forms the urinary bladder and the urethra. The epithelium inside the trigone is initially derived from mesoderm by way of the roots of the ureteric buds. This area is secondarily overgrown by endodermally derived epithelium, which also lines the urinary bladder outside the trigone. A diverticulum of the urogenital sinus, the allantois, projects up into the umbilical cord. It degenerates, leaving behind the urachus.

6. The answer is E (all). *(V A, C)* Fetuses urinate into the amniotic fluid; the urine is hypotonic. They also swallow the amniotic fluid. Therefore, renal agenesis and blockage of the urethra will lead to a reduced volume of amniotic fluid (oligohydramnios), and swallowing disorders, as would be present in an anencephalic fetus, will lead to an increased volume of amniotic fluid (polyhydramnios). Fetal nitrogenous wastes diffuse across the placenta into maternal blood where they are eliminated from the system by way of the maternal kidneys.

7–12. The answers are: 7-B, 8-A, 9-E, 10-D, 11-C, 12-C. *(II B; III A)* The mesonephros (A) functions in fetal urine production before the metanephros is fully formed and functional. Gradually, the mesonephros undergoes regressive changes as the metanephros takes over fetal urine production. The mesonephric duct (B) drains the mesonephros and forms the excurrent duct system for the testis. It also forms a branch called the ureteric bud (C), which forms the ureters, the lining of the renal pelvis and calyces, and the papillary ducts. The metanephric blastema (D) forms the nephrons of the metanephros, including Bowman's capsule, the convoluted tubules, and the loop of Henle. The urogenital sinus (E) is a hindgut diverticulum which forms the urinary bladder and urethra.

17
Development of the Male and Female Reproductive Systems

I. INTRODUCTION

A. Components of the reproductive system

1. The reproductive system consists of the gonads, genital ducts associated with the gonads, and the external genitalia.
2. The **functional anatomy** of the male and female reproductive systems in the adult is described in Chapter 1, sections IV and V, and therefore will not be presented here.

B. The indifferent stage and development of sexual dimorphism

1. The human newborn shows a striking **sexual dimorphism**: the reproductive systems of the male and female are notably different. This sexual dimorphism is augmented further by the development of secondary sexual characteristics at puberty.
2. However, during the embryonic and early fetal periods, there is a preliminary **indifferent stage**, in which the male and female have identical gonads, genital ducts, and external genitalia, regardless of the genetic sex of the individual (Fig. 17-1).
   a. The **genetic sex** of an individual is determined at fertilization and depends entirely upon the individual's complement of sex chromosomes.
   b. The **establishment of physical gender**, however, is the result of a complex interplay of factors that takes place during fetal development.
      (1) These factors include not only the **chromosomal constitution** of the developing fetus, but also several **hormones** and a complex **interaction between tissues**.

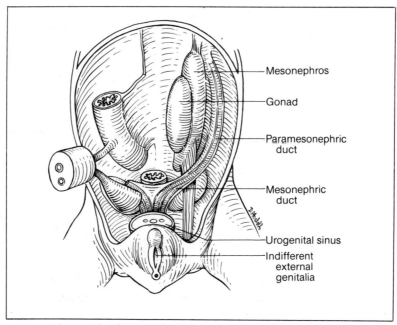

Figure 17-1. The reproductive system at the indifferent stage.

(2) These factors bring about a process of differential growth, differential regression, and fusion of rudiments that creates the strikingly different reproductive systems of the male and female (Table 17-1).
   c. By the fifth month in utero, the male and female gonads are completely differentiated. The genital ducts and external genitalia become differentiated soon after the gonads.
3. As discussed in sections VI and VII, **hormonal and genetic imbalances** can result in **atypical sexual differentiation**, leading to the formation of individuals with anatomically mixed or ambiguous sexual organs and uncertain gender.

II. DEVELOPMENT OF THE GONADS

A. Development of the indifferent gonad

1. The gonads first appear at about the fifth week of development.
   a. The gonad is first evident as a columnar thickening of the epithelial cells lining the coelomic cavity on the medial aspect of the urogenital ridge (see Fig. 17-1).
   b. The basement membrane underlying these columnar cells begins to break down, and cells actively migrate away from the epithelium into urogenital ridge mesenchyme.
   c. Having invaded the condensing mesenchyme in the gonadal primordium, the proliferating coelomic cells then form cords of cells, the **primitive sex cords**, that remain attached for a time to the surface of the gonad.
2. The gonad becomes populated by **primordial germ cells** by the sixth week of development. These cells are the precursors of **spermatogonia** or **oogonia**.
   a. In the early stages, the gonad is composed predominantly of cells derived from the lining of the coelomic cavity.
   b. Soon, however, a second group of cells, the **primordial germ cells**, comes to populate the developing gonad.
      (1) These cells are larger than the original population, have a pale-staining cytoplasm, and exhibit intense **alkaline phosphatase** activity when stained appropriately by histochemical means.
      (2) Primordial germ cells arise in the wall of the yolk sac in an area close to the allantois. They may originate either from endodermal cells or from nearby mesodermal cells.
      (3) The primordial germ cells migrate away from the yolk sac, along the hindgut mesentery, and into the gonadal primordium.

Table 17-1. Developmental Fate of Indifferent-Stage Structures in Male and Female Fetuses*

	Ultimate Structures	
Indifferent-Stage Structures	**Male**	**Female**
Indifferent gonad 　Primordial germ cell 　Coelomic epithelium 　Genital ridge mesenchyme	Testis 　Spermatogonia 　Sertoli cells 　Leydig cells	Ovary 　Oogonia 　Follicular cells 　Thecal cells
Mesonephric tubules	Rete testis, efferent ductules, paradidymis, appendix of epididymis	Rete ovarii, epoophoron, paroophoron
Mesonephric duct	Epididymis, ductus deferens, seminal vesicles and ejaculatory duct	*Gartner's duct*
Paramesonephric duct	*Appendix testis, prostatic utricle*	Uterine tubes, uterus, cervix, proximal 1/3 of vagina
Genital tubercle and urogenital folds	Glans penis, shaft of penis	Clitoris, labia minora
Labioscrotal swellings	Scrotum	Labia majora
Urogenital sinus	Urethra, prostate, bulbourethral glands	Distal 2/3 of vagina

* Structures in italics are rudimentary in the adult.

3. There is something about the environment of the developing gonad that is required for the survival and differentiation of primordial germ cells. This has been shown by experimental studies in the mouse.
   a. If gonadal tissue is transplanted to an ectopic site in the developing kidney, before the primordial germ cells have reached it, then an abnormal gonad lacking sex cells but with genital ducts will arise.
   b. If the gonad is transplanted to an ectopic site after the primordial germ cells have reached it, then a typical gonad complete with sex cells and ducts will develop.

B. **Testicular differentiation**
   1. Before the seventh week of development, the gonad is in the **indifferent stage** (Fig. 17-2); that is, it is not differentiated into a testis or an ovary in spite of the fact that the fetus is genetically male or female.
   2. The gonad becomes recognizable as male by the eighth week, because of various histologic changes:
      a. **Formation of the tunica albuginea**
         (1) Connective tissue elements begin to develop between the primitive sex cords, and the tunica albuginea becomes recognizable as a dense connective tissue capsule around the testis (Fig. 17-3).
         (2) Formation of the tunica albuginea severs the connection between the primitive sex cords and the coelomic epithelium.

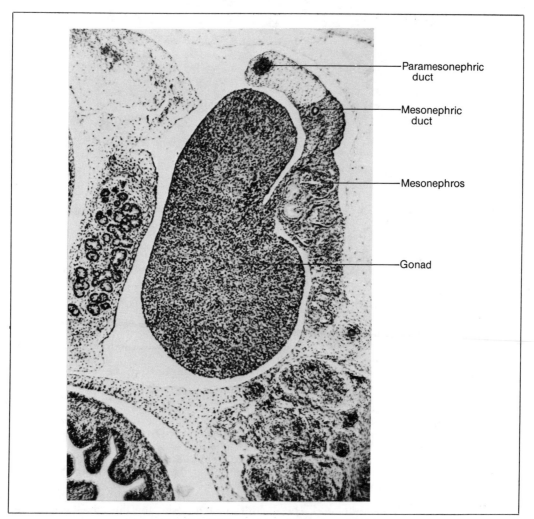

Figure 17-2. The indifferent gonad. (Light micrograph)

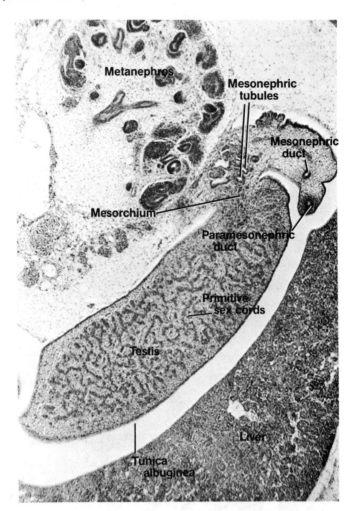

Figure 17-3. The testis soon after it has passed the indifferent stage and has established a tunica albuginea and primitive sex cords. (Light micrograph)

- **b. Formation of the seminiferous tubules and Leydig cells**
  - (1) The **seminiferous tubules** (Fig. 17-4) form from the **primitive sex cords**.
  - (2) The sex cords are composed of supporting (sustentacular) **Sertoli cells** interspersed by quiescent **spermatogonia**.
    - (a) The **Sertoli cells** of the seminiferous tubules are derived from the coelomic epithelium.
    - (b) The **spermatogonia** are derived from the primordial germ cells.
  - (3) In between the sex cords, interstitial cells differentiate into testosterone-secreting **Leydig cells**.
    - (a) These cells are especially prominent in the testis in the second trimester of pregnancy.
    - (b) The **testosterone** from these cells influences the differentiation of the reproductive organs in the male direction.
  - (4) In the fetus and young male child, the primitive sex cords lack lumina and none will appear until puberty, at which time spermatogenesis will begin in earnest.
- **c. Formation of the rete testis**
  - (1) The **primitive sex cords** grow into the **mesorchium** (the mesentery of the testis).
  - (2) In the mesorchium of the developing gonad, the sex cords form into a complex of channels which will later become the **rete testis**.
    - (a) The rete testis is an anastomosing network of channels that empties into the efferent ductules. The ductules connect with the ducts of the epididymis, which in turn connect with the ductus deferens.

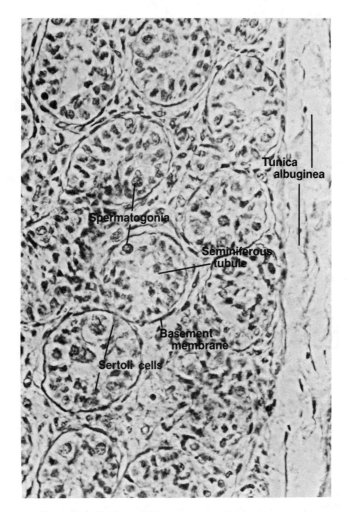

Figure 17-4. Fetal seminiferous tubules. (Light micrograph)

- (b) There is some controversy about the **origin** of the rete testis. Some authors feel that it is derived from mesonephric tubules rather than from the primitive sex cords.
- (3) The **efferent ductules** are derived from mesonephric tubules that form adjacent to the developing testis in the mesonephric mass.
- (4) In the adult, the seminiferous tubules are connected to the rete testis by the **tubuli recti**. In the adult, the tubuli recti are lined by modified Sertoli cells and they are almost certainly derived from the primitive sex cords, as are the seminiferous tubules and the rete testis.

C. **Ovarian differentiation.** The ovary becomes differentiated somewhat later than the testis.
1. The **tunica albuginea** does not become a prominent feature of the early female gonad, although it is present in the adult female. Instead, the coelomic epithelium continues to proliferate.
2. Also, the **primitive sex cords** and an associated network of connecting tubules undergo medullary degeneration in the ovary and the tubular nature of the sex cords is never established. Instead, isolated **nests of cortical oogonia** surrounded by **follicular cells** arise.
    a. The primitive sex cords become broken up into a series of isolated cell clusters.
    b. The primitive sex cords which formed as a result of the primary waves of proliferative activity of the coelomic epithelium occupy the medullary portion of the ovary. These cell clusters degenerate.

c. Meanwhile, a secondary wave of cell clusters arises.
  (1) These result from:
    (a) Continued proliferation and migration of coelomic epithelium
    (b) An interaction between coelomic epithelial cells and primordial germ cells in the gonadal primordium
  (2) These definitive cortical clusters of cells later go on to develop into **follicles** with **granulosa cells** surrounding a central **oogonium**.
d. The **oogonia** are derived from the primordial germ cells, which later proliferate and subsequently differentiate into primary **oocytes**.

3. In the adult female, there are steroid hormone–secreting **thecal cells** that form a highly vascularized shell around the follicles. These cells are located external to the basement membrane of the follicle.
  a. Most embryologists hold that the thecal cells are derived from the mesenchymal stroma of the developing gonadal ridge.
  b. The **thecal cells** are thought to be **homologous** to the interstitial **Leydig cells** in the male, since the Leydig cells are also derived from gonadal ridge mesenchyme and they also secrete steroids.

III. DEVELOPMENT OF THE GENITAL DUCTS

A. Genital ducts in the indifferent stage

1. At the indifferent stage, the genital ducts are alike in both male and female embryos.
2. The genital ducts are paired structures, a **mesonephric (wolffian) duct** and a companion **paramesonephric (müllerian) duct**, associated with the urogenital ridge on each side of the body (see Fig. 17-1).
  a. The **mesonephric (wolffian) duct** arises in situ by canalization of a solid mass of cells in the urogenital ridge. It forms on the lateral edge of the urogenital ridge.
    (1) The mesonephric duct drains the developing mesonephros (see Chapter 16, section II B 6).
    (2) It runs from the cranial to the caudal pole of the mesonephros and then empties into the urogenital sinus.
    (3) The orifice of the mesonephric duct opens into the urogenital sinus near the midline of the body, at a location lateral to the paramesonephric duct orifices.
  b. The **paramesonephric (müllerian) duct** arises as an invagination from the lateral surface of the urogenital ridge.
    (1) The cranial pole of the paramesonephric duct passes through the urogenital ridge lateral to the mesonephric duct.
    (2) It courses toward the midline of the embryo as it proceeds caudally, and crosses the mesonephric ducts before emptying into the urogenital sinus (see Fig. 17-1).
      (a) The separate caudal poles of the paramesonephric ducts fuse during the late indifferent stage.
      (b) The paramesonephric ducts communicate with the urogenital sinus at the **paramesonephric (müllerian) tubercle**.

B. Overview of the fate of the genital ducts

1. The fates of the mesonephric and paramesonephric ducts are radically different in the male and the female (see Table 17-1).
  a. In the **male**, the **mesonephric duct** gives rise to the excurrent ducts for the testis, while the **paramesonephric duct** degenerates almost completely.
  b. In the **female**, the **paramesonephric duct** forms the uterine tubes, uterus, cervix, and part of the vagina, while the **mesonephric duct** degenerates for the most part.
2. In **both sexes**, the **ureteric bud**, a branch of the mesonephric duct, persists as several structures of the urinary system (see Chapter 16, section III).
  a. It becomes the drainage system for the metanephros (the definitive kidney).
  b. Part of the caudal extremity of the ureteric bud becomes incorporated into the trigone of the urinary bladder.

C. Fate of the genital ducts in the male (Fig. 17-5)

1. The genital ducts in the male arise principally from the **mesonephric duct**.
  a. A collection of **mesonephric tubules** drains the nephrons of the mesonephros into the mesonephric duct.

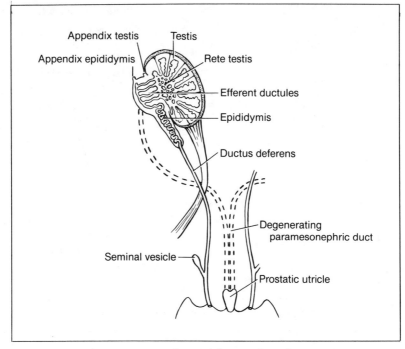

Figure 17-5. Fate of genital ducts in the male.

   (1) As the mesonephros itself undergoes degenerative changes, so the mesonephric tubules cranial and caudal to the gonad regress, giving rise to rudimentary cystic structures of little functional significance.
      (a) The cranial mesonephric tubules become the **appendix of the epididymis**.
      (b) The caudal mesonephric tubules become a collection of closed tubules called the **paradidymis**.
   (2) The mesonephric tubules in close proximity to the gonad persist as the **efferent ductules**, which connect the rete testis to the duct of the epididymis.
   b. The **seminal vesicles** arise as a pair of diverticula from the caudal portion of the mesonephric ducts.
   c. The remainder of the caudal mesonephric duct forms the **duct of the epididymis**, the **ductus (vas) deferens**, and the **ejaculatory ducts**.

  2. The **paramesonephric ducts** in the male degenerate for the most part, persisting only as the **appendix of the testis** and perhaps as the **prostatic utricle**, a small blind-ending diverticulum in the prostatic urethra.

D. Fate of the genital ducts in the female (Figs. 17-6, 17-7, and 17-8; see also Table 17-1)
  1. The genital ducts in the female arise principally from the **paramesonephric ducts**.
     a. The paramesonephric ducts form the **uterine tubes** at their cranial ends.
     b. They come together and fuse caudally to form the **uterus** and **cervix** in the midline of the pelvis (see Fig. 17-7).
     c. There is some controversy concerning the development of the lower portion of the uterus and the vagina. Part of this controversy stems from differences in different animal species and part stems from the difficulty of performing studies on human embryos. We may never know the precise origin of the entire uterus and vagina.
        (1) One common interpretation is as follows:
           (a) The uterine, cervical, and vaginal epithelium come from the uterovaginal primordium. The connective tissue elements of the uterine endometrium and bulk of the myometrium are formed from the mesenchymal cells around the uterovaginal primordium.
           (b) As the uterovaginal primordium grows toward the urogenital sinus (see Fig. 17-8), it is presumed to induce the differentiation of an endodermally derived outgrowth, the solid **vaginal plate**, which develops a lumen secondarily.

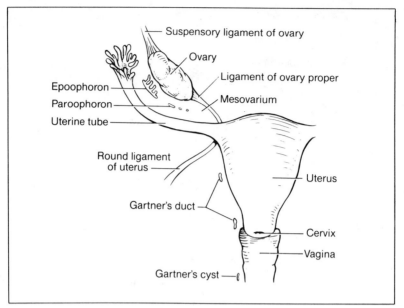

Figure 17-6. Fate of genital ducts in the female.

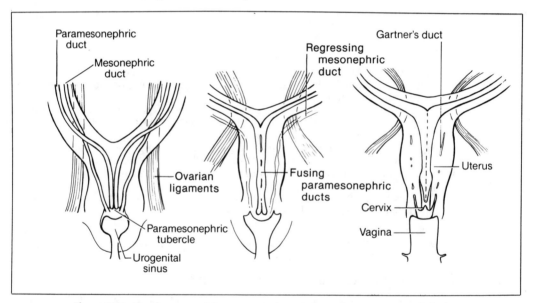

Figure 17-7. Development of the uterus and cervix from the paramesonephric ducts.

  (2) The other (and favored) interpretation is that the uterovaginal primordium and surrounding mesenchyme form the uterus and the superior one-third of the vagina, while the vaginal plate and surrounding mesenchyme form the inferior two-thirds of the vagina.
  d. When the laterally placed paramesonephric ducts come together and fuse to form the uterus, the fusion creates a continuous sheet of mesentery, the **broad ligament**.
     (1) The broad ligament suspends the uterus from the body wall.
     (2) It also divides the lower reaches of the female abdominal cavity into a posterior **rectouterine pouch (of Douglas)** and an anterior **vesicouterine pouch** (Fig. 17-9).

2. The **mesonephric duct** in the female undergoes extensive regression (see Fig. 17-7), but may persist as several **remnants**.

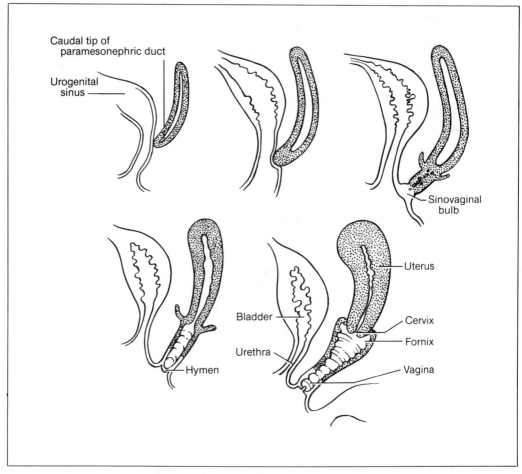

Figure 17-8. Development of the uterus, cervix, and vagina.

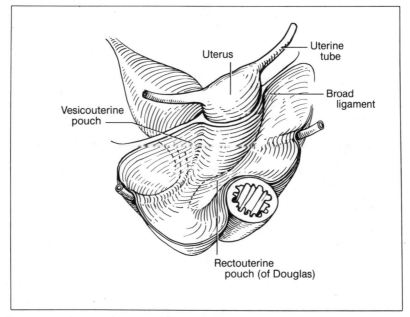

Figure 17-9. Formation of the rectouterine and vesicouterine pouches.

a. The cranial mesonephric tubules may persist as a structure known as the **appendix vesiculosa**.
b. A small group of tubules in the mesovarium known as the **epoophoron** are probably remnants of the mesonephric tubules that form the efferent ductules in males.
c. In a more caudal location, mesonephric duct remnants can be seen as the **paroophoron** in the mesovarium, as **Gartner's duct** in the broad ligament along the wall of the uterus, and as **Gartner's cysts** in the wall of the vagina (see Figs. 17-6 and 17-7).

IV. DEVELOPMENT OF THE EXTERNAL GENITALIA (Fig. 17-10)

A. The external genitalia in the indifferent stage

1. The external genitalia develop from a tubercle and folds of tissue on the external surface of the body.
2. Like the gonads and the genital ducts, the external genitalia also pass through an indifferent stage.
   a. In the indifferent stage of the external genitalia, a small **genital tubercle** can be seen on the outer surface of the body in the midline at the cranial extreme of the urogenital system (see Fig. 17-10).
   b. At first, the **cloaca** (a hindgut derivative) receives both the genitourinary and the gastrointestinal tubes. With the growth of the **urorectal septum**, however, the cloaca is divided into a cranial **urogenital sinus** and a caudal **rectum**.
   c. Similarly, the **proctodeal membrane** is divided into a **urogenital membrane** and an **anal membrane**.
   d. At 6 weeks of development, the urogenital membrane is flanked by two ridges of tissue, the **urogenital folds**.
      (1) The urogenital folds fuse cranially with the genital tubercle and caudally with the anus.
      (2) The paired urogenital folds are flanked laterally by paired **labioscrotal swellings**.

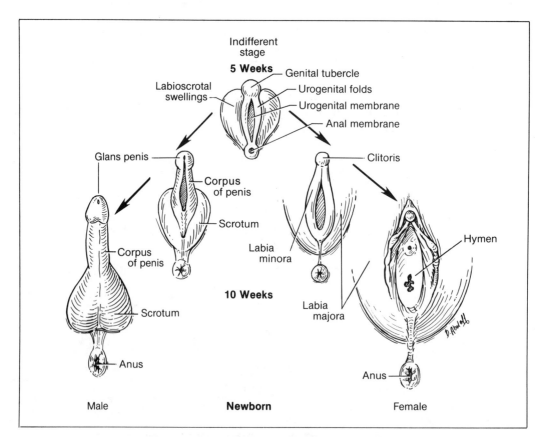

Figure 17-10. Development of the external genitalia.

B. Later sexual differentiation of the external genitalia

1. **Changes by 10 weeks of development** (see Fig. 17-10)
   a. By 10 weeks of development, the external genitalia of the **male** have become somewhat differentiated.
      (1) The genital tubercle has begun to elongate into a **glans penis**.
      (2) The urogenital folds are beginning to fuse to form the **corpus of the penis**.
   b. In the **female**, by contrast, the genital tubercle remains smaller and the urogenital folds do not fuse.

2. **Changes by term** (see Fig. 17-10)
   a. **The newborn male**
      (1) The glans and urethral folds have fused together to form a **penis**.
      (2) The labioscrotal swellings have united into a single **scrotum**.
      (3) Also, the **testes** have usually descended at least partly into the scrotum.
   b. **The newborn female**
      (1) The urogenital folds have grown but not fused, leaving paired **labia minora** flanking the partially perforated urogenital membrane, now known as the **hymen**.
      (2) The labioscrotal swellings also fail to fuse. Instead, they give rise to paired **labia majora**.

V. DESCENT OF THE TESTES

A. The process of testicular descent (Fig. 17-11)

1. As previously described, the testis develops as part of the urogenital ridge on the posterior body wall inside the abdominal cavity.

2. The testis is attached to the **scrotum** by a band of connective tissue known as the **gubernaculum testis**.

3. The testis begins to descend during the third month, with a concomitant shortening of the gubernaculum.

4. Meanwhile, a finger-like extension of the peritoneal cavity, the **processus vaginalis**, extends out into the developing scrotum.

5. The testis now descends across the pubic bone and, by around term, takes up residence in the posterior portion of the scrotum.
   a. The **scrotum** is merely an outpocketing of the body wall.
   b. It contains several layers of fascia and muscle (the **dartos muscle**).

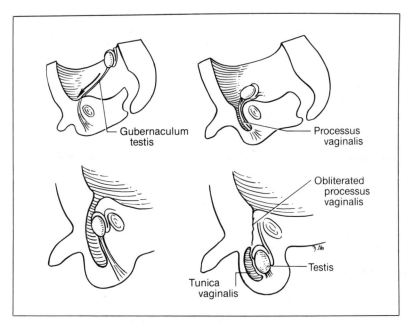

Figure 17-11. Descent of the testis.

6. The **processus vaginalis** becomes closed off from the peritoneal cavity.
    a. It persists as a closed cystic structure that enfolds the anterior and lateral aspects of the testis.
    b. This closed cavity surrounds much of the testis, and its walls form the **tunica vaginalis**.
    c. The former connection between the peritoneal cavity and the processus vaginalis normally becomes obliterated. However, it is a potential pathway for the **herniation** of loops of bowel into the scrotum, a condition which occurs with **congenital inguinal hernia**.

B. **Control of testicular descent**
    1. The descent of the testis is under the control of **testosterone** and **gonadotropins**.
    2. For example, patients with testicular feminization syndrome (see section VII E 1) often have maldescent of the testes.

C. **Maldescent of the testes (cryptorchidism)**
    1. Maldescent is a relatively common congenital anomaly.
    2. All newborn males should be examined for normal testicular descent, because maldescent can have adverse consequences.
        a. Proper descent is essential for complete **fertility**.
            (1) This is so because the temperature of the peritoneal cavity, which is slightly higher than scrotal temperature, is incompatible with normal spermatogenesis.
            (2) If uncorrected, cryptorchidism can cause irreversible **hyaline degeneration** of the seminiferous epithelium and, secondarily, complete sterility.
        b. Malignant tumors of the testis (**seminomas**) are also seen with increased frequency in cryptorchid males.
    3. Milder forms of cryptorchidism can be corrected by administration of hormones. More severe cases may require surgical treatment.

VI. CONTROL OF SEXUAL DIFFERENTIATION

A. **Overview**
    1. A person's **genetic sex** depends on the complement of sex chromosomes, established during fertilization.
        a. Individuals carrying **a complete X chromosome and a Y chromosome** are genetically **male**.
        b. Individuals carrying **two complete X chromosomes** are genetically **female**.
    2. By contrast, the **differences in the functional anatomy** of the gonads and external genitalia, and the development of secondary sexual characteristics during puberty, are all controlled by **hormonal differences** as well as genetic factors. For example, **testosterone**, produced in significant quantities by the fetal testis, helps direct development in a male direction in XY fetuses.
    3. Recent experimental studies in laboratory animals and humans have revealed a number of **genes** that are also important for sex determination.
        a. A gene on the Y chromsome codes for a cell-surface H-Y antigen that is essential for male sexual differentiation.
        b. A testis-determining factor (TDF) gene has also been identified on the Y chromosome.
        c. Males produce a müllerian-inhibiting factor, which suppresses development of the paramesonephric (müllerian) duct.
        d. A gene on the X chromosome codes for a testosterone receptor.
    4. Fetuses with an XX chromosome complement develop into sexually differentiated female fetuses without the aid of these combined genetic and hormonal influences, but two copies of the X chromosome are needed for normal female development, suggesting that female development is also genetically controlled.

B. **Determining genetic sex**
    1. It is possible to determine the genetic sex of an individual in many cases by examination of histologic specimens.
        a. In **females**, one of the two X chromosomes is inactivated and is represented as a bit of heterochromatin that is attached to the nuclear envelope (Fig. 17-12).

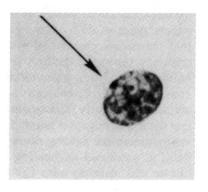

Figure 17-12. Light micrograph of a Barr body (*arrow*). (Reprinted with permission from Simpson JL: *Disorders of Sexual Differentiation: Etiology and Clinical Delineation.* New York, Academic Press, 1976, p 29.)

   (1) This so-called **Barr body** can be observed in many different somatic cells.
   (2) It can be used as a way of counting the number of X chromosomes, since there is one more X chromosome than the number of Barr bodies. For example:
      (a) Cells of normal females show a single Barr body.
      (b) Cells of females with three X chromosomes show two Barr bodies.
   b. The **Y chromosome** can be stained with quinacrine, a fluorescent dye. When appropriately stained cells are viewed in a fluorescent microscope, there is a single **Y body** for each Y chromosome (Fig. 17-13).

2. A more accurate method of studying sex chromosomes, and autosomes as well, is to examine a **karyotype** (see also Chapter 24, section III).
   a. In the preparation of a karyotype, cells from the individual are grown in tissue culture and then arrested at metaphase with colchicine.
   b. The metaphase chromosomes can then be spread out to make the karyotype, allowing an accurate assessment of the morphology of the individual chromosomes, including both autosomes and sex chromosomes.
      (1) The X chromosome is larger than the Y chromosome (Fig 17-14).
      (2) Both are **submetacentric**; that is, the centromere is not exactly in the middle of the chromosome (see Fig. 17-14).

C. **The H-Y (histocompatibility-Y) antigen.** The H-Y antigen is a cell-surface antigen that is thought to be essential for normal testicular differentiation in humans.

   1. Early research showed that female mice would not accept skin grafts from males of the same inbred strain, suggesting that male cells had certain histocompatibility-like cell-surface antigens that were not present in females.
   2. Further studies showed that the H-Y antigen is coded for by genes located in the **short arm of the Y chromosome**.

D. **Testis-determining factor (TDF)**

   1. Recent genetic studies have shown that a small segment of the Y chromosome encodes for a **regulatory protein** called the **testis-determining factor (TDF)** because it is thought to

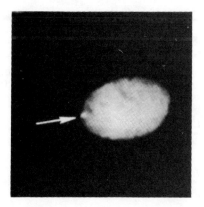

Figure 17-13. Light micrograph of Y chromatin (*arrow*) stained with quinacrine mustard. (Reprinted with permission from Simpson JL: *Disorders of Sexual Differentiation: Etiology and Clinical Delineation.* New York, Academic Press, 1976, p 31.)

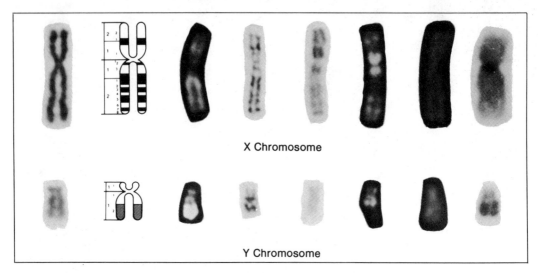

Figure 17-14. Morphologic differences between the X chromosome (*top*) and the Y chromosome (*bottom*) in humans, demonstrated by different staining techniques. (Adapted with permission from de Grouchy J, Turleau C: *Clinical Atlas of Human Chromosomes.* New York, John Wiley, 1977, p 223.)

control sexual differentiation. The TDF region encodes a "finger protein" which interacts with DNA, presumably as a regulator of gene function.

    a. Detailed genetic mapping studies using recombinant DNA technology have shown that some XY males are phenotypically female due to the deletion of the TDF region of the Y chromosome.

    b. Conversely, some XX females are phenotypically male due to the addition of the TDF region to the X chromosome.

2. These results strongly suggest that the TDF region of the Y chromosome is crucial for normal **testicular differentiation**, an event which later controls much of sexual differentiation.

3. The results also suggest that the H-Y antigen may be less important in controlling testicular differentiation.

E. Müllerian-inhibiting substance

1. Another gene product, known as the **müllerian-inhibiting substance** or **antimüllerian hormone**, is secreted by the male gonads, and suppresses the development of the paramesonephric (müllerian) ducts.

2. Because of this role, it too is important for sex determination.

F. Genetic mutations and hormonal control

1. The testosterone receptor

    a. The gene for the testosterone receptor is located on the X chromosome, and certain women are heterozygous for a mutation in the testosterone receptor.

    b. In such heterozygotes, 50% of their XY (genetically male) offspring will be afflicted with the **testicular feminization syndrome** (see section VII E 1 a).

2. Other genes encode the proteins involved in **steroid biosynthesis and metabolism**. A number of different mutations in these genes can occur that would result in defective steroid metabolism, causing aberrant sexual differentiation.

VII. CONGENITAL ABNORMALITIES OF SEXUAL DIFFERENTIATION (Table 17-2)

A. Gonadal agenesis

1. Gonadal agenesis is a relatively rare anomaly. When it occurs, for unknown reasons, the **gonads fail to form**. Consequently, the hormonal influences that promote the development of the genital ducts and external genitalia are absent.

Table 17-2. Common Abnormalities of Sexual Differentiation

Condition	Chromosomal Complement	Gonad	Body Habitus, Genital Ducts, and External Genitalia	Cause
Gonadal agenesis	46, XX or 46, XY	Absent	Either sex; ducts absent or juvenile	Unknown
Gonadal dysgenesis	46, XY	Testis; Leydig cells present, poor development of seminiferous tubules	Female body; ducts hypoplastic and female	Unknown
Turner syndrome	45, XO	Hypoplastic ovary	Female body; poorly developed genital ducts; immature female external genitalia	No H-Y antigen; no X-coded gene products for ovarian development
Klinefelter syndrome	47, XXY	Hypoplastic testis	Male body; normal male genital ducts and external genitalia	Extra copy of X causes abnormal testicular development
Testicular feminization syndrome	46, XY	Hypoplastic testis	Female body; no female genital ducts; abnormal female external genitalia	No androgen receptors
Adrenogenital syndrome	46, XX	Ovary	Female body and genital ducts; masculinized external genitalia	Excess adrenal androgen production due to various enzyme deficiencies

2. Gonadal agenesis is commonly associated with anomalies in the urinary system, suggesting that there is some fundamental, multifactorial teratogenic event affecting not only the gonad, but all the other structures derived from the urogenital ridge.

B. Gonadal dysgenesis

1. Gonadal dysgenesis has been observed in both XX and XY individuals.
2. Some XY patients with gonadal dysgenesis possess the H-Y antigen but nevertheless fail to show normal testicular development.
   a. This finding suggests that other factors besides H-Y antigen are needed for normal testicular differentiation.
   b. The testes in these patients show clumps of Leydig cells and degenerate seminiferous tubules. The genital ducts are hypoplastic but of a female type.
3. **Turner syndrome** is the classic form of gonadal dysgenesis.
   a. Patients with Turner syndrome have a distinctly female but immature body habitus, a broad chest with widely spaced nipples, short stature, and a webbed neck (Fig. 17-15), and have poorly developed ("streak") ovaries (Fig. 17-16).

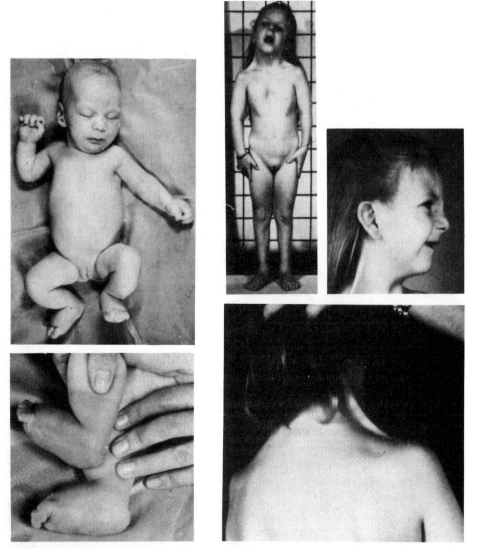

Figure 17-15. Examples of patients with Turner syndrome. Note the lymphedema, especially in the lower extremities, in the newborn infant, and the webbed neck and immature body habitus in the young female. (Reprinted with permission from de Grouchy J, Turleau C: *Clinical Atlas of Human Chromosomes.* New York, John Wiley, 1977, p 231.)

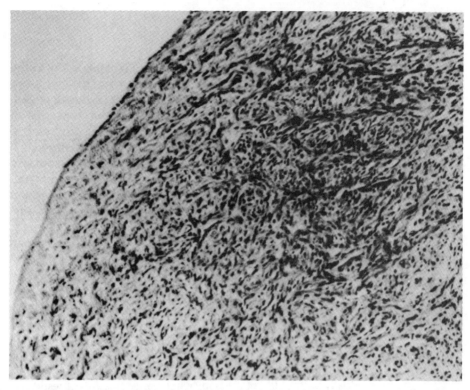

Figure 17-16. Streak ovary of a patient with Turner syndrome. (Light micrograph) Note the lack of normal follicular development. (Reprinted with permission from Simpson JL: *Disorders of Sexual Differentiation. Etiology and Clinical Delineation.* New York, Academic Press, 1976, p 269.)

    b. Such individuals are sterile because of abnormal ovarian development and show poor development of secondary sexual characteristics as well.
    c. The karyotype of such individuals is 45, X; that is, the second sex chromosome is lacking.
        (1) Because of the lack of the H-Y antigen, the gonads and genital ducts develop in a female direction, presumably under the influence of maternal and placental estrogens, but the gonads remain hypoplastic.
        (2) The clinical findings in patients with Turner syndrome are compatible with the idea that each X chromosome carries genes that are required, in some poorly understood fashion, for the normal differentiation of the female gonad.
    d. Mental retardation is also commonly associated with the Turner syndrome, which occurs with a frequency of 1 in 1500 people in the general population.

C. Klinefelter syndrome

    1. Klinefelter syndrome is associated with a distinctly male body habitus (Fig. 17-17); however, patients often show a gynecoid pelvis and gynecomastia.
        a. Affected patients, who are unusually tall and thin, have normal male external genitalia and genital ducts, although cryptorchidism is common.
        b. After puberty, abnormalities in the testes appear, however. The Leydig cells are present but abnormal and there is a degenerative hyalinization of the seminiferous tubules.
    2. Cytogenetic studies show that individuals with Klinefelter syndrome are usually 47, XXY, although they may also be 48, XXXY, and various mosaics can occur.
    3. The incidence of Klinefelter syndrome in the normal population is about 1 in 500; the incidence is much higher than this among mentally defective institutionalized males.

D. Hermaphroditism

    1. A **true hermaphrodite**—that is, one individual containing both ovarian and testicular tissue—is not seen often by the clinician.

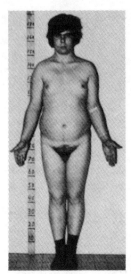 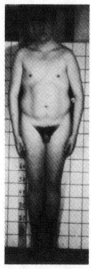 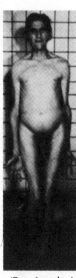 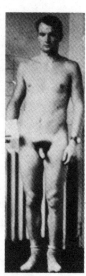

Figure 17-17. Examples of patients with Kleinfelter syndrome. (Reprinted with permission from de Grouchy J, Turleau C: *Clinical Atlas of Human Chromosomes.* New York, John Wiley, 1977, p 245.)

  2. When it occurs, usually the patient is a 46, XX individual with testicular tissue mixed in with ovarian tissue.
     a. The ovarian tissue is usually fairly normal in appearance but the testicular tissue is degenerate.
     b. Female genital ducts are usually present and may be accompanied by male genital ducts, especially on the side of the body where large amounts of testicular tissue are present in the mixed gonad.
  3. The etiology of hermaphroditism is unknown at the present time.

E. **Pseudohermaphroditism**
  1. In **male pseudohermaphroditism**, an individual has male gonads, but the genital ducts, external genitalia, or both are female or ambiguous. Male pseudohermaphroditism is a complex collection of clinical entities caused by several different abnormalities.
     a. The **testicular feminization syndrome** is one type of male pseudohermaphroditism.
        (1) Patients with testicular feminization syndrome have a 46, XY chromosomal complement and develop testes.
           (a) The testes, however, fail to undergo normal descent and usually are located in the inguinal canal or in the labia majora.
           (b) The testes function in the production of androgens and müllerian-inhibiting factor.
           (c) Consequently, the uterine tubes and uterus [which are derivatives of the paramesonephric (müllerian) ducts] are entirely absent, because the production of müllerian-inhibiting factor suppresses the development of the female genital ducts.
        (2) Despite the androgen production, the patient has a distinctly female body habitus (Fig. 17-18) and the external genitalia of a female.
        (3) Some patients with testicular feminization syndrome have been shown to have H-Y antigen but **lack testosterone receptor protein**.
           (a) The consequent **insensitivity to androgens** in various target tissues leads to the development of the female body habitus.
           (b) The lack of testosterone sensitivity also leads to failure of the development of mesonephric duct derivatives, a process known to be testosterone-dependent.
     b. Other male pseudohermaphrodites have **defects in the production of androgens**.
        (1) There are several different classes of enzymatic defects, each blocked at a different step in androgen synthesis.
        (2) The lack of one or more enzymes involved in androgen synthesis may be due to genetic mutations of the structural genes controlling the enzymes synthesizing the hormones.
        (3) In such patients, cryptochid testes and male genital ducts are usually present, but the external genitalia are feminized to greater or lesser degree.

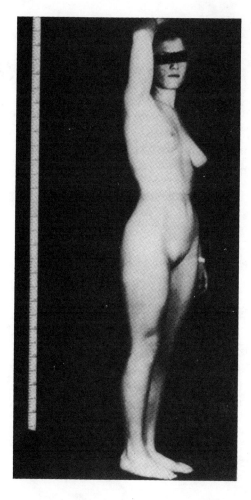

Figure 17-18. Example of a patient with testicular feminization syndrome. (Reprinted with permission from Simpson JL: Male pseudohermaphroditism. Genetics and clinical delineation. *Human Genet* 44:1. New York, Springer-Verlag, 1978, p 20.)

2. In **female pseudohermaphroditism**, an individual has female gonads and genital ducts, but the external genitalia are ambiguous. Female pseudohermaphroditism can also have different causes.
   a. The **adrenogenital syndrome**, caused by **congenital adrenal hyperplasia** (see Chapter 19, section VII), is the most common cause of female pseudohermaphroditism.
      (1) In this anomaly, the patient has a 46, XX chromosome complement and a distinctly female body habitus. The external genitalia, however, are masculinized to a variable degree (see Chapter 19, Fig. 19-6).
         (a) Enlargement of the clitoris and a variable degree of fusion of the labia are common.
         (b) An ovary and female genital ducts are present, without any evidence of masculinization of the genital ducts.
      (2) This condition is due to intrauterine exposure to **abnormally high levels of androgens** because of abnormalities in the fetal adrenal gland.
         (a) Usually, there is a congenital lack of certain adrenal cortical enzymes needed for steroid metabolism. This results in an accumulation of androgens in the fetus.
         (b) The androgenic accumulation usually occurs after the gonads and genital ducts have passed a critical period, but while the developing external genitalia are still sensitive.
   b. **Maternal exposure to androgenic substances** can also cause female pseudohermaphroditism, but this is uncommon.
      (1) Rarely, the mother has a virilizing tumor or other **virilizing endocrine disorder**.
      (2) Maternal **exposure to virilizing drugs** is now an unusual cause, since physicians are alert to the effects of medications in pregnant women.

STUDY QUESTIONS

Directions: Each question below contains five suggested answers. Choose the **one best** response to each question.

1. The development of the mesonephric duct has all of the following characteristics EXCEPT

   (A) the mesonephric duct forms the epididymis
   (B) its differentiation is suppressed by müllerian-inhibiting substance
   (C) its differentiation is testosterone-dependent
   (D) it forms Gartner's duct and cysts
   (E) it forms the ductus deferens

2. Differentiation of a male body habitus can be seen in all of the following circumstances EXCEPT

   (A) 46, XX karyotype with genes for testis-determining factor on the X chromosome
   (B) 47, XXY karyotype
   (C) 46, XY karyotype with H-Y antigen but not the testosterone receptor
   (D) 46, XY normal karyotype
   (E) 48, XXXY karyotype

3. A person with Klinefelter syndrome would have all of the following clinical findings EXCEPT

   (A) undescended testes
   (B) increased risk of seminoma
   (C) hyalinization of the seminiferous epithelium
   (D) a euploid karyotype
   (E) a gynecoid pelvis and gynecomastia

4. All of the following are derived from primordial germ cells EXCEPT

   (A) spermatogonia
   (B) spermatozoa
   (C) epoophoron
   (D) oogonia
   (E) ova

5. A person with a deletion of the gene coding for testis-determining factor from the Y chromosome would have all of the following clinical findings EXCEPT

   (A) a female body habitus
   (B) no epididymis
   (C) H-Y antigen
   (D) no Barr body
   (E) a testis rather than an ovary

6. Normal female development requires all of the following EXCEPT

   (A) at least two X chromosomes
   (B) ovarian follicles
   (C) Leydig cell differentiation
   (D) a normal adrenal gland
   (E) paramesonephric duct derivatives

7. The development of normal male external genitalia requires all of the following EXCEPT

   (A) at least an X and a Y chromosome
   (B) testosterone
   (C) testes
   (D) labioscrotal swellings
   (E) paramesonephric duct derivatives

8. Turner syndrome shows all of the following characteristics EXCEPT

   (A) absence of menses
   (B) numerous ovarian follicles
   (C) webbed neck
   (D) sterility
   (E) 45, X karyotype

9. A patient with Klinefelter syndrome would show which of the following characteristics?

(A) Female body habitus
(B) 47, XXY karyotype
(C) Normal fertility
(D) Female external genitalia
(E) Short, plump appearance

10. A patient with testicular feminization syndrome would show which of the following characteristics?

(A) Male body habitus
(B) 46, XX karyotype
(C) Testes but no seminal vesicles
(D) A rudimentary uterus
(E) Müllerian-inhibiting substance absent

11. All of the following statements about the H-Y antigen are true EXCEPT

(A) it is encoded in DNA on the short arm of chromosome Y
(B) it is required for testicular differentiation
(C) it is present in the testicular feminization syndrome
(D) it is absent in Turner syndrome
(E) it is absent in Klinefelter syndrome

12. All of the following statements about müllerian-inhibiting substance are true EXCEPT

(A) it is produced by the testes
(B) it is lacking in Klinefelter syndrome
(C) it is lacking in Turner syndrome
(D) it is present in testicular feminization syndrome
(E) it suppresses paramesonephric duct development

13. A person with Turner syndrome would show all of the following clinical manifestations EXCEPT

(A) menses
(B) a uterus
(C) a streak ovary
(D) a lack of follicular development
(E) lymphedema and a webbed neck

Directions: Each question below contains four suggested answers of which **one or more** is correct. Choose the answer

A if **1, 2, and 3** are correct
B if **1 and 3** are correct
C if **2 and 4** are correct
D if **4** is correct
E if **1, 2, 3, and 4** are correct

14. The urogenital folds are the origin of which of the following structures?

(1) Body of penis
(2) Glans of clitoris
(3) Labia minora
(4) Labia majora

15. Mesonephric duct derivatives include which of the following structures?

(1) Ductus deferens
(2) Gartner's duct
(3) Ejaculatory duct
(4) Epididymis

SUMMARY OF DIRECTIONS				
A	**B**	**C**	**D**	**E**
1, 2, 3 only	1, 3 only	2, 4 only	4 only	All are correct

16. Paramesonephric duct derivatives include which of the following structures?

(1) Uterine tubes
(2) Uterus
(3) Cervix
(4) Upper portion of the vagina

17. Which pairs of structures represent structures with the same embryologic origin?

(1) Ovarian interstitial glandular tissue and Leydig cells
(2) Penile urethra and lower portion of the vagina
(3) Appendix testis and uterine tubes
(4) Efferent ductules and paroophoron

18. Which of the following cells are derived from coelomic epithelium?

(1) Spermatozoa
(2) Sertoli cells
(3) Theca interna cells
(4) Follicular epithelial cells

19. Which of the following cells are derived from genital ridge mesenchyme?

(1) Theca externa cells
(2) Rete testis
(3) Leydig cells
(4) Granulosa cells

ANSWERS AND EXPLANATIONS

1. The answer is B. [*III C 1, D 2; VI A 2, 3; VII E 1 a (3) (b)*] The mesonephric duct (wolffian duct) forms the excurrent duct system for the testis, including the epididymis and the ductus (vas) deferens. Its differentiation is dependent on testosterone produced in the testes. The testes also produce müllerian-inhibiting substance, which causes regression of the paramesonephric ducts (müllerian ducts) in the male. In the female, the paramesonephric ducts form the uterine tubes, uterus, and upper portion of the vagina, while the mesonephric ducts form remnants called Gartner's duct or Gartner's cysts.

2. The answer is C. (*VI C, D, F; VII C, E 1 a*) If a patient with a 46, XX karyotype carried the gene for the testis-determining factor, there would be complete sex reversal and the patient would be a phenotypically normal male. Patients with Klinefelter syndrome (47, XXY or the rare 48, XXXY) and normal males (46, XY) also have a male body habitus. In most cases, patients with the H-Y antigen will also have a male body habitus. However, patients with a 46, XY karyotype but lacking the testosterone receptor will have the H-Y antigen (because they have a Y chromosome) but will have a female body habitus (because they are insensitive to testosterone). These patients have the so-called testicular feminization syndrome.

3. The answer is D. (*V C 2 b; VII C*) Patients with Klinefelter syndrome are aneuploid; that is, they do not have 46 chromosomes. Their karyotype is 47, XXY. They form testes, but these often fail to descend normally. Long-term exposure of the testis to the higher temperature in the body cavity compared to the lower temperature of the scrotum results in irreversible degenerative changes in the seminiferous epithelium (hyalinization) and an increased risk of malignant transformation of the seminiferous epithelium (seminoma). Patients with Klinefelter syndrome have a male body habitus but often show a gynecoid pelvis and gynecomastia (excessive breast development). They are usually quite tall as well.

4. The answer is C. (*II B, C; III D 2*) Primordial germ cells form all stages of all gametogenic cell lines from the spermatogonia and oogonia to the mature spermatozoa and ova. The epoophoron is a remnant of the mesonephric duct in the female.

5. The answer is E. (*VI D*) The testis-determining factor is encoded by a small portion of the Y chromosome. Under normal circumstances, it directs normal testicular differentiation and thus differentiation in a male direction. When it is deleted, the patient has an XY karyotype, has the H-Y antigen, but lacks testicular differentiation. In fact, such patients differentiate as females with ovaries rather than testes and with no epididymis. There is only one X chromosome and therefore no Barr body. One Barr body is seen in genetically female (XX) persons due to the inactivation of one of the two X chromosomes.

6. The answer is C. (*II B, C; III D; VI A 4; VII E 2*) Two copies of the X chromosome must be present for normal ovarian development to occur. Ovarian follicles produce sex steroids that control menstrual cycles and secondary sexual characteristics. An abnormal fetal adrenal gland can result in abnormally high levels of androgen, causing masculinization of the newborn female's genitalia. Paramesonephric duct derivatives form the uterine tubes, uterus, cervix, and upper portion of the vagina. Leydig cells are androgen-secreting cells in the testis, and are not found in normal females.

7. The answer is E. (*IV A B; VI A, B*) The normal development of the male external genitalia requires at least one X and one Y chromosome although it also occurs in 47, XXY karyotypes as well. Testes and their steroid hormone, testosterone, are also required, but the testosterone receptor must be present as well as the hormone itself. In the male fetus, the labioscrotal swellings will ultimately form the scrotum. Paramesonephric duct derivatives form the female reproductive tract and form only vestigial structures in the male.

8. The answer is B. (*VII B 3*) Turner syndrome is an example of gonadal dysgenesis. A patient with Turner syndrome has a 45, X karyotype. As a result of this genetic anomaly, normal ovaries fail to form. The abnormal ovaries that do form have no follicles in them. Therefore secondary sexual characteristics, which are normally induced by follicular steroids, are also lacking. Sterility, lack of menses, and a webbed neck are all characteristics of patients with Turner syndrome.

9. The answer is B. (*VII C*) Klinefelter syndrome is caused by a 47, XXY karyotype. A tall, thin male body habitus forms, with male external genitalia and genital ducts, but with feminization such as gynecomastia and a gynecoid pelvis. Testicular descent is abnormal in many cases and there is a hyalinization of the seminiferous epithelium, leading to infertility.

10. The answer is C. *(VII E 1 a)* Testicular feminization syndrome, a type of male pseudohermaphroditism, is due to a lack of the testosterone receptor. Patients have a female body habitus but a 46, XY karyotype. Testes are present, but mesonephric duct derivatives such as the seminal vesicles are lacking. The testes produce normal levels of testosterone and müllerian-inhibiting substance, and so there are no paramesonephric duct derivatives such as the uterus.

11. The answer is E. *(VI C)* The H-Y antigen is required for testicular differentiation of the indifferent gonad. It is encoded for by genes in the DNA on the short arm of the Y chromosome. It would therefore be absent in a patient whose karyotype was 45, X (Turner syndrome) but present with a 47, XXY karyotype (Klinefelter syndrome). It would also be present in testicular feminization syndrome, since here the karyotype is 46, XY.

12. The answer is B. *(VI E)* Müllerian-inhibiting substance, a hormone produced by the testis, causes regression of the paramesonephric (müllerian) ducts. Because it is a gene product found in males (i.e., in persons with a Y chromosome), it would be present in a patient with Klinefelter syndrome but lacking in Turner syndrome. It is also present in patients with testicular feminization syndrome.

13. The answer is A. *(VII B 3; Fig. 17-16)* Turner syndrome is caused by lack of the heteromorphic sex chromosome; that is, by a 45, X karyotype. In these patients, ovaries are present but they are abnormal in that they are small streaks of tissue which show a lack of follicular development upon histologic examination. Patients with Turner syndrome have lymphedema in the extremities, a prominent webbed neck, and a lack of development of secondary sexual characteristics such as pubic and axillary hair, breast development, and a growth spurt. These characteristics are all the result of failed ovarian maturation. In addition, since there is no normal cyclic function of the ovary, there is no menstrual cycle and no menses occur.

14. The answer is B (1, 3). *(IV A, B)* The urogenital folds form the body of the penis and the labia minora. The glans of the clitoris, like the glans penis, is derived from the genital tubercle. The labia majora are derived from the labioscrotal swellings.

15. The answer is E (all). *(III B, C, D 2)* The mesonephric duct (wolffian duct) forms the entire excurrent system of the male gonad between the epididymis and the ejaculatory duct. The efferent ductules are derivatives of the mesonephric tubules.

16. The answer is E (all). *(III B, D)* In the female, the paramesonephric duct (müllerian duct) forms the uterine tubes, uterus, cervix, and upper portion of the vagina. In the male, the paramesonephric duct degenerates almost completely, persisting only as the appendix of the testis and perhaps as the prostatic utricle, a small pouch in the prostatic urethra.

17. The answer is E (all). *(II B, C; III C, D)* Genital ridge mesenchyme forms ovarian interstitial glandular tissue and Leydig cells. The urogenital sinus forms the penile urethra and the lower portion of the vagina. The paramesonephric duct forms the appendix testis and the uterine tubes. The mesonephric tubules form the efferent ductules and the paroophoron.

18. The answer is C (2, 4). *(II A, B, C)* The spermatozoa are derived from primordial germ cells. Sertoli cells and follicular epithelial cells are homologous and both are derived from coelomic epithelial cells. The theca interna cells are derived from genital ridge mesenchyme.

19. The answer is B (1, 3). *(II B, C)* Genital ridge mesenchyme forms the hormone-secreting cells of the theca externa and Leydig cells. The rete testis forms from the primitive sex cords or perhaps from the mesonephric tubules. Granulosa cells are cells of the follicular epithelium and are derivatives of the coelomic epithelium.

18
Development of the Face, Oral Cavity, and Pharyngeal Arches

I. INTRODUCTION. This chapter examines the development of the face, the hard and soft palates, and the nasal and oral cavities, including the tongue and salivary glands. The development of the skull is covered in Chapter 9, section IV F, the development of the teeth in Chapter 12, section V, and the development of the eyes and ears in Chapters 20 and 21, respectively.

A. Clinical significance of the face
1. The face has an important role in our everyday behavior.
   a. We use the face not only for recognizing people who are familiar to us but also in nonverbal communication.
   b. Facial expressions can often tell a good deal about a person's mood, revealing joy or anger even when neither emotion is verbally expressed.
2. Besides this everyday role, the face provides useful clues for making clinical judgments in the process of identifying a particular clinical syndrome.
   a. The face can communicate sorrow, pain, and depression to a clinician.
   b. Alterations in facial morphology are highly noticeable, in part because human beings are accustomed to examining faces and use the facial appearance and expressions to learn so much about a person's identity or mood.

B. Overview of embryology of the head and neck
1. The face develops from the **frontal prominence**, the **nasal structures**, and the **first pharyngeal arch**. Involved in this process are a complex series of differential growth events followed by the fusion of several rudiments, providing many possibilities for congenital abnormalities.
   a. The **oral cavity** and the two **nasal cavities** begin as a single cavity.
      (1) The three cavities are separated from one another during embryologic development by the growth of the **nasal septum** and the formation of the **palate**.
      (2) In the adult, all three cavities still join at the **nasopharynx**.
      (3) During the partitioning of the nasal and oral cavities, the **olfactory epithelium**, **nasal sinuses**, and **nasal conchae** are formed.
   b. The **first pharyngeal arch** forms around the oral cavity.
   c. The **tongue** and **salivary glands** also develop in the oral cavity.
2. The **four pharyngeal arches**, with their associated **pouches** and **clefts**, contribute to various structures situated in the head and neck (see Table 18-1).

C. Functions of the tongue and salivary glands. The tongue and salivary glands are extremely important in the ingestion of food.
1. **The tongue**
   a. The tongue is used for moving food about in the oral cavity so that it can be crushed and torn by the teeth.
   b. The tongue also mixes the masticated foodstuffs with saliva.
2. **Saliva** is a complex secretion product from the salivary glands. It contains water, salts, mucus, immunoglobulins, and some digestive enzymes such as **ptyalin**.
   a. The principal function of saliva is to facilitate the formation of relatively small, cohesive balls of food that can be swallowed and transported rapidly down the esophagus into the stomach for further digestion.
   b. However, saliva also plays an immediate role in the digestion of some foods. Starch digestion, for example, begins in the oral cavity, as soon as the tongue has mixed starch-containing foods with the ptyalin of saliva.

II. DEVELOPMENT OF THE FACE

A. Embryonic rudiments of the face

1. The face is formed principally between the fourth and tenth weeks of intrauterine development.
2. The primordia that contribute to the face (Figs. 18-1 and 18-2) are masses of mesenchymal cells covered by a thin layer of skin which is derived from the surface ectoderm.
   a. The **frontal prominence (frontonasal process)** is a mass of tissue that represents the mesenchyme overlying the rapidly growing frontal lobes of the forebrain.
   b. Paired **maxillary swellings** are the cranial portions of the bifurcated first pharyngeal arch.
   c. Paired **mandibular swellings** are the caudal portions of the bifurcated first pharyngeal arch.
3. In the 4-week embryo, the mandibular swellings have met and fused with one another to form a continuous mass of tissue on the lower border of the **stomodeum**, the precursor of the oral cavity.
4. At this early stage, the **oropharyngeal (buccopharyngeal, stomodeal) membrane** is a thin sheet of ectodermal epithelium pressed tightly against a thin sheet of endodermal epithelium without any intervening mesodermally derived mesenchyme.
5. **Beginnings of the human face**
   a. Early in its development, the human face is not recognizably human (see Fig. 18-1). Instead, it looks much like the face of any other early mammalian embryo.

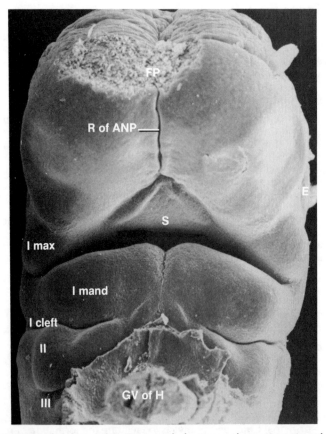

Figure 18-1. The developing face in an early human embryo. (Scanning electron micrograph) *E*, eye; *FP*, frontal prominence; *GV of H*, great vessels of heart; *R of ANP*, remnant of anterior neuropore; *S*, stomodeum; *I max*, first pharyngeal arch, maxillary branch; *I mand*, first pharyngeal arch, mandibular branch; *I cleft*, first pharyngeal cleft; *II*, second pharyngeal arch; *III*, third pharyngeal arch.

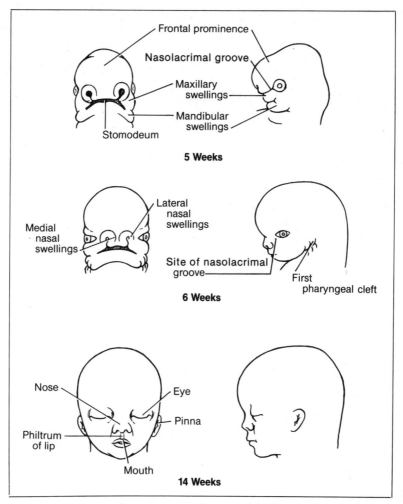

Figure 18-2. Development of the face.

    b. By 4 weeks, **precursors of the nasal cavity and the lens of the eye** have formed.
        (1) Nasal placodes, the precursors of the nasal cavities, have formed bilaterally on the medial aspect of the lower portion of the frontal prominence.
            (a) These paired ectodermal thickenings appear as roughly oval swellings.
            (b) They lie just above the maxillary processes of the first pharyngeal arch.
        (2) Lens placodes, the precursors of the lenses, have formed bilaterally on the lateral aspect of the lower portion of the frontal prominence (see Chapter 20, section II B).
    c. Not until 10 weeks of development does the face of the human fetus become recognizably human.

B. Development of the nose (see Figs. 18-2 and 18-4)
    1. Nasal pits and nasal swellings
        a. Soon after their formation, the nasal placodes begin to sink beneath the surface ectoderm on the frontal prominence, forming **nasal (olfactory) pits** (see section III A). This is due chiefly to mesenchymal growth around the nasal placodes.
        b. As this growth proceeds, C-shaped **nasal swellings** appear. The nasal swellings have a medial portion and a lateral portion that are not joined together on their inferior and medial aspects but instead have a small cleft separating them.
    2. While the nasal swellings are forming, two other events are in progress.
        a. The **eye** is becoming prominent on either side of the head, forming structures that at first project laterally.
        b. The **maxillary swellings** are growing medially. Their medial tips meet and fuse with the

lateral nasal swellings, leaving a shallow **nasolacrimal groove** (see Fig. 18-2).
- (1) The nasolacrimal groove runs from the medial corner of the developing eye into the stomodeum.
- (2) Later, the nasolacrimal groove invaginates and sinks below the surface ectoderm. It becomes a complete closed tube, the **nasolacrimal duct**, which drains tears from the eye into the nasal cavity.

3. After fusing with the lateral nasal swellings, the **maxillary processes** continue to grow medially. They first fuse with the medial nasal swellings and finally with a rhomboidal mass of tissue known as the **intermaxillary segment**.
4. As the maxillary processes grow medially, the **eyes** and **nose** move frontally.
   a. The **eyes** grow into the frontal plane of the face, so that they project forward.
   b. The **nasal swellings** move into the median frontal plane, where the two medial nasal swellings fuse with one another to make a single midline **bridge of the nose**.

C. Development of the mandible and maxilla

1. While the maxillary swellings are fusing with the nasal swellings and the intermaxillary segment (week 7), the **mandibular swellings** are also growing. They fuse with the maxillary swellings along the side of the face lateral to the border of the stomodeum.
2. As the maxillary and mandibular swellings are fusing on their surfaces, dramatic changes are also occurring in the mesenchymal cells deep within.
   a. **Formation of the mandible**
      (1) Within the mandibular swelling, the mandibular process of the first pharyngeal arch differentiates a large bar of cartilage known as **Meckel's cartilage**.
      (2) Mesenchymal cells surrounding Meckel's cartilage begin to form the **mandible** by the complex process of intramembranous bone formation (see Chapter 9, section III C)—that is, without the conversion of Meckel's cartilage to bone.
      (3) Later, Meckel's cartilage degenerates and disappears, but it is not converted into the mandible by endochondral bone formation.
   b. **Formation of the maxilla**
      (1) Within the maxillary swelling, mesenchymal cells in the maxillary processes of the first pharyngeal arch differentiate into the maxilla.
      (2) Again, the bone formation is by intramembranous ossification.
3. Since the mandible and the maxilla are formed from pharyngeal arch mesenchyme by intramembranous ossification, they are part of the **membranous viscerocranium** (see Chapter 9, section IV F 2).

III. DEVELOPMENT OF THE NASAL CAVITIES AND PALATE (Figs. 18-3, 18-4, and 18-5). Formation of the nasal cavities and formation of the oral cavity are intimately linked to one another.

A. Nasal cavities—early morphogenesis

1. The **nasal placodes**, surrounded by the medial and lateral nasal swellings, begin to invaginate dorsally and caudally beneath the developing brain during weeks 5 and 6, to form deep recesses known as **nasal (olfactory) pits**.
   a. The nasal pits form predominantly by rapid growth of the nasal swellings around the nasal placodes.
   b. Formation is also due in part to invagination as the nasal placodes grow dorsocaudally.
2. As the nasal pits deepen, they become the **nasal sacs**.
   a. At first, the two nasal sacs are separated from one another and from the oral cavity by a transient **bucconasal (oronasal) membrane**.
   b. Once the bucconasal membrane breaks down, the separate nasal sacs are in communication with one another and with the oral cavity (see Figs. 18-3 and 18-4).
3. A single medial **nasal septum** soon begins to grow downward from the roof of the nasal cavities (see Fig. 18-3). Once fully formed (by 11 weeks), this septum divides the nasal sacs into a left and a right nasal cavity.

B. The primary palate, intermaxillary segment, and lateral palatine processes

1. As the nasal septum begins to grow, simultaneously a **primary palate** forms from the intermaxillary segment, and right and left **lateral palatine processes** form from the maxillary processes.
   a. The **primary palate** (see Figs. 18-4 and 18-5) is roughly triangular. It forms between the

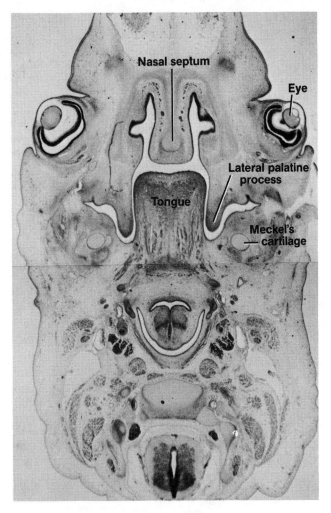

Figure 18-3. The developing nasal and oral cavities in a human embryo. (Light micrograph)

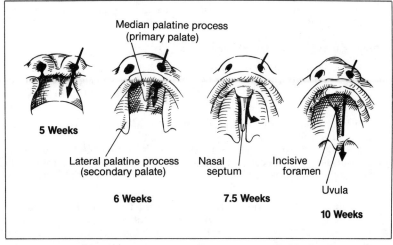

Figure 18-4. Development of the nose, nasal cavities, and palate. *Arrows* indicate the passageway between the nasal cavity and the oral cavity or pharynx.

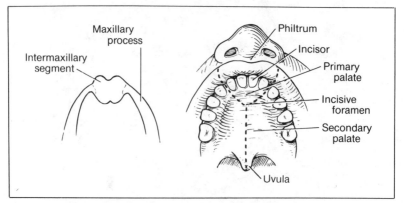

Figure 18-5. Development of the intermaxillary segment.

nasal sacs, from mesenchymal cells in the caudal portion (the **median palatine process**) of the intermaxillary segment.
   b. The **lateral palatine processes (secondary palatal shelves)** are two shelves of tissue that grow ventromedially. They arise from the maxillary processes on the side facing inward toward the nasal and oral cavities (see Figs. 18-3 and 18-4).
  2. The **intermaxillary segment** gives rise to several structures besides the primary palate:
     a. The **philtrum**, the indented fleshy mass of tissue on the middle portion of the upper lip (see Figs. 18-2 and 18-5)
     b. The premaxillary portion of the **maxillary bone**
     c. The two upper medial **incisors**

C. Fusion of the palatine processes and formation of the secondary palate (see Figs. 18-4 and 18-5)
  1. At first, the **tongue** is elevated and lies between the **lateral palatine processes**. These separate flaps of tissue project medially and downward from the maxillary processes in the recesses on either side of the tongue (see Fig. 18-3).
  2. Next, between weeks 6.5 and 7.5, the tongue is depressed and the lateral palatine processes swing upward toward the midline of the roof of the oral cavity, as if they were spring-loaded and under tension.
  3. The **primary palate**, meanwhile, is expanding laterally and posteriorly, essentially by differential growth.
  4. The cranial edges of the lateral palatine processes next fuse with the primary palate and then proceed to fuse with one another along their medial edges in a cranial to caudal sequence. The craniocaudal fusion of the two lateral palatine processes produces the **secondary palate** (week 10).

D. Partitioning of the nasal and oral cavities
  1. While the palatine processes are fusing with one another, the medial **nasal septum** is growing downward from the roof of the nasal cavity (see Fig. 18-4). The septum meets and fuses with the palatine processes, dividing the space into left and right nasal cavities (week 10).
  2. The fusion of the **primary palate** and the **secondary palate** completes the division of the nasal cavities from the oral cavity.
     a. The secondary palate and the medial nasal septum each have a caudal boundary.
     b. Consequently, the oral and nasal cavities remain in direct communication with one another in the **pharynx** near the **uvula**, the most caudal portion of the secondary palate.
  3. In the adult, a **Y-shaped line of fusion** marks the boundary between the median palatine process (the primary palate) and the lateral palatine processes (see Fig. 18-5).
     a. The Y extends in a cranial direction from the **uvula** to the right and left lateral edges of the **philtrum**.
     b. The **incisive foramen** (named for the incisor teeth), which forms at the caudal margin

of the median palatine process, is at the branch in the Y and represents the posterior border of the primary palate.
    c. This **anatomic landmark** becomes significant in classifying clefts of the palate (see section VI A).
  E. **The hard and soft palates**
    1. The entire primary palate and the cranial part of the secondary palate become ossified to form the **hard palate**.
    2. The caudal portion of the secondary palate does not become ossified but retains its fleshy character as the **soft palate** and **uvula**.
  F. **Further changes in the nasal cavities.** While the nasal and oral cavities are being partitioned by the formation of the palate, three other changes occur in the nasal cavities.
    1. The **olfactory epithelium** forms. Two patches of epithelium in the superior portion of each nasal cavity become highly differentiated into the greatly thickened olfactory epithelium.
      a. This differentiation may be due to inductive stimuli received from the olfactory bulbs of the brain.
      b. The olfactory epithelium is a tall, pseudostratified columnar epithelium which forms many **ciliated cells**.
        (1) The cilia that form, however, are not motile. Instead, they become unusually elongated, providing a large surface area for the differentiation of chemoreceptor sites.
          (a) The **chemoreceptors** are proteins in the plasma membrane on the apical surfaces of the olfactory epithelial cells.
          (b) These chemoreceptors respond to different chemical substances in the inspired air.
        (2) The **ciliated cells** are **bipolar neurons**. The basal portion of each ciliated cell sends an axon out of the olfactory epithelium and through the developing ethmoid bone, to synapse with neurons in the **olfactory bulb**.
          (a) The unmyelinated axons are gathered together in bundles that later become the **fila olfactoria (olfactory nerves)**.
          (b) The fila olfactoria penetrate the ethmoid bone via fenestrations in the **cribriform plate**, the part of the ethmoid bone that overlies the olfactory epithelium.
    2. **Paranasal air sinuses** form by ingrowth of the epithelium of the nasal cavities into the surrounding bony tissues.
    3. The **nasal conchae** form. Three groups of mesenchymal cells in the lateral walls of each nasal cavity proliferate extensively, giving rise to three distinct shelves of bone. The shelves grow medially and become elaborately curled to form the **superior, middle, and inferior nasal conchae**.

IV. DEVELOPMENT OF THE TONGUE AND SALIVARY GLANDS

  A. **The tongue**
    1. **Formation of the tongue** (Fig. 18-6)
      a. The tongue begins to form late in the fourth week with the appearance of the **tuberculum impar**, a median tongue bud which forms in the floor of the pharynx just cranial to the rudiment of the thyroid gland.
      b. The **anterior two-thirds** of the tongue forms from two **lateral lingual swellings** that develop on either side of the tuberculum impar.
        (1) The lateral lingual swellings grow rapidly by proliferation of the underlying mesenchyme of the ventromedial portions of the **first pharyngeal arch**.
        (2) The swellings fuse with one another as they overgrow the tuberculum impar. Their line of fusion is the **median sulcus** of the tongue.
      c. The **posterior one-third** of the tongue arises from two structures, the **copula** and the **hypobranchial eminence**.
        (1) The **copula** forms the caudal portion of the **second pharyngeal arch** and the cranial portion of the **third pharyngeal arch**.
        (2) The large **hypobranchial eminence** grows rapidly and soon obliterates the copula, later fusing with the lateral lingual swellings along a line of demarcation represented in the adult by the **terminal sulcus** of the tongue.

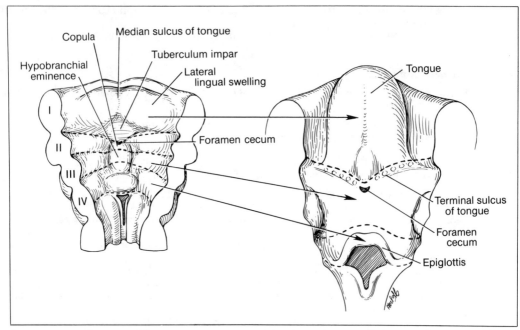

Figure 18-6. Development of the tongue. *Roman numerals* indicate the original pharyngeal arches, and *dotted lines* indicate the approximate boundaries between the arches. Note that the second arch derivatives of the tongue are displaced by third arch derivatives.

2. **Derivations of the tissues of the tongue**
   a. **Blood vessels**, **lymphatics**, and **connective tissue** of the tongue are derived from the appropriate pharyngeal arch mesenchyme.
   b. The **intrinsic muscles** of the tongue arise from the myoblasts that migrate into the tongue from the occipital myotomes.
   c. The **nerve supply** of the tongue comes from several sources.
      (1) Since the muscles of the tongue are derived from occipital myotomes, they receive their motor innervation from the nerve of these myotomes, namely the **hypoglossal nerve** (cranial nerve XII).
      (2) The anterior two-thirds of the tongue, since it is derived from the ventromedial portion of the first pharyngeal arch, receives its sensory nerve supply from the lingual branch of the **trigeminal nerve** (cranial nerve V), the nerve that supplies the first pharyngeal arch.
      (3) The posterior one-third of the tongue, since it is formed partly from the third pharyngeal arch, takes its innervation largely from the **hypoglossal nerve**, although the **superior laryngeal branch of the vagus nerve** (cranial nerve X) supplies the most posterior portion of the posterior third of the tongue.

B. **Development of the salivary glands**
   1. The salivary glands all arise as proliferating epithelial cords of cells that grow into the surrounding mesenchymal masses of the jaws. The epithelial cords branch extensively as they invade the mesenchyme, resulting in the formation of a **collecting duct** and **secretory acini** (Fig. 18-7).
      a. The large **duct** to drain the gland forms first in the proximal portion of the cord.
      b. The many **secretory acini** that produce salivary secretions then form in the distal portions of the epithelial cords.
   2. There are **three major pairs of salivary glands**.
      a. The **parotid salivary glands** are thought to form from epithelial cords that arise anterior to the oropharyngeal membrane and are therefore ectodermally derived.
      b. In contrast, the **submandibular** (or **submaxillary**) and **sublingual salivary glands** are thought to form from epithelial cords that arise posterior to the buccopharyngeal membrane and are therefore endodermally derived.

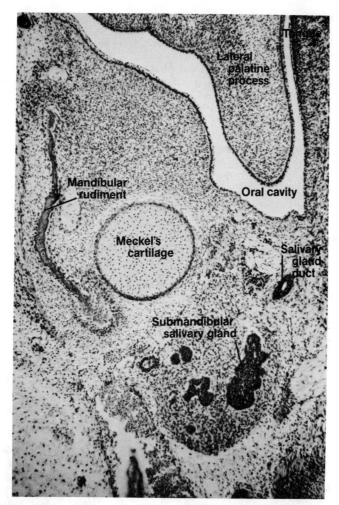

Figure 18-7. Salivary gland, salivary duct, and Meckel's cartilage in the developing lower jaw of the human embryo. (Light micrograph)

V. DEVELOPMENT OF THE PHARYNGEAL ARCHES

A. General features of pharyngeal arch development

1. In humans, the pharyngeal apparatus forms as a series of four distinct masses of mesenchymal tissue on the lateral aspects of the developing head and neck (Fig. 18-8). These four masses become the **four pharyngeal arches**. A rudimentary **fifth arch** becomes fused with the fourth pharyngeal arch.
   a. The mesenchymal tissue masses are invaded by cranial **neural crest cells** which contribute to the later development of mesenchyme in the head and neck.
   b. Each pharyngeal arch is covered on its lateral surface by ectodermally derived epithelium and on its medial surface by endodermally derived epithelium.
2. Between the pharyngeal arches, a series of **pharyngeal pouches, clefts, and membranes** form (Fig. 18-9).
   a. **Four pharyngeal pouches** form on the medial aspects of the pharyngeal arches, and **four pharyngeal clefts** form on the lateral aspects. The first pharyngeal pouch and cleft form between the first and second pharyngeal arches; the second pharyngeal pouch and cleft form between the second and third arches, and so on.
   b. A **pharyngeal membrane** forms at least transiently across each pharyngeal arch.
      (1) The membranes form as a bit of mesenchyme sandwiched between the lateral ectodermally derived pharyngeal cleft epithelium and the medial endodermally derived pharyngeal pouch epithelium.

312 Human Developmental Anatomy

        (2) Only the membrane between the first pharyngeal cleft and pouch persists in the adult, becoming the **tympanic membrane**.
    c. During the fifth week of development, the second pharyngeal arch begins to grow caudally.
        (1) In consequence, the second pharyngeal cleft and membrane and all the other more caudal clefts and membranes are overgrown by the second arch during organogenesis.
        (2) Thus, these structures normally have no representation in the adult. However, they may lead to a variety of **cystic structures** (cervical sinuses or fistulas) in the neck.
  3. Each pharyngeal arch is supplied with its own blood vessel and its own cranial nerve, and its mesenchyme forms muscles and connective tissue elements such as bones, cartilage, and ligaments (Table 18-1).

B. The first pharyngeal arch (mandibular arch) [see Table 18-1]
  1. The bifurcated first pharyngeal arch (the mandibular arch) has a cranial **maxillary branch** and a caudal **mandibular branch**.
  2. Derivatives of the first arch
    a. The first pharyngeal arch contributes to the development of:
        (1) The upper lip (via the intermaxillary segment of the maxillary process)
        (2) The roof of the mouth (via the median palatine process and the lateral palatine processes)
        (3) The maxilla
        (4) The mandible
        (5) The anterior tongue

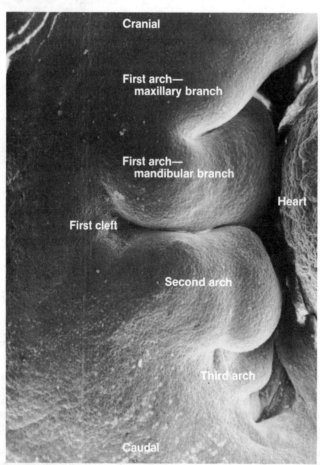

Figure 18-8. Scanning electron micrograph of the pharyngeal apparatus in the same embryo as shown in Figure 18-1.

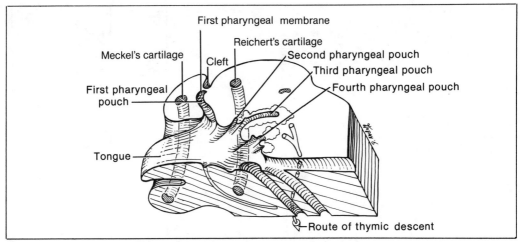

Figure 18-9. Development of the pharyngeal clefts and pouches.

    b. The mandibular arch has a core of mesenchyme that differentiates into Meckel's cartilage (see Figs. 18-7 and 18-9) and the muscles of mastication.
        (1) Meckel's cartilage becomes converted into the malleus and incus (middle ear ossicles; see Fig. 18-10) and forms the ligament of the malleus and the sphenomandibular ligament.
        (2) The **muscles of mastication** include the temporalis, masseter, and mylohyoid muscles, and the anterior belly of the digastric muscle.
  3. Nerve supply. The first arch receives innervation from the maxillary and mandibular branches of the **trigeminal nerve** (cranial nerve V).
  4. Cleft, pouch, and membrane derivatives
    a. The **first pharyngeal cleft** becomes the external auditory meatus.
    b. The **first pharyngeal pouch** becomes the auditory tube.
    c. The boundary between these two recesses, the tympanic membrane, is derived from the **first pharyngeal membrane**.
    d. The **auricle (pinna) of the ear** develops from six mesenchymal masses surrounding the first pharyngeal cleft (i.e., the future external auditory meatus). Three of these masses derive from the caudal border of the **first pharyngeal arch** and three from the cranial border of the **second pharyngeal arch**.

C. The second pharyngeal arch (hyoid arch) [see Table 18-1]
  1. Derivatives of the second arch
    a. The second pharyngeal arch (the hyoid arch) has a core of mesenchyme that forms **Reichert's cartilage** (see Fig. 18-9), which later contributes to (see Fig. 18-10):
        (1) The stapes (a middle ear ossicle)
        (2) The styloid process
        (3) The lesser horn and the upper body of the hyoid bone
        (4) The stylohyoid ligament
    b. The second arch mesenchyme also forms:
        (1) The **muscles of facial expression** (frontalis, orbicularis oculi, orbicularis oris, platysma, and buccinator)
        (2) The stapedius muscle
        (3) The posterior belly of the digastric muscle
  2. Nerve supply. The second arch receives innervation from the branches of the **facial nerve** (cranial nerve VII).
  3. Cleft, pouch, and membrane derivatives
    a. The second pharyngeal **pouch** forms the epithelium of the palatine tonsils, which later become infiltrated by large numbers of lymphocytes to form the **definitive palatine tonsils**.
    b. The caudal overgrowth of the second arch eliminates the second and the more caudal pharyngeal clefts and membranes, so that these have no normal representation in the adult.

Table 18-1. Pharyngeal Apparatus Derivatives

Pharyngeal Arch	Arch Derivatives				Pouch Derivatives	Cleft Derivatives	Nerve Supply
	Muscles	Bone and Cartilage	Other Connective Tissues				
First (mandibular)	Mastication muscles Mylohyoid Anterior belly of digastric Tensor tympani Tensor veli palatini	Meckel's cartilage Mandible Maxilla Premaxilla Zygomatic arch Pinna of ear (anterior) Malleus Incus	Anterior ligament of malleus Sphenomandibular ligament Tympanic membrane (from first pharyngeal membrane)		Auditory tube	External auditory meatus	V (trigeminal)
Second (hyoid)	Facial expression muscles Stapedius Stylohyoid Posterior belly of digastric	Reichert's cartilage Pinna of ear (posterior) Stapes Styloid process Hyoid bone (lesser horn and upper body)	Stylohyoid ligament		Palatine tonsils	None	VII (facial)
Third	Stylopharyngeus	Hyoid bone (greater horn and lower body)	None		Inferior parathyroid Thymus	None	IX (glossopharyngeal)
Fourth and fifth combined	Cricothyroid Levator velum palatini Constrictors of pharynx Intrinsic muscles of larynx	Laryngeal cartilages (cricoid, thyroid, arytenoid, corniculate, cuneiform)	None		Superior parathyroids Thymus Ultimobranchial bodies of thyroid	None	X (superior and recurrent laryngeal branches of vagus)

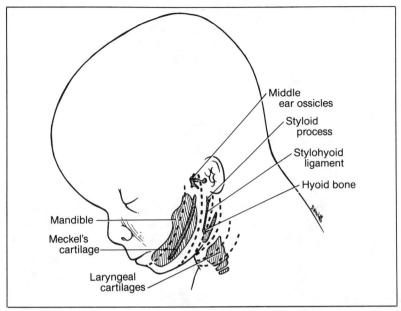

Figure 18-10. Development of pharyngeal arch cartilages. *Dotted lines* indicate the approximate boundaries between the pharyngeal arch derivatives. Note the dual source of the middle ear ossicles: The malleus and incus derive from the first arch by way of Meckel's cartilage; the stapes derives from the second arch by way of Reichert's cartilage.

- **D. The third pharyngeal arch** (see Table 18-1)
    1. **Derivatives of the third arch.** The third pharyngeal arch has a core of mesenchyme that forms muscles such as the stylopharyngeus and bones such as the greater horn and lower part of the body of the hyoid bone.
    2. **Nerve supply.** The third arch receives innervation from the **glossopharyngeal nerve** (cranial nerve IX).
    3. The third pharyngeal pouch becomes bifid.
        a. The anterior portion forms the **inferior parathyroids**.
        b. The posterior portion forms the **epithelial reticular cells of the thymus**. These later become invaded by lymphocytes to form the **definitive thymus gland**.

- **E. The fourth pharyngeal arch** (see Table 18-1)
    1. The fourth pharyngeal arch becomes fused with the rudimentary **fifth arch**.
    2. **Derivatives of the fourth arch.** The fourth arch mesenchyme forms laryngeal cartilage (see Fig. 18-10), the cricothyroid and levator velum palatini muscles, the constrictors of the pharynx, and the intrinsic muscles of the larynx.
    3. **Nerve supply.** The fourth arch structures receive innervation from either the superior laryngeal branch or the recurrent laryngeal branch of the **vagus nerve** (cranial nerve X).
    4. The fourth pharyngeal pouch also becomes bifid.
        a. The anterior portion forms the **superior parathyroids**.
        b. The posterior portion forms the remainder of the **thymic reticular epithelial cells** and the **ultimobranchial bodies**, which become incorporated into the **thyroid**.

VI. CONGENITAL ANOMALIES IN THE HEAD AND NECK

- **A. Clefting anomalies** (Fig. 18-11)
    1. **Cleft lip** and **cleft palate** represent failures of fusion along the Y-shaped intersection of the median palatine process (the primary palate) and the lateral palatine processes.
    2. **Cleft lip**, with or without cleft palate, is the most common congenital birth defect of the orofacial region.

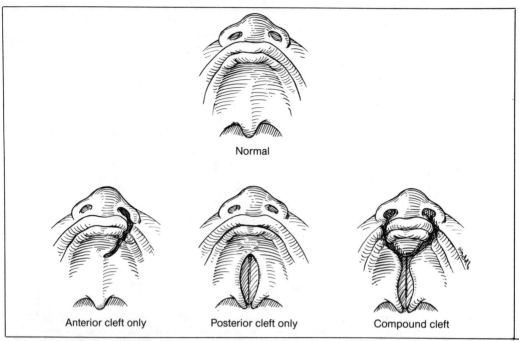

Figure 18-11. Palatal anomalies. (A) Normal palate at term. (B) Anterior cleft. Only the fusion between the posterior border of the primary palate and the anterior border of the secondary palate on the left side is affected. (C) Posterior cleft. Only the fusion between the medial borders of the lateral maxillary processes (secondary palate) is affected. (D) Compound cleft. The entire borders of the median palatine process (primary palate) and lateral palatine processes (secondary palate) have failed to fuse.

3. Many different combinations of facial clefting can occur. One convenient **classification system** for clefting (see Fig. 18-11) has a firm anatomic basis derived from the development of the intermaxillary segment and the lateral palatine processes.
   a. An **anterior cleft** involves only the intermaxillary segment. That is, it occurs from the incisive foramen anteriorly through the palate and the lip to the nasal cavity. Anterior clefts can be unilateral or bilateral.
   b. A **posterior cleft** involves only the fusion of the lateral palatine processes. That is, it occurs posteriorly from the incisive foramen.
      (1) Posterior clefts can be minor, with a cleft in all or a portion of the uvula.
      (2) They may be more serious, extending anteriorly through the soft palate and even into the hard palate.
   c. A **compound cleft** involves the entire line of fusion between the median and lateral palatine processes.
4. Clefting defects occur more frequently in males than in females. **Unilateral cleft lip without cleft palate** accounts for about 80% of all clefts of the lip. It may occur as a relatively minor anomaly which can be corrected with plastic surgery, or it may be only one of a more severe collection of anomalies. In children with trisomy 13 (Patau syndrome), for example, cleft lip, cleft palate, and other anomalies are common.

B. Mandibulofacial dysostosis (Treacher Collins syndrome, first arch syndrome)

1. Mandibulofacial dysostosis is a syndrome that results from maldevelopment of the first pharyngeal arch.
2. Afflicted children have malformations of the face affecting the region under the eye, the zygoma, the ear, the mandible, and the mouth (Fig. 18-12).
3. The syndrome is transmitted as an **autosomal dominant gene** but with **variable penetrance**.
   a. Thus, when parents are unafflicted but have an afflicted child, the syndrome may be due to either of **two genetic patterns**:
      (1) Subclinical presence of the gene in one or both of the parents
      (2) A new, spontaneously arising mutation (a less likely cause)

b. An example of a child with mandibulofacial dysostosis and a detailed pedigree of his family are shown in Figure 18-12.
  (1) In this family, the mode of transmission is clearly compatible with autosomal dominant inheritance rather than with a new mutation.
  (2) The variability in expression of the syndrome in different members of the family is due to variable penetrance of the dominant gene.
c. Mandibulofacial dysostosis is particularly common among Caucasians in Appalachia in the United States. This may be due to the common ethnic heritage or to modest inbreeding among these people.

C. DiGeorge syndrome (see also Chapter 15, section IX A 2)
  1. DiGeorge syndrome results from a developmental defect in the formation of the third and fourth pharyngeal pouches.
    a. Afflicted patients have hypoplastic parathyroid glands and little or no thymic tissue.
    b. Consequently, patients have difficulties with regulation of serum calcium and with the cell-mediated (T cell–dependent) immune system (see Chapter 15, section IV A 2).
    c. Associated cardiovascular defects are seen in many patients.
  2. Craniofacial anomalies are common in patients with DiGeorge syndrome, perhaps due to faulty migration of neural crest cells into the pharyngeal arches.

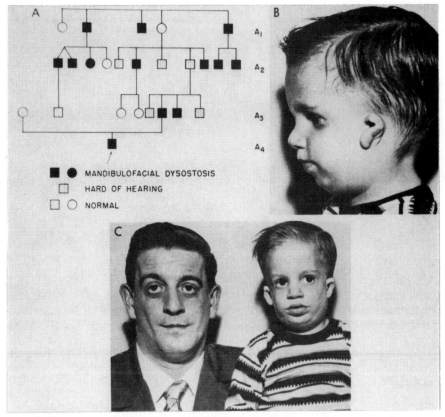

Figure 18-12. Mandibulofacial dysostosis. The *arrow* in the pedigree (*A*) indicates the child shown in *B* and *C*. Both the father and the child (*C*) have this congenital syndrome. (Reprinted with permission from Warkany J: *Congenital Malformations.* Chicago, Year Book, 1971, p 651.)

STUDY QUESTIONS

Directions: Each question below contains five suggested answers. Choose the **one best** response to each question.

1. Which pharyngeal pouches form endocrine tissue?

   (A) First pouch only
   (B) Third pouch only
   (C) First and third pouches
   (D) Second and fourth pouches
   (E) Third and fourth pouches

2. All of the following are characteristics of first arch syndrome (mandibulofacial dysostosis) EXCEPT

   (A) defects in the auricle and external auditory meatus
   (B) mandibular hypoplasia
   (C) mental retardation
   (D) downward-sloping palpebral fissures (eye slits)
   (E) deafness

3. All of the following statements about facial clefts are true EXCEPT

   (A) cleft uvula is a secondary palatal cleft
   (B) cleft hard palate posterior to the incisive foramen without cleft lip is a primary palatal cleft
   (C) cleft lip alone is a primary cleft
   (D) cleft of the lip and hard palate anterior to the incisive foramen is a primary cleft
   (E) clefting is more frequent in males than females

4. Partitioning of the oral and nasal cavities involves all of the following anatomic structures EXCEPT

   (A) the nasal septum
   (B) the nasal conchae
   (C) the primary palate
   (D) the secondary palate
   (E) the tongue

Directions: Each question below contains four suggested answers of which **one or more** is correct. Choose the answer

   A if **1, 2, and 3** are correct
   B if **1 and 3** are correct
   C if **2 and 4** are correct
   D if **4** is correct
   E if **1, 2, 3, and 4** are correct

5. First pharyngeal arch derivatives include which of the following structures?

   (1) Zygomatic arch
   (2) Hyoid bone
   (3) Malleus
   (4) Stapes

6. Second pharyngeal arch derivatives include which of the following structures?

   (1) Stapes
   (2) Styloid process
   (3) Lesser horn (cornu) of hyoid bone
   (4) Mandible

7. First pharyngeal arch derivatives include which of the following structures?

   (1) Maxilla
   (2) Masseter muscle
   (3) Mandible
   (4) Orbicularis oris muscle

8. Third pharyngeal arch derivatives include which of the following structures?

   (1) Lower body of hyoid bone and greater horn (cornu) of hyoid bone
   (2) Stylohyoid ligament
   (3) Stylopharyngeus muscle
   (4) Platysma muscle

9. Second pharyngeal arch derivatives include which of the following muscles?

(1) Buccinator muscle

(2) Orbicularis muscles

(3) Frontalis muscle

(4) Anterior belly of the digastric muscle

Directions: The group of questions below consists of lettered choices followed by several numbered items. For each numbered item select the **one** lettered choice with which it is **most** closely associated. Each lettered choice may be used once, more than once, or not at all.

Questions 10–14

Match each description of a pharyngeal arch derivative below with the appropriate structure shown in the accompanying diagram.

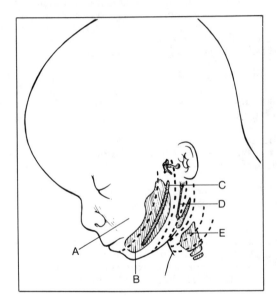

10. This structure forms in the first pharyngeal arch; it is a cartilage that forms the malleus and incus

11. This structure forms in the hyoid arch and gives rise to the stapes

12. This structure is a cartilage in the fourth pharyngeal arch

13. The bones under this structure are derived from the maxillary process lateral to the midline and form the intermaxillary segment in the midline of the face

14. This bone forms around Meckel's cartilage by intramembranous ossification

ANSWERS AND EXPLANATIONS

1. The answer is E. *(V B–E)* The parathyroid glands are endocrine tissue, and they arise from the third and fourth pharyngeal pouches. The first pharyngeal pouch forms the auditory tube. The second pharyngeal pouch forms the palatine tonsils. The third and fourth pharyngeal pouches also contribute to the reticular epithelial cells of the thymus gland. This gland is not traditionally considered to be an endocrine gland. Rather, it is an organ of the immune system.

2. The answer is C. *(VI B)* Mandibulofacial dysostosis in its severe form involves many different structures related to the first arch. Thus, the auricle, the external auditory meatus, and the inner ear ossicles may all be missing, leading to deafness. This deafness may cause a learning deficit, but there is no mental retardation associated with this syndrome. Because of facial dysplasia, there may also be downward-sloping palpebral fissures.

3. The answer is B. *(VI A)* Primary clefts are anterior to the incisive foramen. Secondary clefts are posterior to the incisive foramen. Thus, cleft hard palate would be a secondary palatal cleft. Cleft uvula is secondary, and cleft lip alone is primary. Clefting is more frequent in males than in females.

4. The answer is B. *(III C, D, F 3)* The nasal conchae are shelves that form inside the nasal cavities, but they have no role per se in partitioning of the oral and nasal cavities. For this important morphogenetic process, the nasal septum fuses with the primary and secondary palates. The primary and secondary palates also fuse with one another. Initially, the lateral palatine processes (which comprise the secondary palate) are held apart in the lateral recesses on either side of the tongue, which is at first elevated. When the tongue descends, these processes move upward and come together in the midline, where they fuse with the primary palate and the nasal septum. This fusion completes the division of the right and left nasal cavities from the oral cavity.

5. The answer is B (1, 3). *(V B; Table 18-1)* The first arch forms the zygomatic arch, the maxilla, the intermaxillary segment, and the mandible. The malleus and incus form at the end of Meckel's cartilage, a first arch cartilage. The hyoid bone forms from the second and third arches. The stapes comes from the end of Reichert's cartilage, a second arch derivative.

6. The answer is A (1, 2, 3). *(V C; Table 18-1)* The stapes and lesser horn of the hyoid bone, as well as the upper body of the hyoid bone, are second arch derivatives. The styloid process is also a second arch derivative. The mandible is a first arch derivative.

7. The answer is A (1, 2, 3). *(V B; Table 18-1)* The mandible and maxilla are both first arch derivatives, as is the masseter, one of the muscles of mastication. The orbicularis oris is a muscle of facial expression and therefore a second arch derivative.

8. The answer is B (1, 3). *(V D; Table 18-1)* The greater horn and lower part of the body of the hyoid bone are third arch derivatives, as is the stylopharyngeus muscle. The stylohyoid ligament is a second arch derivative. The platysma muscle, a muscle of facial expression, is also a second pharyngeal arch derivative. Other muscles of facial expression include the orbicularis oris, orbicularis oculi, buccinator, and frontalis muscles.

9. The answer is A (1, 2, 3). *(V B 2 b, C)* The second arch gives rise to the muscles of facial expression, which include the platysma, frontalis, orbicularis, and buccinator muscles. The anterior belly of the digastric muscle is a first arch derivative.

10–14. The answers are: 10-C, 11-D, 12-E, 13-A, 14-B. *(II C 2; III B; V B 2 b, C 1 a, E 2)* The upper lip (A) is derived from the tips of the maxillary processes lateral to the midline and from the intermaxillary segment in the midline. The bones of the primary palate are derived from the intermaxillary segment. The maxillary bones are derived from the maxillary process of the first pharyngeal arch. The mandible (B) forms around Meckel's cartilage (C) by intramembranous ossification. Meckel's cartilage forms the malleus and incus, while Reichert's cartilage (D), which forms in the second (hyoid) arch, forms the stapes. The laryngeal cartilages (E) are fourth arch derivatives.

19
Development of the Endocrine System

I. INTRODUCTION

A. Major glandular components of the endocrine system
1. The endocrine glands of the human body consist of the **pituitary** and **pineal glands, thyroid** and **parathyroid glands, adrenal glands, gonads,** and **pancreatic islet tissues** (Fig. 19-1).
2. The **amine precursor uptake and decarboxylation (APUD) cells** are often considered to be endocrine cells as well.
3. In addition, the **hypothalamus** secretes a number of hormones which regulate the activities of the endocrine glands.

B. Regulation of endocrine function
1. The function of most endocrine organs is under the strict control of the **hypothalamus** and the **pituitary (hypophysis)**.
   a. The **hypothalamus** produces a number of **releasing hormones** that reach the **anterior pituitary (adenohypophysis)** via a hypothalamic–hypophyseal portal system.
      (1) Each hypothalamic releasing hormone stimulates the adenohypophysis to produce a corresponding **trophic hormone**.
      (2) Each trophic hormone then induces its corresponding **endocrine gland** to produce the final hormone that acts on a target organ, thereby regulating fundamental bodily processes—the ultimate goal of the whole cascade.
   b. The hypothalamus is also involved directly in hormone production by the **posterior pituitary (neurohypophysis)**.
2. A **feedback-loop system** regulates hormone production.
   a. When an endocrine gland releases sufficient hormone into the blood stream, the blood level of that hormone depresses the production of hypothalamic releasing hormone and thus of pituitary trophic hormone.
   b. In this way, the endocrine glands are prevented from producing excessive amounts of hormones.

C. Overview of embryology of the endocrine system. The embryology of the endocrine system is quite complex.
1. Origin of endocrine tissue
   a. Endocrine glands can be derived from any of the three primary germ layers.
      (1) The pituitary gland epithelium is derived from the **ectoderm**.
      (2) The endocrine portions of the gonads and the adrenal cortex are derived from the **mesoderm**.
      (3) The thyroid epithelium and the parathyroid glands are derived from the **endoderm**.
   b. The adrenal medulla, the parafollicular C cells of the thyroid gland, some cells of the pancreatic islets of Langerhans, and scattered APUD endocrine cells in the brain, gastrointestinal tract, and respiratory system are all derived from the **neural crest**. Thus, these cells are also **ectodermal** in origin.
2. **Fetal–placental interaction.** The production and metabolism of steroid hormones involves a complex interaction between the fetal endocrine glands and the placenta.

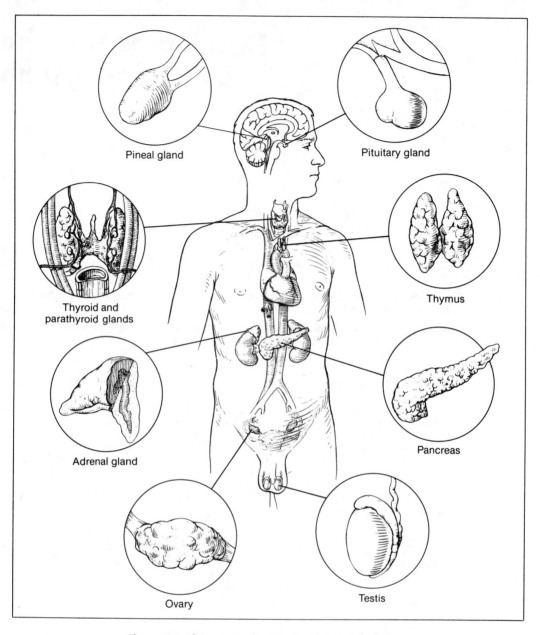

Figure 19-1. The major endocrine glands of the human body.

II. THE PITUITARY GLAND AND THE PINEAL GLAND

A. Components of the pituitary gland

1. The pituitary gland has two main components, the **adenohypophysis** and the **neurohypophysis**.
   a. The **adenohypophysis (anterior lobe)** is subdivided into three parts:
      (1) The pars distalis
      (2) The pars tuberalis
      (3) The pars intermedia
   b. The **neurohypophysis (posterior lobe)** is also subdivided into three parts:
      (1) The median eminence
      (2) The infundibular stem
      (3) The infundibular process (pars nervosa)

2. The **median eminence** is connected to the hypothalamus and is a part of the **tuber cinereum**.
   a. The tuber cinereum constitutes part of the floor of the third ventricle of the brain.
   b. It is poorly developed in humans.
3. Neurons with their cell bodies in brain nuclei located either in or near the tuber cinereum (i.e., in the supraoptic nucleus and the paraventricular nucleus) have axons that terminate in the median eminence and other parts of the neurohypophysis.

B. **Development of the pituitary gland** (Fig. 19-2)
   1. **Origins of the two lobes**
      a. The pituitary develops from two separate rudiments.
         (1) The **neurohypophysis** is derived from the **infundibulum**, a small evagination of the floor of the diencephalon and thus neuroectodermal in origin.
         (2) The **adenohypophysis** is derived from **Rathke's pouch**, an evagination of the roof of the mouth and thus ectodermal in origin.
      b. These two separate rudiments come together during weeks 6 to 8, long before the formation of the bony parts of the sphenoid bone and the secondary palate.
   2. **Development of the infundibulum.** The development of the infundibulum is relatively straightforward.
      a. As the infundibulum grows, it remains connected to the brain.
      b. The infundibulum grows extensively, elongating and eventually giving rise to the **infundibular stem** and **infundibular process**.
   3. **Development of Rathke's pouch.** The development of Rathke's pouch is considerably more complicated.
      a. The connection between the roof of the mouth and Rathke's pouch is rapidly obliterated.
         (1) In certain pathologic cases small strands of pituitary-like cells may be seen in the roof of the mouth.
         (2) Less often in these cases, the pituitary-like cells lie in nests deep within recesses of the sphenoid bone.
      b. In separating from the roof of the mouth, Rathke's pouch becomes a closed vesicle lined by epithelium and closely associated with the infundibulum.
      c. Three changes now occur.
         (1) The anterior portion of this vesicle grows enormously, giving rise eventually to all of the **anterior lobe**.
            (a) The terminology **anterior and posterior lobes** originally arose because the

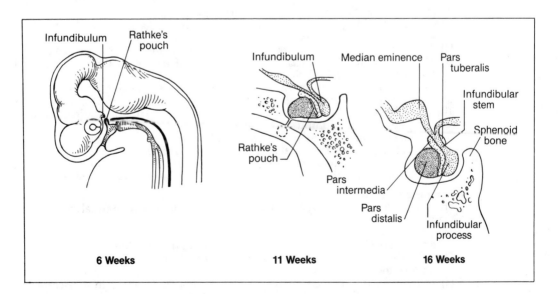

Figure 19-2. Development of the pituitary gland. The *dotted circle* in the central diagram shows the potential site of ectopic pituitary tissue.

pituitary gland can be easily split at a cleft that represents the remnant of the cavity of the vesicle formed from Rathke's pouch.
- (b) The **pars distalis** of the adenohypophysis essentially develops from the anterior wall of this vesicle.
- (2) The posterior wall of the vesicle next fuses with the infundibulum and becomes incorporated into it. This explains the later intimate association between the **pars intermedia** and the **pars nervosa**.
- (3) The walls of the vesicle now grow dorsolaterally to surround the infundibulum nearest the median eminence, forming the **pars tuberalis**.

4. **Histogenesis of the adenohypophysis**
    a. The developing epithelial cells in the pars distalis are arranged in epithelial cords or follicles. These become surrounded by a dense network of capillaries that grow into the gland.
    b. Most of the cells in the pars distalis remain as **chromophobes** but a few differentiate first into **acidophils** (at 8 weeks) and next into **basophils** (at 9 weeks).

5. **Hormone secretion**
    a. The fetal pituitary is known to secrete the following hormones:
       (1) Adrenocorticotropic hormone (ACTH)
       (2) Growth hormone
       (3) Prolactin
       (4) Thyroid-stimulating hormone (TSH)
       (5) Gonadotropins
    b. **Hypothalamic–pituitary relationships**
       (1) The hypothalamus contains thyrotropin-releasing hormone (TRH) and gonadotropin-releasing hormone (GnRH) at 9 weeks, but the hypothalamic–hypophyseal portal system does not develop until 15 weeks.
       (2) During the interval, the hypothalamic hormones may diffuse to the adenohypophysis, or the early secretory activities of hormone-producing cells in the adenohypophysis may be independent of hypothalamic releasing hormones.

C. **Development of the pineal gland.** The pineal gland develops as an evagination from the roof of the brain, much as the infundibulum evaginates from the floor of the brain.

III. THE THYROID GLAND AND THE PARATHYROID GLANDS

A. **The thyroid gland**

1. **Development of the thyroid gland** (Fig. 19-3)
    a. The thyroid gland arises as an endodermal invagination of the floor of the pharynx caudal to the oropharyngeal membrane. It appears near the root of the developing tongue, between the first and second pharyngeal arches.
    b. The thyroid quickly grows ventrally and caudally, becoming somewhat bilobate on its distal end.
       (1) The thyroid for a time remains attached to the pharynx by a **thyroglossal duct**.
       (2) The attachment site of the thyroglossal duct to the root of the tongue is marked by the **foramen cecum** in the adult.
    c. The thyroid, accompanied by the thyroglossal duct, next descends over the second pharyngeal arch derivatives (e.g., the hyoid bone) and comes to rest near the larynx.
    d. The thyroglossal duct then degenerates, leaving an isolated **thyroid rudiment** with two **lobes** connected by an **isthmus**.
       (1) In some persons, there is also a **pyramidal lobe**, projecting cranially in the midline. This is a remnant of the distal part of the thyroglossal duct.
       (2) In fact, **ectopic thyroid tissue** can remain anywhere along the course of the thyroglossal duct, from the root of the tongue to the pyramidal lobe (see Fig. 19-3).

2. **Histogenesis of the thyroid gland**
    a. The thyroid **follicular epithelial cells** are derived from the **endodermal** thyroid diverticulum.
    b. The connective tissue capsule, trabeculae, and blood vessels of the thyroid are derived from **splanchnic mesoderm** surrounding the thyroid diverticulum.
    c. The thyroid tissue fuses with the **ultimobranchial bodies**, which arise in the caudal fourth pharyngeal pouches.
       (1) In humans, the ultimobranchial bodies are not represented in a discrete adult organ. Rather, they fuse with the thyroid rudiment, after becoming infiltrated with cells derived from the neural crest.

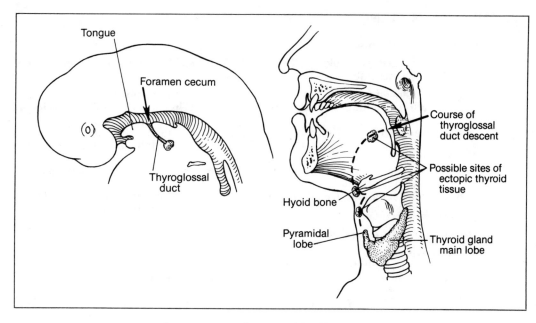

Figure 19-3. Development of the thyroid gland.

- (2) These **neural crest–derived cells** are destined to differentiate into the calcitonin-secreting **parafollicular (C) cells** of the thyroid.
3. **Hormone secretion**
   a. By 11 weeks of development, the thyroid follicular epithelium is differentiated. Iodine trapping occurs, and functional thyroid hormones **thyroxine (T4)** and **triiodothyronine (T3)** are produced.
   b. The fetal adenohypophysis is capable of producing **thyroid-stimulating hormone (TSH)** at 11 weeks. However, the hypothalamic–hypophyseal portal system is not fully functional yet, and so fetal thyrotropin-releasing hormone (TRH) can not be transported from the hypothalamus to the adenohypophysis.
      (1) **TRH** is a small-molecular-weight tripeptide and is readily transported across the placenta. If a pregnant monkey is injected with TRH, there is a sudden rise in TSH in both the mother and her fetus, indicating that TRH is transported across the placenta.
      (2) In contrast, the **TSH** levels in mother and fetus are very different, because TSH, a 28-kDa glycoprotein, is not transported across the placenta. There is some evidence, however, that TRH is synthesized in the placenta.
   c. **T3** and **T4** exert a regulatory effect by blocking TRH synthesis and TSH secretion in the fetus.
   d. **TSH** and **chorionic gonadotropin (hCG)** are structurally related compounds, and hCG has distinct but reduced TSH activity.

B. The parathyroid glands

1. **Development of the parathyroid glands**
   a. The parathyroid glands arise from small collections of cells that form in the cranial portions of the third and fourth pharyngeal pouches.
   b. The **superior parathyroids** arise in the **fourth pharyngeal pouch**.
   c. The **inferior parathyroids** arise in the **third pharyngeal pouch** and migrate along with the thymic rudiments to a position caudal (inferior) to the superior parathyroids.
2. **Histogenesis of the parathyroid glands**
   a. In the early stages of histogenesis, prior to their separation from the pharyngeal pouches, the parathyroid evaginations have cells which are less acidophilic and much larger than the nearby endodermal cells.
   b. These are the predominant cell types until the second half of gestation, when the **chief cells** and **oxyphil cells** characteristic of the adult parathyroid begin to appear.

IV. THE ADRENAL GLANDS

A. Origins of adrenal tissue
1. The adrenal glands develop in the posterior body wall between the urogenital and gastrointestinal mesenteries.
2. They are derived from two separate sources of tissue in the embryo.
   a. The **adrenal medulla** develops from **neural crest cells** (Fig. 19-4), which are **ectodermal** in origin.
      (1) Neural crest cells migrate to the region of formation of the adrenal gland in the body wall near the intraembryonic coelom between the urogenital ridge and the gut mesentery.
      (2) Nests of neural crest derivatives then differentiate into epinephrine- and norepinephrine-secreting cells.
   b. The **fetal** and **definitive adrenal cortices** are formed from **mesodermally derived cells** lining the **intraembryonic coelom** in the region of development of the adrenals.

B. Development of the adrenal cortex
1. **Early development**
   a. Mesothelial cells from the lining of the coelomic cavity become tall and columnar and then migrate into the mesenchyme of the posterior body wall.
   b. The precursors of the cortical cells leave the coelomic epithelium in two distinct waves. The first wave forms the **fetal cortex** and the second wave forms the **definitive cortex**.
   c. Consequently, the fetal cortex is a very thick layer of differentiated cells surrounded by a thin shell of undifferentiated cells representing the rudiment of the definitive cortex (see Fig. 19-4).
2. **Development of the definitive cortex**
   a. The fetal adrenal gland at 4 months is a good deal larger than the fetal metanephric (definitive) kidney.
   b. After 4 months, the fetal cortex begins to regress and the definitive cortex begins to grow.
   c. During the first 6 months of the neonatal period the fetal cortex disappears.
   d. However, the adult pattern of cortical zonation into a **zona glomerulosa**, **zona fasciculata**, and **zona reticularis** is not complete until late in childhood, just before the onset of puberty.
      (1) This transition occurs gradually, with the zona glomerulosa appearing first, at about 30 weeks in the fetus.
      (2) All three layers can be distinguished in a 4-year-old child, but definitive cortical zonation is not seen until age 11 to 15 years, at the onset of puberty.

C. Steroid biosynthesis and secretion during fetal development.
Steroid biosynthesis during fetal development is an extremely complex matter, involving at least the adrenals, pituitary, gonads, and liver of both the mother and fetus. In addition, there is transport and even synthesis of steroids in the placenta.

1. In the **fetal adrenal cortex**, there is evidence of histologic differentiation of steroid-secreting cells as early as the eighth week of development.
   a. At this time, large **acidophilic cells** appear in the fetal cortex.
   b. These cells are laden with lipid droplets and contain an abundance of smooth endoplasmic reticulum and mitochondria with tubular and vesicular cristae. These histologic features are characteristic of cells involved in steroid biosynthesis.
2. Because of the intriguing complementary interaction between the fetus and the **placenta** vis-à-vis steroid biosynthesis, one can properly refer to a **fetoplacental unit** for steroid metabolism (see also section VII D).
   a. Because the fetal cortex lacks 3-β-hydroxysteroid dehydrogenase activity, steroids must be synthesized from **placental progesterone**.
      (1) The placenta produces progesterone in large quantities after the maternal corpus luteum of pregnancy regresses.
      (2) Some of this progesterone reaches the fetal adrenal cortex where it serves as a precursor of cortisol, corticosterone, androgens, and aldosterone.
   b. The fetal liver and adrenal cortex can also synthesize **dehydroepiandrosterone sulfate (DHEAS)**, which can then be converted to **estrogens** in the placenta.

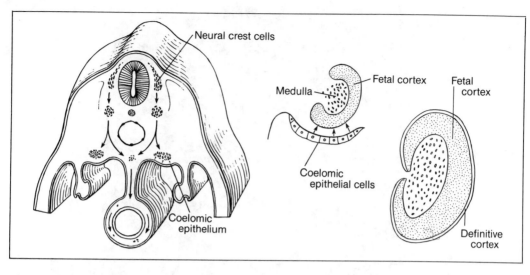

Figure 19-4. Migration of neural crest cells and development of the adrenal gland. *Arrows* indicate the routes of migrating cells. Neural crest cells destined to become the adrenal medulla migrate toward the intraembryonic coelom, and mesothelial cells leave the coelomic epithelium in two waves. The first wave forms the fetal cortex and the second wave forms the definitive cortex around the fetal cortex.

    3. **Gonadal steroid synthesis** also takes place in the fetus.
        a. The **Leydig cells** of the testis are highly developed and active in the male fetus, producing **testosterone** for male development.
        b. The ovarian **thecal cells**, which secrete **estrogen**, are thought to be homologous to the Leydig cells.
        c. The Leydig cells and thecal cells arise from mesodermally derived urogenital ridge mesenchyme (see Chapter 17, sections II A, B 2 b, and C 3).

V. THE ENDOCRINE PANCREAS

    A. **Origins of pancreatic endocrine tissue**
        1. The chief endocrine pancreatic **islets of Langerhans** (Fig. 19-5) are derived from the same source as the exocrine pancreatic tissue and the ductwork of the pancreas, namely the dorsal and ventral **pancreatic buds** (see Chapter 13, section III B).
        2. The **alpha and beta cells** form from endodermally derived cells that arise as branches of the primitive ducts of the pancreas and subsequently become detached from these ducts.
        3. The **C** and **delta (D) cells** form from **neural crest**.

    B. **Histogenesis**
        1. The first cells to differentiate in the islets of Langerhans are called **argyrophilic cells**.
           a. These subsequently differentiate into precursors of the **glucagon-secreting alpha cells** in week 10.
           b. The alpha cells begin to secrete glucagon during the third month.
        2. Precursors of **insulin-secreting beta cells** appear in week 13 and become functional during the fourth month.
        3. The placenta is impermeable to insulin, and consequently the fetal pancreatic insulin must serve the fetus.

VI. DIFFUSE HORMONE-SECRETING CELLS

    A. **Characteristics of APUD cells**
        1. In addition to having discrete endocrine organs, the human body is also equipped with at least twenty different varieties of **hormone-secreting cells** scattered throughout the brain, the respiratory system, and the digestive system.

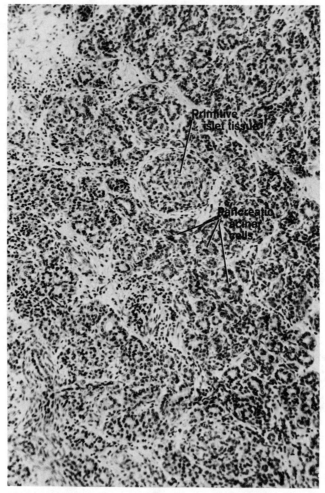

Figure 19-5. The developing human pancreas. (Light micrograph)

    2. Usually, these cells are isolated from one another and secrete **peptide hormones** that have **localized effects** rather than systemic effects.

    3. A few examples of the cells of this system will illustrate its complexity.
        a. **G (gastrin) cells** are found in the mucosa of the pyloric stomach and duodenum. These cells secrete the polypeptide hormone **gastrin**, which controls acid secretion in the stomach.
        b. **EC (enterochromaffin) cells** in the stomach secrete **serotonin**.
        c. **D (delta) cells** in the islets of Langerhans, stomach, and small intestines secrete the polypeptide hormone **somatostatin**.

B. Nomenclature

    1. Some investigators have called this collection of endocrine cells the **amine precursor uptake and decarboxylation (APUD) cells** and others have called them the **gastroenteropancreatic (GEP) cells**.

    2. Recent research has shown that neither name is completely appropriate.
        a. Not all of these cells take up and decarboxylate amine precursors.
        b. The cells are not restricted to the digestive system, since they are found throughout the brain and in the respiratory system.

    3. Furthermore, some of these cells, strictly speaking, are not even endocrine cells, because they do not release their secretions into the blood. Rather, their hormones sometimes interact with adjacent epithelial cells.

    4. Consequently, some investigators have decided to call these cells **paracrine cells**.

C. Embryology of APUD cells

1. While the functions of many of these cells and their hormones are not well worked out, many of the cells in this complex and far-flung collection have recently been shown to be **neural crest derivatives**.

2. Further experimental studies will probably clarify this system from both a functional and an embryologic standpoint.

VII. THE PLACENTA AS AN ENDOCRINE ORGAN

A. Endocrine function of the placenta.
The placenta is a complex endocrine organ of considerable importance to the developmental physiology of pregnancy. The placenta serves three important **endocrine functions for the fetus**.

1. The placenta **transports** certain hormones or hormone precursors.

2. The placenta **secretes** hormones of its own, including chorionic gonadotropin, chorionic somatomammotropin, and progesterone.

3. The placenta **metabolizes** certain hormones and hormone precursors for steroid biosynthesis.

B. Chorionic gonadotropin (hCG)

1. Chorionic gonadotropin is a glycoprotein with a molecular weight of 37 kDa.

2. It has an α subunit and a β subunit.
   a. The α **subunit** of hCG is very similar to the α subunits of glycoprotein hormones produced by the basophils of the adenohypophysis, namely luteinizing hormone (LH), follicle-stimulating hormone (FSH), and thyroid-stimulating hormone (TSH).
   b. The β **subunit** of hCG is peculiar to hCG. Therefore, it can be used to raise antibodies which are in turn useful for identifying and measuring hCG by radioimmunoassay (RIA).

3. As its name implies, hCG stimulates the corpus luteum of the ovary of the pregnant woman to produce **progesterone**.
   a. The syncytiotrophoblast begins synthesis and secretion of hCG very early in pregnancy and hCG secretion maintains the corpus luteum.
   b. Chorionic gonadotropin secretion continues throughout pregnancy. Secretion is maximal during the first trimester, and later declines.

C. Chorionic somatomammotropin (hCS)

1. Chorionic somatomammotropin is a growth-hormone–like peptide with a molecular weight of 22 kDa. It resembles prolactin closely as well.
   a. This hormone is often called **human placental lactogen (hPL)** because of its putative effects on the development of the mammary glands during pregnancy.
   b. It has also been called **placental growth hormone** because of its resemblance to pituitary growth hormone (**somatotropin**).

2. Chorionic somatomammotropin has several **physiologic effects**.
   a. It has a mild somatotropic activity, so that it stimulates the epiphyseal plates.
   b. There is some evidence to suggest that hCS has a stimulatory effect on the mammary glands.
   c. Its primary effect may be in its metabolic effects on glucose metabolism and lipolysis.

D. Placental steroidogenesis (see also section IV C)

1. The placenta is extremely active in steroid biosynthesis. Pregnant women excrete large quantities of progesterone and estrogens in their urine.

2. The production and metabolism of steroid hormones involves a complex **interaction between the fetal endocrine glands and the placenta**. This interaction is so intimately coupled that these functions together can be considered as a **fetoplacental unit**.
   a. The placenta can take **cholesterol** from maternal serum and convert it into **progesterone**.
      (1) This progesterone can serve as a precursor for steroid synthesis in the fetal adrenal cortex.
      (2) The fetal cortex can not synthesize steroids de novo because it lacks 3-β-hydroxysteroid dehydrogenase activity.

b. The placenta can not synthesize **estrogens** from acetate or cholesterol.
  (1) However, it can aromatize derivatives of **dehydroepiandrosterone sulfate (DHEAS)** into estrogens.
  (2) The fetal adrenal cortex and fetal liver supply the DHEAS for placental estrogen synthesis.

VIII. CONGENITAL ADRENAL HYPERPLASIA (ADRENOGENITAL SYNDROME)

A. Pathogenesis

1. There are several congenital disorders in which the lack of certain enzymes for steroid biosynthesis results in adrenal hyperplasia and, in females, ambiguous external genitalia.

2. For example, the enzyme **21-hydroxylase** converts 11-deoxycortisol to **cortisol**. A deficiency of this enzyme results in a decreased production of fetal adrenal cortisol.
  a. Cortisol regulates ACTH production by the adenohypophysis through a negative feedback mechanism. Therefore, a **lack of cortisol** results in **excessive ACTH secretion** and, consequently, in chronic ACTH stimulation of the adrenal cortex.
  b. As a result, there is an **overproduction of adrenal androgens** in a female fetus, which will result in masculinization of external genitalia (Fig. 19-6).

B. Effects in the newborn

1. **Congenital adrenal hyperplasia** (**adrenogenital syndrome**; see also Chapter 17, section VII E 2) is the most common cause of ambiguity in the female external genitalia.

2. In this syndrome, often there is enlargement of the clitoris, partial fusion of the labio-scrotal swellings, and sometimes a displacement of the urethral orifice into a male-like location.

3. Patients have normal gonadal development into an ovary, and paramesonephric duct derivatives are present.

4. Because of the lack of cortisol and other mineralocorticoids, fluid and electrolyte balance may be abnormal in newborn infants with congenital adrenal hyperplasia.

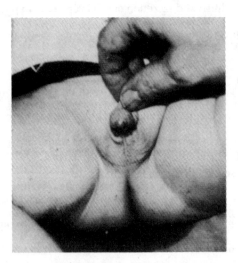 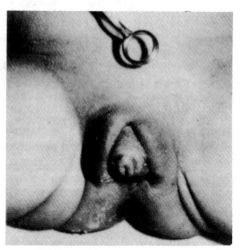

Figure 19-6. External genitalia of two female siblings with 21-hydroxylase deficiency. Lack of this enzyme causes masculinization due to congenital adrenal hyperplasia. (Reprinted with permission from Summitt RL: Differential diagnosis of genital ambiguity in the newborn. *Clin Obstet Gynecol* 15:112–140, 1972.)

STUDY QUESTIONS

Directions: Each question below contains five suggested answers. Choose the **one best** response to each question.

1. APUD (paracrine) cells include all of the following cell types in the human body EXCEPT

   (A) alpha (A) cells in the pancreatic islets of Langerhans
   (B) delta (D) cells in the pancreatic islets of Langerhans
   (C) G cells in the stomach
   (D) EC cells in the stomach
   (E) D cells in the stomach

2. The embryology of the parathyroid glands is correctly described by all of the following statements EXCEPT

   (A) the superior parathyroids are derived from the fourth pharyngeal pouch
   (B) the inferior parathyroids are derived from the third pharyngeal pouch
   (C) the superior parathyroids and palatine tonsils are derived from the same pharyngeal pouch
   (D) the inferior parathyroids descend along with the thymic rudiment
   (E) the parathyroid glands differentiate functional chief cells during the second half of gestation

Directions: Each question below contains four suggested answers of which **one or more** is correct. Choose the answer

    A   if **1, 2, and 3** are correct
    B   if **1 and 3** are correct
    C   if **2 and 4** are correct
    D   if **4** is correct
    E   if **1, 2, 3, and 4** are correct

3. True statements about thyroid gland origins include which of the following?

   (1) Thyroid follicular epithelial cells are ectodermal derivatives
   (2) Parafollicular cells are ectodermal derivatives
   (3) The connective tissue in the thyroid is an endodermal derivative
   (4) The pyramidal lobe is a remnant of the thyroglossal duct

4. True statements about the origins of the parathyroid glands include which of the following?

   (1) Their epithelial cells are endodermal derivatives
   (2) The superior parathyroids develop from the fourth pharyngeal pouch
   (3) The inferior parathyroids develop from the same rudiment as the thymus
   (4) The inferior parathyroids develop from the third pharyngeal pouch

5. Rathke's pouch forms which of the following pituitary structures?

   (1) The pars nervosa
   (2) The pars intermedia
   (3) The median eminence
   (4) The pars distalis

6. Cells of the endocrine pancreas originate in which of the following ways?

   (1) Alpha cells come from the pancreatic buds
   (2) Beta cells come from the pancreatic rudiment
   (3) C cells come from the neural crest
   (4) Delta cells come from the pancreatic buds

SUMMARY OF DIRECTIONS				
A	**B**	**C**	**D**	**E**
1, 2, 3 only	1, 3 only	2, 4 only	4 only	All are correct

7. True statements about the adrenal gland include which of the following?

(1) The fetal cortex is a mesodermal derivative
(2) The fetal cortex undergoes extensive growth and then regresses
(3) The definitive cortex develops extensively after birth
(4) The adrenal medulla is a neural crest derivative

8. Cells of the APUD (amine precursor uptake and decarboxylation) system have which of the following characteristics?

(1) They are derived from neural crest cells
(2) They are widely distributed throughout the body
(3) They are involved in control of gastrointestinal function
(4) They are absent from the pancreas

9. The role of the placenta as an endocrine organ includes which of the following features?

(1) The placenta does not secrete glycoproteins
(2) The α subunit of placental chorionic gonadotropin is similar to that of luteinizing hormone
(3) The placenta can synthesize estrogens from cholesterol
(4) Chorionic somatomammotropin stimulates the mammary glands and the epiphyseal plate

10. Congenital adrenal hyperplasia is characterized by which of the following features?

(1) Adrenocorticotropic hormone (ACTH) production is suppressed
(2) Cortisol synthesis is abnormal because of a lack of 21-hydroxylase activity
(3) There is feminization of male external genitalia
(4) There is masculinization of female external genitalia

Directions: The group of questions below consists of lettered choices followed by several numbered items. For each numbered item select the **one** lettered choice with which it is **most** closely associated. Each lettered choice may be used once, more than once, or not at all.

Questions 11–15

Match each of the descriptive statements below with the type of endocrine organ or tissue that it best describes.

(A) Thyroid gland

(B) Pituitary gland

(C) Parathyroid gland

(D) Adrenal cortex

(E) Adrenal medulla

11. This structure contains ectodermally derived cells not originating in the neural crest

12. This structure contains neural crest derivatives and, during descent of its rudiments, may leave ectopic tissue in the root of the tongue or near the hyoid bone

13. The major parenchymal cells of this structure are mesodermally derived

14. The major functional cells of this structure are derived from the coelomic epithelium

15. This structure is formed by an outpocketing of the roof of the mouth and a downgrowth of the floor of the brain

ANSWERS AND EXPLANATIONS

1. The answer is A. *(V A; VI A 3)* APUD (amine precursor uptake and decarboxylation) cells are widely distributed throughout the human body. Many of these cells have recently been shown to be neural crest derivatives. Delta cells in the islets of Langerhans secrete somatostatin and are neural crest derivatives considered to be APUD cells. G (gastrin) cells, D (delta) cells, and EC (enterochromaffin) cells in the stomach are also APUD cells. The chromaffin cells in the adrenal medulla are neural crest derivatives; they secrete epinephrine or norepinephrine and are also considered to be APUD cells. The alpha cells of the islets of Langerhans are not APUD cells. The alpha cells secrete glucagon and are derived from the dorsal and ventral pancreatic buds (endoderm).

2. The answer is C. *(Chapter 18 V C 3, E 4; Chapter 19 III B)* The inferior parathyroid glands are derived from the third pharyngeal pouch and the superior parathyroid glands are derived from the fourth pharyngeal pouch. The palatine tonsils are derived from the second pharyngeal pouch. The third and fourth pouches also form parts of the thymus gland. The inferior parathyroids descend extensively with the thymic rudiments. During the first half of gestation, the parathyroids contain undifferentiated acidophilic cells; these differentiate into chief and oxyphil cells during the second half of gestation.

3. The answer is C (2, 4). *(III A 1 d, 2)* Thyroid follicular epithelial cells arise posterior to the oropharyngeal membrane and are therefore endodermal derivatives. Parafollicular cells come from the neural crest, which is an ectodermal derivative. The connective tissue in both the thyroid and the parathyroid is derived from mesoderm. The thyroglossal duct degenerates to a greater or lesser extent. This variable degeneration explains the variable morphology of the pyramidal lobe, since this lobe is derived from the hypoglossal duct.

4. The answer is E (all). *(I C 1; III B)* The parathyroid glands are derived from the endodermal lining of the third and fourth pharyngeal pouches. These pouches also contribute to the thymus gland. Most of the thymus comes from the third pouch; as it descends, it carries the third-pouch parathyroids to an inferior position below the superior fourth-pouch parathyroids.

5. The answer is C (2, 4). *(II A 1, B 3)* Rathke's pouch forms the adenohypophysis, which includes the pars distalis, pars intermedia, and pars tuberalis. The infundibulum forms the neurohypophysis, which includes the infundibular stem, the infundibular process, and the median eminence.

6. The answer is A (1, 2, 3). *(V A, B; VI A 3)* The pancreatic alpha and beta cells secrete glucagon and insulin, respectively. They are the chief cells of the islets of Langerhans and as such develop from both the ventral and dorsal pancreatic rudiments, along with the pancreatic acinar cells and ducts of the pancreas. The C and D (delta) cells of the pancreas are paracrine cells arising in neural crest.

7. The answer is E (all). *(IV A 2, B)* The adrenal cortex arises as a result of two waves of proliferation of coelomic epithelial cells (which are mesodermal derivatives). The fetal cortex arises first, undergoes substantial growth and regression prior to birth, and is gradually replaced by the definitive cortex. The adrenal medulla is a modified sympathetic ganglion and arises from the neural crest.

8. The answer is A (1, 2, 3). *(VI A, B, C)* The amine precursor uptake and decarboxylation (APUD) system is derived from cells of the neural crest. Cells of this system are widely dispersed throughout the body. Several kinds of APUD cells are involved in the regulation of gastrointestinal function. Cells of the APUD system are present in the pancreas as C and D (delta) cells.

9. The answer is C (2, 4). *(VII B 1, 2, C 2, D 2 b)* The placenta secretes the glycoprotein hormone chorionic gonadotropin (hCG). The α subunit of hCG is similar to the α subunits of hormones secreted by the basophilic gonadotrophs and lactotrophs of the adenohypophysis. The placenta also secretes chorionic somatomammotropin (hCS), which has lactogenic properties and a growth hormone–like activity. The placenta can not make estrogens from cholesterol. Instead, it converts other steroid precursors, such as dehydroepiandrosterone sulfate (DHEAS), into estrogens.

10. The answer is C (2, 4). *(VIII A, B)* In congenital adrenal hyperplasia, cortisol biosynthesis is reduced because of an enzymatic deficiency. As a result of decreased cortisol synthesis, production of adrenocorticotropic hormone (ACTH) is elevated. This results in overproduction of androgens, which in turn results in masculinization of female external genitalia. Congenital adrenal hyperplasia is the leading cause of masculinization of external genitalia in genetically female individuals.

11–15. The answers are: 11-B, 12-A, 13-D, 14-D, 15-B. (*I C; II B; III A 1 d, 2 c, B; IV A, B*) The thyroid gland (A) forms from an endodermal diverticulum arising at the base of the tongue. The C cells of the thyroid gland are neural crest derivatives (and thus ectodermal). As the thyroid descends to its normal position, it sometimes leaves behind ectopic tissue in the tongue or over the hyoid bone. The pituitary gland (B) contains only ectodermally derived parenchymal cells. It arises from Rathke's pouch (in the roof of the mouth) and from the infundibulum (in the floor of the brain). The parathyroid glands (C) are derived from the third and fourth pharyngeal pouches, along with the thymus. The mesodermally derived epithelial lining of the intraembryonic coelom between the urogenital ridge and the gut mesenteries is the source of the steroid-secreting cells of the adrenal cortex (D). The adrenal medulla (E) is a neural crest derivative.

20
Development of the Eye

I. INTRODUCTION

A. Basic anatomy (Fig. 20-1)

1. Three tunics surround the eyeball:
   a. A **fibrous coat** consists of:
      (1) The fibrous **sclera**, visible as the white of the eye, where it is covered by a vascular conjunctiva
      (2) The transparent **cornea**
   b. The **uvea**, a primarily vascular coat, is composed of:
      (1) The **iris**, the pigmented muscular structure around the pupil
      (2) The **ciliary body**, which suspends the **lens** and controls its shape
      (3) The **choroid**, which lies between the retina and the sclera and contains many capillaries
   c. The **retina** has two major components:
      (1) The **neural retina**, which contains the photoreceptors—**rods** and **cones**—and other neurons and glia
      (2) The **pigmented retina**, behind the neural retina, which absorbs stray light

2. These outer layers surround three chambers:
   a. The **anterior chamber**, between the cornea and the iris, and the **posterior chamber**, between the iris and the lens, both contain the thin, watery **aqueous humor**.
   b. The **vitreous body**, within the eyeball, behind the lens, contains the transparent, gelatinous **vitreous humor**.

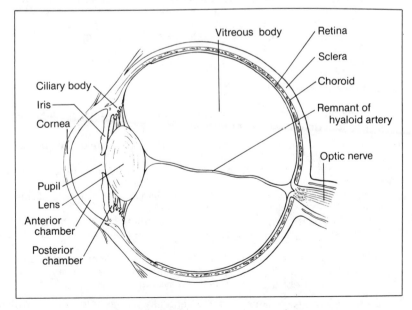

Figure 20-1. Basic anatomy of the adult eye.

3. The **limbus** lies at the juncture of the cornea and the sclera.
   a. Near the limbus is the **ciliary body**, which regulates the shape of the **lens**.
   b. The limbus contains structures that regulate the **flow of aqueous humor**:
      (1) The ciliary body is covered by the **ciliary epithelium**, which secretes the aqueous humor into the **posterior chamber**, from which it flows into the **anterior chamber** via the pupil.
      (2) The aqueous humor flows out of the anterior chamber, through the **trabecular meshwork**, and into the **canal of Schlemm**.
      (3) The canal of Schlemm drains the aqueous humor from the anterior chamber back into the venous system. If this drainage is impaired, **glaucoma** results.
         (a) The blocked outflow of aqueous humor increases the intraocular pressure, which in turn obstructs the blood flow to the retina.
         (b) Retinal ischemia ensues, resulting in blindness.

B. Basic functional anatomy
   1. Functional mechanisms of the eye
      a. The eye is an elegantly constructed **transducer**.
         (1) It turns light into electrical impulses in the **retina**.
         (2) It then transmits these electrical impulses along the **optic nerve** centrally into the brain for processing as visual information.
      b. In addition, the eye has a mechanism for the formation of focused, sharp images on the retina. This involves three **refractive media**:
         (1) The **cornea**
         (2) The **lens**
         (3) The **vitreous body**
   2. Functional anatomy of vision
      a. a. Light first passes through the transparent **cornea** and the **anterior chamber** of the eye.
      b. It then passes through the **iris**, a variable diaphragm.
         (1) The aperture of the iris, the **pupil**, automatically expands or shrinks by the contraction of smooth muscle fibers in the iris.
         (2) Changes in the level of light in the environment and in distance from the subject of inspection serve as stimuli for the automatic changes in the iris.
      c. After passing through the iris and the **posterior chamber**, the light passes through the **lens**.
         (1) A change in the shape of the lens alters its radius of curvature and focal length.
         (2) The refraction of light rays by the lens accommodates the eye for near or far vision.
      d. The light then traverses the **vitreous body (humor)** and strikes the **retina**.
         (1) Here the light evokes an **action potential** in cells that synapse with the **cones** and **rods** (the **photoreceptors**).
         (2) Nerve impulses are then carried to the brain via the **optic nerve**.

II. EARLY MORPHOGENESIS OF THE EYE

A. **Origins of the optic vesicle.** The **optic vesicle** is the precursor of the **optic cup**, which eventually goes on to form the **retina** of the eye.
   1. The eye develops from a lateral evagination of the wall of the **diencephalon**, a subdivision of the prosencephalon (forebrain).
      a. This eye rudiment, known as the **optic groove**, first appears before the cranial portion of the neural tube has closed.
      b. The eye rudiment gives rise to the **optic vesicle** after the closure of the cranial neural plate.
         (1) The name **optic vesicle** is somewhat misleading because the optic vesicle is really still just an outpocketing of the wall of the brain rather than a cystic vesicular structure.
         (2) The optic vesicle is attached to the wall of the diencephalon by an **optic stalk**.
         (3) The optic vesicle and optic stalk have a lumen that is continuous with the lumen of the remainder of the central nervous system.
   2. The **optic vesicle** grows laterally and eventually comes into contact with the surface ectoderm.

B. Formation of the lens placode and optic cup (Figs. 20-2 and 20-3)
  1. After contact between the optic vesicle and the surface ectoderm, there is a **reciprocal inductive interaction** between these two tissues.
     a. The optic vesicle induces the overlying surface ectoderm to form the rudiment of the lens.
        (1) The overlying surface epithelium is first induced to form a thickening known as the **lens placode**.
        (2) The lens placode then invaginates and becomes detached from the overlying epithelium to form a true closed cystic structure, the **lens vesicle** (see Fig. 20-3).
     b. The lens placode and lens vesicle in turn induce the optic vesicle to become invaginated into an **optic cup** (see Fig. 20-3).
  2. The optic vesicle and optic cup remain attached to the wall of the brain by the **optic stalk** (see Fig. 20-2), which eventually develops into the **optic nerve**.

C. The choroid fissure and the hyaloid vessels
  1. Early in its formation, the optic cup is invaginated by a ventral **choroid fissure** (see Fig. 20-2).
  2. The choroid fissure becomes deeply invaginated into the optic stalk, providing a recess for the developing **hyaloid artery and vein**.
     a. These blood vessels pass along the optic stalk and optic cup through the developing vitreous body to the lens vesicle (see Fig. 20-2).
     b. Eventually, the choroid fissure completely encloses the hyaloid vessels, which have grown forward through the optic stalk and cup to form the blood supply for the vitreous body and the lens.
        (1) The choroid fissure fuses along most of the length of the optic stalk.
        (2) Thus, the hyaloid vessels become completely surrounded by head mesenchyme and neural tissue of the optic stalk.

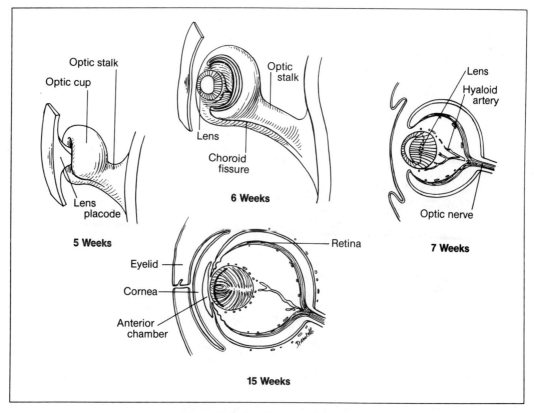

Figure 20-2. Development of the eye.

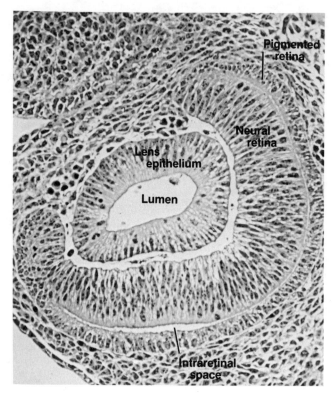

Figure 20-3. The optic cup and lens vesicle. (Light micrograph)

III. DEVELOPMENT OF THE RETINA

A. Formation of the two-layered retina (Figs. 20-3 and 20-4)

1. The invagination of the optic vesicle causes the optic cup to fold back upon itself. This produces a **double-layered optic cup**.
2. The walls of the optic cup are destined to undergo an impressive differentiation into a complex multilayered structure specialized for receiving photons of light and for creating electrical impulses as a result of light stimulation.
    a. The inner layer of the optic cup (nearest the vitreous body) eventually develops into the **neural retina**, the part of the retina that contains photoreceptors (the rods and cones) and transduces light energy into electrical activity.
    b. The outer layer of the optic cup eventually becomes the **pigmented retina**, which prevents stray light from striking the neural retina.
    c. Between the two layers is an **intraretinal space** (see Figs. 20-3 and 20-4). The intraretinal space is at first continuous with the lumen of the brain.

B. Histogenesis of the pigmented retina. The histogenesis of the pigmented retina is relatively uncomplicated.

1. The pigmented retina develops from the outer layer of the optic cup.
    a. It becomes pigmented by the accumulation of **melanosomes** synthesized directly in the retinal cells.
    b. In contrast, melanosomes in the skin accumulate in the stratum basale after they are synthesized in melanocytes and transported into the cells in the stratum basale.
2. The pigmented retina prevents stray light from striking the cones and rods of the neural retina.
3. The pigmented retinal cells also show **phagocytic activity** and are important in the turnover of effete membrane components from the outer segments of the cones and rods.

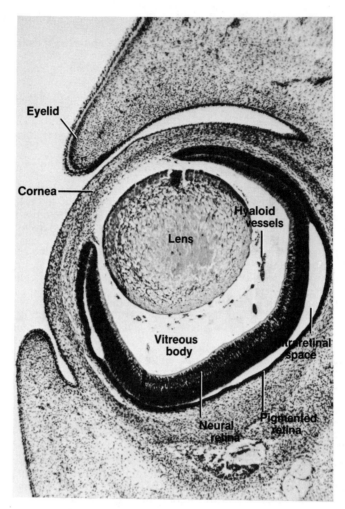

Figure 20-4. The developing eye of a mouse embryo approximately equivalent to a 6-week human embryo. (Light micrograph)

C. **Histogenesis of the neural retina.** The histogenesis of the neural retina is a good deal more complicated.
   1. **The two-layered early neural retina**
      a. Differentiation of the neural retina begins near the optic stalk and progresses peripherally toward the front of the eye.
      b. Soon after its formation, the inner layer of the optic cup is a fairly unremarkable pseudostratified neuroepithelium (see Chapter 11, section II A).
      c. At first, the neural retina has two layers (Fig. 20-5):
         (1) A **nucleated layer** near the pigmented retina
         (2) A **region of cell processes** but free from nuclei
      d. These zones of the neural retina are completely homologous to the **mantle and marginal layers**, respectively, of the developing neural tube (see Chapter 11, section II C).
         (1) The cells in the nucleated layer divide and differentiate into **neuroblasts**.
         (2) Some of these neuroblasts migrate away from the initial nucleated layer and establish a second neuroblastic layer.
   2. **The three-layered neural retina.** By 3 months, the neural retina has a distinctly three-layered appearance, with an **outer neuroblastic layer**, an **inner neuroblastic layer**, and a **non-nucleated inner fiber layer**.

a. At this stage, the outer neuroblastic layer contains nuclei of differentiating **rods and cones**.
   (1) The rods and cones are homologous to the **ependymal cells** that line the ventricles of the brain. These ependymal cells are often ciliated.
   (2) The **outer segments** of the rods and cones, which contain the **photoreceptor pigments**, develop from modified cilia.
b. The inner neuroblastic layer at this stage contains nuclei of differentiating **bipolar and ganglion cells**.

3. **The definitive layering of the neural retina**
   a. By 6 months, immature rods and cones are visible, and the definitive layering of the retina is more or less established.
   b. Proceeding inward from the pigmented retina toward the vitreous body, these layers are as follows:
      (1) An **outer nuclear layer** that contains primarily the nuclei of rods and cones
      (2) An **outer plexiform layer** that contains two types of cell processes:
         (a) Photoreceptor cell processes projecting away from the rods and cones
         (b) Bipolar cell processes projecting toward and synapsing with the processes of the rods and cones
      (3) An **inner nuclear layer** that predominantly contains the cell bodies and nuclei of bipolar cells
      (4) An **inner plexiform layer** containing processes that connect bipolar cells with ganglion cells
      (5) A **ganglion cell layer** containing cell bodies of ganglion cells
      (6) An **optic nerve fiber layer** containing axons from ganglion cells that project through the optic nerve into the lateral geniculate body of the brain

4. **Blood supply of the neural retina**
   a. The neural retina is an avascular epithelium.
   b. It receives nutrients by diffusion from the **retinal artery** and blood vessels deep to the pigmented retina in the choriocapillary layer of the uvea (the **choroid**).

D. **Postnatal development of the retina**
   1. Behavioral studies in human newborn infants suggest that their visual perception is significantly immature.
   2. Recent observations suggest that at least part of this immaturity is due to anatomic immaturity of the **fovea centralis** of the neural retina, the site of maximum visual acuity.
      a. The **fovea centralis** is an area of the retina where the outer cone segments are exposed to incoming light rays with a minimum of interference from overlying structures. The photoreceptive pigments are located in the **outer cone segments** of the fovea.
      b. In an adult human, the cones in the fovea are unusually long and densely packed together. In addition, the nuclei of bipolar and ganglion cells attaching to foveal cones have migrated out of the fovea centralis, so that the entire retina is thinned. This has the effect of reducing the diffracting structures that light must pass through before striking the outer segments of the foveal cones.
      c. In newborn human infants, the fovea shows significant immaturity, marked by extremely short cones with poorly developed outer segments, and only partial migration of cell nuclei of bipolar cells and ganglion cells away from the fovea (Fig. 20-6).
   3. By about one year after birth, the human fovea has become more mature, and behavioral studies indicate that visual acuity in a one-year-old child is considerably better than in a newborn infant.

E. **Establishment of retinotectal projections**
   1. The **optic stalk** develops into the **optic nerve**.
      a. Axons from the **ganglion cell layer** of the neural retina grow away from the retina and along the optic stalk to the brain.
         (1) As the nerve fibers grow out from the retina, the lumen of the optic stalk is obliterated and the **optic nerve** forms.
         (2) Derivatives of the hyaloid vessels (i.e., the retinal artery) continue to pass through the optic nerve to supply blood for the retina.
      b. The nerve fibers growing toward the brain reach the **optic chiasm**. Here, some fibers continue to grow toward the ipsilateral (same) side of the brain, while others grow toward the contralateral (opposite) side of the brain.

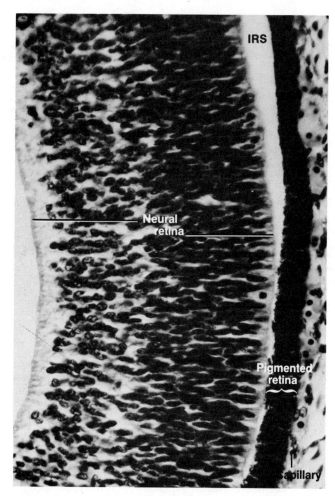

Figure 20-5. Histogenesis of the retina. (Light micrograph) *IRS,* intraretinal space.

    c. The axons of ganglion cells from the retina project to the **lateral geniculate nucleus** in very precisely arranged maps that allow for great precision in optical perception and in actions directed by the coordination between the sense of sight and voluntary motor centers in the cerebral cortex.
 2. The **control of the growth of these nerve fibers** is a major topic of research interest in developmental neurobiology.
    a. There is little doubt that nerve fibers from the retina find their way to the proper areas within the brain by precisely regulated **axon migration**. The nature of the guidance system is unknown at the present time but there can be little doubt that it exists.
    b. Studies have been performed to determine when in development the nerve fiber outgrowth is specified and to examine the control of nerve fiber outgrowth and nerve fiber projection.
    c. Experimental work with the visual system of lower vertebrates is the basis for the conviction that nerve fiber outgrowth is a precisely controlled affair.
        (1) For example, if an amphibian optic nerve is severed, a new one will regenerate that maps (judged by behavioral and electrophysiologic measurements) to the correct areas of the brain.
        (2) If an eye is removed, rotated through 180°, and then replaced, the optic nerve fibers will still regenerate to the proper optic centers in the brain. However, since the eye is rotated, the animal's behavior will be radically altered and the animal will aim downward at food objects located above it.
        (3) Nerve fibers may migrate along pathways that contain chemical signals in them to guide the locomotory organelles of cells. In chick embryos, it has been shown that

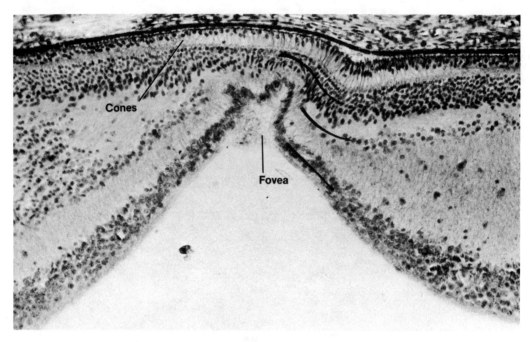

Figure 20-6. The fovea centralis of a newborn human infant. (Light micrograph) The nuclei in the ganglion cell layer, inner nuclear layer, and outer nuclear layer are migrating away from the fovea centralis, as indicated by the *arrows*. (Reprinted with permission from Abramov I, et al: The retina of the newborn human infant. *Science* 217:265-267, 1982.)

       there is a **chemical gradient** on the cell surface which may control cell migration to a particular destination in the brain.
    d. All in all, this is a promising area of research, and in the future scientists may be able to provide a detailed chemical explanation for the control of the migration of axons of ganglion cells from the retina to the brain.

F. Development of the anterior retina
    1. The retina is divided from front to back into two components separated by a circular landmark with a serrated edge, the **ora serrata**.
        a. The **pars optica**, the component posterior to the ora serrata, is sensitive to light.
        b. The component anterior to the ora serrata has no photoreceptors. This anterior component has two parts:
            (1) The **pars ciliaris** lies over the ciliary body.
            (2) The **pars iridica** lies over the posterior surface of the iris.
    2. The pars ciliaris and pars iridica have two distinct layers, just as in the rest of the retina.
        a. On the **ciliary body**, the outer layer is pigmented and the inner layer is nonpigmented.
            (1) The nonpigmented layer and the pigmented layer face one another on their apical surfaces.
            (2) They have a basement membrane on the side facing the lens and on the side facing the sclera.
        b. On the **posterior surface of the iris,** the pars iridica consists for a time of two layers of cells which are again apically apposed and covered on each basal surface by a basement membrane.
            (1) The **inner (posterior) layer of cells** keeps its epithelial character and becomes a **pigmented epithelium**.
            (2) The **outer (anterior) layer of cells** thins at the margin of the iris and differentiates into the **pupillary sphincter muscles**.
                (a) In this unusual case, the smooth muscle arises from an ectodermally derived structure, the outer layer of the optic cup.
                (b) All other smooth muscle in the body arises from mesodermally derived tissue.

G. The intraretinal space

1. When the optic cup invaginates to form the neural and the pigmented layers of the retina, an **intraretinal space** is created (see Figs. 20-3, 20-4, and 20-5).
2. In the adult, the intraretinal space is obliterated. The cones and rods become intimately associated with the pigmented retinal cells, as the outer rod segments are deeply embedded in recesses in the pigmented retinal cells.
3. Nevertheless, the intraretinal space persists as a **potential space**.
   a. A sharp blow to the head such as a prize fighter might receive can cause a **retinal detachment**, thus recreating the intraretinal space.
   b. As stated earlier, the neural retina is an avascular epithelium. When the neural retina is detached from the pigmented retina, the neural retina will become separated from its blood supply and can eventually undergo irreversible degenerative changes leading to blindness.

IV. DEVELOPMENT OF OTHER STRUCTURES OF THE EYE

A. Development of the sclera and choroid

1. The optic cup forms in the milieu of the mesenchyme of the head and eventually becomes surrounded by a dense capsule of mesenchymal cells.
2. This capsule develops into the **sclera** and the **choroid coat** of the eyeball.
   a. The **choroid layer** is rich in blood vessels.
   b. The **sclera**, a dense fibrous connective tissue capsule, forms a protective layer around the delicate retina. The anterior portion of the sclera develops into the clear **cornea**.

B. Development of the cornea.
The transparent cornea has a microscopic anatomy much different from the rest of the sclera.

1. The cornea is covered on its **anterior surface** by a stratified squamous **corneal epithelium** derived from surface ectoderm.
2. On its **posterior surface** is **endothelium** that continues on to cover the strands of the **trabecular meshwork**, and lines the vascular channel that leads into the **canal of Schlemm**.
3. Soon after the formation of the anterior epithelium and the posterior endothelium, **mesodermal fibroblasts** migrate into the space between the epithelium and endothelium and form the corneal stroma.
   a. These fibroblasts begin to secrete proteoglycans and collagen fibrils.
   b. It is thought that the secretion of the proteoglycans and the action of fibroblasts is important for organizing the collagen fibrils into **orthogonally arranged layers of fibrils**.
   c. Without this orthogonal arrangement, the cornea does not become transparent.

1. After the **lens placode** invaginates due to the inductive stimulation received from the optic vesicle, the lens forms a closed **lens vesicle** (see Fig. 20-3).
2. The lens vesicle is made up of a **continuous closed sheet** of epithelial cells.
   a. Soon after its initial formation, the posterior cells begin to elongate and grow toward the anterior wall of the lens vesicle (see Fig. 20-2).
   b. As they do so, they begin to obliterate the lumen of the lens vesicle.
   c. The lens continues to grow in diameter because cells on the periphery of the lens divide and then migrate toward the center of the lens as they elongate.
   d. Eventually, the elongated posterior cells lose their nuclei and are converted into membrane-delimited sacs.
      (1) These sacs are filled with an extraordinarily high concentration of lens-specific proteins called **crystallins**.
      (2) The highly modified remnants of the lens epithelial cells are called **lens fibers**.
   e. Thus, the fully formed lens has only an anterior epithelium as a covering. The posterior epithelium has been converted into lens fibers, highly modified crystallin-filled cells without nuclei.
3. The mesenchymal cells surrounding the optic cup at first form a **pupillary membrane** over the anterior surface of the lens. This structure degenerates secondarily.
4. The lens is supplied with nutrients for a time by the **hyaloid artery**. The hyaloid vessels reach the central portion of the optic cup via the choroid fissure.

D. Development of the anterior chamber, iris, and aqueous humor

1. The **anterior chamber** of the eye develops by cavitation of the extracellular spaces behind the cornea and in front of the lens (see Figs. 20-2 and 20-4).
   a. The anterior chamber of the eye forms by a simple cavitation in the mesenchyme, much like the formation of a blood vessel or synovial joint cavity.
   b. The cavity has as its anterior boundary the **corneal endothelial layer**, and its lumen is continuous with the spaces of the **trabecular meshwork** and the **canal of Schlemm**.
   c. The **corneal endothelium** is continuous with the endothelium covering the trabecular meshwork and lining the canal of Schlemm.
2. The optic cup gives rise to the epithelium covering the ciliary body and the posterior surface of the iris (i.e., the pars ciliaris and pars iridica of the retina).
3. Interestingly enough, however, the anterior surface of the **iris** is never covered by an epithelium.
4. The stromal fibroblasts of the iris are bathed directly in the **aqueous humor**.
   a. This fluid is produced behind the lens from the epithelium coating the ciliary body.
   b. It drains from the anterior chamber of the eye through the canal of Schlemm.

E. Development of the vitreous body

1. Before the choroid fissure fuses, mesenchymal cells migrate through the choroid fissure and fill the space between the lens and the neural retina with a loose meshwork of cells.
2. These cells differentiate into **hyalocytes**, cells which secrete a highly hydrated extracellular matrix that contains proteoglycans and collagen, known as the **vitreous body**.
3. The **vitreous body** is a semisolid, gelatinous structure that has several functions:
   a. It serves as a support for the neural retina.
   b. It probably allows free diffusion of nutrients throughout the inner chamber of the eye.
   c. It serves as part of the refractive media of the eye, so essential for image formation.

V. DEVELOPMENT OF THE OCULAR ADNEXA.
The **ocular adnexa** are the **accessory structures** that form around the eyeball and support its function. The eyelids, the lacrimal and tarsal (meibomian) glands, and the tear ducts are all part of the adnexa.

A. Development of the eyelids

1. The eyes are initially not covered by eyelids.
2. The eyelids develop in the seventh week as folds of the surface skin (see Fig. 20-4) which rapidly grow over the surface of the eyeball.
   a. By the ninth week the eyelids have fused with one another, leaving a complete union of the epidermis over the eyes.
   b. By the fifth month, however, there is a breakdown of the fusion and the eyelids open secondarily.
3. Small **hairs** and associated modified **sebaceous and sweat glands** form on the eyelids. Like hairs and associated glands in the rest of the body, these structures arise as surface invaginations from the epidermis of the fetal skin.

B. Development of lacrimal glands and ducts

1. In the medial portions of the upper eyelids, a series of invaginations grow and fuse to form the **lacrimal glands**.
2. The **nasolacrimal duct** forms along the point of fusion between the maxillary processes and the lateral nasal processes (see Chapter 18, section II B 2).
   a. The nasolacrimal duct begins as a thickening of the surface epidermis.
   b. This thickening sinks beneath the surface of the epidermis and becomes secondarily canalized, resulting in the formation of a duct between the eye and the nasal cavity.
3. The **tarsal (meibomian) glands** are modified sebaceous glands formed by ectodermal surface invagination.

VI. CONGENITAL ANOMALIES IN OCULAR DEVELOPMENT.
Major developmental anomalies restricted to the ocular system are extremely rare, but ocular defects are associated with other abnormalities in many congenital birth defect syndromes.

A. Gross anomalies

1. **Anophthalmia** (lack of eyes) and **microphthalmia** (small eyes) are closely related abnormalities in ocular development.
   a. Both are due to defective growth and development of the **optic vesicle** and **optic cup**.
   b. Since there is an inductive interaction between optic vesicle and lens placode, when there is true anopthalmia, there would be no lens, no eye, no optic nerve, and no optic chiasma.

2. Rarely, there is an extreme abnormality in the development of the face that is known as **cyclopia**.
   a. In many such cases, the eyes are fused to a variable extent in the middle of the face.
   b. In the most extreme cases, known as **true cyclopia**, there is a single median eye with a proboscis of sorts over the fused eyes.

3. A **coloboma** is a cleft that persists in tissues derived from the optic cup; it is present when the **choroid fissure** fails to fuse.
   a. A coloboma usually involves the inferior and medial portions of the iris.
   b. It may also involve the same portion of the retina.

4. In some instances, the **pupillary membrane** fails to break down, leaving a lacework of cellular strands over the pupil that can interfere with normal vision.

B. Ocular abnormalities seen in metabolic and chromosomal disorders

1. **Congenital corneal opacities** can be caused by inborn errors of metabolism; for example, **Hurler syndrome**.

2. **Congenital lens opacities (congenital cataracts)** have several causes:
   a. Infectious disease, most notably **rubella infection** during pregnancy
   b. Chromosomal anomalies, such as **trisomy 21 (Down syndrome)**
   c. Inborn errors of metabolism, such as **galactosemia**

3. **Trisomy 13 (Patau syndrome)** involves microphthalmia and many other defects (see Chapter 23, section II B 3).

4. **Tay-Sachs disease** leads to degenerative changes in the brain and other parts of the central nervous system, including the neural retina.

STUDY QUESTIONS

Directions: The groups of questions below consist of lettered choices followed by several numbered items. For each numbered item select the **one** lettered choice with which it is **most** closely associated. Each lettered choice may be used once, more than once, or not at all.

Questions 1–6

For each description of a component of the eye below, choose the appropriate lettered structure shown in the accompanying diagram.

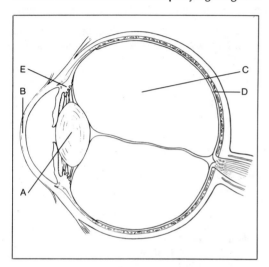

1. This structure forms by the migration of mesenchymal cells through the choroid fissure

2. This structure is induced to form in epithelium by the optic vesicle

3. This structure has a posterior endothelium formed much like vascular endothelium

4. This structure is derived from the optic cup; it contains neuroblast derivatives that differentiate from a pseudostratified epithelium

5. This structure is covered by two layers of optic vesicle derivatives without differentiated neurons or photoreceptors

6. The stroma of this structure differentiates from fibroblasts; its anterior epithelium is derived from surface ectoderm

Questions 7–10

Match each description of a developmental process below with the appropriate embryonic rudiment.

(A) Optic vesicle
(B) Lens vesicle
(C) Both
(D) Neither

7. This structure forms the vitreous body

8. This structure develops as a result of inductive interaction

9. This structure forms the pigmented retina

10. This structure differentiates into an adult structure rich in crystallins

ANSWERS AND EXPLANATIONS

1–6. The answers are: 1-C, 2-A, 3-B, 4-D, 5-E, 6-B. (*II B; III A 2, C 1, F 2; IV B, C, D 1, E*) The lens (*A*) is induced to form from surface ectoderm by the optic vesicle. The cornea (*B*) is covered anteriorly by an epithelium derived from surface ectoderm and posteriorly by an endothelium derived from mesenchyme. Between these two epithelial layers, fibroblasts differentiate into the corneal stroma. The vitreous body (*C*) forms from mesenchymal cells that invade the optic cup through the choroid fissure. The retina (*D*) has two major subdivisions, the neural retina and the pigmented retina; both develop from the optic cup. The neural retina is like the rest of the nervous system in that it starts as a pseudostratified epithelium and forms neuroblasts. The retinal neuroblasts differentiate into retinal neurons such as ganglion cells. The ciliary body (*E*) is covered by a non-neuronal retina derived, like the rest of the retina, from the optic vesicle.

7–10. The answers are: 7-D, 8-C, 9-A, 10-B. (*II A, B 1; III B 1; IV C 2, E*) The vitreous body is derived from mesenchymal fibroblasts that differentiate into hyalocytes. There is a reciprocal inductive interaction involved in eye formation: The optic vesicle induces the lens placode and lens vesicle, and the lens vesicle induces the invagination of the optic vesicle to form the optic cup. The optic cup in turn forms the neural retina and the pigmented retina. The lens contains high concentrations of crystallins and is derived from the lens vesicle.

21
Development of the Ear

I. INTRODUCTION

A. General features of the ear

1. The ear has two major **sensory functions**:
   a. Hearing
   b. Balance
2. The ear is composed of a group of specialized **mechanoreceptors** that convert sound vibrations and movements of the head into action potentials.
3. The ear also has associated structures to collect sound from the environment and transmit vibrations to the mechanoreceptors.

B. Components of the ear (Fig. 21-1)

1. The **external ear** is composed of the **auricle**, or **pinna** (the visible part of the ear), and the **external auditory meatus** (the ear canal).
2. The **middle ear** contains the auditory **ossicles**.
   a. The middle ear connects with the **auditory (eustachean) tube**, which in turn empties into the nasopharynx.
   b. The **tympanic membrane (eardrum)** separates the middle ear from the external ear.
3. The **inner ear** contains two organs, one for hearing and one for balance.
   a. The **cochlea**, which contains the **organ of Corti**, functions in **hearing**.
   b. The **vestibular apparatus** functions in **balance** by detecting movement of the head.

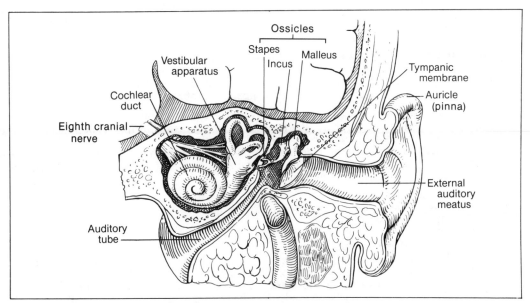

Figure 21-1. Basic anatomy of the human ear.

(1) The vestibular apparatus consists of three structures:
    (a) The **semicircular canals**
    (b) The **saccule**
    (c) The **utricle**
(2) These structures contain specialized neuroepithelium for detection of movement of the head.

II. THE EXTERNAL EAR

A. Histology of the external ear

1. The **auricle (pinna)** contains a large amount of elastic cartilage and is covered by skin with hairs, sebaceous glands, and a few eccrine sweat glands.
2. The elastic cartilage extends partway along the external auditory meatus.
3. The **external auditory meatus** penetrates the temporal bone.
4. The epithelium lining the external auditory meatus is similar to the skin of the auricle, but its sebaceous glands are especially large and it has **ceruminous glands**, a highly modified variety of apocrine sweat glands, which produce the **cerumen (wax)** of the ear.

B. Formation of the auricle

1. The auricle forms from the fusion of six separate hillocks of tissue that arise around the **first pharyngeal cleft**.
    a. Three hillocks arise cranial to the cleft, at the lateral end of the first pharyngeal arch, and three arise caudal to the cleft, at the lateral end of the second pharyngeal arch.
    b. These hillocks are proliferations of mesenchymal cells covered over by a thin layer of ectodermally derived embryonic skin.
2. The rudiments of the auricle ascend with respect to the eye as the mandible grows.
3. Minor anomalies in the shape of the auricle are very common and are of psychological significance only. In congenital anomalies involving abnormal facial development, the auricles and external auditory meatus may be low-set (see section V B).

C. Formation of the external auditory meatus

1. The external auditory meatus forms from the **first pharyngeal cleft** and therefore its stratified squamous epithelium is ectodermally derived.
2. The epithelial cells lining the meatus proliferate extensively around the ninth week and eventually produce a solid **meatal plug**.
    a. This plug disintegrates and canalizes later in the fetal period.
    b. If the meatal plug fails to degenerate, no meatus will form and the patient will have a hearing deficit.

III. THE MIDDLE EAR AND TYMPANIC MEMBRANE

A. Anatomy of the middle ear.
The middle ear is made up of the tympanic cavity, the ossicles, the auditory (eustachian) tube, and the tympanic membrane.

1. The **tympanic cavity** is an irregular cavity in the temporal bone.
    a. Its lateral boundary lies at the tympanic membrane and its medial boundary is at the bony wall of the inner ear. Anteriorly, it is continuous with the auditory tube.
    b. The tympanic cavity is lined by a simple squamous epithelium except near the tympanic membrane and the beginning of the auditory tube, where it is lined by a ciliated cuboidal or columnar epithelium.
2. **The middle ear ossicles**
    a. The middle ear contains three auditory ossicles:
        (1) The **malleus** (hammer)
        (2) The **incus** (anvil)
        (3) The **stapes** (stirrup)
    b. These three ossicles form a chain to conduct vibrations from the **tympanic membrane** to the **oval window**, the entry to the inner ear.
        (1) The **malleus** attaches to the medial side of the tympanic membrane.
        (2) The **incus** connects the malleus to the stapes.
        (3) The **stapes** attaches to the oval window of the scala vestibuli.

c. The ossicles are supported by miniature ligaments and are covered by reflections of the simple squamous epithelium of the middle ear cavity.
3. **The auditory tube**
   a. The auditory tube projects anteromedially from the middle ear to open in the nasopharynx.
      (1) The portion near the middle ear is surrounded by the temporal bone.
      (2) The portion near the nasopharynx is partially surrounded by a spiral of elastic cartilage.
   b. The mucosa of the auditory tube within the temporal bone has a low ciliated columnar epithelium. Nearer the nasopharynx this gives way to a pseudostratified layer with tall columnar ciliated cells, some goblet cells, and mucous glands.
   c. The lamina propria in the more medial portion of the tube is also thicker and may be extensively infiltrated with lymphocytes, which may even form discrete patches called the **tubal tonsils (of Gerlach)**. These tonsils arise by lymphoid infiltration of the lamina propria.
   d. The auditory tube is usually closed, but the pharyngeal orifice becomes patent during yawning and swallowing, equalizing the pressure in the tympanic cavity with that of the outside world.
4. **The tympanic membrane** (eardrum)
   a. The tympanic membrane forms the outer wall of the middle ear. The malleus is attached to its inner (medial) surface.
   b. On its **medial side**, the tympanic membrane is covered by a simple **squamous epithelium**. The medial epithelium is continuous with the epithelial lining of the middle ear cavity and the auditory tube connecting the middle ear to the nasopharynx.
   c. On its **lateral side** the tympanic membrane is covered by a thin **stratified squamous epithelium**. This thin layer is continuous with the lining of the external auditory meatus, but it lacks glands and hairs.
   d. Sandwiched between these two layers is a **connective tissue domain** with radially arranged collagenous fibers and a layer of circularly arranged fibers, elastic fibers, and fibroblasts.
   e. The **anterosuperior quadrant (Shrapnell's membrane)** has no connective tissue.

B. **Origin and development of the middle ear cavities** (Fig. 21-2)
   1. Both the **tympanic cavity** and the **auditory tube** form from the **first pharyngeal pouch** (see Fig. 21-2).
   2. This endodermally derived diverticulum of the pharynx grows laterally and expands considerably on its distal extremity. It grows around the developing ossicles and coats them with a continuous sheet of epithelium that also invades the tympanic cavity.
   3. The remainder of the tympanic cavity is covered by a layer of epithelium also derived from the first pharyngeal pouch, and the same is true for the entire length of the auditory tube.

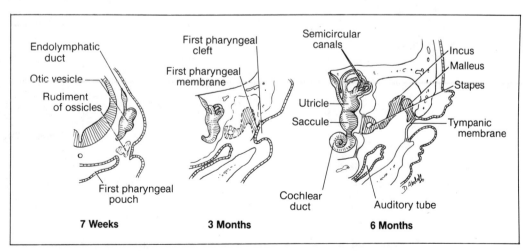

Figure 21-2. Development of the middle ear and inner ear.

C. Origin of the middle ear ossicles (see Fig. 21-2)

1. The **malleus** (including its anterior ligament) and the **incus** come from the first pharyngeal arch cartilage (Meckel's cartilage).
2. The **stapes** comes from the second pharyngeal arch cartilage (Reichert's cartilage).

D. Origin and development of the tympanic membrane (see Fig 21-2)

1. The tympanic membrane develops from the **first pharyngeal membrane**.
2. The **lateral epithelium** is ectodermally derived, like the lining of the external auditory meatus.
3. The **medial epithelium** is endodermally derived, like the lining of the middle ear cavity and auditory tube.
4. The thin fibrous **connective tissue domain** in the tympanic membrane is derived from head mesenchyme.

IV. THE INNER EAR

A. Anatomy and histology of the inner ear

1. General features
a. The inner ear is responsible for converting motion into electrical impulses, subserving our senses of hearing, motion, and body position.
b. The inner ear is composed of a complex closed space, the **membranous labyrinth**, which is bounded everywhere by an epithelium.
  (1) This membranous labyrinth exists inside a bony cavity known as the **bony labyrinth** in the petrous portion of the temporal bone.
  (2) The membranous labyrinth completely surrounds a compartment filled with a fluid known as **endolymph**.
  (3) A second compartment exists between the membranous labyrinth and the bony labyrinth. This compartment is filled with a different fluid medium, known as **perilymph**.

2. The vestibular apparatus
a. Three **semicircular canals** radiate from the **vestibule**, a chamber in the bony labyrinth. The semicircular canals are filled with **endolymph**, and each canal has a dilation, the **ampulla**, at its vestibular end.
b. The **utricle** and **saccule** are dilations of the membranous labyrinth within the vestibule. The utricle and saccule also contain **endolymph**.
c. Vibrations in the vestibular apparatus cause action potentials to be generated and transmitted centrally along the **vestibular division of the vestibulocochlear (acoustic) nerve (cranial nerve VIII)**.

3. The cochlear apparatus
a. The **bony cochlea** consists of two **perilymphatic ducts** that spiral around a central **modiolus**.
  (1) The **scala vestibuli** begins at the **oval window**, which abuts the footplate of the stapes in the middle ear.
  (2) The **scala tympani** ends at the **round window**.
b. The **cochlear duct (scala media)** is a spiraling diverticulum of the membranous labyrinth located between the scala vestibuli and the scala tympani.
  (1) The cochlear duct is filled with **endolymph**.
  (2) The cochlear duct contains the **organ of Corti**, which is bathed in the endolymph.
  (3) Vibrations in the organ of Corti, induced by sounds that enter the ear and stimulate the oval window, cause action potentials to be generated and transmitted centrally along the **cochlear nerve**, the **auditory division of the vestibulocochlear nerve**.

4. Sensory receptors of the inner ear
a. The membranous labyrinth has six striking modifications to its epithelial wall.
b. These six **neuroepithelia** are the locations of the mechanoreceptors that convert motion into electrical impulses, which then travel to the brain via the vestibular and cochlear divisions of cranial nerve VIII.
c. The six neuroepithelial sites are as follows:
  (1) The **three dilated ampullae** each contain a patch of neuroepithelium called the **crista ampullaris**.

(a) These patches of neuroepithelium are equipped with **hair cells** whose apical projections are embedded in an extracellular secretion product known as the **cupula**.
(b) Movement of the endolymphatic fluid within the semicircular canals stimulates the cupula, deforms the apical projections on the hair cells, and sets off action potentials.
(2) In the **utricle** and the **saccule** are two other patches of neuroepithelium called **maculae**.
(a) The maculae also have **hair cells** with apical projections. These are embedded in an amorphous extracellular material known as the **otolithic membrane**, which in turn contains calcified granules known as **otoliths**.
(b) Movements of the head stimulate movements of the otoliths, and these then deform the hair cell processes, triggering off action potentials.
(3) The sixth and by far most complicated patch of neuroepithelium is the **organ of Corti**, in the wall of the cochlear duct.
(a) The organ of Corti also contains **hair cells** that can trigger action potentials.
(b) Hair cells in different regions respond maximally to vibrations of differing frequencies, allowing the perception of different sounds.

5. A long, sac-like diverticulum of the membranous labyrinth, the **endolymphatic sac**, is not lined by any neuroepithelium and has no striking innervation. Endolymph is resorbed here.

B. **Development of the membranous labyrinth** (Figs. 21-2 and 21-3)
1. The entire membranous labyrinth develops from a single rather simple **auditory (otic) placode**, which appears at about 3 weeks. Between 3.5 and 4.5 weeks the auditory placode invaginates and becomes a closed **otocyst** (**otic vesicle;** see Fig. 21-2), which is detached from the surface ectoderm.
2. The otocyst now becomes somewhat elongated, sends out a bud, the **endolymphatic duct**, and becomes subdivided into a **vestibular pouch (utricular portion)** and a **cochlear pouch (saccular portion)** [see Fig. 21-3].
   a. The **vestibular pouch** becomes indented in several places and its walls collapse upon one another.
      (1) Some tissue in the middle of these collapsed diverticula is resorbed, creating the loops of the **semicircular canals**.
      (2) The **cristae ampullares** and **macula utriculi** differentiate in the vestibular pouch.
   b. The **cochlear pouch** elongates and grows into a spiral (see Fig. 21-3). A thin constriction arises at the base of this spiral, separating the **saccule** from the **cochlear duct**.

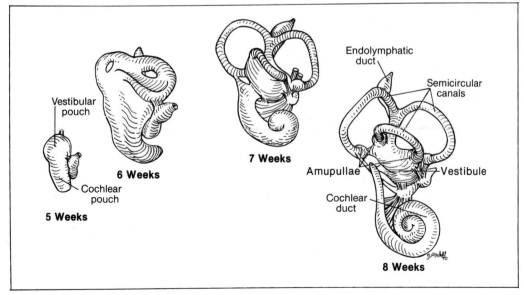

Figure 21-3. Development of the membranous labyrinth.

3. Next, the **neuroepithelium** of the macula sacculi and the organ of Corti differentiate.
   a. Differentiation of the neuroepithelium begins at the base of the cochlea and proceeds toward the apex.
      (1) The outgrowth of nerve fibers from the eighth cranial nerve probably stimulates the regional differentiation of the neuroepithelial patches inside the membranous labyrinth.
      (2) Ganglionic **neuroblasts** also migrate to the growing spiral of the cochlear duct and become arranged in a **spiral ganglion** along its course. These neuroblasts eventually send out dendrites which innervate the **hair cells** and pass axons into the acoustic nuclei of the brain.
   b. The **cristae** and **maculae** differentiate during the seventh week.
   c. Differentiation of the more complex **organ of Corti** (Fig. 21-4) begins somewhat later, around the tenth week of development. By week 24, the organ of Corti is more or less completely formed and in a functional state comparable to that of the adult.

C. **Development of the bony labyrinth**
   1. The membranous labyrinth is surrounded by a loose mesenchyme and a more compact mesenchymal condensation.
      a. The loose mesenchyme degenerates, leaving a cavity around the membranous labyrinth.
      b. The more compact mesenchymal condensation differentiates first into cartilage and subsequently into the petrous part of the temporal bone, thus forming the bony labyrinth.
   2. A space filled with **perilymph** appears between the bony labyrinth and the membranous labyrinth.

V. **CONGENITAL ANOMALIES OF THE EAR.** Congenital anomalies of the development of the ear as isolated phenomena are not common, other than the minor developmental abnormalities seen in auricular development.

   A. **Minor external auricular variations.** Slightly abnormal shapes in the external ear are fairly common but not very important clinically, aside from potential psychological problems related to cosmetic features of the ear.

   B. **The external ear in chromosomal anomalies**
      1. In certain congenital anomalies involving abnormal development of the face, the placement or shape of the auricles and external auditory meatus may be unusual.

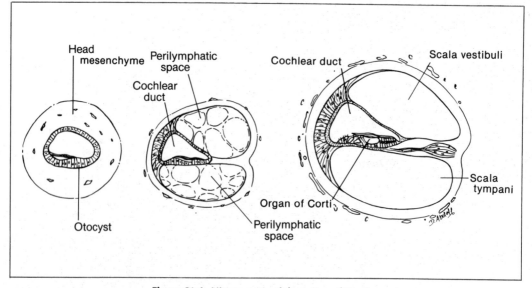

Figure 21-4. Histogenesis of the organ of Corti.

2. Consequently, close examination of the position and shape of the external ear is useful in diagnosing certain syndromes. For example:
   a. In **Down syndrome (trisomy 21), Patau syndrome (trisomy 13), and Edwards syndrome (trisomy 18)** [Fig. 21-5], there are striking alterations in the shape of the auricle.
   b. The position of the external auditory meatus and auricle is abnormally low-set in cases of **mandibulofacial dysostosis** (first arch syndrome; Treacher Collins syndrome—see Chapter 18, section VI B). In some of these patients, the entire external auditory meatus may be lacking.

C. **Etiology of congenital hearing deficits.** Among children in special schools for the care of deafness, 60% of the cases are thought to be due to prenatal, and often genetic, causes.
   1. For example, a **prenatal rubella infection**, especially during the seventh and eighth weeks of pregnancy, can result in a failure of differentiation of the organ of Corti and therefore congenital deafness.
   2. Most documented **genetic causes** of congenital deafness are due to recessive mutations.
      a. In some of these cases, the mutation somehow results in an absence of the neuroepithelium in the cochlear duct and macula sacculi.
      b. Perhaps the differentiation of derivatives of the cochlear pouch is affected by a genetic lesion that alters the outgrowth of nerve fibers from the branches of the eighth cranial nerve.

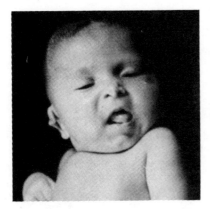
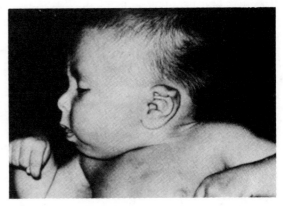

Figure 21-5. Typical abnormality of the auricle in a child with trisomy 18 (Edwards syndrome). Note the low position of the auricle with respect to the eye and the flattened appearance of the top of the auricle. (Reprinted with permission from de Grouchy J, Turleau C: *Clinical Atlas of Human Chromosomes.* New York, John Wiley, 1977, p 167.)

STUDY QUESTIONS

Directions: Each question below contains five suggested answers. Choose the **one best** response to each question.

1. Morphologic abnormalities of the ear are often observed under all of the following circumstances EXCEPT

(A) congenital rubella infections
(B) Down syndrome
(C) Klinefelter syndrome
(D) genetically normal children
(E) Edwards syndrome

2. The otocyst gives rise to all of the following kinds of epithelial tissues EXCEPT

(A) the medial epithelium lining the tympanic membrane
(B) the cristae ampullares
(C) the macula sacculi
(D) the macula utriculi
(E) the organ of Corti

3. The first pharyngeal arch or first pharyngeal cleft contributes to all of the following components of the adult ear EXCEPT

(A) ceruminous glands
(B) the epithelial lining of the external auditory meatus
(C) the lateral epithelium of the tympanic membrane
(D) the auricle
(E) the stapes

Directions: The group of questions below consists of lettered choices followed by several numbered items. For each numbered item select the **one** lettered choice with which it is **most** closely associated. Each lettered choice may be used once, more than once, or not at all.

Questions 4–9

Match each of the following origins of structures in the adult ear with the appropriate lettered structure in the accompanying diagram.

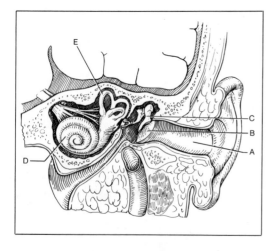

4. This structure develops from the vestibular pouch

5. This structure develops from the cochlear pouch

6. This structure develops from the first pharyngeal membrane

7. This structure develops from the first pharyngeal arch

8. This structure develops from the first pharyngeal cleft

9. This structure develops from the posterior portion of Meckel's cartilage along with the anterior ligament of the malleus

ANSWERS AND EXPLANATIONS

1. The answer is C. *(V A, B, C)* The ear is normal in Klinefelter syndrome. Congenital rubella infections often result in destruction of the organ of Corti, with consequent deafness. The auricle is characteristically abnormal in Down syndrome and Edwards syndrome. It can also be abnormal in genetically normal children; this minor abnormality might be caused by physical effects such as a hand compressed against the developing ear in utero.

2. The answer is A. *(III B; IV A 4, B)* The medial lining of the tympanic membrane, the epithelial lining of the middle ear cavity, and the epithelial lining of the auditory tube are all derived from the first pharyngeal pouch. The otocyst forms the entire epithelial lining of the membranous labyrinth. This closed layer of epithelial cells differentiates six patches of specialized neuroepithelial transducers. These six patches include three cristae ampullares (one for each of the three semicircular canals), two maculae (one in the saccule and one in the utricle), and one organ of Corti (in the cochlear duct).

3. The answer is E. *(II B, C; III C, D)*. The first pharyngeal arch and cleft make an important contribution to the development of the external ear. The anterior half of the auricle comes from the first arch. The external auditory meatus and the external (lateral) surface of the tympanic membrane are lined (or covered) by an epithelium derived from the first cleft. The ceruminous glands are invaginations of this epithelium and are also derived from the first cleft. The malleus and incus are first arch derivatives but the stapes is a second arch derivative.

4–9. The answers are: 4-E, 5-D, 6-B, 7-C, 8-A, 9-C. *(II C; III C, D 1; IV B 2; Chapter 18 Table 18-1)* The external auditory meatus (A) forms from the first pharyngeal cleft. The tympanic membrane (B) forms from the first pharyngeal membrane. The malleus (C) and its anterior ligament form from the posterior portion of the first pharyngeal arch cartilage, also called Meckel's cartilage. The cochlear duct (D) forms from the cochlear pouch. The semicircular canals (E) form from the vestibular pouch.

22
Normal Labor and Delivery

I. CLINICAL TOOLS FOR ASSESSING FETAL DEVELOPMENT

A. Clinical assessment of developmental stages. Often, an obstetrician will need to know the **gestational age** of a pregnancy, because therapeutic modalities and medical indications for both the mother and the embryo or fetus can change, depending upon the age of the embryo or fetus.

1. **Calculation of gestational age**
   a. Clinically, the **gestational age (menstrual age)** is calculated from the date of the **last menstrual period (LMP)**. For example, obstetricians routinely speak of a 20-week pregnancy taken from the LMP.
   b. Using this clinical system, human gestation covers **40 weeks from LMP to delivery**.
   c. By contrast, the embryologist calculates **developmental age** from the time of conception (i.e., fertilization), which occurs about 2 weeks after the LMP. Thus, the fetus in a 20-week LMP pregnancy is at a developmental age of 18 weeks, and human gestation covers **38 weeks from fertilization to delivery**.

2. **Size of the fetus as an indication of age**
   a. For determining the developmental stage of an embryo or fetus, its **length** provides a major clue.
      (1) Early embryos, before flexion has occurred, are measured for their greatest length; that is, the distance between the cranial and caudal ends of the embryo.
      (2) Once the basic body plan has been established, the length from the crown of the skull to the base of the buttocks is usually taken as a measurement of size. This so-called **crown–rump length** is usually a reliable measure of the age of the embryo, assuming that normal development has occurred.
      (3) Once the limbs begin to develop, obstetricians can measure a **crown–heel length**.
   b. Naturally, **other criteria** such as the development of limbs or facial characteristics are also helpful in determining the true age of the fetus.

B. Sonography (diagnostic ultrasound)

1. **General features of sonography**
   a. Obstetricians have recently developed several new procedures for visualizing and observing the fetus. **X-rays** are **not routinely used** because their ionizing radiations pose unacceptable mutagenic risks for the fetus (see Chapter 23, section IV A).
   b. **Diagnostic ultrasound (sonography)** was developed as a benign, noninvasive technique for visualizing the fetus in order to determine its size, observe the position of the placenta, and detect many different congenital anomalies in utero.
      (1) Sonography is one of the most powerful new techniques available to help the obstetrician make definitive diagnoses of the presence of congenital birth defects prior to birth.
      (2) The chief **advantages** of sonography are that it is noninvasive and it carries no known risk to either the mother or fetus.
      (3) Furthermore, the data gathered can often mean a great deal to the life of the fetus and mother.
   c. Many examples of sonograms can be found throughout this book.

2. **How sonography works**
   a. Pulses of high-frequency sound are generated in a piezoelectric transducer that is applied to the maternal abdomen.
      (1) These pulses pass through the skin and into maternal and fetal tissues.

(2) The pulses are reflected from the tissues in greater or lesser degree, depending on the differences in density between different anatomic structures.
   b. In the intervals between pulses, the piezoelectric transducer is in the **receiving mode** and is stimulated by the reflected **echoes** from deep tissues.
      (1) The transducer converts these echoes into electrical impulses.
      (2) The electrical impulses are amplified and are then converted into an **image** by the electronic circuitry of the ultrasound machine.
   c. This basic technique can be modified in several different ways that allow one to measure the dimensions of structures, create cross-sectional images of organs, and detect fetal movements, for example of the limbs or the heart.
3. **Uses of sonography**
   a. Sonography is of immense clinical value in the following situations:
      (1) Early detection of pregnancy and location of the gestational sac and placenta
      (2) Identification of multiple pregnancies or conjoined twins
      (3) Measurement of fetal size, amniotic sac, and placenta; serial measurements can be used to indicate growth rates
      (4) Guidance of amniocentesis
      (5) Determination of cranial and abdominal diameters to identify microcephaly, hydrocephalus, and anencephaly
      (6) Detection of many congenital anomalies such as polycystic kidneys, intestinal obstructions, omphalocele, neural tube defects, and limb malformations
      (7) Detection of fetal demise
   b. **Specific examples of uses**
      (1) If sonography demonstrates that a woman is carrying an anencephalic fetus with no chance of survival after birth, the parents might elect to terminate the pregnancy to spare them the anguish of a hopelessly deformed child.
      (2) If sonography indicates that a woman is carrying a fetus with a surgically correctable congenital defect such as gastroschisis or omphalocele, the obstetrician can then arrange for delivery in a setting where first-class pediatric surgeons are on hand to perform the surgery.

C. **Amniocentesis.** Amniocentesis is another technique which has recently been added to the obstetrician's tools for assessing the fetus and dealing with birth defects.

1. **Technique**
   a. A needle attached to a syringe is inserted through the abdominal wall, through the uterine wall, through the decidua and fetal membranes, and into the amniotic sac.
   b. The insertion of the needle can be guided by ultrasonography in order to minimize the risk of harming either the placenta or the fetus.
   c. **Amniotic fluid**, which contains free-floating **fetal cells**, is collected into the syringe and can then be subjected to a variety of biochemical and cytogenetic tests.
2. There are **risks** to this procedure, including:
   a. Injury to the fetus or placenta
   b. Premature induction of labor
   c. Introduction of infection
3. **Uses of amniocentesis**
   a. **Indications for use**
      (1) Amniocentesis should be performed routinely on all pregnant women over 35 years of age. It is at this age that the risk of carrying a fetus with a congenital anomaly outweighs the risk of the amniocentesis.
      (2) Amniocentesis is also strongly indicated when congenital anomalies were present in previous pregnancies or for sex determination when the family history suggests that the parents may be carriers of an X-linked genetic disorder.
   b. **Disorders detectable by amniocentesis** (see also Chapter 23, section VI)
      (1) **Cytogenetic analysis** of the cells in amniotic fluid can identify Down syndrome and other trisomies, and anomalies of sex chromosomes such as Kleinfelter syndrome or Turner syndrome.
      (2) **Biochemical analysis** of amniotic fluid can reveal neural tube defects and determine the stage of lung development.
         (a) Elevated α-**fetoprotein** strongly suggests the presence of a neural tube defect.
         (b) The concentration of **surfactant** can be used as an indicator of fetal lung maturity.
      (3) Many **congenital metabolic disorders** can also be detected by amniocentesis. A few examples are as follows:

(a) Disorders of lipid metabolism (e.g., Tay-Sachs disease)
(b) Disorders of mucopolysaccharide metabolism (e.g., Hurler syndrome)
(c) Disorders of carbohydrate metabolism (e.g., Pompe disease)
(d) Disorders of purine metabolism (e.g., Lesch-Nyhan syndrome)

II. NORMAL LABOR AND DELIVERY

A. General considerations

1. **At term**—that is, at the end of 38 weeks from conception (40 weeks from the last menstrual period)—normal **labor** begins.
   a. **Labor** is the process whereby the smooth muscle contractions of the uterus and cervix become rhythmic and progressively more forceful.
   b. The events of labor result in dilation of the cervix and ejection of the fetus from the uterine cavity.
   c. Labor is completed when the newborn baby and placenta are **delivered** by expulsion from the uterus.

2. **Role of prostaglandins and other hormones in labor**
   a. The exact mechanism of the onset of labor is not well understood but prostaglandins play an important role in the initiation and maintenance of uterine and cervical smooth muscle contractions.
      (1) Fetal membranes and the decidua are rich in the enzyme **prostaglandin synthetase**, and the amniotic fluid and peripheral blood of women in labor both contain elevated levels of prostaglandins.
      (2) **Arachidonic acid** is an essential precursor for prostaglandin synthesis.
         (a) Arachidonic acid is available as a fatty acid esterified to phosphatidyl ethanolamine (PE).
         (b) When certain phospholipases are released from destabilized lysosomes, it is thought that these phospholipases cleave arachidonic acid from PE.
      (3) The cleavage of arachidonic acid produces an increase in prostaglandin concentration as a result of prostaglandin synthetase activity.
      (4) The prostaglandins then induce smooth muscle contraction and labor (Fig. 22-1).
   b. There is also evidence that the fetal hypothalamic–hypophyseal axis, the fetal adrenal glands, and estrogens all play a role in the initiation of labor.
      (1) For example, in anencephalic fetuses, the hypophysis and adrenal cortex are usually markedly underdeveloped.
      (2) When the fetus is anencephalic, there is often a concomitant delay in the onset of labor at term.

B. Early signs of labor

1. Near the end of pregnancy, the most obvious clinical indication of the imminent onset of labor is a **change in the shape of the uterus**. The height of the uterine fundus is decreased because the lower uterine segment changes its shape.

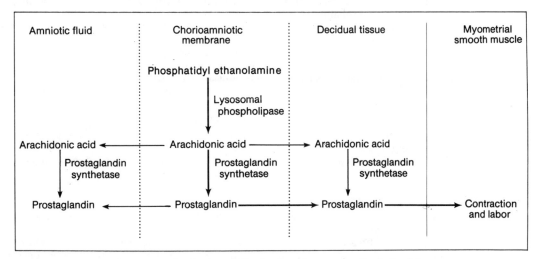

Figure 22-1. Synthesis and distribution of prostaglandin during labor.

2. Also, the **fetus descends** in the uterus so that the head becomes engaged in the pelvic inlet.
3. There is also a simultaneous decrease in the volume of amniotic fluid.
4. One reliable indicator of the imminent onset of labor is the **release of the cervical mucus plug** along with a small amount of **bleeding**, sometimes referred to as **"show"** or **"bloody show."** Normally, labor will begin in earnest within a few hours to days after this event.
5. **False labor** may also be experienced before the onset of true labor. False labor is usually manifested as short and irregular uterine contractions felt principally in the groin and lower abdomen.

C. "Labor pains"
1. In contrast to false labor, **authentic labor** consists of longer and more regular **uterine contractions**.
   a. These are felt first at the fundus of the uterus and then radiating over the body of the uterus and into the lower back.
   b. Once contractions of labor have begun in earnest, they gradually increase in regularity and duration.
      (1) At first, contractions occur at intervals of about 10 minutes but soon the intervals may decrease to as little as 1 minute.
      (2) The duration of contractions is between 30 and 90 seconds but usually they last about 60 seconds.
2. Labor pain may be **caused** by several factors:
   a. Transient uterine and cervical hypoxia
   b. Stretching and compression of nerve fibers
   c. Stretching of the uterus, cervix, and uterine coverings
3. **Blood flow in the placenta** is altered during uterine contractions.
   a. During a contraction, perfusion of the placenta is markedly decreased because of compression of uterine arteries.
   b. Between contractions, however, the uterine arteries open, allowing free perfusion of the intervillous spaces of the placenta.

D. Normal sequence of labor
1. The early signs of labor, before uterine contractions are regular and before cervical dilation has begun, are sometimes called the **latent phase of labor**.
2. Labor itself is traditionally divided into three **stages**.
   a. The **first stage of labor** begins when contractions are regular and intense enough to cause recognizable dilation of the cervix. It ends when cervical dilation is complete.
      (1) The chorioamniotic membrane surrounding the fetus usually ruptures during the first stage of labor, releasing about 250 ml of clear, watery amniotic fluid.
      (2) When this fluid is stained green or brown due to fetal defecation of **meconium**, this is often a reliable indicator of **fetal distress** due to the rigors of labor.
   b. The **second stage of labor** begins when cervical dilation is complete and ends when the fetus has been delivered.
      (1) At this stage, the placenta is still attached to the wall of the uterus.
      (2) The umbilical cord still attaches the external fetus to the internal placenta, so that the fetal circulation is still dependent upon the placenta.
   c. The **third stage of labor** begins when the fetus is delivered and ends when the placenta has been delivered.
3. Some obstetricians also refer to a **fourth stage of labor**.
   a. Contractions of uterine smooth muscle continue after the delivery of the placenta.
   b. These contractions serve to shrink the uterus.
   c. They also aid in closing off uterine blood vessels, which may bleed for a short time after the separation of the placenta from the uterine wall.

E. Normal sequence of delivery
1. During normal head-first delivery (Fig. 22-2), the **head of the fetus** is forced through the birth canal by uterine contractions.
   a. During labor, the **fetal skull** is quite deformable, due to the fact that the bones forming the vault of the skull are not fully ossified, especially at the sutures between skull bones.

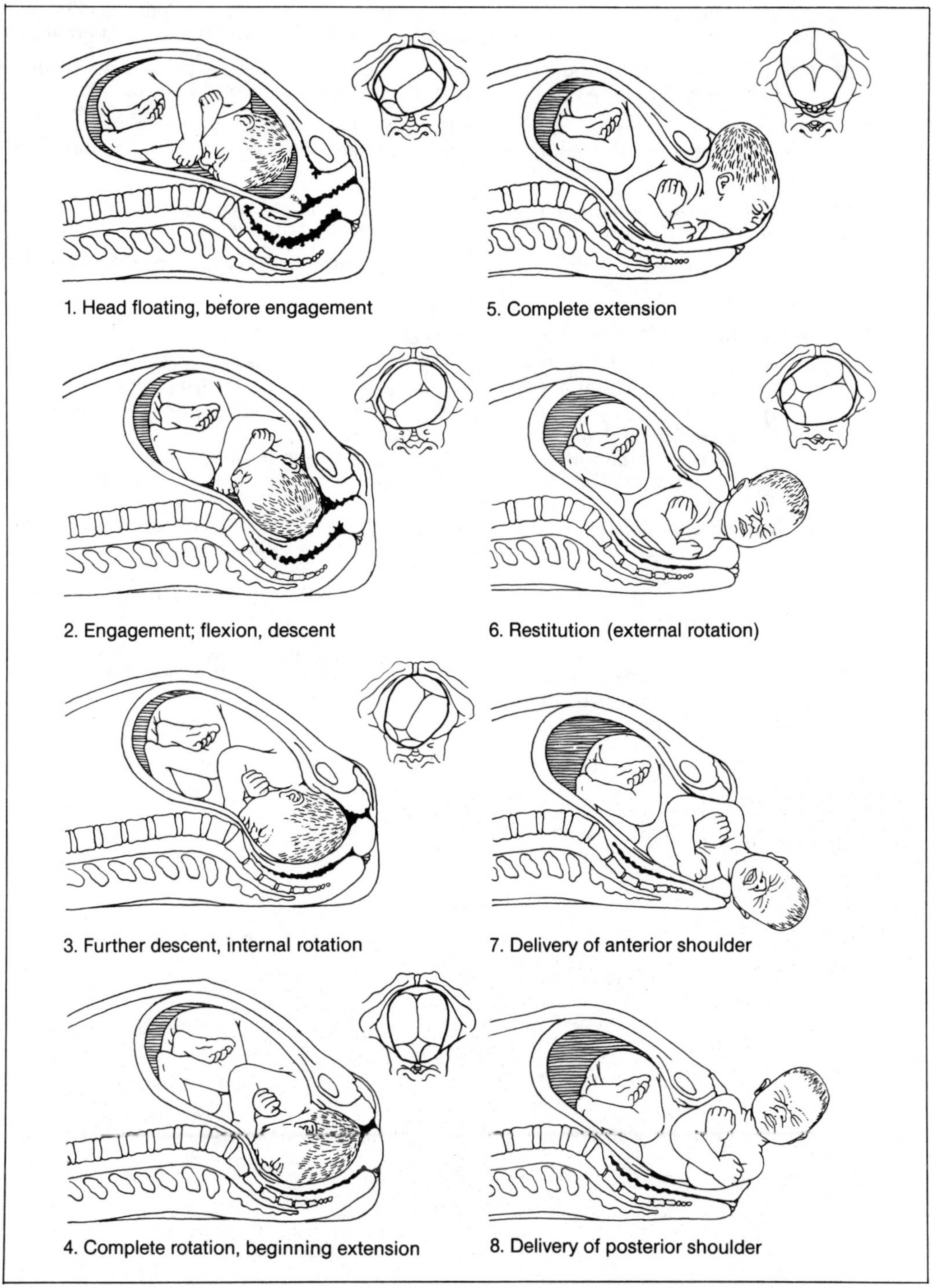

1. Head floating, before engagement
2. Engagement; flexion, descent
3. Further descent, internal rotation
4. Complete rotation, beginning extension
5. Complete extension
6. Restitution (external rotation)
7. Delivery of anterior shoulder
8. Delivery of posterior shoulder

Figure 22-2. Normal labor. (Redrawn from Pritchard J, MacDonald P: *Williams Obstetrics*, 16th ed. New York, Appleton-Century-Crofts, 1980, p 397.)

  b. As a result of this incomplete ossification, there is great flexibility, allowing overlap of the bones so that the skull is strikingly molded into an elongated shape as it passes through the birth canal.
  c. Within hours after birth, however, the skull resumes its normal, more rounded shape.

2. The **shoulders** are delivered next. Usually, the anterior shoulder is delivered first so that the shoulder does not become lodged under the symphysis pubis of the maternal pelvis.
3. After delivery of the shoulders, uterine contractions (aided by the mother's pushing) spontaneously expel the **rest of the fetus**, completing the second stage of labor.
4. The distended uterus now quickly contracts by elastic recoil and smooth muscle contraction. This decreases the volume of the placenta and expels the maternal blood from the placenta back into the maternal and fetal circulation.
5. The placenta then separates from the uterine wall. The placenta carries some maternal decidual tissue with it, but the rest remains in the wall of the uterus.
6. Finally, the **placenta**, with the remainder of the **umbilical cord**, is expelled, completing the third stage of labor.

F. **Common complications of labor and delivery**
  1. Normal labor and delivery can be complicated in a number of ways.
     a. The baby may present itself in the birth canal feet first (the **"breech" position**).
        (1) It is occasionally possible to rotate a fetus in the uterine cavity by **external cephalic conversion** so that it is presented head first.
        (2) This is a difficult maneuver which may entangle the fetus in the umbilical cord. Also, labor may not progress at its normal rate, leaving the mother too exhausted for the rigors of delivery.
     b. With **cord prolapse**, the umbilical cord protrudes through the cervix ahead of the fetus. In this instance, or when the fetus becomes **entangled in the cord**, the blood supply to the fetus will be compromised and the fetus may die.
     c. In **cephalopelvic disproporti0on**, the fetal head is too large or the pelvis is too small to allow facile delivery.
  2. Many of these complications can be anticipated by ultrasonography. They can then be dealt with by **cesarean section**, in which an incision is made in the abdominal wall and the uterine wall to allow extraction of the fetus from the uterus.

STUDY QUESTIONS

Directions: Each question below contains five suggested answers. Choose the **one best** response to each question.

1. Ultrasound can be used for all of the following purposes EXCEPT

   (A) to detect Down syndrome
   (B) to detect neural tube defects
   (C) to measure skull size
   (D) to guide amniocentesis by visualizing the fetus and placenta
   (E) to locate the placenta

2. All of the following statements concerning the role of prostaglandin in labor are true EXCEPT

   (A) prostaglandin induces uterine smooth muscle contraction
   (B) prostaglandin synthetase increases maternal blood prostaglandin levels
   (C) a decrease in arachidonic acid causes prostaglandin to increase in maternal blood
   (D) lysosomal enzymes cleave arachidonic acid from phospholipids
   (E) phosphatidyl ethanolamine cleavage produces a prostaglandin precursor

Directions: Each question below contains four suggested answers of which **one or more** is correct. Choose the answer

   A if **1, 2, and 3** are correct
   B if **1 and 3** are correct
   C if **2 and 4** are correct
   D if **4** is correct
   E if **1, 2, 3, and 4** are correct

3. Amniocentesis can detect which of the following conditions?

   (1) Inborn errors of metabolism
   (2) Numerical chromosomal anomalies
   (3) Neural tube defects
   (4) Immature fetal lungs

Directions: The group of questions below consists of lettered choices followed by several numbered items. For each numbered item select the **one** lettered choice with which it is **most** closely associated. Each lettered choice may be used once, more than once, or not at all.

Questions 4–8
Match each characteristic below with the appropriate phase or stage of labor.

(A) The latent phase of labor
(B) The first stage of labor
(C) The second stage of labor
(D) The third stage of labor
(E) The fourth stage of labor

4. Delivery of the placenta
5. Uterine contractions after expulsion of the placenta
6. Weak and irregular uterine contractions
7. Regular contractions and cervical dilation
8. Complete cervical dilation and fetal expulsion

ANSWERS AND EXPLANATIONS

1. The answer is A. (*I B 3*) Ultrasound provides images of fetal structure and the location of the placenta in a safe, noninvasive fashion. Ultrasound by itself would not be useful for detection of Down syndrome, although ultrasound can be used to guide the sampling needle during amniocentesis, and the sample thus obtained could be used for karyotype analysis, which in turn could detect Down syndrome. Neural tube defects often show up on ultrasonography. The technique can also be used to measure skull size.

2. The answer is C. (*II A 2*) Phosphatidyl ethanolamine (PE) contains a fatty acid called arachidonic acid. Lysosomal phospholipase would release arachidonic acid from PE. Arachidonic acid is a precursor of prostaglandin. The enzyme that converts arachidonic acid to prostaglandin is known as prostaglandin synthetase. When arachidonate levels in maternal blood increase, prostaglandin synthetase increases the prostaglandin levels. Subsequently, the prostaglandin stimulates uterine and cervical smooth muscle contraction, which is important during labor.

3. The answer is E (all). (*I C 3*) In amniocentesis, a sample of amniotic fluid and fetal cells is collected. The amniotic fluid can then be subjected to biochemical analysis and the cells can be cultured for karyotype analysis. Biochemical studies on the cells can detect many inborn errors of metabolism. Karyotype analysis would determine if there are numerical chromosomal anomalies. Neural tube defects would be strongly suggested if the amniotic fluid contained elevated levels of α-fetoprotein. Maturity of the fetal lungs could be determined from a measurement of surfactant in amniotic fluid. Amniocentesis is indicated in all pregnant women aged 35 or older and would probably also be indicated in a younger woman when other evidence suggests a problem that can be identified by amniocentesis—for example, a sex-linked disorder that might be passed on to offspring.

4–8. The answers are: 4-D, 5-E, 6-A, 7-B, 8-C. (*II D*) During the latent phase of labor, contractions are weak and irregular. Once true labor begins, contractions become regular and the cervix dilates during the first stage of labor, the fetus is delivered during the second stage of labor, and the placenta is delivered during the third stage of labor. Some obstetricians consider the postdelivery stage, during which uterine contractions decrease the size of the uterus, to be the fourth stage of labor.

23
Etiology of Congenital Birth Defects

I. INTRODUCTION

A. Overview

1. Congenital birth defects can be described as any structural or functional defect that arose due to aberrant developmental processes prior to birth or immediately after birth.
2. Congenital defects range from **gross structural defects** such as anencephaly or cleft palate to **molecular structural defects** such as the altered hemoglobin β chain in sickle cell anemia.
3. Some congenital birth defects are known to have a strictly **genetic basis** (see Chapter 24).
   a. Some genetic defects are known to result from alterations in DNA structure. These defects are often single point mutations resulting in single amino acid substitutions, such as the above-mentioned altered hemoglobin β chain in sickle cell anemia.
   b. Other congenital genetic defects are due to alterations in the number of chromosomes (monosomy or trisomy), translocation or deletion of fragments of chromosomes, or duplication of selected regions of chromosomes.
4. A few **environmental factors** have been clearly implicated as the etiologic agent in congenital birth defects.
   a. Certain infectious agents, notably rubella virus, cytomegalovirus, and *Toxoplasma*, are known to cause congenital birth defects (see section III).
   b. Ionizing radiation in high doses is also known to cause congenital birth defects (see section IV).
   c. Certain drugs, such as thalidomide and alcohol, are known to cause birth defects, and a host of others are suspected teratogenic agents (see section V).
5. Most congenital birth defects have an unknown etiology or are known to result from a complex but poorly understood interplay between heredity and environment.
6. In some interesting medical cases, the pregnant mother has a disease that predisposes the fetus to a congenital anomaly even though the mother and fetus may not share the disease. For example, women with **diabetes mellitus** may give birth to obese children with congenital musculoskeletal disorders.
   a. Diabetic women are known to have a number of obstetric problems, most notably unusually large babies and babies with a substantially increased risk of congenital anomalies.
   b. The **caudal regression syndrome**, which involves congenital musculoskeletal anomalies in the pelvis and legs, is seen more frequently in fetuses of diabetic mothers.

B. Incidence trends

1. The overall frequency of congenital defects is about 7% of all births. Many of these defects are trivial in nature but others are serious enough to warrant medical attention.
2. Table 23-1, taken from a recent World Health Organization report on congenital defects, shows the relative frequency of some common multifactorial congenital malformations.
   a. Many gross structural defects show wide variation of occurrence in certain ethnic groups. Notice in Table 23-1, for example, the differences in the frequency of neural tube defects in different ethnic groups.
   b. When members of an affected ethnic group emigrate from the homeland, the differences in frequency may persist only partially.

Table 23-1. Approximate Frequency of Some Common Multifactorial Malformations

Condition	Frequency per 100,000 Births	Location
Anencephaly	400	Northern Ireland
	200	England
	80	Japan
	50	West Africa
Myelomeningocele	250	England
	30	Japan
	20	Nigeria
Heart malformations (all types)	600	England, Sweden, N. America
Cleft lip (with or without cleft palate)	300	Japan
	100	England, Denmark, N. America
	40	Nigeria
Talipes equinovarus	400	New Zealand (Maoris)
Pyloric stenosis	300	England, Sweden

Data from Bickel M, et al: Genetic disorders—Prevention, treatment, and rehabilitation. *WHO Tech Rep Ser* 497 Annex 1: *Frequency of Genetic Disorders*, 1980.

  (1) For example, neural tube defects are more frequent among Irish people in Ireland than among Irish people in the United States.
  (2) However, Irish people in the United States still have a higher frequency of neural tube defects than Black people in the United States.
 3. These and many other similar epidemiologic findings point to the conclusion that both heredity and environment contribute to the frequency of birth defects.

II. CHROMOSOMAL NUMERICAL AND STRUCTURAL ANOMALIES AND CONGENITAL BIRTH DEFECTS

  A. General considerations
   1. One common cause of congenital birth defects is an abnormality in the number of chromosomes.
      a. Numerical disorders of autosomes are described below and in Chapter 24, section VI.
      b. Numerical disorders of the sex chromosomes are described in Chapter 17, section VII and Table 17-2.
   2. Numerical chromosomal anomalies are thought to arise by nondisjunction during meiosis (see Chapter 2, section VII B).
   3. Table 23-2 shows the relative frequency of a number of different congenital developmental defects known to be due to anomalies in chromosome number.

  B. Trisomies. In this chapter are presented the clinical features and karyotypes of the three most common trisomies. Recurrence risks and the rare translocation variants of these trisomies are discussed in Chapter 24, section VI.
   1. **Down syndrome (trisomy 21)**
      a. Trisomy 21, or Down syndrome, is the most common numerical anomaly.
      b. A karyotype of a patient with trisomy 21 is shown in Figure 23-1.
      c. An example of a child with Down syndrome is shown in Figure 23-2.
         (1) Clinically, trisomy 21 is a pleiotropic anomaly causing characteristic facial defects and mental retardation.
         (2) A simian palmar crease, oblique palpebral fissures (eye slits) and epicanthal folds of skin at the bridge of the nose, a protruding tongue, and a broad chest are typical findings (see Fig. 23-2).
         (3) Cardiovascular defects occur in a large number of afflicted children. The life span is usually shortened.
   2. **Edwards syndrome (trisomy 18)**
      a. An example of the karyotype of infants afflicted with trisomy 18, or Edwards syndrome, is shown in Figure 23-3.

Table 23-2. Approximate Frequency of Some Chromosomal Aberrations

Condition	Frequency per 100,000 Births
Down syndrome (trisomy 21)	
In general population	140
When mother is over age 40	1000
Edwards syndrome (trisomy 18)	20
Patau syndrome (trisomy 13)	10
XXX Genotype	50
XXY Genotype (Klinefelter syndrome)	80
XYY Genotype	100
XO Genotype (Turner syndrome)	8

Data from Bickel M, et al: Genetic disorders—Prevention, treatment, and rehabilitation. *WHO Tech Rep Ser* 497 Annex 1: *Frequency of Genetic Disorders*, 1980.

b. Examples of infants with Edwards syndrome are shown in Figure 23-4.
  (1) Clinically, infants with Edwards syndrome are born of a normal term pregnancy.
  (2) The newborn infants are unusually small and abnormally thin, with loose skin due to a failure of accumulation of subcutaneous adipose tissue. The infants have flexed hands and feet and low-set ears (see Fig. 23-4). The occipital lobe is also unusually prominent in these children.
  (3) Cardiovascular, gastrointestinal, and musculoskeletal defects are also commonly seen in children with Edwards syndrome and they are invariably profoundly mentally retarded.

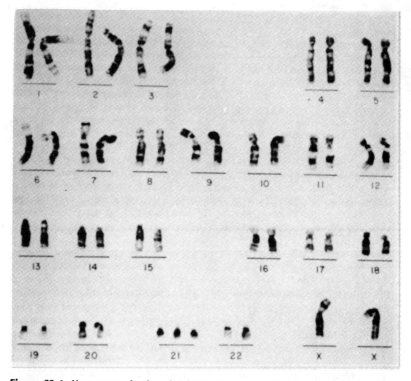

Figure 23-1. Karyotype of a female child with trisomy 21 (Down syndrome). (Reprinted with permission from Simpson JL, et al: *Genetics in Obstetrics and Gynecology.* New York, Grune and Stratton, 1982, p 57.)

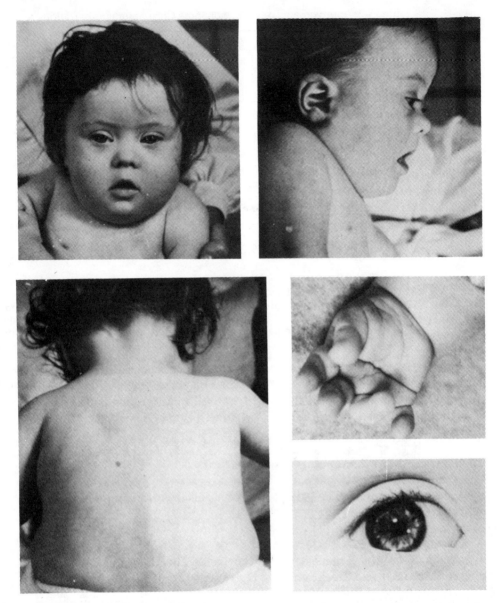

Figure 23-2. Clinical features of Down syndrome. (Reprinted with permission from de Grouchy J, Turleau C: *Clinical Atlas of Human Chromosomes.* New York, John Wiley, 1977, p 195.)

      c. Children afflicted with this syndrome rarely live past the first year after birth.
  3. Patau syndrome (trisomy 13)
      a. An example of the karyotype of infants afflicted with trisomy 13, or Patau syndrome, is shown in Figure 23-5.
      b. Examples of infants afflicted with Patau syndrome are shown in Figure 23-6.
          (1) Clinically, Patau syndrome is characterized by absence or gross reduction of the eyes (microphthalmia) and other ocular defects such as coloboma, cloudy corneas, or cyclopia.
          (2) Other clinical abnormalities are also commonly seen, including:
              (a) Cleft lip, cleft palate, and abnormal development in nasal structures

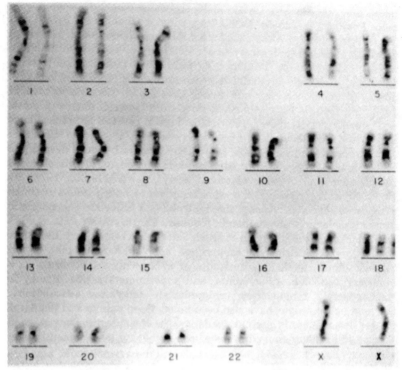

Figure 23-3. Karyotype of a female child with trisomy 18 (Edwards syndrome). (Reprinted with permission from Simpson JL, et al: *Genetics in Obstetrics and Gynecology.* New York, Grune and Stratton, 1982, p 69.)

- (b) Polydactyly, manual flexion and pedal extension, and hypoplastic finger and toe nails
- (c) Various gross defects in the brain
- (d) Cardiovascular defects
- (e) Abnormalities in the urogenital system

c. Afflicted children show severe mental retardation and usually die soon after birth.

C. Other chromosomal anomalies

1. Many other congenital defects are known to be caused by more subtle alterations in the karyotype less dramatic than duplication or absence of a chromosome.
   a. For example, the **cri du chat syndrome** results from a deletion of the short arm of chromosome 5.
   b. In this syndrome, which is relatively rare, microcephaly, mental retardation, cardiovascular defects, and a peculiar, cat-like cry are present in the afflicted child.
2. As cytogeneticists have become more adept at examining the human karyotype, they have discovered a whole host of minor syndromes due to deletions or duplications of small segments of various chromosomes.
3. About 25% of all spontaneously aborted fetuses show some form of gross structural abnormality in the karyotype, including triploidy, monosomy of a number of different autosomes, ring chromosomes, and so forth.
4. In children born alive with congenital anomalies, only about 4% show chromosomal anomalies, although this number is sure to increase with increasing sophistication in cytogenetic analysis.

III. INFECTIOUS AGENTS AND CONGENITAL BIRTH DEFECTS

A. Rubella virus

1. Rubella virus causes the formerly common childhood disease known as German measles.

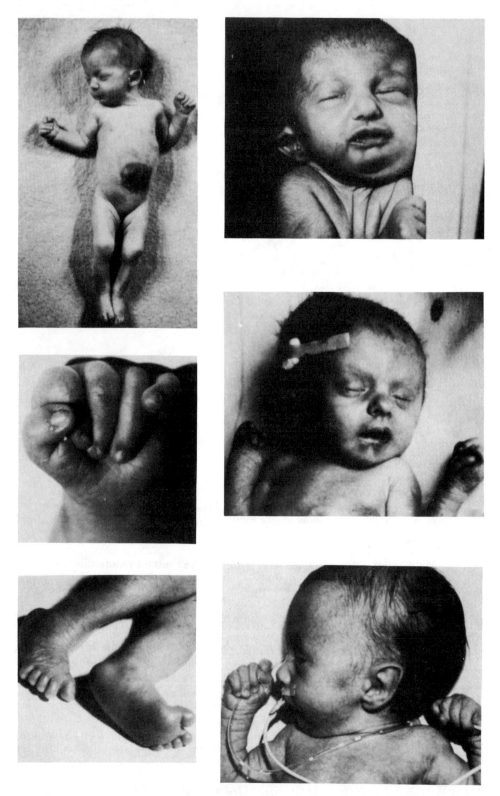

Figure 23-4. Clinical features of Edwards syndrome. (Reprinted with permission from de Grouchy J, Turleau C: *Clinical Atlas of Human Chromosomes.* New York, John Wiley, 1977, p 163.)

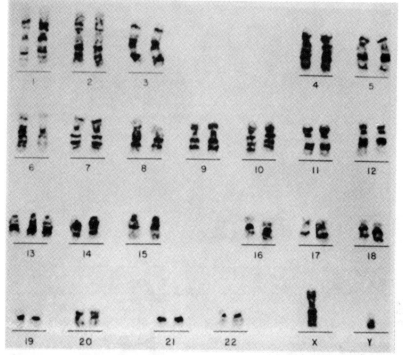

Figure 23-5. Karyotype of a male child with trisomy 13 (Patau syndrome). (Reprinted with permission from Simpson JL, et al: *Genetics in Obstetrics and Gynecology*. New York, Grune and Stratton, 1982, p 67.)

    a. The virus has been clearly established as a teratogenic agent.
    b. The rubella virus in the infected mother invades the placenta and crosses into the fetal environment.

2. Among children whose mothers were infected with rubella during their pregnancy, there is a striking increase in congenital birth defects. The incidence and type of defects depend upon the **stage of infection**.
    a. With rubella infections in the **first trimester**, about 15% of children born alive show congenital anomalies.
    b. Rubella infections during the **fourth to eighth weeks** of pregnancy—the end of the period of major organogenesis—result in the most severe abnormalities.
    c. Infections that occur **after the first trimester** are considerably less dangerous.

3. The following conditions are observed in children affected by rubella virus in utero:
    a. Cataracts
    b. Patent ductus arteriosus and other cardiovascular abnormalities
    c. Hearing defects
    d. Mental retardation
    e. Intrauterine growth retardation

4. Attenuated rubella virus vaccine is now administered to all preschool children, usually in the first year after birth or as a condition for admission into public schools.
    a. This public health measure has effectively eliminated rubella as an infectious disease and as a major cause of congenital birth defects.
    b. Nevertheless, it is likely that rubella will continue to be a minor public health problem for the foreseeable future.
        (1) Since rubella is a highly contagious disease, all health professionals should be aware of the possibility of contacting patients with infectious rubella and then transmitting it to pregnant women in the hospital or in their homes.
        (2) Since the virus is known to be teratogenic, physicians should be alert to preventing the spread of this agent to pregnant women when it is encountered in other patients.

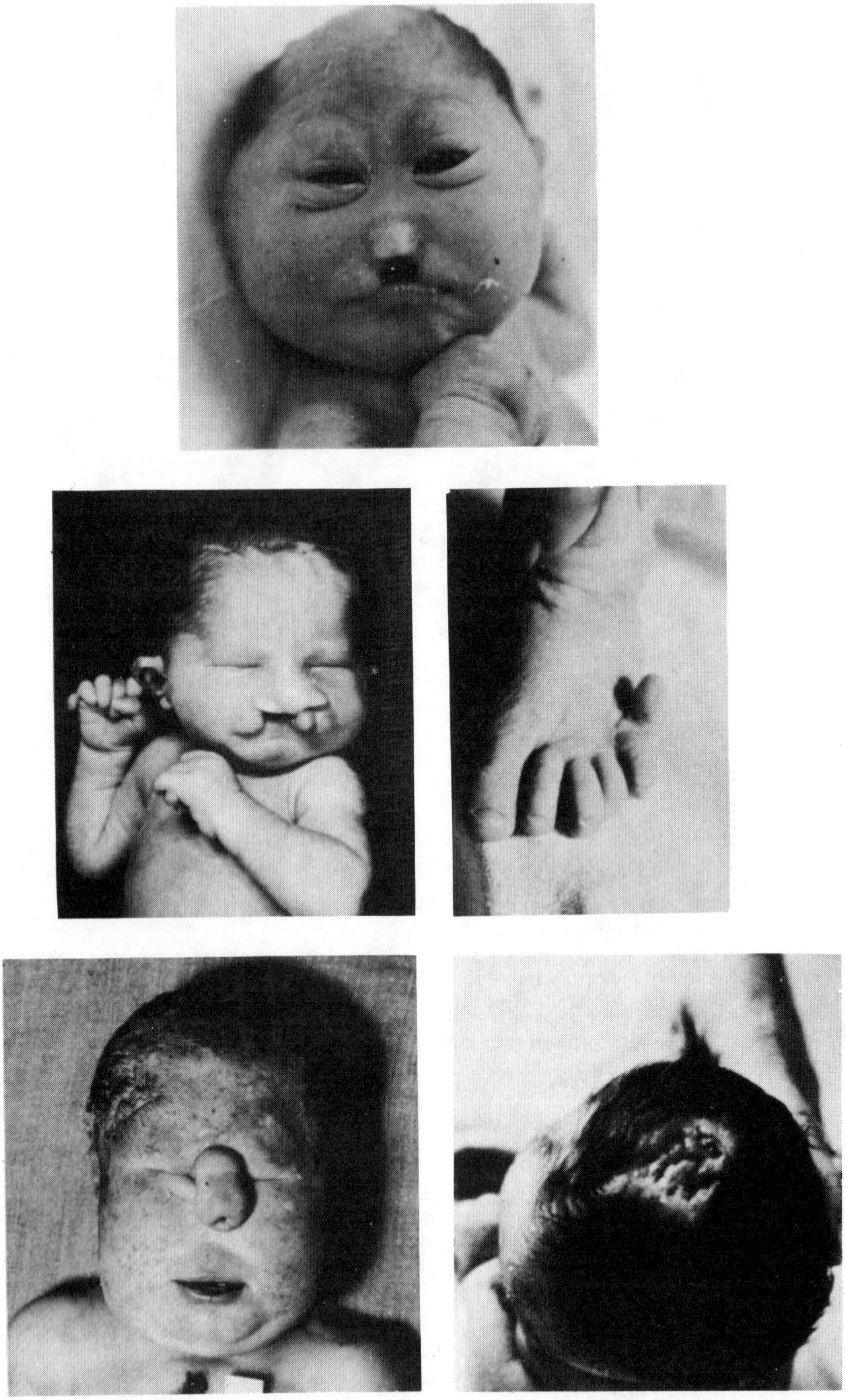

Figure 23-6. Clinical features of Patau syndrome. (Reprinted with permission from de Grouchy J, Turleau C: *Clinical Atlas of Human Chromosomes.* New York, John Wiley, 1977, p 131.)

B. Cytomegalovirus

1. Cytomegalovirus (CMV) infection in utero is known to cause a condition in newborn children known as **cytomegalic inclusion disease**.
   a. This disorder is characterized chiefly by developmental defects in the central nervous system.
      (1) The brain and consequently the entire head are often abnormally small. The brain ventricles may be outlined on x-ray examination by characteristic periventricular calcifications.
      (2) Mental retardation is common.
   b. Jaundice and hepatomegaly may also occur with this disease.
2. Cytomegalovirus infection is widespread but asymptomatic in the adult population, and many pregnant women are infected with cytomegalovirus, although not all infected women give birth to children with congenital defects.
   a. About 1% of all pregnant women have an intrauterine cytomegalovirus infection.
   b. Of these, 5% to 10% give birth to children who show symptoms of cytomegalovirus infection at birth.

C. Herpes simplex virus

1. There is considerable controversy about whether or not herpes simplex virus is teratogenic. The most recent findings suggest that it is not important as a teratogenic agent.
2. Whether or not it is teratogenic, it is an increasingly serious problem because of the potentially disastrous effects of **congenital herpes infection**. This is transmitted from an infected mother to the newborn as the infant passes through the birth canal.
   a. Almost half of all newborns with herpes venereal infection will die.
   b. Therefore, pregnant women with active genital herpes infections are invariably delivered by cesarean section.
3. This disease will undoubtedly become a more serious problem with the continued spread of herpes simplex virus in men and women of reproductive competence.

D. Toxoplasma

1. *Toxoplasma gondii* is a protozoan organism that can infect pregnant women, cross the placenta, invade fetal tissues, and cause congenital malformations, primarily in the developing brain and ocular systems.
   a. *Toxoplasma gondii* infections result in mental retardation, microphthalmia, chorioretinitis, hydrocephalus, and microcephaly.
   b. Calcifications are also sometimes seen around the choroid plexus.
2. *Toxoplasma* infections in pregnant women are quite common and usually are without overt symptoms, thus making it difficult to estimate the incidence of congenital defects.
3. It is not known why some children of infected mothers show symptoms and others do not.

IV. TERATOGENIC EFFECTS OF IONIZING RADIATION

A. X-Irradiation

1. When x-rays were first developed as a diagnostic tool, their harmful effects on fetuses were unknown.
2. Studies were performed by Goldstein and Murphy in 1929. They examined 106 women given therapeutic radiation doses during their pregnancies.
   a. Of the children in this study born alive, 51% were born unhealthy, although not all of the malformations were considered to be caused by the radiation.
   b. Nevertheless, the children of these pregnancies included 14 with microcephaly, 2 with hydrocephaly, 1 with Down syndrome, and 3 with skeletal defects.
   c. This was an obvious increase in the incidence of malformations over what would be encountered normally in women who were not exposed to x-rays.
3. Numerous experiments performed on animals have established that x-rays can cause birth defects and that the sensitivity of the fetus to damage from ionizing radiation varies with developmental stage.
   a. For example, mouse embryos are killed by relatively low doses of radiation during early cleavage, become less sensitive during implantation and gastrulation, and become more sensitive again during the period of organogenesis.

b. The specific type of congenital anomaly caused by a specific dose of radiation varies, depending upon the developmental stage of the irradiated fetus.
   (1) In rat embryos irradiated at 9 days of development, anencephaly, encephalocele, and anopthalmia are commonly observed.
   (2) In rat embryos irradiated at 20 days after fertilization or soon after birth, defects are largely restricted to the cerebellum.
   (3) This observation is partially related to two facts:
      (a) Different parts of the brain are formed by cellular proliferation events at different times during development.
      (b) **Mitotic cells** are more susceptible to radiation damage than cells in interphase.

B. Ionizing radiation from nuclear weapons

1. Human beings were exposed to massive doses of ionizing radiation at the end of World War II when the United States dropped atomic bombs on Hiroshima and Nagasaki in Japan.
2. The devastating effects on pregnant women in these cities point impressively to the serious effects of ionizing radiation on human fetuses.
   a. The exact number of women who were pregnant at that time is, of course, not known, because many were in the initial portions of their pregnancies and may not have been aware of the fact that they were pregnant.
   b. Among those known to be pregnant, many showed spontaneous abortions soon after the bomb blast. The newborn mortality rate was also unusually high after the attack.
   c. Microcephaly and mental retardation were seen in the offspring of many women irradiated during weeks 7 through 15 of gestation.
3. We can only hope that human beings will never be exposed again to the high levels of radiation encountered in a nuclear attack.

C. Low-level ionizing radiation and other environmental pollution

1. There is great controversy over the effects of low-level ionizing radiation on pregnant women.
   a. Human beings are naturally exposed to low doses of ionizing radiation, due primarily to cosmic rays and natural radionuclides present in the environment.
   b. We may never know the precise details of the dose–response curves for radiation-induced teratogenesis in humans.
   c. There is little doubt, however, that human exposure to low-level ionizing radiation will have no effects at best and slight deleterious effects at worst.
2. Advocates of nuclear power minimize the dangers to humans of increasing radiation loads. Opponents of nuclear power, on the other hand, may forget that the waste products released from more conventional modes of power generation are also not without health hazards.
3. The cost–benefit analysis of political decisions about power generation generally ignore the problem of teratogenesis because there are no solid numerical data to show precisely what the risk is.
   a. The unavailability of precise data should not be taken to mean that the risk is insignificant, merely that it is unknown.
   b. A prudent society would decide to conserve energy and thereby decrease heat pollution, air pollution, and radiation pollution of the environment.

V. TERATOGENIC EFFECTS OF DRUGS

A. General considerations

1. Some drugs are used medically and others socially in our culture. Either type can sometimes have disastrous consequences for newborn fetuses, as the examples below will show.
2. Physicians prescribing drugs for pregnant women need to be alert to the fact that they are prescribing drugs for two patients.
3. They must also be sensitive to the pregnant woman's use of social drugs, especially cigarettes and alcohol.

B. **Medications**
 1. **Thalidomide**, an antinausea agent and mild sedative, is perhaps the most notorious teratogenic drug.
    a. Experimental animal studies indicated that thalidomide was not teratogenic, but when clinical use of the drug became widespread in Europe, there was a sudden increase in the frequency of amelia and phocomelia (absence of all or the greater part of one or more limbs).
       (1) These limb defects were extremely rare before thalidomide use.
       (2) The sudden increase in their frequency prompted clinicians to make a careful examination of prenatal histories, which soon revealed a common thread of thalidomide ingestion.
    b. When the thalidomide use was discontinued, the incidence of amelia and phocomelia decreased to its former low level.
 2. **Antimitotic drugs**
    a. **Aminopterin**, a folic acid antagonist, has been implicated in a number of cases of birth defects, and the use of this and other antimetabolites should be avoided in pregnant women.
    b. Antimetabolites probably exert their teratogenic effects by altering cell division in the developing embryo.
 3. **Drugs acting on the central nervous system**
    a. **Phenytoin (diphenylhydantoin)**, an anticonvulsant that is used to treat epilepsy, is a teratogen.
    b. **Phenothiazines** and **lithium**, used in treatment of psychosis, are also suspected teratogens, as is the widely used antianxiety drug **diazepam**.
 4. **Aspirin.** Large doses of aspirin are thought to be teratogenic.
 5. **Steroid hormones.** A number of steroids have been implicated as having teratogenic potential.
    a. **Synthetic progestins** have a masculinizing effect on the external genitalia of female embryos.
       (1) Synthetic progestins which have been used to avert spontaneous abortion have shown this effect.
       (2) **Birth control pills** contain progestins and therefore also can have a masculinizing effect.
          (a) Thus birth control pills should be avoided in pregnant women.
          (b) Before birth control pills are prescribed, it should be established that the patient is not pregnant.
    b. Another synthetic steroid, **diethylstilbestrol (DES)** has been shown to cause an increased frequency of gynecologic cancers in the daughters of women treated with DES during pregnancy to avert threatened abortion.

C. **Social drugs**
 1. Two widely used social drugs, alcohol and nicotine, are known to have deleterious effects on the fetus.
    a. **Alcohol**
       (1) There is no doubt that consumption of large amounts of ethanol during pregnancy causes abnormalities in human development.
          (a) Children from chronic alcoholic mothers show a striking group of abnormalities known as **fetal alcohol syndrome (FAS)**.
             (i) These include abnormalities in the central nervous system such as microcephaly and mental retardation.
             (ii) Children with fetal alcohol syndrome are also smaller in stature and exhibit a complex of minor facial malformations involving the eyes, maxilla, and upper lip.
          (b) Recent experimental studies reveal defects in the development of the central nervous system in mice treated with single high doses of ethanol.
       (2) While there is considerable controversy concerning the effects of moderate and light drinking during pregnancy, the AMA Council on Scientific Affairs since 1983 has recommended complete abstinence from alcohol for pregnant women.
    b. **Nicotine.** Cigarette smoking has not been shown per se to cause congenital birth defects. However, it is a well established fact that cigarette smokers have smaller babies and a higher infant mortality rate.

2. **Other social drugs**
   a. **Cannabis** use has not been shown to cause congenital birth defects, but cannabis has not been shown to be free from deleterious effects either.
   b. Similarly, **LSD (lysergic acid diethylamide)**, **PCP** (phenylcyclohexyl piperidine; **phencyclidine**), **cocaine**, and **heroin** are not known to be free of teratogenic effects.
3. The use of all these superfluous social drugs should be discouraged in pregnant women.

Table 23-3. Some Inherited Metabolic Disorders Detectable in the Midtrimester of Pregnancy

Disorders of lipid metabolism
   Fabry's disease
   Gaucher's disease, infantile and adult types
   G_{M1} gangliosidosis types I and II
   G_{M2} gangliosidosis types I (Tay-Sachs disease), II (Sandhoff disease), and III
   G_{M3} gangliosidosis
   Metachromatic leukodystrophy, infantile, juvenile, and adult types
   Niemann-Pick disease, types A, B, and C

Disorders of carbohydrate or glycoprotein metabolism
   Fucosidosis
   Galactokinase deficiency
   Galactosemia
   Glucose-6-phosphate dehydrogenase (G6PD) deficiency
   Glycogen storage disease, types II (Pompe disease), III (Forbes disease), IV (Andersen disease), VI (Hers disease), and VIII (phosphorylase kinase deficiency)

Disorders of mucopolysaccharide (MPS) metabolism
   Hurler syndrome (MPS I-H)
   Hunter syndrome (MPS II)
   Sly syndrome (β-glucuronidase deficiency; MPS VII)

Disorders of amino acid and organic acid metabolism
   Arginase deficiency
   Cystinosis
   Maple syrup urine disease, severe and intermittent types

Miscellaneous disorders
   Adenosine deaminase deficiency
   Congenital adrenal hyperplasia
   Cystic fibrosis
   Hypophosphatasia
   Lesch-Nyhan syndrome
   Xeroderma pigmentosum

Data from Burton BK, Nadler HL: Antenatal diagnosis of metabolic disorders. *Clin Obstet Gynecol* 24:1041, 1981.

VI. ANTENATAL DIAGNOSIS OF CONGENITAL ANOMALIES

A. General considerations

1. Due to recent advances in medical technology, physicians have an increased ability to detect a host of congenital anomalies.

2. **Amniocentesis** (see also Chapter 22, section I C) allows the collection of amniotic fluid and fetal cells. Biochemical and cytogenetic analysis of this fluid or of cells cultured from it can then rule out a large number of congenital anomalies or make a firm diagnosis of an anomaly.

3. Many of these diseases are fatal or extremely debilitating. The ability to detect congenital defects in utero presents the parents with the opportunity to terminate the pregnancy or prepare themselves for the birth of a child with a birth defect.
   a. If the parents elect to have the afflicted child, psychological and medical preparations can be made in advance of the birth.
   b. Diagnosis in advance allows the obstetrician to prepare for a potentially difficult delivery and alerts the neonatologist to be prepared to deal with medical problems that may arise as a result of congenital birth defects.

B. Congenital diseases detectable by techniques based on amniocentesis

1. **Neural tube defects.** α-Fetoprotein screening of amniotic fluid along with sonography can detect many neural tube defects in utero (see Chapter 5, section VI B).

2. **Aneuploidy**
   a. It is possible to prepare a karyotype from cultured fetal cells obtained from the amniotic fluid or biopsied from the fetus.
   b. Careful karyotype analysis can then rule out or diagnose any of the chromosomal numerical anomalies such as Down syndrome and other trisomies.

3. **Inherited metabolic disorders**
   a. At present, more than 70 different metabolic disorders can be detected in midtrimester pregnancies. Table 23-3 lists some representative examples.
   b. A combination of techniques is employed, including adult screening, enzymatic analysis of amniotic fluid, and cytogenetic and biochemical analysis of cells cultured from amniotic fluid.
      (1) For example, **Tay-Sachs disease** is a genetic disorder involving glycolipid metabolism. It is a fatal disease in the homozygous condition, involving progressive neurologic degeneration.
      (2) Tay-Sachs disease is an autosomal recessive disorder carried by about 4% of individuals in the American Jewish population. Heterozygous adult carriers can be identified by a serum hexosaminidase assay, and if this assay suggests that the fetus is at risk, a hexosaminidase assay can then be performed on cultured fetal cells collected from amniotic fluid.

STUDY QUESTIONS

Directions: Each question below contains five suggested answers. Choose the **one best** response to each question.

1. Drugs known to be teratogenic to the fetus include all of the following EXCEPT

   (A) aminopterin
   (B) alcohol
   (C) birth control pills
   (D) phenytoin
   (E) heroin

2. All of the following statements about the effects of microorganisms are true EXCEPT

   (A) herpes simplex virus is a known teratogen
   (B) rubella virus is a known teratogen
   (C) cytomegalovirus is a known teratogen
   (D) *Toxoplasma* is probably a teratogen
   (E) herpes simplex infections during birth are often fatal to the newborn

3. All of the following statements concerning Down syndrome are true EXCEPT

   (A) it is most frequently caused by a translocation
   (B) it can be caused by trisomy of chromosome 21
   (C) its recurrence risk is related to maternal age
   (D) the patient invariably has mental retardation
   (E) it shows a dramatic increase in frequency with maternal age

Directions: Each question below contains four suggested answers of which **one or more** is correct. Choose the answer

   A if **1, 2, and 3** are correct
   B if **1 and 3** are correct
   C if **2 and 4** are correct
   D if **4** is correct
   E if **1, 2, 3, and 4** are correct

4. True statements about Patau syndrome include which of the following?

   (1) Microphthalmia is common
   (2) Mental retardation is rare
   (3) Cleft palate is common
   (4) A normal life span is common

5. True statements about cri du chat syndrome include which of the following?

   (1) It is an example of aneuploidy
   (2) Cardiovascular anomalies are common
   (3) Mental retardation is rare
   (4) It involves a deletion of part of chromosome 5

6. True statements about the teratogenic effects of ionizing radiation include which of the following?

    (1) Low doses are known to be harmless
    (2) X-rays are safe to use on pregnant women after the first trimester
    (3) Women in Nagasaki had few spontaneous abortions after the atomic bomb blast
    (4) Microcephalic and mentally retarded newborn infants were seen in unusually high frequency after the atomic bomb blasts in Japan

7. Fetal alcohol syndrome causes which of the following characteristics?

    (1) Midfacial hypoplasia
    (2) Short stature
    (3) Mental retardation
    (4) Obesity

8. The effects of rubella virus on developing fetuses include which of the following?

    (1) Blindness
    (2) Deafness
    (3) Mental retardation
    (4) Intrauterine growth retardation

9. Edwards syndrome shows which of the following characteristics?

    (1) Most cases are caused by trisomy 18
    (2) The incidence is related to maternal age
    (3) Infants are small for gestational age
    (4) Mental retardation and prominent occiput are common features

ANSWERS AND EXPLANATIONS

1. The answer is E. (*V B 2 a, 3 a, 5 a, C 1 a, 2 b*) Teratogenic drugs are those known to cause structural defects in utero. Aminopterin inhibits cell division and is therefore a known teratogen. Alcohol in large doses is known to have deleterious effects on the fetus; the effects of smaller doses are not certain. Synthetic progestins, including those in birth control pills, are known teratogens. Phenytoin is an anticonvulsant, and like certain other drugs active on the central nervous system, it is known to be teratogenic. Heroin crosses the placenta and causes addiction of the fetus, but it is not a well established teratogenic agent.

2. The answer is A. (*III A, B, C, D*) Herpes simplex is not thought to be a teratogenic virus. However, neonatal herpes simplex infections are fatal in about 50% of all infected newborns. Rubella has been definitely established as a teratogen. Cytomegalovirus causes teratogenic effects on the developing nervous system in some cases. *Toxoplasma* is also a suspected teratogen, although it is difficult to establish this from epidemiologic data because *Toxoplasma* infections are so common.

3. The answer is A. (*Chapter 23 II B 1; Chapter 24 VI B*) Down syndrome is the most common trisomy seen in humans. The overall incidence is approximately 1 in 800 live births. Down syndrome is caused by trisomy of chromosome 21 in 95% of the cases; about 5% of the cases are due to a translocation of most of chromosome 21. Because the meiotic metaphase in oogenesis is increasingly prolonged as a woman ages, the frequency of nondisjunction increases dramatically with maternal age. Therefore, the incidence of Down syndrome (and of all other trisomies) increases with advancing maternal age. There is also a less pronounced paternal age effect. Patients with Down syndrome usually have an IQ in the 60–80 range, and their life expectancy is decreased.

4. The answer is B (1, 3). (*II B 3*) Patau syndrome, or trisomy 13 (47, +13), is characterized by microphthalmia and other ocular defects, cleft lip and palate, facial defects, profound mental retardation, and death soon after birth, with individuals rarely living even one year.

5. The answer is C (2, 4). [*Chapter 23 II C 1; Chapter 24 III D 2 d (1) (a)*] Cri du chat syndrome is due to a deletion of the short arm of chromosome 5. The number of chromosomes is 46, and the syndrome is therefore not an example of aneuploidy. Infants born with cri du chat syndrome have cardiovascular defects, mental retardation, and microcephaly. The characteristic sound these children make when crying gave the syndrome its name.

6. The answer is D (4). (*IV A, B, C*) Ionizing radiation is known to cause congenital birth defects. X-rays could cause abnormalities of the developing brain after the first trimester of pregnancy. Victims of the bomb blasts in Japan showed significant increases in the incidence of spontaneous abortions. Of the children born alive, many more than usual had microcephaly and mental retardation.

7. The answer is A (1, 2, 3). (*V C 1 a*) Fetal alcohol syndrome is seen in children of women who were chronic alcoholics during pregnancy. Children with fetal alcohol syndrome show midfacial hypoplasia, intrauterine growth retardation and therefore short stature, and intellectual deficits. Since the effects of moderate drinking during pregnancy are uncertain, currently it is felt that even moderate alcohol consumption in pregnancy is contraindicated.

8. The answer is E (all). (*III A*) Rubella virus infections in pregnant women can cause congenital anomalies in their offspring. Congenital defects are centered in the nervous system and can include blindness, deafness, and mental retardation, but intrauterine growth retardation is also seen.

9. The answer is E (all). (*Chapter 23 II B 2; Chapter 24 VI A 2*) In 80% of the cases, Edwards syndrome is due to trisomy 18 (47, +18), and is thus an example of aneuploidy, or abnormal numbers of chromosomes in the karyotype. However, Edwards syndrome can also be caused by translocation. Since the trisomy cases are caused by nondisjunction, there is an increase in frequency with maternal age. Infants with Edwards syndrome are born of a normal term pregnancy, but are unusually small and thin. Mental retardation and prominent occiput are common features of Edwards syndrome.

24
Medical Genetics and Related Birth Defects

I. INTRODUCTION

A. Incidence and causes of genetic defects

1. Up to 7% of all live births involve some sort of congenital abnormality. A much larger percentage of all conceptions end before the birth of a live child, often because the embryo or fetus is fatally affected by a congenital abnormality.

2. Many congenital abnormalities are caused by **genetic defects** of varying complexity. Genetic defects are of several **types**:
   a. Some congenital genetic abnormalities are caused by **numerical abnormalities** or **abnormal rearrangements of the karyotype**, such as:
      (1) Extra copies of the entire chromosomal complement (**polyploidy**)
      (2) Addition or deletion of particular chromosomes (**aneuploidy**)
      (3) Losses of small parts of chromosomes (**deletions**)
      (4) Transfers of small parts of one chromosome to another chromosome (**translocations**)
   b. Other genetic abnormalities are caused by **point mutations** affecting a single genetic locus or a small number of loci. These mutations may be autosomal dominant or recessive, or X-linked dominant or recessive.
   c. Still other congenital genetic abnormalities are **polygenic lesions** or **multifactorial lesions**—the last-named caused by a poorly understood complex of genetic and environmental components.

3. Physicians are now aware of numerous well characterized clinical entities representing all these abnormalities with different degrees of genetic complexity.
   a. The fantastic scientific advances that have been made in the field of molecular genetics in the last three decades have led to a truly exponential growth in the number of diseases that are now understood on a genetic basis.
   b. For example, in 1959 there were 412 identified disease entities that were known to be due to mendelian traits in humans. By 1978, this number had increased to 2811.

4. Many congenital genetic defects are quite rare, but others are among the most common of all congenital abnormalities, such as trisomy 21 (Down syndrome).

B. Diagnosis of genetic defects

1. The correct diagnosis of a genetically determined congenital abnormality often requires great diagnostic skill and careful evaluation of cytogenetic and biochemical data as well as data gathered from physical and psychological examination of the patient.

2. Diagnosis is often greatly aided by **karyotype analysis** (see section III).
   a. Great advances in medical genetics have been made possible in recent years with the advent of chromosome banding techniques.
   b. It is now possible to detect not only numerical chromosomal abnormalities but also deletions, translocations, and inversions of very small fragments of particular chromosomes by karyotype analysis.

C. The physician's responsibilities after diagnosis of genetic disease. Once a correct diagnosis of a genetically determined congenital abnormality is made, there are three major responsibilities that the physician will face.

1. First, the physician must treat the afflicted patient, using a variety of techniques that may range from corrective surgery to special diets.

2. Second, the physician must console the parents of the afflicted child. Many parents will not understand the cause of the congenital defect and will feel shame, guilt, or depression over giving birth to an abnormal offspring.
3. In addition to providing psychological support for the parents, the physician must also advise the parents about the risk of recurrence of the disease in a subsequent pregnancy.

D. Genetic counseling

1. It is the job of the obstetrician or perinatologist to make an accurate diagnosis of genetically determined congenital abnormalities so that he or she can then offer intelligent advice in the form of genetic counseling to the parents of the afflicted infant.
   a. Genetic counseling is best done by a professional who is trained in this field and has access to complex cytogenetic and biochemical diagnostic techniques.
   b. However, all physicians involved with pregnant women and newborn children should have some understanding of modern molecular genetics, if for no other reason than that the attending physician should know when further genetic studies are indicated.
2. Giving proper advice requires great sophistication in some cases. For example, a single clinical entity such as Down syndrome can occur by two very different genetic mechanisms, and the risk of recurrence depends on both parental age and the exact genetic mechanism underlying the disease (see section VI B).
3. The advice that a physician will give will often require the preparation of a **pedigree** (see Figs. 24-2, 24-3, and 24-4) in order to understand the transmission of a given disease in the close relations of the afflicted infant.
   a. Preparing a pedigree involves gathering a detailed family history. This can be a difficult task often because the family members of an afflicted child are not trained observers of human appearance or human behavior.
   b. Whenever possible, the genetic counselor should make first-hand observations of family members in order to establish an accurate pedigree.

II. DNA AND PROTEIN SYNTHESIS

A. Genes and DNA structure

1. **Genes** are specific sequences of **deoxyribonucleic acid (DNA)** which are contained on **chromosomes**, in the cell **nucleus**.
2. **DNA** is a macromolecule composed of two intertwined **helical strands**.
   a. The strands contain:
      (1) A sugar, **deoxyribose**
      (2) Phosphate groups
      (3) Nitrogen-containing bases of four varieties:
         (a) Two kinds of purines, **adenine** and **guanine**
         (b) Two kinds of pyrimidines, **thymine** and **cytosine**
   b. On the two intertwined helical strands, the purines of one strand are strongly **linked**, via hydrogen bonding, with the pyrimidines of the opposite strand.
      (1) The purine **adenine** of one strand is linked with the pyrimidine **thymine** of the opposite strand, forming **A-T base pairs**.
      (2) The purine **guanine** of one strand is linked with the pyrimidine **cytosine** of the opposite strand, forming **G-C base pairs**.
   c. The formation of these complementary A-T and G-C base pairs is of fundamental importance for DNA replication (self-duplication).
   d. The opposite strands of DNA are **complementary** to one another, and this complementarity assures accurate self-duplication of specific nucleotide sequences when DNA strands become uncoiled and replicated during the S (synthesis) phase of mitosis.
3. The essence of structural differences between different genes lies in the specific nucleotide sequences found in each gene. The **nucleotide sequence** of a DNA molecule is what determines the **specific amino acid sequences** in **proteins**, which are the ultimate **gene products** in a differentiated cell.

B. DNA replication and protein synthesis

1. **Transcription**
   a. During transcription, the DNA double helix becomes uncoiled due to the action of the enzyme **RNA polymerase**, and a complementary **messenger RNA molecule (mRNA)** is produced in multiple copies.

- **b.** The mRNA molecule contains a single strand of nucleotides, and the nucleotide sequence is complementary to the DNA strand that is read during transcription.
- **c.** This mRNA molecule makes its way to **cytoplasmic ribosomes**.
  - **(1)** If the protein is destined for **intracellular utilization**, the ribosomes are free in the cytoplasm as **polysomes**. A polysome is merely a group of ribosomes bound together into a unit by a long strand of mRNA.
  - **(2)** If the protein is destined for **extracellular secretion**, the ribosomes are bound to the membranes of the **rough endoplasmic reticulum (RER)**.

2. **Translation**
   - **a.** The mRNA bound to ribosomes is now translated into a specific protein with the aid of another kind of RNA known as **transfer RNA (tRNA)**.
     - **(1)** There are a large number of different tRNAs, one or more for each amino acid found in proteins.
     - **(2)** Each specific tRNA has two **recognition sites** on it.
       - **(a)** One recognition site is specific for a particular amino acid.
       - **(b)** The other site is specific for a three-base-long nucleotide sequence, known as a **codon**, in mRNA.
   - **b.** During translation, a strand of ribosome-bound mRNA is read from one end to the other in three-nucleotide units (codons) by a series of tRNA molecules that have been coupled to specific amino acid molecules.
   - **c.** Simultaneously, peptide bonds are formed and a nascent chain of growing amino acid sequences appears near the ribosome to be read off into the cytoplasm of the cell engaged in protein synthesis (for polysomes) or transported into the lumen of the RER.

III. CHROMOSOMES AND KARYOTYPES

A. Basic chromosome structure

1. The DNA sequences of genes are structurally integrated into long strands of DNA and protein, which are then coiled in a complex and poorly understood fashion into the structures known as **chromosomes** contained within the nucleus of the cell.
2. Much of the DNA in a chromosome apparently does not code for specific gene sequences, but instead may have a regulatory function, a structural function, or spacer functions.
3. The proteins associated with chromosomes are probably important for structural integrity of the chromosomes and may also serve to protect and regulate genetic function.

B. Chromosome complement (karyotype)

1. Each species has a specific chromosome complement, consisting usually of a certain number of **autosomes** and a pair of **sex chromosomes**, which in mammals are usually structurally different in the two sexes.
2. Human beings have 22 pairs of **homologous autosomes** and 2 **sex chromosomes**. In females the sex chromosomes are **homomorphic (XX)** and in males they are **heteromorphic (XY)**.
3. Thus, the entire normal human chromosome complement, or **karyotype**, consists of **46 chromosomes** (Fig. 24-1).

C. Preparation of a karyotype for analysis

1. With the advent of tissue culture techniques and the discovery that colchicine could arrest mitosis at metaphase, the science of human cytogenetics took a great leap forward.
2. It became possible to obtain bits of tissue from patients after birth or in utero (via **amniocentesis** or **chorionic villus sampling**), grow these tissues into large numbers of cells in vitro, arrest dividing cells at metaphase, and then by use of hypotonic tissue culture media and squashing techniques, to spread out all of the metaphase chromosomes and photograph them with a light microscope.
   - **a.** At first, cytogeneticists had a difficult time in discriminating among all of the different chromosomes because many were very similar in size, length of chromatids, and position of the centromere along the chromosome.
   - **b.** Thus, the chromosomes were initially assigned to several large groups containing more than one pair of chromosomes. These groupings were based largely on the size of chromosomes and position of the centromere.

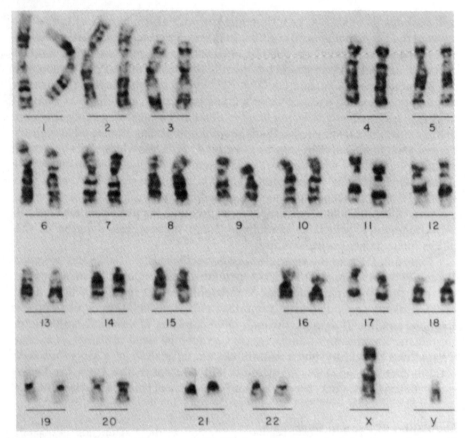

Figure 24-1. Karyotype of a normal human male (46, XY) demonstrated by the G-banding technique. (Reprinted with permission from Simpson JL, et al: *Genetics in Obstetrics and Gynecology*. New York, Grune and Stratton, 1982, p 6.)

3. Further advances were made when cytogeneticists developed **banding techniques** based on the differential uptake of certain dyes along the length of chromosomes.
   a. Each chromosome was found to have a characteristic banding pattern when stained with appropriate dye mixtures.
   b. One common banding technique, known as **G-banding**, involves salt treatment of a "chromosome squash" followed by Giemsa staining. The G-banding technique was used to prepare the karyotype shown in Figure 24-1.
4. Once each chromosome could be unambiguously distinguished from all other chromosomes, rapid advances in the diagnosis of cytogenetic disease could be made.

D. Karyotype nomenclature

1. To avoid confusion, a precise nomenclature system has been developed to encompass all possible modifications of the human karyotype and to provide a convenient shorthand notation for describing abnormal karyotypes (Table 24-1). The basic elements of the nomenclature system were developed at the Paris Conferences in 1971 and 1975.
2. The entire chromosome complement of a patient can be described conveniently and unambiguously using the established shorthand notation.
   a. For example, the **entire chromosome complement** is written by stating the total number of chromosomes, then a comma, and the sex chromosome complement. Thus, **normal males** are written 46, XY and **normal females** are written 46, XX.
   b. If **sex chromosomes** are added or deleted, an appropriate modification is made.
      (1) For example, in **Klinefelter syndrome**, there is an **extra X chromosome** along with the usual XY male constitution. Therefore, the shorthand for this syndrome would be 47, **XXY**.
      (2) Similarly, in **Turner syndrome** one of the two **X chromosomes is missing**, and this is designated as **45, X**.

Table 24-1. Symbols Used in Karyotype Nomenclature

Description or Alteration	Symbol
Centromere of chromosome	cen
Short arm of chromosome	p
Long arm of chromosome	q
Isochromosome	i
Addition of an autosome	+
Deletion of an autosome	−
Deletion of part of a chromosome	del
Translocation of part of a chromosome	t
Reciprocal translocation of part of a chromosome	rcp
Chromosomal mosaicism	/*
Ring chromosome	r
Chromosome with two centromeres (dicentric)	dic
Duplication of a segment of a chromosome	dup
Inversion of a segment of a chromosome	inv

*The diagonal line is used to separate cell lines in mosaicism.

- c. If **autosomes** are added or deleted, the addition is indicated by a + and the deletion is indicated by a −.
  - (1) Thus, **Down syndrome (trisomy 21)** is designated **47, XY, +21** in a **male** and **47, XX, +21** in a **female**.
  - (2) Similarly, **Edwards syndrome (trisomy 18)** is designated **47, XY, +18** in a **male** and **47, XX, +18** in a **female**.
- d. More complex and subtle alterations in the karyotype, such as **deletions, translocations**, or **mosaicism**, can also be designated with this method.
  - (1) Each chromosome has short arms and long arms (see Fig. 24-1); in the standard shorthand, these are designated **p** and **q**, respectively. Subfragments of the **p (short) arms** and **q (long) arms** can be identified and numbered on the basis of their banding patterns.
    - (a) For example, **cri du chat syndrome** involves a deletion of a variable amount of the distal tip of the short arm of chromosome number 5.
    - (b) Thus, for a child with cri du chat syndrome, **46, XY, del (5p14)** unambiguously designates a male child in whom the 14 region of the short arm of the fifth chromosome and everything distal to this band is completely deleted from the chromosome.
  - (2) Chromosomal **mosaics** are individuals who have two or more different kinds of chromosomal composition in different cells. In the standard shorthand system, the designations for the different cell lines are separated by a slash.
    - (a) For example, in **Klinefelter syndrome**, various **mosaics** can occur.
    - (b) Thus, for a child with Klinefelter syndrome, **47, XXY/48, XXXY** unambiguously designates a child with mosaicism who has **two cell lines**: one cell line has one extra X chromosome, and the other has two extra X chromosomes.

E. Numerical errors in the chromosomal complement

1. Numerical errors involving only one chromosome result from the **loss (monosomy)** or the **gain (trisomy)** of a **single chromosome**, most often due to **meiotic nondisjunction** (see Chapter 2, section VII B).
2. **Polyploidy** involves integral multiples of the usual number of chromosomes, such as **three full sets (triploidy)** or **four full sets (tetraploidy)** of chromosomes instead of the usual **two pairs (diploidy)**.
   - a. Polyploidy can result from a number of mechanisms, including perhaps polyspermy, diploidy of the male or female pronucleus, fertilization of the first polar body, or abnormal early division in the zygote.
   - b. Most polyploid fetuses are spontaneously aborted but 46/69 mosaics and fetuses with

69 chromosomes have been born. In both instances, there is severe mental retardation, multiple congenital defects, and a poor prognosis for life beyond infancy.

IV. PRINCIPLES OF MENDELIAN TRANSMISSION

A. Linkage

1. The principles of mendelian inheritance are well understood based on the independent assortment of genes located on different chromosomes.
2. If two different genes are located on the same chromosome, they are said to be **linked**.
3. Each autosome is paired with an identical homologous partner.
    a. During meiosis, paired homologs may exchange genetic material, leading to differential distribution of different genetic combinations to different gametes (see Chapter 2, section I B 2).
    b. Thus, linked genes can recombine by crossing over during meiosis.

B. Mutations and mendelian inheritance

1. **Mutant genes**
    a. A **mutant gene** is distinguished from its **wild-type (normal) allele** when a new characteristic (i.e., a new **phenotype**) appears in a population of freely interbreeding animals.
    b. A mutant gene is either dominant or recessive.
        (1) With a **dominant gene**, the mutant phenotype is expressed in all progeny carrying at least one chromosome with the mutation. That is, the mutant phenotype will be expressed in both **heterozygotes** and in **mutant homozygotes**.
        (2) With a **recessive gene**, the mutant phenotype will only be expressed in **mutant homozygotes**, and not in heterozygotes or wild-type homozygotes.

2. **Autosomal dominant inheritance**
    a. If one parent carries a single autosomal dominant mutation (i.e., is heterozygous) and the other parent is a wild-type homozygote (Fig. 24-2), then 50% of the offspring, regardless of sex, will be heterozygous for the gene and will express the gene in addition to passing it on to their progeny. The remaining 50% of the progeny will be homozygous wild-type and will neither express the mutation nor will they pass it on to their progeny.

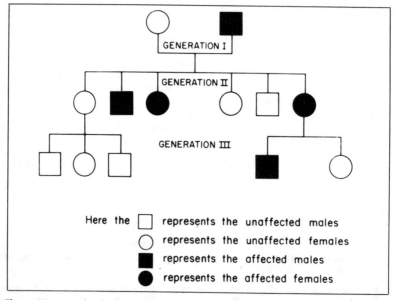

Figure 24-2. Mode of transmission of an autosomal dominant mutation. The father carries only one copy of the mutant gene and thus is heterozygous; the mother is wild-type homozygous. (Reprinted with permission from *Principles and Practice of Clinical Gynecology*. Edited by Kase NG and Weingold AB. New York, John Wiley, 1983, p 206.)

b. This relationship has been proven to be precisely true in many experiments using peas, *Drosophila*, and other well characterized genetic systems. In human beings, however, the situation is usually not so simple.

3. **Autosomal recessive inheritance**
   a. If a mutation is an autosomal recessive trait and **both parents** are **heterozygous carriers** of the gene (Fig. 24-3), then theoretically 25% of their offspring will be affected by the mutation, 25% will be wild-type homozygotes, and the remaining 50% will be unaffected heterozygous carriers, capable of passing the mutation on to their progeny. In clinical practice, families are often too small for this theoretic ratio to be reached.
   b. When a **heterozygous** autosomal recessive (**carrier**) **parent** mates with a **homozygous wild-type parent**, then none of the children will exhibit the mutant phenotype but 50% will be carriers and 50% will be normal wild-type homozygotes.
   c. When **both parents** are **homozygous** for a recessive autosomal mutation, then all their children will also be homozygotes, will express the mutant phenotype, and will pass the gene on to future generations.

4. Mutant autosomal genes are usually expressed equally in male and female offspring. However, the expression of certain autosomal genes involves gamete function, and this can distort sex ratios so that in offspring the trait is expressed more often in one sex than in the other.

5. **Sex-linked inheritance.** If the mutation is sex-linked—that is, carried on the sex chromosomes—then the situation can be a good deal more complicated (Fig. 24-4).
   a. As a general rule, most sex-linked mutations are carried on the X chromosome, since very few genes are located on the largely heterochromatinized Y chromosome.
   b. Sex-linked mutations, of course, can also be dominant or recessive.
   c. The phenotypic expression of X-linked dominant and recessive mutations in progeny is directly related to the sex chromosome constitution and therefore the genotypic sex of the offspring (see Fig. 24-4).

C. Clinical problems in determining inheritance patterns

1. In clinical practice, it is usually impossible to make such clear-cut distinctions as those diagrammed above because most genes show less than 100% penetrance; thus, an individual may be carrying a dominant gene in a heterozygous condition that **does not gain phenotypic expression** due to **incomplete penetrance**.
2. Furthermore, many congenital birth defects are known not to follow a simple mendelian inheritance pattern but instead behave as if they are either **polygenic** (due to many genes

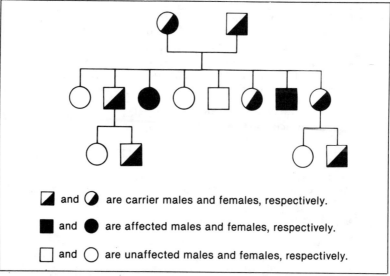

Figure 24-3. Mode of transmission of an autosomal recessive mutation. Both mother and father are heterozygous for the mutation. (Adapted from *Principles and Practice of Clinical Gynecology*. Edited by Kase NG and Weingold AB. New York, John Wiley, 1983, p 206.)

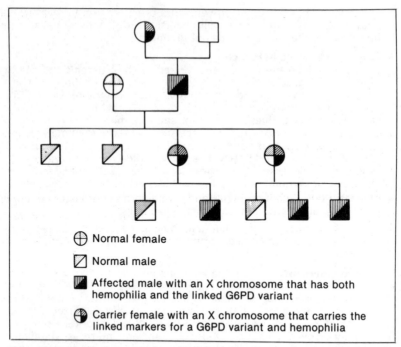

Figure 24-4. Mode of transmission of X-linked mutations such as hemophilia and a variant G6PD (glucose-6-phosphate dehydrogenase) enzyme. (Reprinted with permission from *Principles and Practice of Clinical Gynecology*. Edited by Kase NG and Weingold AB. New York, John Wiley, 1983, p 207.)

summed together) or **multifactorial** (due to an interaction between genome and environment). Practically speaking, many congenital birth defects can not be classified unambiguously as polygenic or multifactorial.

V. MENDELIAN DISORDERS—SOME COMMON EXAMPLES

A. Hemoglobinopathies

1. **Hemoglobin** is a tetrameric molecule composed of a variety of globin chains, each specified by a different gene. The predominant adult form of hemoglobin, **hemoglobin A (HbA)**, is composed of two α chains and two β chains (written as $\alpha_2\beta_2$).
2. Several common hemoglobinopathies are transmitted as simple mendelian traits.
   a. In **sickle cell anemia**, an autosomal recessive trait, valine replaces the normal glutamic acid in the sixth amino acid position of the β chains, resulting in abnormal erythrocyte morphology, anemia due to excessive erythrocyte destruction, and many other clinical consequences.
      (1) About 10% of all Blacks in the United States are heterozygotes for the sickle gene, due to the fact that a heterozygote is protected partially from malaria.
      (2) When heterozygous carriers mate, 25% of their offspring will be unaffected, 50% will be heterozygous carriers, and 25% will suffer from sickle cell anemia.
   b. The **thalassemias** are also caused by autosomal recessive mutations. In these diseases, the hemoglobin chains are correct in amino acid sequence but are synthesized in unbalanced quantities. The α-thalassemias affect the α chains of hemoglobin, and the β-thalassemias affect the β chains.

B. Phenylketonuria (PKU)

1. Phenylketonuria (PKU) is an autosomal recessive mutation caused by deficiencies in the enzyme responsible for metabolizing phenylalanine, namely **phenylalanine hydroxylase**.
   a. An affected fetus in a normal mother will accumulate phenylalanine in the blood stream and tissues. This results in progressive neurologic damage to the infant after birth, but this damage can be minimized by special dietary restrictions.
   b. Fetuses in mothers with PKU will show mental retardation, microencephaly, and perhaps cardiovascular defects unless the maternal diet is modified to eliminate phenylalanine from it.

2. Newborns are presently screened routinely for PKU in most hospitals.

C. Cystic fibrosis

1. Cystic fibrosis is the most common lethal genetic disease among Caucasians, occurring in about 1 in 2000 newborns. It is transmitted as an autosomal recessive mutation.
2. In cystic fibrosis, there are abnormalities in the secretion products of the glands in the respiratory system and the skin.

D. Other examples of single-gene defects

1. **Adult polycystic kidney disease** is an autosomal dominant trait that is usually not manifested until well into adult life but it is one of the leading causes of renal failure in our country.
2. **Marfan syndrome, achondroplasia,** and several forms of **osteogenesis imperfecta** are also transmitted as autosomal dominant mendelian traits.

VI. NUMERICAL CHROMOSOME ABNORMALITIES—SOME COMMON EXAMPLES

A. General considerations

1. Three of the most commonly encountered **aneuploidies** in human beings are 47, +21 (Down syndrome, trisomy 21), 47, +18 (Edwards syndrome, trisomy 18), and 47, +13 (Patau syndrome, trisomy 13).
2. For all these chromosomal anomalies, there is a striking increase in frequency of occurrence with increasing maternal age (Fig. 24-5). The data in Figure 24-5 have not been corrected for a paternal age effect but the implications are quite clear nevertheless.

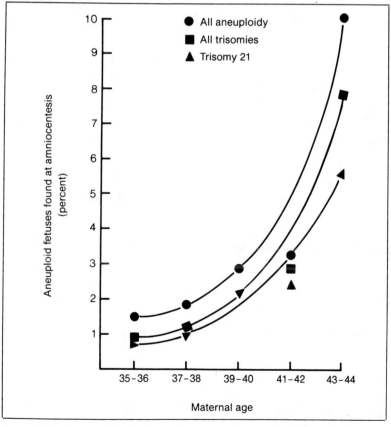

Figure 24-5. Age-specific risk that amniocentesis will demonstrate an aneuploid fetus. (Redrawn from Simpson JL, et al: *Genetics in Obstetrics and Gynecology.* New York, Grune and Stratton, 1982, p 103.)

3. In most centers at the present time, women aged 35 years and older are monitored by **amniocentesis** and **cytogenetic screening**, unless there is some specific contraindication for the amniocentesis.
   a. As described in Chapters 22 and 23, amniotic fluid and the fetal cells contained in it can be used for both biochemical and cytogenetic studies.
   b. In many cases of congenital anomalies, this allows a reliable prenatal diagnosis, especially when the obstetrician is aided by diagnostic sonography.
4. In the case of the commonly encountered numerical anomalies, **genetic counseling** of the parents is relatively straightforward, assuming that a correct clinical diagnosis of the afflicted child has been made and this diagnosis has been supported by karyotype analysis of the child and, in some cases, of both parents as well.

B. **Recurrence risk in Down syndrome**
   1. The clinical entity known as Down syndrome exemplifies the importance of karyotype analysis in predicting recurrence risk and thus its importance in genetic counseling.
      a. Down syndrome can be due either to 47, +21 or to several different translocation possibilities, usually 46, t (14q;21q).
      b. The **risk of recurrence** is considerably different for these two cytogenetically different manifestations of a single clinical syndrome.
         (1) In the former instance, the **proband** (afflicted child) is simply **trisomic for chromosome 21**. Here, the risk that Down syndrome will recur in another child born later is probably quite close to the risk of occurrence after maternal age is taken into consideration.
         (2) In the latter case, the proband has the long arm of chromosome 21 translocated to the long arm of chromosome 14 (**translocation Down syndrome**). Even though the proband is clinically very like the proband with simple trisomy 21, the risk of recurrence is much different.
            (a) In some cases when the proband is **46, t (14q;21q)**, one **parent** may be **45, t (14q;21q)**, and in this instance the recurrence risk theoretically would be 33%.
            (b) In actuality, however, the risk appears to be considerably less than 33%. For unknown reasons, it is more like 10% if the mother carries the translocation and 2% to 3% if the father carries it.
   2. The clinician should search for translocation Down syndrome when the clinical features of the syndrome are detected in probands born to young mothers, since the occurrence risk of 47, +21 Down syndrome in younger women is relatively low.
   3. In clinical practice, about 95% of all infants with Down syndrome will prove to be 47, +21, while the remaining cases will be due to a translocation, including the 46, t (14q;21q) type.

C. **Recurrence risk in other major chromosomal numerical anomalies**
   1. **Edwards syndrome**
      a. About 80% of the probands with Edwards syndrome are **47, +18 (trisomy 18)**, and the remaining 20% are either mosaics or translocations.
      b. It appears that the recurrence risk for this syndrome is about 1%.
   2. **Patau syndrome**
      a. About 80% of the probands with Patau syndrome are **47, +13 (trisomy 13)**, and the remaining 20% are translocations.
      b. The recurrence risk is somewhere around 1%.
         (1) The recurrence rate is negligible if the proband is 47, +13 (due to the low frequency of occurrence in the first place).
         (2) The recurrence rate is slightly higher than 1% if one or both of the parents are translocation carriers.

VII. DEFECTS PRESUMED TO BE POLYGENIC OR MULTIFACTORIAL

A. **Neural tube defects**
   1. As stated earlier, often it is not possible to distinguish between defects caused by a combination of several mutations and defects caused by an interaction between genome and environment—that is, between defects that are polygenic and defects that are the result of multifactorial inheritance.
   2. For example, the **frequency** of neural tube defects such as anencephaly or myelomeningocele varies greatly in different ethnic groups (see Chapter 23, Table 23-1), suggesting that

there is a subtle interplay between heredity and environment in the etiology of neural tube defects.
  a. The incidence is as high as 1% in some parts of Wales and Northern Ireland, and is much lower among Blacks in the United States.
  b. Welsh and Irish people in America show an increased incidence in comparison to American Blacks. However, the incidence is lower for Irish in America than for Irish in Ireland.
3. The **recurrence risk** of neural tube defects is also different in different populations.
  a. The recurrence risk in the British Isles is taken to be about 5% after one afflicted child and about 12% after two afflicted siblings.
  b. The comparable figures for the United States are estimated to be about 2% and 5% respectively.

B. **Other congenital anomalies caused by multifactorial inheritance**
  1. Many other common congenital anomalies are caused by multifactorial inheritance, including:
    a. Cleft lip and cleft palate
    b. Cardiovascular anomalies
    c. Tracheoesophageal fistula
    d. Pyloric stenosis
    e. Omphalocele
    f. Horseshoe kidney
    g. Bladder exstrophy
    h. Cryptorchidism
    i. Hip dysplasia
  2. These congenital anomalies have a recurrence risk of 1% to 5% when a single proband is afflicted.

VIII. THE FUTURE AND THE HOPE OF CORRECTING GENETIC DEFECTS

A. **Recent scientific advances.** In the last three decades, there has been revolutionary scientific progress in understanding genetic function as the result of studies conducted in lower life forms.
  1. Only 36 years after the publication of Watson and Crick's paper outlining the molecular basis for genetic transmission, scientists have learned how to map genes to the level of individual nucleotide resolution.
  2. They have been able to synthesize large genes in vitro.
  3. They have also controlled the transmission of genes from one organism into another.
    a. Recently, a genetic trait was transferred into early mouse embryos in vitro.
    b. These altered embryos were then transplanted into foster mothers, where there was clear evidence of expression of the transduced genes.

B. **Techniques for correction of genetic defects**
  1. **In vitro fertilization**
    a. At this writing, thousands of children have been born as a result of in vitro fertilization (see Chapter 4, section IX).
    b. It is only a matter of time before it will be possible to do a complex genetic analysis of prospective parents to identify those who are likely to give birth to genetically abnormal offspring.
    c. These parents could have normal children by serving as surrogate parents for genetically normal zygotes.
  2. **Genetic manipulation**
    a. In the not too distant future, it will also be possible to predict genetic lesions in zygotes and correct them with appropriately directed genetic vectors.
    b. Perhaps, for example, the gene for sickle cell anemia or phenylketonuria could be specifically removed from the genome and replaced by synthetic genes capable of synthesizing normal proteins and thus curing the genetic lesion in offspring.
    c. These possibilities are not the stuff of science fiction, because similar experiments are currently being performed with success in laboratory animals.
      (1) For example, the genes for growth hormone have been transferred into genetically

dwarfed mouse embryos and these corrected embryos have then been transferred to female mice.
(2) Normal offspring have resulted from such manipulations.
d. In animal husbandry, embryo transfer and surrogate motherhood are already being used to improve meat production, speed, and strength of domestic animals.
e. It will only be a matter of time before certain human traits can be propagated and other traits eliminated from the human gene pool. For example, it might be possible to remove cancer susceptibility genes or the genes controlling aggressive behavior from the human gene pool.

C. Ethical problems
1. It should be clear from the above discussion that the scientific possibilities have already outstripped our ethical sophistication.
    a. Scientists are racing forward with the technology of genetic engineering. Surrogate parenting is technologically feasible but complex ethical and legal questions, still to be resolved, complicate matters.
    b. Simultaneously, major world religions flatly denounce this new technology as immoral and unethical.
    c. Even worse, world political leaders continue to push the technology of nuclear annihilation and stockpile weapons capable of ending all human life on the planet with the touch of a button while at the same time ignoring the enormous potential for correcting many diseases by way of genetic engineering.
2. The **ethical issues** that will surround the application of genetic engineering technology to human beings are indeed most complex, as a few **examples** will show:
    a. Why should we spend resources on improving parts of the human gene pool while much of the human race is malnourished or starving to death?
    b. Is correction of phenylketonuria more desirable than dealing with drug addiction or schizophrenia?
    c. Who will decide which human traits are to be propagated and which are to be eliminated?
    d. What are the long-term consequences of manipulation of the human genome?
    e. Who is responsible for the birth of a child with a new congenital defect following efforts to correct another defect?
3. The scientists and medical practitioners of the future will be faced with difficult ethical decisions in this regard.
4. We need to establish a list of priorities for the betterment of the human race, after we have solved the obvious problem of our own extermination by nuclear weapons.
    a. Population control and the use of genetic engineering to improve the food supply may eventually help to solve problems of overpopulation and malnutrition.
    b. Then we could begin the fascinating task of improving the human species that has evolved so far without significant human intervention.

STUDY QUESTIONS

Directions: Each question below contains four suggested answers of which **one or more** is correct. Choose the answer

- A if **1, 2, and 3** are correct
- B if **1 and 3** are correct
- C if **2 and 4** are correct
- D if **4** is correct
- E if **1, 2, 3, and 4** are correct

1. Autosomal dominant mutations show which of the following patterns of expression?

   (1) Expressed in all progeny if either parent carries the gene
   (2) Expressed in 50% of male children
   (3) Expressed in 50% of female children
   (4) Expressed in 75% of progeny if both parents are heterozygotes

2. Autosomal recessive mutations show which of the following patterns of expression?

   (1) Expressed in 25% of progeny if both parents are heterozygotes
   (2) Expressed in 25% of progeny if one parent is homozygous wild-type and one parent is heterozygous
   (3) Expressed in none of the progeny if one parent is homozygous recessive and one parent is homozygous wild-type
   (4) Expressed in none of the progeny if both parents are heterozygotes

3. Which of the following would be caused by a single-gene defect?

   (1) Cleft lip
   (2) Phenylketonuria
   (3) Neural tube defects
   (4) Achondroplasia

4. Anomalies caused by multifactorial inheritance include which of the following?

   (1) Adult polycystic kidney disease
   (2) Cystic fibrosis
   (3) Marfan syndrome
   (4) Horseshoe kidney

5. Which of the following congenital anomalies would show increased incidence with increased maternal age?

   (1) Down syndrome
   (2) Treacher Collins syndrome
   (3) Patau syndrome
   (4) Sickle cell anemia

Directions: The group of questions below consists of lettered choices followed by several numbered items. For each numbered item select the **one** lettered choice with which it is **most** closely associated. Each lettered choice may be used once, more than once, or not at all.

Questions 6-10

Match each of the descriptions below with the type of congenital anomaly that it best describes.

(A) Phenylketonuria

(B) Sickle cell anemia

(C) β-Thalassemia

(D) Down syndrome

(E) Neural tube defect

6. Caused by aneuploidy

7. Caused by a single-gene substitution of valine for glutamic acid in hemoglobin β chains

8. A multifactorial congenital anomaly

9. Characterized by accumulation of phenylalanine in blood

10. Characterized by reduced synthesis of hemoglobin β chains

ANSWERS AND EXPLANATIONS

1. The answer is D (4). *(IV B 2)* Autosomal dominant genes are expressed in all progeny only if both parents are homozygotes. Autosomal dominant expression has no relationship to the sex of progeny, as sex-linked traits do. If both parents are heterozygotes for an autosomal dominant gene, then 25% of the progeny would be homozygous wild-type, 50% would be heterozygotes (expressed), and 25% would be homozygous mutant (expressed). Therefore, 75% of the progeny would have expression of the gene.

2. The answer is B (1, 3). *(IV B 3)* If both parents are heterozygotes for an autosomal recessive mutation, 25% of the progeny would be homozygous mutants (expressed), 50% would be heterozygous (not expressed), and 25% would be homozygous wild-type (not expressed). If one parent is homozygous wild-type and one parent is heterozygous, none of the progeny would express the recessive mutation. If one parent is homozygous recessive and the other is homozygous wild-type, none of the progeny would receive two doses of the gene. If both of the parents were heterozygotes, 25% of the progeny would be homozygous mutants and would show expression of the recessive mutation.

3. The answer is C (2, 4). *(V B, D 2; VII A, B 1 a)* Many congenital birth defects are caused by a poorly understood multifactorial mechanism. Traits caused by a multifactorial mechanism are due to a subtle interplay between heredity and the environment. Cleft lip and neural tube defects are caused by multifactorial inheritance. Phenylketonuria and achondroplasia are caused by single-gene defects. The inheritance of such defects follows simple mendelian laws.

4. The answer is D (4). *(V C, D; VII B 1 f)* Of the disorders listed in the question, only horseshoe kidney is caused by multifactorial inheritance. In horseshoe kidney, there is a single kidney shaped like a horseshoe. This is due to fusion of the caudal portions of the metanephric kidneys, resulting in a single kidney with fusion at the caudal pole rather than two separate kidneys. Adult polycystic kidney disease, cystic fibrosis, and Marfan syndrome are all caused by single-gene defects.

5. The answer is B (1, 3). *(Chapter 18 VI B; Chapter 24 V A 2; VI A 1, 2)* Down syndrome and Patau syndrome are aneuploid conditions due to nondisjunction, which usually shows an increase in frequency with maternal age. Treacher Collins syndrome (first arch syndrome, mandibulofacial dysostosis) is caused by an autosomal dominant mutation, and sickle cell anemia is caused by an autosomal recessive mutation. Mutations that behave in a simple mendelian manner do not show striking increases in frequency with maternal age.

6–10. The answers are: 6-D, 7-B, 8-E, 9-A, 10-C. *(V A 2, B; VI A 1; VII A)* Phenylketonuria (A) is a genetic disease caused by an autosomal recessive mutation affecting phenylalanine hydroxylase activity. Because of this enzymatic deficiency, phenylalanine accumulates in blood and tissue fluids. Sickle cell anemia (B) is caused by a single gene affecting the amino acid sequence in the globin gene of hemoglobin. β-Thalassemia (C) is caused by a single gene affecting the rate of globin synthesis in hemoglobin. Down syndrome (D) is caused in 95% of the cases by trisomy of chromosome 21, resulting in aneuploidy or an abnormal number of chromosomes. About 5% of the cases of Down syndrome are caused by translocation and patients therefore have a normal number of chromosomes. Neural tube defects (E) such as spina bifida or anencephaly are caused by multifactorial inheritance.

Challenge Exam

Introduction

One of the least attractive aspects of pursuing an education is the necessity of being examined on what has been learned. Instructors do not like to prepare tests, and students do not like to take them.

However, students are required to take many examinations during their learning careers, and little if any time is spent acquainting them with the positive aspects of tests and with systematic and successful methods for approaching them. Students perceive tests as punitive and sometimes feel that they are merely opportunities for the instructor to discover what the student has forgotten or has never learned. Students need to view tests as opportunities to display their knowledge and to use them as tools for developing prescriptions for further study and learning.

A brief history and discussion of the National Board of Medical Examiners (NBME) examinations (i.e., Parts I, II, and III and FLEX) are presented in this preface, along with ideas concerning psychological preparation for the examinations. Also presented are general considerations and test-taking tips as well as how practice exams can be used as educational tools. (The literature provided by the various examination boards contains detailed information concerning the construction and scoring of specific exams.)

National Board of Medical Examiners Examinations

Before the various NBME exams were developed, each state attempted to license physicians through its own procedures. Differences between the quality and testing procedures of the various state examinations resulted in the refusal of some states to recognize the licensure of physicians licensed in other states. This made it difficult for physicians to move freely from one state to another and produced an uneven quality of medical care in the United States.

To remedy this situation, the various state medical boards decided they would be better served if an outside agency prepared standard exams to be given in all states, allowing each state to meet its own needs and have a common standard by which to judge the educational preparation of individuals applying for licensure.

One misconception concerning these outside agencies is that they are licensing authorities. This is not the case; they are examination boards only. The individual states retain the power to grant and revoke licenses. The examination boards are charged with designing and scoring valid and reliable tests. They are primarily concerned with providing the states with feedback on how examinees have performed and with making suggestions about the interpretation and usefulness of scores. The states use this information as partial fulfillment of qualifications upon which they grant licenses.

Students should remember that these exams are administered nationwide and, although the general medical information is similar, educational methodologies and faculty areas of expertise differ from institution to institution. It is unrealistic to expect that students will know all the material presented in the exams; they may face questions on the exams in areas that were only superficially covered in their classes. The testing authorities recognize this situation, and their scoring procedures take it into account.

Scoring the Exams

The diversity of curriculum necessitates that these tests be scored using a criteria-based normal curve. An individual score is based not only on how many questions were answered correctly by a specific student but also on how this one performance relates to the distribution of all scores of the criteria group. In the case of NBME, Part I, the criteria group consists of those students who have completed 2 years of medical training in the United States and are taking the test for the first time and those students who took the test during the previous four June sittings.

Since this test has been constructed to measure a wide range of educational situations, the mean, or average, score generally can be achieved by answering 64% to 68% of the questions correctly. Passing the exam requires answering correctly 55% to 60% of the questions. The competition for acceptance into medical school and the performance levels necessary to stay in school are so high that many students who have always achieved these high levels naturally assume they must perform in a similar fashion and attain equivalent scores on the NBME exams. This is not the case. In fact, among students who are accustomed to performing at levels exceeding 80% to 90%, fewer than 4% taking these tests perform at that high level. Unrealistically high personal expectations leave students psychologically unprepared for these tests, and the anxiety of the moment renders them incapable of doing their best work.

Actually, **most students have learned quite well**, but they fail to display this learning when they are tested because they do not understand the construction, purpose, or scoring procedures of board exams. It is imperative that they understand that they are **not** expected to score as well as they have in the past and that the measurement criteria is group performance, not only individual performance.

While preparing for an exam, it is important that students learn as much as they can about the subject they will be tested on as well as prepare to discover just how much they may not know. Students should study to acquire knowledge, not just to prepare for tests. **For the well-prepared candidate, the chances of passing far exceed the chances of failing.**

Materials Needed for Test Preparation

In preparation for a test, many students collect far too much study material only to find that they simply do not have the time to go through all of it. They are defeated before they begin because either they cannot get through all the material leaving areas unstudied, or they race through the material so quickly that they cannot benefit from the activity.

It is generally more efficient for the student to use materials already at hand; that is, class notes, one good outline to cover or strengthen areas not locally stressed and for quick review of the whole topic, and one good text as a reference for looking up complex material needing further explanation.

Also, many students attempt to memorize far too much information, rather than learning and understanding less material and then relying on that learned information to determine the answers to questions at the time of the examination. Relying too heavily on memorized material causes anxiety, and the more anxious students become during a test, the less learned knowledge they are likely to use.

Positive Attitude

A positive attitude and a realistic approach are essential to successful test taking. If concentration is placed on the negative aspects of tests or on the potential for failure, anxiety increases and performance decreases. A negative attitude generally develops if the student concentrates on "I must pass" rather than on "I can pass." "What if I fail?" becomes the major factor motivating the student to **run from failure rather than toward success**. This results from placing too much emphasis on scores rather than understanding that scores have only slight relevance to future professional performance.

The score received is only one aspect of test performance. Test performance also indicates the student's ability to use information during evaluation procedures and reveals how this ability might be used in the future. For example, when a patient enters the physician's office with a problem, the physician begins by asking questions, searching for clues, and seeking diagnostic information. Hypotheses are then developed, which will include several potential causes for the problem. Weighing the probabilities, the physician will begin to discard those hypotheses with the least likelihood of being correct. Good differential diagnosis involves the ability to deal with uncertainty, to reduce potential causes to the smallest number, and to use all learned information in arriving at a conclusion.

This same thought process can and should be used in testing situations. It might be termed **paper-and-pencil differential diagnosis**. In each question with five alternatives, of which one is correct, there are four alternatives that are incorrect. If deductive reasoning is used, as in solving a clinical problem, the choices can be viewed as having possibilities of being correct. The elimination of wrong choices increases the odds that a student will be able to recognize the correct choice. Even if the correct choice does not become evident, the probability of guessing correctly increases. Just as differential diagnosis in a clinical setting can result in a correct diagnosis, eliminating incorrect choices on a test can result in choosing the correct answer.

Answering questions based on what is incorrect is difficult for many students since they have had nearly 20 years experience taking tests with the implied assertion that knowledge can be displayed only by knowing what is correct. It must be remembered, however, that students can display knowledge by knowing something is wrong, just as they can display it by knowing something is right. **Students should begin to think in the present as they expect themselves to think in the future**.

Paper-and-Pencil Differential Diagnosis

The technique used to arrive at the answer to the following question is an example of the paper-and-pencil differential diagnosis approach.

A recently diagnosed case of hypothyroidism in a 45-year-old man may result in which of the following conditions?

(A) Thyrotoxicosis
(B) Cretinism
(C) Myxedema
(D) Graves' disease
(E) Hashimoto's thyroiditis

It is presumed that all of the choices presented in the question are plausible and partially correct. If the student begins by breaking the question into parts and trying to discover what the question is attempting to measure, it will be possible to answer the question correctly by using more than memorized charts concerning thyroid problems.

- The question may be testing if the student knows the difference between "hypo" and "hyper" conditions.
- The answer choices may include thyroid problems that are not "hypothyroid" problems.
- It is possible that one or more of the choices are "hypo" but are not "thyroid" problems, that they are some other endocrine problems.
- "Recently diagnosed in a 45-year-old man" indicates that the correct answer is not a congenital childhood problem.
- "May result in" as opposed to "resulting from" suggests that the choices might include a problem that **causes** hypothyroidism rather than **results from** hypothyroidism, as stated.

By applying this kind of reasoning, the student can see that choice **A**, thyroid toxicosis, which is a disorder resulting from an overactive thyroid gland ("hyper") must be eliminated. Another piece of knowledge, that is, Graves' disease is thyroid toxicosis, eliminates choice **D**. Choice **B**, cretinism, is indeed hypothyroidism, but it is a childhood disorder. Therefore, **B** is eliminated. Choice **E** is an inflammation of the thyroid gland—here the clue is the suffix "itis." The reasoning is that thyroiditis, being an inflammation, may **cause** a thyroid problem, perhaps even a hypothyroid problem, but there is no reason for the reverse to be true. Myxedema, choice **C**, is the only choice left and the obvious correct answer.

Preparing for Board Examinations

1. **Study for yourself.** Although some of the material may seem irrelevant, the more you learn now, the less you will have to learn later. Also, do not let the fear of the test rob you of an important part of your education. If you study to learn, the task is less distasteful than studying solely to pass a test.

2. **Review all areas.** You should not be selective by studying perceived weak areas and ignoring perceived strong areas. This is probably the last time you will have the time and the motivation to review **all** of the basic sciences.

3. **Attempt to understand, not just to memorize, the material.** Ask yourself: To whom does the material apply? When does it apply? Where does it apply? How does it apply? Understanding the connections among these points allows for longer retention and aids in those situations when guessing strategies may be needed.

4. Try to **anticipate questions that might appear on the test.** Ask yourself how you might construct a question on a specific topic.

5. **Give yourself a couple days of rest before the test.** Studying up to the last moment will increase your anxiety and cause potential confusion.

Taking Board Examinations

1. In the case of NBME exams, be sure to **pace yourself** to use the time optimally. As soon as you get your test booklet, go through and circle the questions numbered 40, 80, 120, and 160. The test is constructed so that you will have approximately 45 seconds for each question. If you are at a circled number every 30 minutes, you will be right on schedule. A 2-hour test will have 150–170 questions and a 2½-hour test will have approximately 200 questions. You should use all of your allotted time; if you finish too early, you probably did so by moving too quickly through the test.

2. **Read each question and all the alternatives carefully** before you begin to make decisions. Remember the questions contain clues, as do the answer choices. As a physician, you would not make a clinical decision without a complete examination of all the data; the same holds true for answering test questions.

3. **Read the directions for each question set carefully.** You would be amazed at how many students make mistakes in tests simply because they have not paid close attention to the directions.

4. It is not advisable to leave blanks with the intention of coming back to answer the questions later. Because of the way board examinations are constructed, you probably will not pick up any new information that will help you when you come back, and the chances of getting numerically off on your answer sheet are greater than your chances of benefiting by skipping around. If you feel that you must come back to a question, mark the best choice and place a note in the margin. Generally speaking, it is best not to change answers once you have made a decision, unless you have learned new information. Your intuitive reaction and first response are correct more often than changes made out of frustration or anxiety. **Never turn in an answer sheet with blanks**. Scores are based on the number that you get correct; you are not penalized for incorrect choices.

5. **Do not try to answer the questions on a stimulus–response basis.** It generally will not work. Use all of your learned knowledge.

6. **Do not let anxiety destroy your confidence.** If you have prepared conscientiously, you know enough to pass. Use all that you have learned.

7. **Do not try to determine how well you are doing as you proceed.** You will not be able to make an objective assessment, and your anxiety will increase.

8. **Do not expect a feeling of mastery** or anything close to what you are accustomed. Remember, this is a nationally administered exam, not a mastery test.

9. **Do not become frustrated or angry** about what appear to be bad or difficult questions. You simply do not know the answers; you cannot know everything.

Specific Test-Taking Strategies

Read the entire question carefully, regardless of format. Test questions have multiple parts. Concentrate on picking out the pertinent key words that might help you begin to problem solve. Words such as "always," "all," "never," "mostly," "primarily," and so forth play significant roles. In all types of questions, distractors with terms such as "always" or "never" most often are incorrect. Adjectives and adverbs can completely change the meaning of questions—pay close attention to them. Also, medical prefixes and suffixes (e.g., "hypo-," "hyper-," "-ectomy," "-itis") are sometimes at the root of the question. The knowledge and application of everyday English grammar often is the key to dissecting questions.

Multiple-Choice Questions

Read the question and the choices carefully to become familiar with the data as given. Remember, in multiple-choice questions there is one correct answer and there are four distractors, or incorrect answers. (Distractors are plausible and possibly correct or they would not be called distractors.) They are generally correct for part of the question but not for the entire question. Dissecting the question into parts aids in discerning these distractors.

If the correct answer is not immediately evident, begin eliminating the distractors. (Many students feel that they must always start at option A and make a decision before they move to B, thus forcing decisions they are not ready to make.) Your first decisions should be made on those choices you feel the most confident about.

Compare the choices to each part of the question. **To be wrong**, a choice needs to be incorrect for only part of the question. **To be correct**, it must be **totally** correct. If you believe a choice is partially incorrect, tentatively eliminate that choice. Make notes next to the choices regarding tentative decisions. One method is to place a minus sign next to the choices you are certain are incorrect and a plus sign next to those that potentially are correct. Finally, place a zero next to any choice you do not understand or need to come back to for further inspection. Do not feel that you must make final decisions until you have examined all choices carefully.

When you have eliminated as many choices as you can, decide which of those that are left has the highest probability of being correct. Remember to use paper-and-pencil differential diagnosis. Above all, be honest with yourself. If you do not know the answer, eliminate as many choices as possible and choose reasonably.

Multiple True-False Questions

Multiple true-false questions are not as difficult as some students make them. These are the questions in which you must mark:

- A if **1, 2, and 3** are correct,
- B if **1 and 3** are correct,
- C if **2 and 4** are correct,
- D if only **4** is correct, or
- E if **all** are correct.

Remember that the name for this type of question is multiple true–false and then use this concept. Become familiar with each choice and make notes. Then concentrate on the one choice you feel is definitely incorrect. If you can find one incorrect alternative, you can eliminate three choices immediately and be down to a fifty–fifty probability of guessing the correct answer. In this format, if choice 1 is incorrect, so is choice 3; they go together. Alternatively, if 1 is correct, so is 3. The combinations of alternatives are constant; they will not be mixed. You will not find a situation where choice 1 is correct, but 3 is incorrect.

After eliminating the choices you are sure are incorrect, concentrate on the choice that will make your final decision. For instance, if you discard choice 1, you have eliminated alternatives A, B, and E. This leaves C (2 and 4) and D (4 only). Concentrate on choice 2, and decide if it is true or false. Rereading and concentrating on choice 4 only wastes time; choice 2 will be the decision maker. (Take the path of least resistance and concentrate on the smallest possible number of items while making a decision.) Obviously, if none of the choices is found to be incorrect, the answer is E (all).

Comparison-Matching Questions

Comparison-matching questions are also easier to address if you concentrate on one alternative at a time. Choose option:

- A if the question is associated with **(A) only**,
- B if the question is associated with **(B) only**,
- C if the question is associated with **both (A) and (B)**, or
- D if the question is associated with **neither (A) nor (B)**.

Here again, the elimination of obvious wrong alternatives helps clear away needless information and can help you make a clearer decision.

Single Best Answer–Matching Sets

Single best answer–matching sets consist of a list of words or statements followed by several numbered items or statements. Be sure to pay attention to whether the choices can be used more than once, only once, or not at all. Consider each choice individually and carefully. Begin with those with which you are the most familiar. It is important always to break the statements and words into parts, as with all other question formats. **If a choice is only partially correct, then it is incorrect.**

Guessing

Nothing takes the place of a firm knowledge base, but with little information to work with, even after playing paper-and-pencil differential diagnosis, you may find it necessary to guess at the correct answer. A few simple rules can help increase your guessing accuracy. Always guess consistently if you have no idea what is correct; that is, after eliminating all that you can, make the choice that agrees with your intuition or choose the option closest to the top of the list that has not been eliminated as a potential answer.

When guessing at questions that present with choices in numerical form, you will often find the choices listed in an ascending or descending order. It is generally not wise to guess the first or last alternative, since these are usually extreme values and are most likely incorrect.

Using the Challenge Exam to Learn

All too often, students do not take full advantage of practice exams. There is a tendency to complete the exam, score it, look up the correct answers to those questions missed, and then forget the entire thing.

In fact, great educational benefits can be derived if students would spend more time using practice tests as learning tools. As mentioned earlier, incorrect choices in test questions are plausible and partially correct or they would not fulfill their purpose as distractors. This means that it is just as beneficial to look up the incorrect choices as the correct choices to discover specifically why they are incorrect. In this way, it is possible to learn better test-taking skills as the subtlety of question construction is uncovered.

Additionally, it is advisable to go back and attempt to restructure each question to see if all the choices can be made correct by modifying the question. By doing this, four times as much will be learned. By all means, look up the right answer and explanation. Then, focus on each of the other choices and ask yourself under what conditions they might be correct? For example, the entire thrust of the sample question concerning hypothyroidism could be altered by changing the first few words to read:

"Hyperthyroidism recently discovered in. . . . ."

"Hypothyroidism prenatally occurring in. . . . ."

"Hypothyroidism resulting from. . . . ."

This question can be used to learn and understand thyroid problems in general, not only to memorize answers to specific questions.

The Challenge Exam that follows contains 180 questions and explanations. Every effort has been made to simulate the types of questions and the degree of question difficulty in the various licensure and qualifying exams (i.e., NBME Parts I, II, and III and FLEX). While taking this exam, the student should attempt to create the testing conditions that might be experienced during actual testing situations. Approximately 1 minute should be allowed for each question, and the entire test should be finished before it is scored.

Summary

Ideally, examinations are designed to determine how much information students have learned and how that information is used in the successful completion of the examination. Students will be successful if these suggestions are followed:
- Develop a positive attitude and maintain that attitude.
- Be realistic in determining the amount of material you attempt to master and in the score you hope to attain.
- Read the directions for each type of question and the questions themselves closely and follow the directions carefully.
- Guess intelligently and consistently when guessing strategies must be used.
- Bring the paper-and-pencil differential diagnosis approach to each question in the examination.

- Use the test as an opportunity to display your knowledge and as a tool for developing prescriptions for further study and learning.

National Board examinations are not easy. They may be almost impossible for those who have unrealistic expectations or for those who allow misinformation concerning the exams to produce anxiety out of proportion to the task at hand. They are manageable if they are approached with a positive attitude and with consistent use of all the information the student has learned.

Michael P. O'Donnell

QUESTIONS

Directions: Each question below contains five suggested answers. Choose the **one best** response to each question.

1. All of the following are true statements about liver development EXCEPT

    (A) the liver parenchymal cells are derived from the liver diverticulum
    (B) hepatic duct epithelial cells are derived from splanchnic mesoderm
    (C) the hepatic sinusoidal endothelium is derived from vitelline and umbilical vessels
    (D) rapid growth of the liver causes the liver to fill much of the peritoneal cavity during early gastrointestinal development
    (E) the liver is a hematopoietic organ after the yolk sac

2. All of the following statements about neurulation are true EXCEPT

    (A) neural crest cells leave the neuroectoderm before neural tube closure
    (B) neural plate tissue invaginates to form a neural groove
    (C) the notochord and paraxial mesoderm induce neural plate formation
    (D) the neural crest induces the formation of neural arches
    (E) the neural groove closes into a neural tube

3. All of the following are characteristics of α-fetoprotein EXCEPT

    (A) it is a fetal blood protein
    (B) it is elevated in the maternal serum if the fetus has an open neural tube defect
    (C) it is elevated in the amniotic fluid if the fetus has an open neural tube defect
    (D) it is present in fetal cerebrospinal fluid
    (E) it can be used for definitive diagnosis of neural tube defects without other tests

4. All of the following adult or embryonic structures are derivatives of the second pharyngeal arch system EXCEPT

    (A) the masseter muscle
    (B) the orbicularis oculi muscle
    (C) Reichert's cartilage
    (D) the stapes
    (E) the lesser horn of the hyoid bone

5. The primordial germ cells differentiate into many distinct cell types in a sexually mature adult. These cell types include all of the following EXCEPT

    (A) spermatids
    (B) polar bodies
    (C) ova
    (D) Sertoli cells
    (E) spermatogonia

6. Respiratory distress syndrome is characterized by all of the following EXCEPT

    (A) it is a leading cause of death in premature infants
    (B) it results from premature maturation of type II cells
    (C) it is caused by an insufficiency of surfactant
    (D) babies with this syndrome would have abnormally low amounts of lecithin in lung lavages
    (E) it would be very likely to occur in a 25-week fetus

7. All of the following are true statements about the rotation of the gut tube EXCEPT

    (A) the first rotation of the stomach elongates the dorsal mesogastrium
    (B) the second rotation of the stomach carries the greater omentum into its location in the frontal plane
    (C) the initial rotation of the midgut loop brings the cecal bud superior to the cranial limb of the midgut
    (D) the entire counterclockwise rotation of the midgut loop occurs while it is herniated into the umbilical cord
    (E) in all, the midgut loop undergoes a 270° counterclockwise rotation

8. All of the following statements concerning gametogenesis are true EXCEPT

    (A) there are more male gametes than female gametes
    (B) meiosis in males is completed in the testes
    (C) meiosis in females is completed just before ovulation
    (D) the secondary oocyte contains a diploid amount of DNA
    (E) the second polar body is a haploid cell

Questions 9–11

Examine the accompanying karyotype, and then answer the following questions concerning this karyotype.

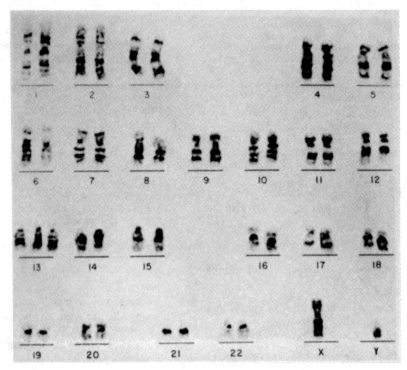

9. Which clinical syndrome is most often associated with this particular karyotype?

(A) Down syndrome
(B) Edwards syndrome
(C) Patau syndrome
(D) Turner syndrome
(E) Klinefelter syndrome

10. Which shorthand designation would be an appropriate description of this karyotype?

(A) 47, XY, +21
(B) 47, XY, +13
(C) 47, XY, +18
(D) 47, XXY
(E) 45, X

11. Which of the following symptoms is associated with this disease but is not a prominent feature of other chromosomal anomalies?

(A) Mental retardation
(B) Shortened life span
(C) Cleft lip and palate
(D) Broad trunk and flat nose
(E) Prominent occiput

12. All of the following statements about the decidua are true EXCEPT

(A) the decidua basalis becomes part of the definitive placenta
(B) the decidua limits syncytiotrophoblast invasion
(C) the decidua parietalis forms part of the wall of the uterine cavity
(D) the decidua vera forms from fusion of the decidual capsularis and the decidua parietalis
(E) most of the decidual tissue remains in the uterus and is resorbed after birth

13. Mandibulofacial dysostosis exhibits all of the following characteristics and clinical findings EXCEPT

(A) mandibular hypoplasia
(B) autosomal dominant inheritance
(C) deafness
(D) auricular anomalies
(E) mental retardation

14. All of the following statements about neurulation are true EXCEPT

(A) failure of the neural groove to close can result in neural tube defects
(B) Neurulation precedes gastrulation
(C) the lumen of the neural tube persists as the brain ventricles
(D) the neural plate results from thickening of ectoderm
(E) the ectoderm lateral to the neural plate forms epidermis

15. All of the following statements about embryonic and fetal urine production are true EXCEPT

(A) the pronephros forms copious hypertonic urine
(B) the mesonephros forms hypotonic urine
(C) polyhydramnios can be due to fetal swallowing disorders
(D) fetuses urinate into the amniotic fluid
(E) oligohydramnios can be due to renal agenesis

16. Rh isoimmunization shows all of the following characteristics EXCEPT

(A) it is usually more severe in second and third pregnancies than in the first pregnancy
(B) it occurs because the fetus mounts an immunologic response to maternal decidual antigens
(C) it leads to destruction of fetal red blood cells
(D) it is seen with an Rh-negative mother
(E) it is a common cause of erythroblastosis fetalis

17. All of the following are features of heart development EXCEPT

(A) the heart is the first organ to begin its physiologic function
(B) the angiogenetic cell clusters giving rise to the heart originate cranial to the oropharyngeal membrane
(C) the ventral mesocardium breaks down after heart looping
(D) the myoepicardial mantle forms cardiac myocytes
(E) the cardiac endothelium is derived from mesenchyme

18. All of the following adult or embryonic structures are derivatives of the first pharyngeal arch system EXCEPT

(A) the lateral palatine processes
(B) the palatine tonsils
(C) the maxilla
(D) Meckel's cartilage
(E) the intermaxillary segment

19. All of the following statements concerning spermatogenesis are true EXCEPT

(A) it ends at about age 55 years
(B) spermatogonia are present prior to puberty
(C) spermatozoa are present after puberty
(D) primary spermatocytes contain paired homologs
(E) spermatids are haploid cells with haploid DNA

20. The frequency of neural tube defects shows all of the following relationships EXCEPT

(A) higher frequency in Irish than in Blacks
(B) higher frequency in Boston than in Dublin
(C) higher frequency in Massachusetts than in California
(D) higher frequency in the United Kingdom than in the United States
(E) higher frequency in Connecticut than in Florida

Questions 21–22

Examine the accompanying karyotype, and then answer the following questions concerning this karyotype.

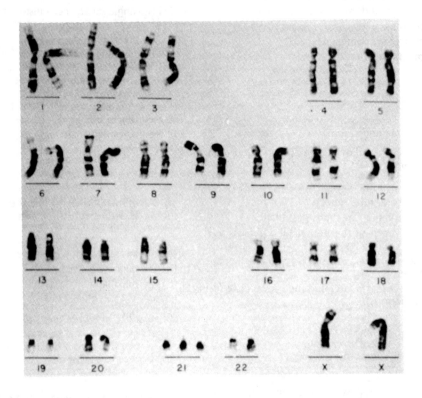

21. The patient with this karyotype would be likely to exhibit all of the following physical or clinical signs EXCEPT

(A) mental retardation
(B) a testis
(C) a shortened life span
(D) a protruding tongue
(E) a simian palmar crease

23. The syncytiotrophoblast shows all of the following features EXCEPT

(A) an abundance of rough endoplasmic reticulum
(B) a scanty Golgi apparatus
(C) many mitochondria
(D) few intercellular junctions between syncytial cells
(E) many cytoplasmic transport vesicles and vacuoles

22. Which shorthand description of this karyotype is most appropriate?

(A) 45, X
(B) 46, XX
(C) 46, XY
(D) 47, XX, +21
(E) 47, XXY

Directions: Each question below contains four suggested answers of which **one or more** is correct. Choose the answer

- A if **1, 2, and 3** are correct
- B if **1 and 3** are correct
- C if **2 and 4** are correct
- D if **4** is correct
- E if **1, 2, 3, and 4** are correct

24. Which of the following pairs of cells share the same embryologic origin?

(1) Leydig cells and thecal cells
(2) Spermatogonia and follicular epithelial cells
(3) Oogonia and spermatozoa
(4) Sertoli cells and polar bodies

25. Ectodermal derivatives include which of the following?

(1) Enamel of teeth
(2) Epidermis
(3) Fingernails
(4) Cardiovascular endothelium

26. The developmental fate of the third pharyngeal arch is correctly described by which of the following statements?

(1) It is innervated by the glossopharyngeal nerve
(2) If forms the anterior belly of the digastric muscle
(3) It forms part of the hyoid bone
(4) It forms the posterior belly of the digastric muscle

27. True statements concerning limb buds include which of the following?

(1) The apical ectodermal ridge induces mesenchymal differentiation
(2) Limb bud mesenchyme forms bone and ligaments
(3) Cell death contributes to digit formation
(4) The hindlimb buds arise after the forelimb buds

28. The notochord shows which of the following characteristics?

(1) It forms the annulus fibrosus
(2) It forms the nucleus pulposus
(3) It persists in the vertebral bodies in adults
(4) It is restricted to the embryonic axis cranial to the primitive node

29. Neural crest derivatives include which of the following?

(1) Schwann cells
(2) Neurons in dorsal root ganglia
(3) Neurons in sympathetic ganglia
(4) Neurons in the spinal cord

30. The developing parathyroid glands are correctly characterized by which of the following statements?

(1) The inferior parathyroids arise from the cranial portion of the third pharyngeal pouch
(2) The superior parathyroids arise from the caudal portion of the third pharyngeal pouch
(3) The parathyroid glands can be variable in location and number
(4) Their oxyphil cells begin to appear by the tenth week

31. True statements concerning the intraembryonic coelom include which of the following?

(1) It is the precursor of the body cavities
(2) It extends cranial to the oropharyngeal membrane prior to head flexion
(3) Its caudal components contribute to the peritoneal cavity
(4) It is in communication with the extraembryonic coelom early in development

32. True statements concerning type II alveolar cells in the developing lungs include which of the following?

(1) Type II cells differentiate from cells in the respiratory diverticulum
(2) They secrete chiefly sphingomyelin
(3) Their state of differentiation can be estimated clinically
(4) They begin to secrete surfactant during the twentieth week of development

SUMMARY OF DIRECTIONS				
A	B	C	D	E
1, 2, 3 only	1, 3 only	2, 4 only	4 only	All are correct

33. Gastrulation shows which of the following characteristics?

(1) It precedes neurulation
(2) It brings the inductor of the CNS under the precursor of the CNS
(3) It establishes the axis of bilateral symmetry
(4) It involves very little cell migration

34. Components of the membranous viscerocranium include which of the following bones of the adult skull?

(1) The mandible
(2) The frontal bone
(3) The maxilla
(4) The parietal bone

35. True statements concerning development of the heart include which of the following?

(1) The septum primum partially partitions the atria
(2) The ostium secundum is a hole in the septum primum
(3) The foramen ovale is a hole in the septum secundum
(4) The endocardial cushions take part in ventricular septation

36. Herpes simplex virus causes widespread venereal disease in men and women of reproductive age. True statements concerning the effects of this virus on the fetus include which of the following?

(1) It has been clearly established as a teratogenic agent
(2) It causes cardiovascular defects
(3) It causes mental retardation
(4) It is often fatal to fetuses infected during birth

37. True statements concerning the syncytiotrophoblast include which of the following?

(1) It is formed by the cytotrophoblast
(2) It is a syncytium derived from the embryoblast
(3) It is formed by cytotrophoblastic cell fusion
(4) It forms the inner lining of the yolk sac

38. Clinical characteristics of Klinefelter syndrome include which of the following?

(1) Hyalinization of seminiferous epithelium
(2) Normal Leydig cell function
(3) Gynecoid pelvis
(4) Euploidy (46 chromosomes)

39. Mesodermal derivatives include which of the following?

(1) Red blood cells
(2) Lymphocytes
(3) Smooth muscle
(4) Mesothelium

40. Embryonic rudiments that contribute to the development of the diaphragm include which of the following?

(1) Septum transversum
(2) Dorsal mesoesophagus
(3) Muscular ingrowth from the body wall
(4) Ventral mesogastrium

41. True statements concerning the central nervous system (CNS) include which of the following?

(1) It is a highly modified epithelium
(2) It contains mesodermal derivatives
(3) A basement membrane surrounds the CNS in the embryo
(4) Cell division plays an important role in CNS morphogenesis

42. The intermaxillary segment forms which of the following adult structures?

(1) The incisors
(2) The philtrum
(3) The primary palate
(4) The nasal conchae

43. True statements concerning cri du chat syndrome include which of the following?

(1) It is caused by a deletion of the long arm of chromosome 5
(2) It is an example of euploidy
(3) It is associated with an IQ of about 90
(4) It is associated with cardiovascular defects

44. The embryologic development of the metanephros is characterized by which of the following events?

(1) The metanephric blastema forms Bowman's capsule
(2) The ureteric bud forms the proximal convoluted tubules
(3) The ureteric bud forms the papillary ducts
(4) The ureteric bud forms the distal convoluted tubules and loop of Henle

45. Neural crest derivatives include which of the following?

(1) Adrenal medullary cells
(2) Melanocytes
(3) Enterochromaffin cells
(4) Dorsal root ganglion neurons

46. Characteristics of Edwards syndrome include which of the following?

(1) Markedly shortened life span
(2) Cleft lip and palate
(3) Prominent occiput
(4) A normal IQ

47. True statements concerning intramembranous ossification include which of the following?

(1) The frontal bone forms in this way
(2) Many facial bones form in this way
(3) No cartilage model is formed
(4) There is no osteoclastic activity

48. True statements concerning adverse effects of viruses include which of the following?

(1) Rubella virus causes congenital deafness
(2) Herpes simplex has been clearly established as a teratogenic agent
(3) Cytomegalovirus causes mental retardation
(4) Rubella causes first arch syndrome

49. The developing thyroid gland is correctly characterized by which of the following statements?

(1) It contains endodermally derived follicular epithelial cells
(2) It contains neural crest derivatives
(3) Ectopic thyroid tissue may be found in the root of the tongue
(4) The thyroglossal duct forms the pyramidal lobe

50. Which of the following organ pairs both contain some endodermal derivatives?

(1) Thymus—duodenum
(2) Pancreas—brain
(3) Stomach—liver
(4) Skin—trachea

51. Drugs clearly established to be teratogenic include which of the following?

(1) Diazepam
(2) Phenytoin
(3) Lithium
(4) Heroin

52. True statements concerning the umbilical vein include which of the following?

(1) It drains oxygenated blood from the placenta
(2) It flows into the sinus venosus
(3) It forms the ductus venosus
(4) It degenerates on the left between the liver and heart

53. The development of the eye is correctly described by which of the following statements?

(1) The inner layer of the optic cup forms the ganglion cell layer of the retina
(2) The internal limiting membrane is the basement membrane of the neural retina
(3) The outer layer of the optic cup forms the pigmented retina
(4) The pupillary sphincter muscles are derived from head mesenchyme

54. Endodermal derivatives include which of the following?

(1) Epithelial lining of the stomach
(2) Smooth muscle in the stomach
(3) Epithelial lining of the gallbladder
(4) Epithelial lining of the peritoneal cavity

SUMMARY OF DIRECTIONS				
A	B	C	D	E
1, 2, 3 only	1, 3 only	2, 4 only	4 only	All are correct

55. Complications of severe congenital diaphragmatic hernia include which of the following?

(1) Pulmonary hypoplasia
(2) Cardiac anomalies
(3) An enlarged thoracic cavity
(4) Inability to swallow

56. Glioblast derivatives include which of the following?

(1) Ependymal cells
(2) Oligodendroglia
(3) Microglia
(4) Astrocytes

57. The developing adrenal glands are correctly characterized by which of the following statements?

(1) The adrenal medulla is a neural crest derivative
(2) The definitive cortex forms from the fetal cortex
(3) The definitive cortex forms the zona glomerulosa
(4) The fetal cortex is superficial to the definitive cortex

58. Components of the cartilaginous neurocranium include which of the following bones of the adult skull?

(1) The base of the occipital bone
(2) The petrous temporal bone
(3) The sphenoid bone surrounding the pituitary gland
(4) The ethmoid bone

59. True statements concerning ionizing radiation include which of the following?

(1) Little clear experimental evidence exists showing that x-rays are teratogenic
(2) High levels of gamma radiation cause spontaneous abortions
(3) Low levels of gamma radiation are known to be safe
(4) Women irradiated in Hiroshima gave birth to increased numbers of children with microcephaly and mental retardation

60. True statements concerning gastrulation include which of the following?

(1) The epiblast forms ectoderm
(2) Mesoderm forms from invagination of epiblast cells
(3) Mesodermal cells migrate laterally from the primitive streak after invagination
(4) The notochord forms from the caudal movement of the primitive node

61. True statements concerning ectopic pregnancies include which of the following?

(1) Fully 95% of ectopic pregnancies are found in the fallopian (uterine) tubes
(2) Ectopic pregnancy can occur in the abdominal cavity
(3) Tubal pregnancies can rupture, leading to life-threatening internal bleeding
(4) A woman with gonorrhea and a woman never infected with gonorrhea would be equally likely to have an ectopic pregnancy

62. The development of the cornea is correctly described by which of the following statements?

(1) The anterior corneal epithelium is derived from surface ectoderm
(2) The posterior corneal endothelium is derived from head mesenchyme
(3) The corneal stroma is derived from mesoderm
(4) Corneal fibroblasts are responsible for corneal transparency

63. Neuroepithelial derivatives include which of the following?

(1) Pyramidal neurons in the cerebrum
(2) Oligodendroglial cells
(3) Purkinje cells in the cerebellum
(4) Protoplasmic astrocytes

64. True statements concerning early human development include which of the following?

(1) Cleavage occurs in the fallopian (uterine) tubes
(2) The morula stage precedes breakdown of the zona pellucida
(3) Implantation occurs after breakdown of the zona pellucida
(4) The blastocyst cavity appears after implantation

65. The developing pituitary gland is correctly characterized by which of the following statements?

(1) The infundibulum forms cells of the pars intermedia
(2) Rathke's pouch forms cells of the pars distalis
(3) Rathke's pouch forms cells in the median eminence
(4) The infundibulum forms cells in the pars nervosa

66. The congenital cardiovascular defect known as tetralogy of Fallot shows which of the following anatomic features?

(1) Pulmonary artery stenosis
(2) Overriding aorta
(3) Ventricular septal defect
(4) Left ventricular hypertrophy

67. True statements concerning the development of the auricle include which of the following?

(1) First pharyngeal arch mesenchyme makes a contribution
(2) Second pharyngeal arch mesenchyme makes a contribution
(3) The auricle is abnormal in Down syndrome and first arch syndrome
(4) The auricle is abnormal in Edwards snydrome

68. Children afflicted with severe fetal alcohol syndrome have which of the following characteristics?

(1) Midfacial hypoplasia
(2) Small stature
(3) Mild mental retardation
(4) A reduced philtrum

69. The developing islets of Langerhans are correctly characterized by which of the following statements?

(1) Insulin-secreting cells are derived from the dorsal pancreatic bud
(2) Glucagon-secreting cells are derived from the ventral pancreatic bud
(3) Somatostatin-secreting cells are derived from the neural crest
(4) Pancreatic D cells are derived from the same rudiment as pancreatic acinar cells

70. The developing adrenal glands are correctly characterized by which of the following statements?

(1) Adult zonation appears at puberty
(2) The medulla forms from the first wave of coelomic epithelial migration
(3) The fetal cortex undergoes extensive regression after birth
(4) The definitive cortex arises from a wave of neural crest cell migration

71. True statements concerning somite derivatives include which of the following?

(1) The sclerotomes form ligaments supporting the vertebral bodies
(2) The dermomyotomes form the intercostal muscles
(3) The dermomyotomes form dense irregular connective tissue
(4) The sclerotomes form the nucleus pulposus of the intervertebral disks

72. True statements concerning human fertilization include which of the following?

(1) It occurs in the uterine (fallopian) tubes
(2) It causes a change in the zona pellucida
(3) It leads to the completion of meiosis in the oocyte
(4) It leads to reformation of a diploid zygote nucleus

73. The neural crest forms which of the following endocrine cells?

(1) Enteroendocrine (APUD) cells
(2) Cells of the adrenal medulla
(3) C cells of the thyroid gland
(4) Alpha cells in the islets of Langerhans

Directions: The groups of questions below consist of lettered choices followed by several numbered items. For each numbered item select the **one** lettered choice with which it is **most** closely associated. Each lettered choice may be used once, more than once, or not at all.

Questions 74–77

Match each description of developmental fate below with the appropriate portion of the early human blastocyst pre-embryo.

(A) Embryoblast
(B) Trophoblast
(C) Both
(D) Neither

74. Forms the cytotrophoblast and syncytiotrophoblast
75. Forms the epiblast and hypoblast
76. Derived from the zygote
77. Forms the placenta and chorion

Questions 82–85

Match each of the statements about the developmental fate of layers of the optic cup with the most appropriate layer.

(A) Inner layer of optic cup
(B) Outer layer of optic cup
(C) Both
(D) Neither

82. This layer forms pigmented epithelial cells
83. This layer forms the photoreceptors in the fovea centralis
84. This layer forms the blood supply of the retina
85. This layer forms the pigmented retina

Questions 78–81

Match each of the descriptions below with the appropriate structure in the accompanying diagram of the indifferent external genitalia.

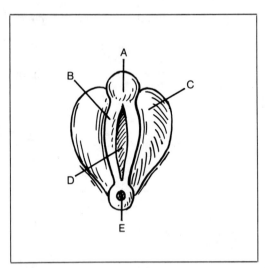

Questions 86–88

Match each description of a component of the embryonic heart below with the appropriate lettered structure in the accompanying diagram.

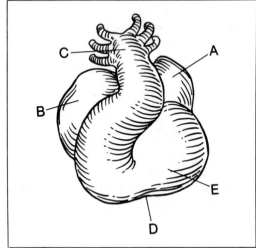

78. This structure forms the body of the penis in males
79. This structure forms the labia majora in females
80. This structure forms the hymen in females
81. This structure forms the scrotum in males

86. This structure receives the right horn of the sinus venosus
87. This sulcus marks the site where the muscular portion of the interventricular septum forms
88. This structure forms the root of the aorta

Questions 89-93

For each morphologic or functional description of a component of the placenta below, choose the appropriate lettered structure in the accompanying diagram.

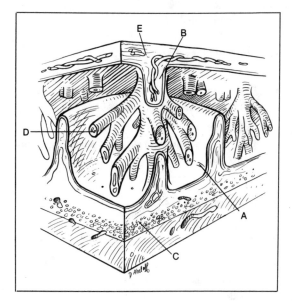

89. This structure is the decidual plate and is penetrated by maternal blood vessels

90. This structure is the intervillous space and contains maternal red blood cells

91. This structure is the chorionic plate and receives the insertion of the umbilical cord

92. This tissue column interconnects the chorionic and decidual plates

93. These structures are chorionic villi and are coated by syncytiotrophoblast

Questions 94-96

For each component of the adult lung listed below, select the embryonic rudiment that forms it.

(A) Respiratory diverticulum
(B) Splanchnic mesoderm
(C) Both
(D) Neither

94. A lobar bronchus

95. Type II cells in the lung

96. Tracheal smooth muscle

Questions 97-102

For each description below of the anatomy or function of a structure in the development of the nervous system, choose the appropriate embryonic structure.

(A) Marginal layer
(B) Mantle layer
(C) Ependymal layer
(D) Lumen of neural tube
(E) External limiting membrane

97. This structure contains many neuronal cell bodies

98. This structure is the basement membrane for the neuroepithelium

99. This structure lines ventricles

100. This structure develops into the white matter which contains much myelin

101. This structure becomes the central canal of the spinal cord and the ventricles of the brain

102. This structure becomes highly modified to form the cuboidal epithelium of the choroid plexus

Questions 103-107

Match each functional description of a gametogenic cell with the kind of gametogenic cell it best describes.

(A) Primordial germ cell
(B) Primary oocyte
(C) Primary spermatocyte
(D) Secondary oocyte
(E) Secondary spermatocyte

103. A tetraploid cell produced by the millions after puberty

104. A cell that has a diploid amount of DNA and undergoes an equal cytoplasmic division to form spermatids

105. A cell that has a diploid amount of DNA and undergoes unequal cytoplasmic divisions

106. A cell that is derived from the yolk sac and forms spermatogonia

107. A cell that has a tetraploid amount of DNA and can be arrested in meiosis I for 40 years or more

Questions 108-112

Match each of the descriptions below with the appropriate structure in the accompanying diagram of the developing urogenital system at the indifferent stage.

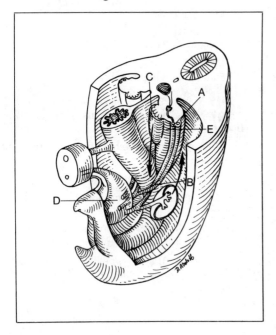

108. This structure forms the appendix epididymis in males

109. This structure forms the cervix in females

110. This structure secretes müllerian-inhibiting substance

111. This structure contributes to the development of the upper third of the vagina

112. This structure fails to differentiate in patients with testicular feminization syndrome because it lacks sensitivity to testosterone

Questions 113-116

Match each structure of the adult ear listed below with its derivation.

(A) Cochlear pouch
(B) Vestibular pouch
(C) Both
(D) Neither

113. Macula sacculi

114. Membranous labyrinth

115. Semicircular canals

116. Perilymphatic space

Questions 117-120

Match the symptoms below with the neural tube defect that is most likely to be the cause.

(A) Lumbar spina bifida with an open neural tube defect
(B) Anencephaly
(C) Both
(D) Neither

117. Elevated maternal serum α-fetoprotein

118. Defects in bone formation

119. Degenerative nervous tissue

120. Gross mental retardation and death soon after birth

Questions 121-122

Match each of the descriptions below with the appropriate structure.

(A) Liver
(B) Pancreas
(C) Both
(D) Neither

121. Contains parenchymal cells derived from gut tube diverticula

122. Contains connective tissue elements derived from the septum transversum

Questions 123-126

Match each of the descriptions below with the embryonic structure that it best describes.

(A) Liver diverticulum
(B) Midgut
(C) Dorsal pancreatic rudiment
(D) Cloaca
(E) Vitelline duct

123. This hindgut derivative receives the excurrent ducts of the reproductive and urinary systems

124. This structure forms at the junction between the foregut and the hindgut and differentiates into glucagon-secreting islet tissue

125. This structure forms the ileum and ascending colon

126. This structure forms endocrine and exocrine tissue as it grows into the septum transversum

Questions 127–129

Match the lettered arch in the accompanying diagram of the aortic arches with the most appropriate adult vascular derivatives described below.

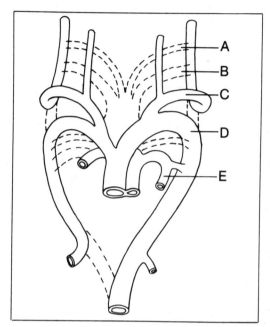

127. Forms the proximal root of the external carotid artery

128. Forms the ductus arteriosus and the pulmonary arteries

129. Forms the maxillary artery

Questions 130–134

Match each of the descriptions below with the appropriate embryonic structure.

(A) Ductus venosus
(B) Foramen ovale
(C) Septum transversum
(D) Pleuroperitoneal membrane
(E) Septum primum

130. This opening is a shunt allowing blood to pass from right to left in the fetal heart

131. Blood from the umbilical vein flows through the liver in this channel

132. This structure forms most of the central portion of the diaphragm and also contributes to the capsule of the liver

133. The ostium secundum forms in this flap of tissue

134. This vessel forms the ligamentum venosum after birth

Questions 135–140

For each description below of a component of a bone developing by endochondral ossification, choose the appropriate lettered area in the accompanying photomicrograph.

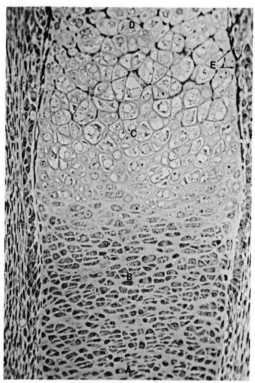

135. Bony collar of ossified tissue

136. Zone of active chondrocyte mitotic cell division

137. Zone where chondrocytes are degenerating and the cartilage matrix is becoming calcified

138. Zone of cartilage hypertrophy

139. Zone where osteoblasts are depositing a layer of osteoid

140. Region where ossification first occurs

Questions 141-144

For each description below of a component of the developing urinary system, select the appropriate structure in the accompanying diagram.

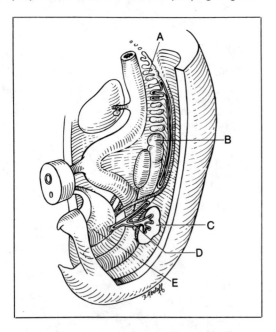

141. This structure degenerates without ever becoming functional in urine production

142. This structure forms convoluted tubules in the adult kidney

143. This structure forms the ureter and the major and minor calyces

144. This structure degenerates, but a branch of its duct forms the ureter

ANSWERS AND EXPLANATIONS

1. The answer is B. *(Chapter 13 I B 1; III A 1, 2 b, 3)* Hepatic duct epithelial cells, as well as all other luminal epithelial cells of the exocrine portion of the liver and pancreas, are derived from the liver diverticulum or pancreatic buds. The splanchnic mesoderm forms the connective tissue, smooth muscle, and blood vessels in the wall of the hepatic ducts. The liver is active in hematopoiesis after the yolk sac and before the bone marrow. This hematopoiesis occurs in the liver sinusoids, blood vessels derived from vitelline and umbilical blood vessels passing through the septum transversum.

2. The answer is D. *(Chapter 5 IV A, B)* During neurulation, the neural plate invaginates to form the neural groove. Next, the neural groove rolls up into a closed neural tube. Just before fusion of the dorsal edges of the neural tube, neural crest cells emigrate from the neuroepithelium. There is reciprocal induction during neurulation. The notochord and paraxial mesoderm induce neural plate and neural tube formation. In turn, the neural tube induces the bony neural arches to form from sclerotome-derived mesenchymal cells.

3. The answer is E. *(Chapter 5 VI B)* α-Fetoprotein is a fetal blood protein that is also present in cerebrospinal fluid. With open neural tube defects, it leaks into the amniotic fluid and then makes its way into the maternal circulation. Elevated maternal serum levels are suggestive of a neural tube defect but can also be associated with other congenital anomalies (e.g., omphalocele). Therefore, ultrasonography is required for the correct differential diagnosis of neural tube defects when maternal serum α-fetoprotein levels are elevated.

4. The answer is A. *(Chapter 18 V B 2 b, C; Table 18-1)* The second pharyngeal arch (hyoid arch) forms the muscles of facial expression (e.g., orbicularis oris and orbicularis oculi). Bones formed in the second arch include the upper body of the hyoid bone and the stapes, the third of the middle ear ossicles. Second arch derivatives are innervated by the facial nerve. Reichert's cartilage is a transitory embryonic cartilage formed in the second pharyngeal arch. The muscles of mastication (e.g., the masseter) are first arch derivatives.

5. The answer is D. *(Chapter 2 II B; Chapter 17 II A 2, B 2)* Primordial germ cells arise in the yolk sac. They migrate to the gonadal primordia where they differentiate into either spermatogonia or oogonia. Spermatogonia then differentiate into spermatocytes, spermatids, and spermatozoa during spermatogenesis. Oogonia differentiate into oocytes, ova, and polar bodies during meiosis. Sertoli cells are derived from the coelomic epithelial cells that cover the gonadal primordium and migrate into the gonadal primordium, where they become associated with primordial germ cells to form primitive sex cords. These coelomic epithelial cells form Sertoli cells in males and follicular epithelial cells in females.

6. The answer is B. *(Chapter 14 V A, B)* Respiratory distress syndrome (RDS) is the leading cause of death of premature infants. This clinical entity is caused by immaturity of the type II surfactant-secreting cells in the alveolar epithelium. Premature infants born before adequate numbers of type II cells have differentiated (i.e., before about 35 weeks) have a significantly increased probability of having RDS. RDS is also sometimes called hyaline membrane disease because the lung surfaces become coated with a hyaline membrane.

7. The answer is D. *(Chapter 13 II C 4, D 1; IV C 2, 3)* The rotations of the stomach are critically involved in the morphogenesis of the greater omentum. The first rotation elongates the dorsal mesogastrium to form the greater omentum, and the second rotation brings the greater omentum into the frontal plane. Midgut loop rotation involves a total of 270° counterclockwise rotation. The initial 90° rotation occurs during physiologic herniation. The final phases of midgut loop rotation occur as the midgut loop is drawn back into the peritoneal cavity after its normal physiologic herniation.

8. The answer is C. *(Chapter 2, IV A 1, B 2; V B)* Gametogenesis is the process of formation of the gametes (ova and spermatozoa). This process occurs in the gonads (ovaries and testes). There are millions of gametes produced every day in males but only one every month in females. In males, meiosis is completed in the testes. In females, meiosis is not completed until the second polar body is cast off from the secondary oocyte, and that is triggered by fertilization. The secondary oocyte is produced in the female just before ovulation, when the first polar body and a secondary oocyte are produced from a primary oocyte.

9–11. The answers are: 9-C, 10-B, 11-C. *(Chapter 23 II B 3))* The karyotype accompanying the questions is that of a male with Patau syndrome (trisomy 13). The appropriate shorthand designation for this karyotype would be 47 (an extra chromosome), XY (male), +13 (trisomy 13). Midfacial defects such as cleft lip and palate, microphthalmia, and nasal abnormalities are most often associated with this syndrome.

12. The answer is E. (*Chapter 7 V A, B*) Decidual tissue is derived from endometrial stromal cells. Decidual cells are large, polygonal acidophilic cells with an abundance of cytoplasmic glycogen. In some poorly understood fashion, decidual tissue limits the invasiveness of the syncytiotrophoblast. As its name implies, the decidual tissue is shed along with the placenta at birth. The decidua basalis forms opposite the implantation site and becomes part of the definitive placenta. The decidua parietalis lines the uterine cavity. The decidua capsularis surrounds the implantation site opposite the decidua basalis. As the embryo grows, it obliterates the uterine lumen and the decidua capsularis fuses with the decidua parietalis to form the decidua vera.

13. The answer is E. (*Chapter 18 VI B*) Mandibulofacial dysostosis (first arch syndrome, Treacher Collins syndrome) involves developmental anomalies in first pharyngeal arch derivatives. Thus the mandible, the maxilla, and the malleus and incus are all often abnormal in this syndrome. Mental capacity is normal in patients with mandibulofacial dysostosis. In many cases, mental retardation may be suspected because of the deafness that often occurs in mandibulofacial dysostosis due to developmental defects in the external auditory meatus and the malleus and incus. The auricle may also be abnormal because the first pharyngeal arch contributes to the anterior components of the auricle. Mandibulofacial dysostosis is caused by an autosomal dominant mutation.

14. The answer is B. (*Chapter 5 IV A, B*) Gastrulation brings the notochord and paraxial mesoderm (the neural inducers) underneath the ectoderm. Neurulation is caused by gastrulation-dependent induction and thus must occur after gastrulation. Neural induction leads to thickening of the ectoderm in the neural plate. Lateral to the neural plate, surface ectoderm forms epidermis. The lumen of the neural tube persists as the central canal of the spinal cord and the brain ventricles. Neural tube defects result from poor closure of the neural tube and perhaps faulty neural arch induction.

15. The answer is A. (*Chapter 16 II A 5, B 7; V C*) The pronephros is not functional in human embryos; the mesonephros is the first renal structure involved in urine formation. The fetus urinates into the amniotic fluid and then swallows the amniotic fluid so that fetal nitrogenous wastes can be absorbed through the fetal gastrointestinal tract, enter the fetal circulation, and then be eliminated across the placenta. If a fetus cannot swallow properly (e.g., because of anencephaly or esophageal atresia), the fetus will urinate into the amniotic fluid but not swallow it, leading to an increased volume of amniotic fluid, a condition known as polyhydramnios. Conversely, in renal agenesis, there is no fetal urine production and thus there is a decrease in the volume of amniotic fluid, a condition called oligohydramnios.

16. The answer is B. (*Chapter 15 VIII A, B*) Rh isoimmunization is seen in Rh-negative mothers carrying Rh-positive fetuses. Fetal blood cells enter the maternal circulation and are recognized as foreign antigens. This leads to a production of maternal antibodies which cross the placenta and subsequently destroy fetal red blood cells. Rh isoimmunization is usually more severe after the first pregnancy. This is due to the fact that the mother produces memory B cells against fetal antigens during the first pregnancy, and these cells then mount an immune response to the fetal antigens in subsequent pregnancies.

17. The answer is C. (*Chapter 10 I B; II A, C 1, 2, 4, D 1*) Angiogenetic cell clusters arise in mesenchyme all over the embryo. Those arising cranial to the oropharyngeal membrane give rise to the endocardial portion of the heart tubes. A myoepicardial mantle also forms around the endocardial tubes, giving rise to the cardiac muscle cells (myocytes) of the definitive myocardium. Those angiogenetic cell clusters arising elsewhere give rise to other blood vessels and to blood cells. The heart begins to beat early in the fourth week, and a few days later there is definite circulation of blood cells. The dorsal mesocardium breaks down during the looping of the heart tube within the pericardial cavity. In the development of the heart, no ventral mesocardium is ever formed.

18. The answer is B. (*Chapter 18 V B, C 3; Table 18-1*) The first pharyngeal arch (mandibular arch) forms the maxilla and the lateral palatine processes (secondary palatal precursors), which grow from the maxilla. The intermaxillary segment and Meckel's cartilage are also formed in the first pharyngeal arch. First arch derivatives are innervated by the trigeminal nerve. The palatine tonsils are second pharyngeal arch derivatives. They have an epithelial component derived from the second pharyngeal pouches (endoderm), whereas their lymphocytes, plasma cells, and macrophages are all mesodermally derived.

19. The answer is A. (*Chapter 2, V A, B*) Spermatogenesis is the process of production of spermatozoa. It occurs in the seminiferous tubules of the testes. There is a gradual decrease in sperm count with advanced age, but spermatogenesis is a continuous process in men from puberty until death. Spermatogonia are present before puberty, but they do not begin to differentiate into spermatozoa until puberty. Primary spermatocytes are tetraploid cells containing paired bivalents (homologous chromosomes). They form secondary spermatocytes (as a result of meiosis I), which in turn form haploid spermatids (as a result of meiosis II). Next, spermatids undergo a complex cytomorphogenesis (during spermiogenesis) to form spermatozoa.

20. The answer is B. (Chapter 5 VI A 2; Chapter 23 I B 2; Table 23-1; Chapter 24 VII A) Neural tube defects are partially caused by unknown environmental influences and partially caused by genetic factors. Neural tube defects are unusually common among Caucasians in the United Kingdom, and especially among the Irish and Welsh. In contrast, Blacks in the United States have a very low incidence of neural tube defects. In the United States, these birth defects occur more frequently in the Northeast but decline in frequency as one moves south or west. These epidemiologic observations may well be a reflection of the distribution of people with ethnic backgrounds predisposing them to neural tube defects. For example, there are more Irish people and fewer Black people in the Northeast than in the Southeast.

21–22. The answers are: 21-B, 22-D. (Chapter 23 II B 1)) The karyotype accompanying the questions is that of a female patient with trisomy 21 (Down syndrome). This karyotype has two X chromosomes, and therefore the patient would be female. The appropriate shorthand designation for this karyotype would be 47 (one extra chromosome), XX (female), +21 (trisomy 21). Since the patient is female, she would not have a testis. All of the other findings described in question 21 are characteristics of patients with Down syndrome.

23. The answer is B. (Chapter 7 IV B) The syncytiotrophoblast has a complex ultrastructure suitable to its many different cellular functions. For example, the syncytiotrophoblast synthesizes and secretes a glycoprotein hormone (chorionic gonadotropin) and thus has an abundance of rough endoplasmic reticulum (for protein synthesis) and an abundant Golgi apparatus (for protein glycosylation). There are also many mitochondria to provide adenosine triphosphate (ATP) for protein synthesis, for the active transport of solutes, and for the movement of maternal immunoglobulin G (IgG) by membrane-bound vesicles across the placenta. There are also strong intercellular tight junctions and desmosomes between syncytial cells.

24. The answer is B (1, 3). (Chapter 2 II B; Chapter 17 II A 2, B 2, C) Leydig cells and thecal cells come from the genital ridge mesenchyme. Sertoli cells and follicular epithelial cells come from the coelomic epithelium. The primordial germ cells, which give rise to all of the cells in the gametogenic cell lines (spermatogonia, which become spermatozoa in males, and oogonia, which become ova and polar bodies in females), are derived from the yolk sac and migrate to the developing gonads.

25. The answer is A (1, 2, 3). (Chapter 5 V B 2, D 2) The ectoderm is the outermost of the three primary germ layers. It forms the outer surface covering of the body, including the epidermis and epidermal appendages such as fingernails. It also forms the anterior lining of the oral cavity and forms enamel on teeth. In addition, the ectoderm forms the central nervous system and the far-ranging derivatives of the neural crest. Endothelium is the simple squamous epithelium lining the cardiovascular system and it is a mesodermal derivative.

26. The answer is B (1, 3). (Chapter 18 V B 2 b, C 1 b, D; Table 18-1) The third pharyngeal arch is innervated by the glossopharyngeal nerve and forms the lower body of the hyoid bone. The third pharyngeal pouches contribute to the development of the thymus gland. They also are involved in the formation of the inferior parathyroid glands. The digastric muscle is derived from the first arch (anterior belly) and the second arch (posterior belly).

27. The answer is E (all). (Chapter 9 V B) The limb buds follow the embryonic pattern of development in a cranial to caudal sequence. Thus, the forelimb buds appear before the hindlimb buds. The limb buds consist of an apical ectodermal ridge, ectodermal cells, and a core of mesenchyme. The apical ectodermal ridge is essential for inducing mesenchymal differentiation. The ectodermal cells form the epidermis on the limb. The limb bud mesenchyme forms muscles, bones, tendons, and ligaments in the limb. Digital rays are sculptured into digits by selective cell death.

28. The answer is C (2, 4). (Chapter 5 III A; V F) The notochord forms from the epiblast during gastrulation. It is a mass of tissue lying in the axis of bilateral symmetry of the pre-embryo cranial to the regressing primitive node (Hensen's node). The notochord forms the nucleus pulposus of the intervertebral disks. Its remnant in embryonic vertebral bodies disappears in the adult. The annulus fibrosus is formed by connective tissues derived from the sclerotomes of somites.

29. The answer is A (1, 2, 3). (Chapter 11 I C; IV A, B) The neural crest makes important contributions to the autonomic nervous system, including the sympathetic ganglia and the myenteric plexus. It also forms the pseudounipolar neurons of the dorsal root (sensory) ganglia. The satellite (glial) cells here, such as Schwann cells, are also neural crest derivatives. Neurons in the spinal cord proper are derived from neuroepithelium-derived neuroblasts rather than from the neural crest.

30. The answer is B (1, 3). (*Chapter 19 III B*) The hormone-secreting cells of the parathyroid glands are derived from endodermal pharyngeal pouch cells. The chief and oxyphil cells that are characteristic of the adult parathyroid do not appear until the second half of gestation. The superior parathyroid glands come from the cranial fourth pouches. The inferior parathyroids come from the cranial third pouches and migrate to a position caudal (inferior) to the superior parathyroids. The complex embryology accounts for the possibility of a variable position and number of parathyroid glands.

31. The answer is E (all). (*Chapter 6 II C 6; Chapter 8 I B 1; II A 3, 4, B*) The intraembryonic coelom is the precursor of the body cavities. Initially, the intraembryonic coelom is in broad communication with the extraembryonic coelom. It extends along the lateral flanks of the embryo all the way to the oropharyngeal membrane. This cranial component eventually forms the pericardial cavity. The middle component of the intraembryonic coelom forms the pleural cavities, and the caudal component forms the peritoneal cavity.

32. The answer is B (1, 3). (*Chapter 14 IV C 2 b; V A, B*) Type II cells secrete surfactant, a lipoprotein chiefly containing lecithin. Type II cells differentiate first around 25 weeks in utero from epithelial cells derived from the respiratory diverticulum. By 35 weeks, there is a population of type II cells adequate to support normal respiration. Because the secreted surfactant makes its way into the amniotic fluid, the state of type II cell differentiation, and therefore the degree of fetal lung maturity, can be assessed by sampling amniotic fluid and measuring its lecithin content. In threatened premature delivery, type II cell differentiation can sometimes be accelerated by administration of steroids to the mother.

33. The answer is A (1, 2, 3). (*Chapter 5 II A 1, B; III B*) Cell migration is a cardinal feature of gastrulation. Gastrulation is a complex morphogenetic process which precedes neurulation and flexion. During gastrulation, the anterior, posterior, cranial, and caudal orientations, and the axis of bilateral symmetry are defined by the formation of appropriate structures. Gastrulation also brings the inductors of the central nervous system (CNS), the notochord and paraxial mesoderm, underneath the ectoderm so that a neural plate can form. During neurulation, which occurs after gastrulation, the neural plate rolls up into a neural tube. Flexion then leads to the establishment of the basic vertebrate body plan.

34. The answer is B (1, 3). (*Chapter 9 IV F 2 a*) The membranous viscerocranium arises from pharyngeal arch mesenchyme by intramembranous ossification. It forms many of the bones of the face, including the mandible and maxilla. The frontal and parietal bones form part of the vault of the skull which surrounds the brain. As such, they are part of the membranous neurocranium.

35. The answer is E (all). (*Chapter 10 III A 2; IV A*) Atrial septation is accomplished by formation of the septum primum, which has a hole in it called the ostium secundum, and the septum secundum, which has a hole in it called the foramen ovale. During fetal life, the atrial septum functions as a one-way valve that allows blood to pass from the right to the left atrium. The valve normally closes at birth. Ventricular septation is accomplished by growth of the endocardial cushions (forming the membranous interventricular septum) and the wall of the ventricle (forming the muscular interventricular septum).

36. The answer is D (4). (*Chapter 23 III C*) Herpes simplex virus is not thought to be a teratogenic virus. However, children born vaginally to women who are actively shedding herpes virus have a 50% mortality rate. This increased mortality rate is due to the fact that the T cell system is not fully functional at birth. Consequently, these children will have extremely severe herpes simplex infections that are often fatal.

37. The answer is B (1, 3). (*Chapter 4 V B; VII C 1*) The syncytiotrophoblast is a syncytial layer derived by proliferation and fusion of cytotrophoblastic cells. It is derived from the trophoblast, not the embryoblast. The inner lining of the yolk sac comes from the hypoblast, one of the two layers of the bilaminar disk embryo, which is entirely derived from the inner cell mass (embryoblast). During implantation, the syncytiotrophoblast forms an invasive tissue which aids implantation of the conceptus. It does this in part by secreting proteolytic enzymes that degrade endometrial stroma and blood vessels.

38. The answer is B (1, 3). (*Chapter 17 VII C*) Klinefelter syndrome (47, XXY) is an example of aneuploidy. Because of the single Y chromosome, despite the abnormal number of X chromosomes, a testis forms with normal numbers of Leydig cells. After puberty, however, the Leydig cells prove abnormal. Testicular descent often fails to occur, leading to hyalinization of the seminiferous epithelium. The pair of X chromosomes results in mild gynecomastia and a gynecoid pelvis.

39. The answer is E (all). (*Chapter 5 V D*) The mesoderm is the middle primary germ layer. It lies between ectoderm on the outside and endoderm on the inside. Mesoderm forms most of the body's general connective tissues (e.g., loose areolar connective tissue in the lamina propria and dense irregular connective tissue in the dermis) and specialized connective tissues (e.g., cartilage, bone, blood cells, and fat). Mesoderm also forms all of the cardiovascular system and the bulk of the visceral smooth muscle. Mesothelium is the name for the simple squamous epithelium lining serous cavities in the body (pericardial, pleural, and peritoneal cavities), and it is a mesodermal derivative.

40. The answer is A (1, 2, 3). (*Chapter 8 IV; V B 3*)The diaphragm is derived mostly from the septum transversum but also from the dorsal mesentery of the esophagus, the pleuroperitoneal membranes, and muscular ingrowth from the body wall. The ventral mesogastrium develops from the septum transversum and contributes to the lesser omentum and the falciform ligament. It does not play a role in the development of the diaphragram.

41. The answer is E (all). (*Chapter 11 II A, B*) The central nervous system (CNS) consists of the brain and spinal cord. Both develop from the neuroepithelium. In the embryo, the neural plate has a typical basement membrane. This comes to lie external to the neuroepithelium (as the external limiting membrane) when the neural tube forms. The neuroepithelium proliferates extensively, forming neuroblasts (precursors of all CNS neurons) and glioblasts (precursors of some CNS glia). The CNS microglia are mesodermally derived.

42. The answer is A (1, 2, 3). (*Chapter 18 III B 2*) The intermaxillary segment is a small mass of mesenchyme lying between the medial tips of the maxillary division of the first pharyngeal arch. This portion of the first pharyngeal arch is important in the formation of the primary palate and soft tissues adjacent to it. The intermaxillary segment forms the central upper lip (philtrum), primary palate, and incisors. It also forms a portion of the maxillary bone. The nasal conchae form in the maxillary processes in close association with the lateral palatine processes.

43. The answer is C (2, 4). (*Chapter 23 II C 1*) Cri du chat syndrome is an example of euploidy (normal number of chromosomes). It is caused by a deletion of the short arm of chromosome 5. The syndrome is associated with profound IQ deficits (50 or less) and cardiovascular defects but a normal life span. Infants with cri du chat syndrome often have elongated skulls, a characteristic facial appearance, and a cat-like cry.

44. The answer is B (1, 3). (*Chapter 16 III A, B*) The entire definitive (metanephric) kidney is formed by the metanephric blastema and the ureteric bud. These two rudiments cooperate in the formation of the definitive kidney by a reciprocal inductive interaction. The metanephric blastema is induced by the ureteric bud to form all of the glomerulus, the proximal and distal convoluted tubules, and the loop of Henle. The branching of the ureteric bud is stimulated by the metanephric blastema. The ureteric bud forms the ureters, the major and minor calyces, the papillary ducts, and the collecting tubules.

45. The answer is E (all). (*Chapter 5 V C*) The cells of the neural crest separate from the neuroectoderm during neurulation and become dispersed widely throughout the body. These cells constitute a pluripotent cell population capable of differentiating into a vast array of different types of cells. Neural crest cells form the adrenal medulla, melanocytes, enterochromaffin cells, dorsal root ganglia, and Schwann cells. In addition, the neural crest contributes to many structures in the head, such as the meninges, the dentin-secreting odontoblasts in teeth, and the osteocytes of jaw bones.

46. The answer is B (1, 3). (*Chapter 23 II B 2*) Edwards syndrome is caused by trisomy of chromosome 18. Children usually die soon after birth, before it is possible to perform IQ tests, but they are profoundly mentally retarded. A prominent occiput and rocker-bottom feet are associated with this syndrome. Facial clefts are associated with Patau syndrome (trisomy 13).

47. The answer is A (1, 2, 3). (*Chapter 9 III C*) Intramembranous ossification is very similar to endochondral ossification except that no cartilage model of the bone is formed. In both types of bone formation, osteoblasts form bone and osteoclasts degrade it during growth and remodeling. During intramembranous ossification, small spicules of bone form first and then fuse with one another to form larger and larger plates of bone. The vault of the skull, including the frontal bone, is formed in this way. Many facial bones, such as the maxilla and the mandible, are also formed by this mode of bone formation.

48. The answer is B (1, 3). (*Chapter 23 III A, B, C*) Rubella virus causes German measles. It is also a teratogenic virus. Rubella virus attacks developing neuroepithelial structures and can result in blindness and deafness because it affects the differentiation of the sensory epithelia. Mental retardation is also seen in some children of rubella-infected mothers. Rubella does not cause first arch syndrome; that is caused by an autosomal dominant mutation. Herpes simplex virus has not been clearly established as a teratogenic virus. Neonatal venereal herpes infections are fatal to newborns in 50% of the cases, however.

49. The answer is E (all). (Chapter 19 III A) The thyroid gland develops from an endodermally derived diverticulum that arises at the root of the tongue and gives rise to the follicular epithelial cells. The calcitonin-secreting C cells (parafollicular cells) of the thyroid are neural crest derivatives. The thyroid gland rudiment descends along the trachea and remains connected to its site of origin for a time by a thyroglossal duct. This duct eventually degenerates but can persist as either ectopic thyroid tissue or as a pyramidal lobe of variable extent.

50. The answer is B (1, 3). (Chapter 5 V G) Many organs have tissues derived from several germ layers. All gastrointestinal organs have an endodermally derived luminal epithelium. The thymus contains reticular epithelial cells that are endodermally derived (from pharyngeal pouches). The brain is mostly derived from ectoderm but does have some mesodermally derived microglia. It has no known endodermal derivatives. The skin has ectodermally derived epidermis and mesodermally derived dermis but no endodermal derivatives.

51. The answer is A (1, 2, 3). (Chapter 23 V B, C) Teratogens are agents that cause structural defects in the developing embryo or fetus. The first three drugs in the question have been clearly established as having teratogenic potential. Heroin addicts have children who share their addiction at birth and may also carry human immunodeficiency virus (HIV) infections, but they do not have congenital anomalies in increased frequency. Other so-called recreational drugs such as marijuana, PCP (phencyclidine), and cocaine are also probably not teratogenic.

52. The answer is E (all). (Chapter 10 II E 2; VI D; VII A 1) The umbilical veins are paired structures early in development. They drain oxygenated blood from the placenta, through the liver, and into the sinus venosus. As the left sinus venosus degenerates, the portion of the left umbilical vein between the liver and the heart degenerates. This explains why there is only one umbilical vein in the term umbilical cord.

53. The answer is A (1, 2, 3). [Chapter 11 II A 1; Chapter 20 III A, B 1, C 1, 3 b, F 2 b (2)] The inner layer of the optic cup is a pseudostratified neuroepithelial layer with a basement membrane (the internal limiting membrane). This layer forms the neural retina, which later differentiates into rods and cones and other neurons and glia, including the ganglion cell layer. The outer layer of the optic cup forms the pigmented retina. The pupillary sphincter muscles are formed from ectodermal cells of the outer layer of the optic cup. These muscles are the only ectodermally derived smooth muscles in the body; all other smooth muscle arises from mesodermally derived tissue.

54. The answer is B (1, 3). (Chapter 5 V D 1, 3, E 1) The endoderm is the innermost of the three primary germ layers. It forms the epithelial lining of the gastrointestinal (GI) tract and respiratory system. Thus, for example, the epithelial cells lining the stomach and small intestine are endodermal derivatives. Similarly, the epithelial lining of pulmonary alveoli and the trachea are also endodermal derivatives. The smooth muscles of the entire GI tract, including the stomach, come from splanchnic mesoderm. The epithelial lining of the peritoneal cavity is mesodermally derived mesothelium

55. The answer is A (1, 2, 3). (Chapter 8 VI B) In congenital diaphragmatic hernia, the embryonic rudiments that form the diaphragm fail to fuse properly. As a result, an opening in the diaphragm allows loops of small intestine to herniate into the left thoracic cavity, displacing the heart and lungs. The displacement results in hypoplasia of the left lung and developmental anomalies in the heart and great vessels. The affected infant may appear normal at first and is able to swallow food. However, the infant becomes cyanotic and short of breath after feeding because the bowel loops compress the lungs as the infant feeds, making breathing difficult. Close inspection reveals an enlarged thoracic cavity and a relatively small abdominal cavity. Congenital diaphragmatic hernia is often fatal, especially in cases of extreme pulmonary hypoplasia.

56. The answer is C (2, 4). (Chapter 11 II B 4, 5) All of the cell types listed in the question are glial cells. Glioblasts are important for the formation of some types of glial cells but not all of them. The ependymal cells are derived directly from nonproliferating cells of the neuroepithelium. Microglial cells are macrophage-like cells in the brain and come from mesoderm like all other elements of the mononuclear phagocyte system. The oligodendroglial cells are glioblast derivatives; they are responsible for the formation of myelin in the central nervous system. Astrocytes are also glioblast derivatives. They have close associations with blood vessels and with the glia limitans at the peripheral portions of the central nervous system.

57. The answer is B (1, 3). *(Chapter 19 IV A, B)* The adrenal medulla is a neural crest derivative. The adrenal cortex forms from two distinct waves of proliferation and migration of coelomic epithelial cells. The first wave forms a fetal cortex and the second wave forms the definitive cortex superficial to the fetal cortex. The fetal cortex eventually forms the deep cortex (zona reticularis) while the definitive cortex forms the superficial cortex (zona glomerulosa and zona fasciculata).

58. The answer is E (all). *(Chapter 9 IV F 1 b)* The cartilaginous neurocranium is formed by endochondral ossification (i.e., by way of a pre-existing cartilage model). The cartilaginous neurocranium forms a bony complex at the base of the brain. It also forms the capsules which surround the eye, inner ear, and olfactory epithelium. The base of the occipital bone, the petrous temporal bone, the sphenoid around the pituitary, and the ethmoid bone are all components of the cartilaginous neurocranium.

59. The answer is C (2, 4). *(Chapter 23 IV A, B, C)* X-rays are clearly teratogenic. High levels of gamma radiation can cause spontaneous abortions, and even low levels are thought to be deleterious. Victims of the atomic bomb blasts had many spontaneous abortions and children born with microcephaly and mental retardation.

60. The answer is E (all). *(Chapter 5 II B)* Gastrulation is the process whereby the bilaminar disk pre-embryo is converted into a trilaminar pre-embryo. Gastrulation begins in the bilaminar disk with the formation of the primitive streak. This invagination site in the epiblast is a place where epiblast-derived cells migrate medially toward the primitive streak, invaginate through it, and then migrate laterally in a movement which results in the establishment of the intraembryonic mesoderm. The notochord grows in a cranial direction from the primitive node (Hensen's node), which is regressing caudally in the primitive streak.

61. The answer is A (1, 2, 3). *(Chapter 7 IX A 1)* An ectopic pregnancy is a pregnancy in which the implantation site and gestational sac are located outside the main cavity of the uterus. Most ectopic pregnancies (95%) are found in the fallopian tubes, but they can also occur at extrauterine sites such as the abdominal cavity or the cervical os. If a tubal pregnancy ruptures, it is associated with intense pain, shock, and potentially fatal blood loss. Gonorrhea and bacterial pelvic inflammatory diseases can disrupt normal function in the uterine tubes and often lead to an increased risk of ectopic pregnancies.

62. The answer is E (all). *(Chapter 20 IV B, D)* The corneal epithelium (on the anterior surface) is derived from surface ectoderm. The corneal endothelium (on the posterior surface) is a mesodermal derivative coming from head mesenchyme. Mesenchymal fibroblasts (which are mesodermal derivatives) form the corneal stroma. These fibroblasts secrete a special extracellular matrix which aligns the collagen fibers orthogonally in the stroma. The orthogonal alignment of the fibrils is in turn responsible for corneal transparency.

63. The answer is E (all). *(Chapter 11 II A, B 2, 3)* The neuroepithelium is a proliferative layer that forms neuroblasts and glioblasts. The proliferative activity of the neuroepithelium produces the fantastically complex array of cells in the brain and spinal cord. The neuroblasts form all central nervous system neurons, including pyramidal neurons and Purkinje cells. The glioblasts differentiate into several kinds of glial cells, such as oligodendroglia and astrocytes.

64. The answer is A (1, 2, 3). *(Chapter 4 IV A, B)* Cleavage is initiated by fertilization. It begins soon after fertilization and occurs as the conceptus passes down the uterine tubes to the uterus. Early cleavages are equal. By repeated mitotic divisions, they create 2, 4, 8, and 16 blastomeres in short order. The repeated rounds of cell division create a solid ball of cells, called the morula. Next, a blastocyst cavity forms, followed by hatching from the zona pellucida and, finally, by implantation.

65. The answer is C (2, 4). *(Chapter 19 II A, B)* The pituitary gland arises from two rudiments, the infundibulum, which forms the neurohypophysis, and Rathke's pouch, which forms the adenohypophysis. The neurohypophysis consists of the infundibular stem and process and the median eminence. The adenohypophysis consists of the pars distalis, pars intermedia, and pars tuberalis.

66. The answer is A (1, 2, 3). *(Chapter 10 VIII B 3)* The tetralogy of Fallot is a complex congenital cardiovascular anomaly. It is probably the result of an abnormal partitioning of the ventricular outflow tracts. Thus, the aorta is placed more toward the right ventricle (overriding aorta), and there is pulmonary artery stenosis. Right (not left) ventricular hypertrophy is present and results from the pulmonary artery stenosis. Ventricular septal defects are also characteristic of the tetralogy of Fallot. Patent ductus arteriosus is present in some cases, converting the tetralogy into the pentalogy of Fallot. Tetralogy of Fallot is compatible with life but is associated with cyanosis at birth, great fatigue after mild exertion, and stunted growth. Dr. Helen B. Taussig, a noted pediatric surgeon at Johns Hopkins Medical School, pioneered pediatric cardiovascular surgical procedures to correct the defect.

67. The answer is E (all). (*Chapter 21 II B; V B*) The auricle, or pinna, is the expanded, sound-gathering component of the external ear. It leads into the external auditory meatus. The auricle forms from ectoderm-covered mesenchymal masses at the tips of the first and second arches. These masses surround the first pharyngeal cleft, which forms the external auditory meatus. Abnormalities in the shape of the auricle are found in all three syndromes mentioned in the question. Down and Edwards syndromes are caused by trisomy; first arch syndrome (also called mandibulofacial dysostosis, or Treacher Collins syndrome) is an autosomal dominant trait with variable penetrance.

68. The answer is E (all). (*Chapter 23 V C 1*) Alcohol in chronic high doses has been well established as a teratogenic drug. Experimental studies suggest that excessive alcohol consumption by the mother has a serious effect on embryonic neural crest cell migration during development of the pharyngeal arch system. Fetal alcohol syndrome involves midfacial hypoplasia, short stature, and mental retardation. The philtrum is also hypoplastic in these children.

69. The answer is A (1, 2, 3). (*Chapter 17 III B 6; Chapter 19 V A, B; VI A 3 c*) Pancreatic islet tissue contains insulin-secreting alpha cells (A cells) and glucagon-secreting beta cells (B cells) derived from both the dorsal and ventral pancreatic rudiments. They also contain C and D cells that are derived from a different embryonic rudiment, the neural crest. D cells secrete somatostatin; similar cells are found in the stomach and small intestines.

70. The answer is B (1, 3). (*Chapter 19 IV A, B*) Only the medulla of the adrenal gland is a neural crest derivative. The adrenal cortex is a mesodermal derivative. The fetal cortex undergoes extensive regression after birth. The adult zonation pattern is not established until puberty.

71. The answer is A (1, 2, 3). (*Chapter 6 II B 1; Chapter 9 II B 3; IV B 3; IV C 1, 2*) The somites are divided into sclerotomes and dermomyotomes. The sclerotomes form the vertebral bodies and neural arches, the annulus fibrosus of the intervertebral disks (but not the nucleus pulposus, which is a notochordal derivative), and ligaments supporting the vertebral column. Each dermomyotome becomes divided into a dermatome and a myotome. The myotomes form segmental muscles, including the intercostal muscles. The dermatomes form the dense irregular connective tissue of the dermis.

72. The answer is E (all). (*Chapter 4 II B 3, III A 3, C*) Fertilization encompasses the penetrating of the ovum by a spermatozoon and the subsequent events leading to the initiation of development. Fertilization is thought to occur in the ampullary portion of the fallopian (uterine) tubes. It is also suspected that an ovum is only viable for 12 to 24 hours after ovulation. The second polar body, marking the completion of meiosis in the female, is not formed until after fertilization. Fertilization introduces a haploid male pronucleus into the egg cytoplasm, where it fuses with the haploid female pronucleus to establish a single diploid zygote nucleus. Fertilization also results in chemical changes in the zona pellucida which prevent polyspermy, and it leads directly to the first cleavage.

73. The answer is A (1, 2, 3). (*Chapter 19 V A; VI A, C*) The alpha and beta cells of the pancreatic islet tissue are endodermal derivatives. They arise from the dorsal and ventral pancreatic rudiments, just like the pancreatic acinar cells which form the exocrine secretory units of the pancreas. The neural crest gives rise to the so-called amine precursor uptake and decarboxylation (APUD) cells, the adrenal medulla, and the parafollicular (C) cells of the thyroid gland. The C and D cells of the pancreatic islets are also thought to be neural crest derivatives. The thyroid follicular epithelial cells come from an endodermal diverticulum which arises at the root of the tongue.

74–77. The answers are: 74-B, 75-A, 76-C, 77-B. (*Chapter 4 IV C; V B*) The fertilized egg, or zygote, gives rise to a morula, which in turn develops into a blastocyst. The embryoblast, or inner cell mass, is a loose collection of blastomeres bordering the blastocoele of the blastocyst. The trophoblast is an epithelial layer making up the wall of the blastocyst and surrounding the embryoblast. Thus, the zygote gives rise to both the embryoblast and the trophoblast. The trophoblast forms the cytotrophoblast and the syncytiotrophoblast; later in development, it forms the extraembryonic membranes such as the chorion and the bulk of the placenta as well. The epiblast and hypoblast are the two layers of the bilaminar disk-stage pre-embryo, and as such, like other structures comprising the body of the developing pre-embryo, are derived from the embryoblast.

78–81. The answers are: 78-B, 79-C, 80-D, 81-C. (*Chapter 17 IV A, B*) At the indifferent stage of genital development, the external genitalia are alike in both sexes. As a result of sexual differentiation, the genital tubercle (A) forms the glans penis and glans clitoris. The urogenital folds (B) form the body of the penis and the labia minora. The labioscrotal swellings (C) form the scrotum and the labia majora. The urogenital membrane (D) forms the hymen. (E) labels the anus.

82–85. The answers are: 82-B, 83-A, 84-D, 85-B. [*Chapter 20 II B, C; III A, B 1, C 2 a, 4, E 1 a (2), F*] The optic cup consists of two epithelial layers. The inner layer forms the neural retina and the outer forms the pigmented retina. Posterior to the ora serrata, the neural retina consists of photoreceptors (rods and cones) and neurons (e.g., bipolar neurons and ganglion cells) and a complex collection of glial cells. Posterior to the ora serrata, the pigmented retina consists of a single layer of pigmented epithelial cells. Anterior to the ora serrata, on the iris, the pars iridica retinae has two layers of pigmented epithelium, derived from both the inner and outer layers of the optic cup. The blood supply for the retina comes from the retinal artery, a remnant of the hyaloid artery. The retina is also nourished by diffusion from the choroid layer, a derivative of head mesenchyme surrounding the optic cup.

86–88. The answers are: 86-B, 87-D, 88-C. (Chapter 10 II F, G) The left and right sinus venosi empty into the left (A) and right (B) atria, respectively. The aortic sac (C) receives the ventricular output, and later it becomes the root of the aorta. The muscular portion of the interventricular septum forms at the small sulcus (D). The membranous portion of the interventricular septum forms from endocardial cushions and bulbar ridges. The precursor of the left ventricle (E) is also labelled in the diagram.

89–93. The answers are: 89-C, 90-A, 91-E, 92-B, 93-D. (Chapter 7 VI A, B) The placenta consists of a decidual plate (C) facing the endometrium and a chorionic plate (E) facing the fetus. The decidual plate and chorionic plate are fused at the margins of the discoid placenta. These two plates are interconnected by cytotrophoblastic cell columns (B). Large numbers of chorionic villi (D) project away from them into the intervillous space (A). Maternal blood vessels end on the decidual plate and pour maternal blood into the intervillous space. Maternal blood directly bathes the chorionic villi. Thus, the human placenta is said to be a hemochorial placenta.

94–96. The answers are: 94-C, 95-A, 96-B. (Chapter 14 III C) The definitive trachea, bronchi, and the lungs themselves are all derived from two embryonic rudiments. The first of these, the respiratory diverticulum, forms epithelial cells lining the lumen of the entire respiratory system, including the alveolar epithelial cells (type I squamous cells and type II surfactant-secreting cells). The second rudiment, the splanchnic mesoderm, forms cartilage, smooth muscle, connective tissues, and blood vessels in the trachea, bronchi, and lungs.

97–102. The answers are: 97-B, 98-E, 99-C, 100-A, 101-D, 102-C. (Chapter 11 I B 1, 2; II A 1, B 5 b, c) The central nervous system (CNS) has a lumen (D) which later forms the central canal of the spinal cord and the ventricles of the brain. This lumen is surrounded by an ependymal layer (C). Some ependymal cells lining the walls of the third and fourth ventricles differentiate into the epithelial cells of the choroid plexus, the site of cerebrospinal fluid production. The ependymal layer is surrounded by a mantle layer (B), the precursor of gray matter. The mantle layer, which contains many neuronal cell bodies, is in turn surrounded by a marginal layer (A), the precursor of white matter, which contains many myelinated nerve processes. The entire CNS is surrounded by an external limiting membrane (E) that is the basement membrane of the neuroepithelium.

103–107. The answers are: 103-C, 104-E, 105-D, 106-A, 107-B. (Chapter 2 II B; IV B; V B) The primordial germ cells are diploid proliferative cells derived from the wall of the yolk sac. They differentiate into diploid spermatogonia and oogonia. Primary spermatocytes are tetraploid cells that are produced in vast quantities by mitosis of spermatogonia in the male after puberty. The proliferation of spermatogonia and production of primary spermatocytes continue until death. Primary oocytes are tetraploid cells which are arrested in meiosis I from their time of formation (before birth) until ovulation at some time later, up to the menopause. Secondary oocytes are diploid cells that undergo unequal cytoplasmic divisions to produce small polar bodies and ova. Secondary spermatocytes are diploid cells that undergo equal cytoplasmic divisions to form spermatids which subsequently differentiate into spermatozoa during spermiogenesis.

108–112. The answers are: 108-A, 109-B, 110-C, 111-B, 112-A. (Chapter 17 III A, C, D; VI E; VII E 1 a) The mesonephric duct (A) and associated mesonephric tubules form the excurrent duct system of the male gonad, including the appendix epididymis. The appendix testis comes from the paramesonephric duct (B), as do the uterine tubes, uterus, cervix, and upper third of the vagina in females. The gonads (C) secrete müllerian-inhibiting substance in the male. In testicular feminization syndrome, the patient is genetically male but phenotypically female due to a lack of the testosterone receptor. Since the differentiation of mesonephric duct derivatives are testosterone-dependent in males, these are lacking in testicular feminization syndrome. The urogenital sinus (D) and the mesonephron (E) are structures in the developing urinary tract.

113–116. The answers are: 113-A, 114-C, 115-B, 116-D. (Chapter 21 IV B, C) The otocyst forms the entire epithelial lining of the membranous labyrinth. By differential growth, the otocyst forms two subdivisions, called the cochlear pouch and the vestibular pouch. The former forms the cochlear duct and the macula sacculi. The latter forms the macula utriculi and semicircular canals. Both contribute to the membranous labyrinth. The perilymphatic spaces develop around the membranous labyrinth by cavitation in head mesenchyme.

117–120. The answers are: 117-C, 118-C, 119-C, 120-B. (*Chapter 5 VI A 3, B*) Maternal serum α-fetoprotein is usually elevated in all severe neural tube defects. Failure of closure of the neural tube usually results in a concomitant failure of neural tissue to differentiate properly and also a failure of bone induction over the defective neural tissue. Thus, both open spina bifida and anencephaly involve faulty formation of the neural arches or the vault of the skull, since these bony structures surround the CNS. Both severe spina bifida and anencephaly usually also have degenerative changes in neural tissue. Individuals with spina bifida have normal mental capacity and a reasonable life expectancy. In anencephalic fetuses, there is no formation of the cerebral hemispheres and death invariably occurs soon after birth.

121–122. The answers are: 121-C, 122-A. (*Chapter 13 III A, B*) The liver parenchymal cells arise from the liver diverticulum. The pancreatic acinar cells and islet tissue form from the dorsal and ventral pancreatic buds. All three are formed from diverticula of the primitive gut tube at the boundary between the foregut and the midgut. The liver diverticulum grows into the septum transversum. Only the liver contains blood vessels and connective tissue elements derived from septum transversum mesenchyme.

123–126. The answers are: 123-D, 124-C, 125-B, 126-A. (*Chapter 13 I B 6; III A, B; IV A 2; V C 2*) The site where the liver diverticulum (A) and the pancreatic buds (C) arise is the boundary between the foregut and the midgut. The liver diverticulum (A) forms the epithelial parenchymal cells, which have both an endocrine and an exocrine function. The pancreatic buds (C) form part of the pancreas, including the islets of Langerhans. The midgut (B) forms the distal small intestine, including most of the duodenum, all of the jejunum, and all of the ileum, as well as the ascending and proximal transverse colon. The cloaca (D) is a hindgut derivative which receives the excurrent ducts of the urinary and reproductive systems. The vitelline duct (E) is a midgut diverticulum which projects into the umbilicus and serves as the axis of rotation of the midgut loop along with the superior mesenteric artery.

127–129. The answers are: 127-C, 128-E, 129-A. (*Chapter 10 V C*) The first aortic arch (A) forms the maxillary artery. The second aortic arch (B) forms the stapedial artery. The third aortic arch (C) forms the common carotid and proximal external carotid arteries. The fourth aortic arch (D) forms part of the arch of the aorta and parts of the subclavian artery. The fifth aortic arch is rudimentary in humans. It forms no adult structures. The sixth aortic arch (E) forms the pulmonary arteries and the ductus arteriosus.

130–134. The answers are: 130-B, 131-A, 132-C, 133-E, 134-A. (*Chapter 8 IV A 1; Chapter 10 III A; VI D; VII C*) The septum transversum (C) is a ventral mass of mesenchyme which contributes to a large portion of the diaphragm. It also contributes to the liver, including the hepatic blood vessels and connective tissues in the capsule and central mass. The pleuroperitoneal membranes (D) contribute to the lateral parts of the diaphragm; they do not contribute to the liver. The ductus venosus (A) passes through the liver and conducts placental blood from the umbilical vein to the inferior vena cava. After birth, the ductus venosus degenerates into a fibrous cord in the liver called the ligamentum venosum. The septum primum (E) is the first flap of tissue formed during atrial septation. Just before the septum primum fuses with the endocardial cushions, an ostium secundum forms in its upper portion. The foramen ovale (B) is a hole in the septum secundum, and along with the ostium secundum it forms a right-to-left shunt through the atrial portion of the heart.

135–140. The answers are: 135-E, 136-B, 137-D, 138-C, 139-E, 140-E. (*Chapter 9 III D*) During endochondral bone formation, a cartilage model grows by cell division in the zone of proliferation (B). Just below this zone of proliferation, one finds a resting zone of chondrocytes (A). The formation of the first ossified tissue, a bony collar (E), causes the formation of a zone of hypertrophy (C). These hypertrophic cells eventually degenerate, leaving behind a zone of cartilage degeneration and calcification (D). Hematopoiesis and bone formation occur within the marrow cavity, which will form after complete cartilage degeneration. The embryonic cartilage model persists in the fully grown adult only at the articular surface (not shown).

141–144. The answers are: 141-A, 142-C, 143-D, 144-B. (*Chapter 16 II A, B 6 d; III A 2, B 1, 2*) The pronephros (A) degenerates without ever becoming active in urine production. The mesonephros (B) forms after the pronephros and also degenerates. The ureteric bud (D), however, forms as a branch from the mesonephric duct and later leads to the formation of everything in the urinary system from the urinary collecting tubules to the urinary bladder. The metanephric blastema (C) forms everything in the kidneys between the glomeruli and the collecting tubules. The cloaca (E) is divided by the urorectal septum into the rectum and the urogenital sinus, a precursor of the urinary bladder.

Index

Note: Page numbers in *italics* denote illustrations; those followed by (t) denote tables; those followed by Q denote questions; and those followed by E denote explanations.

A

Abdominal cavities, 115
Accessory nerve, 183
Achondroplasia, 137–138, 139, 141Q, 144E, 393
Acidophilic cells, 324, 326
Acrocephaly, 139
Acrosome, 8, 25, 28Q, 47
ACTH, see Adrenocorticotropic hormone
Actin, 5, 136
α-Actinin, 5, 136
Adenine, 386
Adenohypophysis, 67, 181, 202, 228, 321, 322, 323, 324, 325, 329
Adenoid tonsils, 252
Adenosine triphosphate, 25, 103
Adipocytes, multilocular, 38
Adipose tissue, 40, 68
Adrenal cortex, 326, 329, 330, 333Q, 335E
Adrenal gland, 321, 326–327, *327*, 332Q, 334E
Adrenal medulla, 68, 326, 333Q, 335E
Adrenocorticotropic hormone, 103, 202, 324, 330
Adrenogenital syndrome, 293(t), 297, 330
Adult polycystic kidney disease, 393
Afferent nuclei, 182–183
Agenesis
  pulmonary, 8
  renal, 8, 272–273
Alar laminae, 171, *172*, 175, 178, 182, 187Q, 190E
Alar plate, 171, 173–174, 187Q, 190E, 189Q, 190E
Albinism, 202, 204Q, 205E
Alcohol, and birth defects, 369, 379
Aldosterone, 326
Alkaline phosphatase, 280
Allantois, 82, 85, 90E, 219, 270–271, 274
Alpha cells, 327
Alveolar cells, 231
Alveolar ducts, 225
Alveoli, 226
Amastia, 202, 204Q, 205E
Amelia, 139, 379
Ameloblasts, 200
Amelogenesis imperfecta, 202
Amine precursor uptake and decarboxylation cells, 321, 327, 328, 329, 331Q, 332Q, 334E
Amino acids, 103, 386
Aminopterin, 379
Amniocentesis, 71, 220, 233, 255, 257, 362–363, 367Q, 368E, 381, 387, 393, 394
Amnion, 33, 50, 55, 87, 93
  folding of, 80
  growth of, 6, 84, *85*
  lateral body folds of, 84, 85, *86*, 90E
Amniotic cavity, 53–54, 55
Amniotic fluid, 71, 233, 235, 255, 272, 362, 364, 381, 394

Ampulla
  of inner ear, 354, 355
  of ovary, 12
Anal canal, 67, 69, 219
  abnormalities of, 221
Anal membrane, 219, 288
Anal valves, 219
Anatomic planes, 2, *2*
Anatomic terms, 14Q
  defined, 1–2, *2*
Anchoring villi, 111Q, 114E
Androgen, 197, 296, 297, 326, 330
Anencephaly, 1, 70, *70*, 71, 72, 73, 272, 362, 363, 369, 378, 394
  incidence of, 370(t)
Aneuploidy, 381, 385, 393
  risk of, with increasing maternal age, 393, 397Q, 399E
Angiogenesis, 82, 83
Angiogenetic cell clusters, 82, 146
Ankle, 36
Annular pancreas, 220
Annulus fibrosus, 133
Anophthalmia, 347, 378
Anterior, 2
Anterior chamber, 337, 338, 346
Anterior intestinal portal, 87, 207
Anterior nares, 227
Anterior retina, 344
Antigen–antibody complexes, 240
Antimetabolites, 379
Antimitotic drugs, 379
Antimüllerian hormone, 292
Antrum, 22
Anus, 207
Aorta, 158
Aortic arches, 148, 153–156, *154*, 155(t), 163Q, 165E
Aorticopulmonary septum, 153
Aortic root, 148
Aortic sac, 153, 154, 155(t)
Aortic trunk, 153, 155
Aortic valves, 153
Apical ectodermal ridge, 9, 134, *136*
Apocrine sweat glands, 191, 196
Aponeuroses, 68
Appendicitis, 218
Appendicular skeleton, 134
Appendix, 215, 217, 218
Appendix vesiculosa, 288
APUD cells, see Amine precursor uptake and decarboxylation cells
Aqueduct of Sylvius, 182
Aqueous humor, 337, 338, 346
Arachidonic acid, 363
Arachnoid membrane, 172
Argyrophilic cells, 327
Arrector pili muscle, 197
Arteries, see *specific types*
Ascending colon, 215, 217
Aspirin, 379
Asthma, 242

Astroblasts, 170
Astrocytes, 170
Astroglia, 170
A-T base pairs, 386
Atelectasis, 233
Atlas, 133
Atresia
  duodenal, 220
  esophageal, 220, 272
  foregut, 220
  of oogonia and oocytes, 20, 21
  rectal, 221
  tricuspid, 161
Atrial septal defect, 160, 161
Atrial septation, 149–150, *149*
Atrioventricular canals, 151
Atrioventricular valves, 153
Atrium, 147, 148, 150–151, 158, 163Q, 164E
Auditory meatus, 67
Auditory placode, 355
Auditory tube, 69, 351, 352, 353
Auricle, 313, 351, 352
Auricular hillocks, 36
Autonomic nervous system, 174, 207
Autosomal dominant inheritance, 390–391, *390*
Autosomal recessive inheritance, 391, *391*
Autosomes, 387, 389
Axial skeleton, 130–134, *133*
Axis of bilateral symmetry, 64
Axons, 170, 171, 172, 173, 175, 178
Azygos vein, 157

B

Balance, 351
Banding techniques, 388
Barr body, 291, *291*
Basalis, 13
Basal laminae, 171, 172, 176, 178, 182, 183, 187Q, 190E
Basal plate, 171, 173–175, 187Q, 190E
Basal stem cells, 201
Basophils, 324
B cell differentiation, 247, *247*, 248–249
B cells, 246, 247–248, 260Q, 261E
Beta cells, 327
Bilaminar disk stage, 33, *34*, 54, 62, *62*, 116
Bilateral renal agenesis, 272–273
Bile, 220
Bile duct, 212, 214, 215
Biliary apparatus, 69, 207, 213, 214
Biliary tract, 208
Bilirubin, 103–104, 254, 255
Bipolar cells, 342
Birth control pills, 26, 103, 379
Birth defects, see Congenital anomalies; Congenital birth defects; *specific types*
Bivalents, 19, 26

437

Bladder, 68, 69, 160, 219, 263, 265, 269–272, 275Q, 277E
anomalies of, 274
Bladder exstrophy, 274, *274*, 395
Blastocoele, 46, 49, 59E
Blastocyst, 33, *34*, 46, 49, 50, *51*, 52, 57E, 59E, 58Q, 93
Blastoderm, 55, 62
Blastomeres, 46, 49, *49*
Blastopore, 62
Blindness, 338, 345
Blood cells, 68, 82
Blood islands, 82, *82*, 83, 88Q, 90E, 146
Blood supply, maternal, to conceptus, 53
Blood transfusion, intrauterine, 255
Blood vessels, 68, 82, 83, 84, 145, 197
"Bloody show," 364
B lymphocytes, 242, 248, 252
Body cavities, 81–82, 115–118
Body folds, 80, 84–85
Body plan, establishment of, 79–82
Bohr effect, 102
Bone marrow, 68, 83, 239, 244, 248, 249, 252
Bone marrow stem cells, 248
Bones, 8, 68, 125, 127–130, 141Q, 144E
abnormal formation of, 138
Bony cochlea, 354
Bony collar, 129, 142Q, 144E
Bony labyrinth, 354, 356
Bowman's capsule, 264, 265, 266, 267
Bowman's glands, 228
Bradykinin, 158, 162Q
Brain, 64, 65, 67, 68, 69, 84, 167, 176, *177*, 178, 324, 327, 328
Brain damage, 254
Brain microglia, 68
Brain ventricles, 167
Brain vesicles, 167, 176
Breast, 202
Breast milk, 242, 252–253, 259Q, 261E
Breech position, 366
Broad ligament, 12, 286
Bronchi, 208, 225, 228–230
Bronchioles, 225
Brown fat, 38
Buccinator muscle, 313
Bucconasal membrane, 227, 306
Buccopharyngeal membrane, 55, 227
Bulbar ridges, 153
Bulbourethral glands, 10, 16E
Bulbus cordis, 147, 148, 153, 161
Bursa of Fabricius, 247, 248, 249

C

Calcium, 103
Calyces, 263, 267, 268
Canalicular stage, of pulmonary development, 231, *231*, 233
Canal of Schlemm, 338, 345, 346
Cancer
gynecologic, 379
of placenta, 106
Cannabis, 380
Cardiac jelly, 147, 148
Cardiac muscle, 68, 136, 145, 153
Cardiac myocytes, 84
Cardiac primordium, 62–63
Cardiac valves, 153
Cardiogenesis, 83, 90E
Cardiovascular defects
with cri du chat syndrome, 373
with DiGeorge syndrome, 256, 317
with Down syndrome, 370
with Edwards syndrome, 371
from multifactorial inheritance, 395
with Patau syndrome, 373
from phenylketonuria, 392
from rubella virus, 375

Cardiovascular system, 68, 84, 145–161
congenital anomalies of, 160–161, 162Q, 164E
Cartilage, 8, 68, 125, 126–127, 129, 130, 135, 141Q, 144E, *315*, 319Q, 320E
Cartilage calcification, 142Q, 144E
Cartilage matrix, 129
Cartilage proteoglycan, 5
Carotid arteries, 155
Cataracts
congenital, 347
from rubella virus, 375
Cauda equina, 175
Caudal, 1
Caudal regression syndrome, 369
Cecal bud, 218, 223Q, 224E
Cecum, 215, 217, 218
Celiac arteries, 156, 208, 210
Cell-mediated immune response, 246
Cementoblasts, 200
Cementum, 200
Central nervous system, 6, 8, 35, 67, 167–186
congenital abnormalities of, 185–186
defects in, from cytomegalic inclusion disease, 377
drugs acting on, 379
ependymal layer of, 171
induction of, 64–65
mantle layer of, 170–171, 173, 178
marginal layer of, 171, 173, 178
teratogenic effect on, 37
Central nervous system inductor, 64
Central nervous system primordium, 64, 65
Centromeres, 20, 24
Cephalopelvic disproportion, 366
Cerebellar cortex, *184*
Cerebellar plate, 183
Cerebellar rudiment, 183
Cerebellum, 167, 178, 182, 183–184, 186, 188Q, 190E
Cerebral cortex, 179, *181*
Cerebral hemispheres, 167, 176, 178, 179
Cerebrospinal fluid, 175, 179, 185
Cerebrum, *179*, 188Q, 190E
Cerumen, 352
Ceruminous glands, 352
Cervical dilation, 367Q
Cervical flexure, 36, 176
Cervical mucus plug, 364
Cervix, 12, 13, 16E, 284, 285, *286*, *287*, 363
Cesarean section, 138, 233, 255, 366, 377
Chemoreceptors, 309
Chemotherapy, 106
Chiasmata, 19, 20
Cholesterol, 329, 330
Chondrification, 126, *127*
Chondroblasts, 8, 125, 127, 129
Chondrocytes, 3, 5, 8, 127, 129, 133, 142Q, 144E
Chondrodystrophy, 137–138
Chondrogenesis, 126–127
Chondroitin sulfate, 125
Chordae tendineae, 153
Chordamesodermal inductor, 61
Chordamesodermal mass, 64
Chorioadenoma destruens, 106
Chorioamnionic membrane, 33
Choriocarcinoma, 106
Chorion, 33, 35, 54, 55, 82, 87, 93, 96, 97
Chorion frondosum, 97, 100
Chorionic gonadotropin, 26, 99, 106, 325, 329
Chorionic plate, 98
Chorionic shell, 94, 145
Chorionic somatomammotropin, 329
Chorionic villi, 84, 94–95, 96, *96*
Chorionic villus sampling, 387
Chorion laeve, 97
Chorioretinitis, 377
Choroid, 337, 342, 345
Choroid fissure, 180, 185, 339, 346, 347

Choroid plexus, 178, 179, 180, 185
Chromatids, 19, 24
Chromophobes, 324
Chromosome complement, numerical errors in, 389–390
Chromosomes, 24, 279, 386, 387
abnormal number of, 26, 48, 160, 347, 369, 370, 370(t), 393–394
haploid, 28Q
preservation of number of, 17, 18
sex, 18, 291, 362, 387, 388
in sexual differentiation, 290, 291, *292*
Cilia, 13, 228, 309
Ciliary body, 337, 338, 344, 346, 348Q, 349E
Cisterna chyli, 249
Clavicles, 134
Cleavage, 46, 49–50, 377
in in vitro fertilization, 56
Clefting anomalies, 315–316, *316*, 318Q, 320E
see also Cleft lip; Cleft palate
Cleft lip, 1, 315, 316, 372, 395
incidence of, 370(t)
Cleft palate, 1, 121, 315, 316, 369, 372, 395
incidence of, 370(t)
Clitoris, 12
Cloaca, 218, 219, 270, 288
Cloacal membrane, 55, 207, 219
Cloverleaf skull syndrome, 139
Cocaine, 380
Cochlea, 351
Cochlear apparatus, 354
Cochlear duct, 354, 356, 357, 358Q, 359E
Cochlear nerve, 354
Cochlear pouch, 355, *355*, 356, 357
Codon, 387
Coelomic duct, 116
Coeloms, communication between intraembryonic and extraembryonic, 43E
Collagen, 5, 125, 148, 201, 202
Collecting tubules, 264, 265, 267, 268
Coloboma, 347, 372
Colon, see Ascending colon; Descending colon; Transverse colon
Colostrum, 242, 252
Columnar cells, 201
Common cardinal veins, 156–157
Common excretory bud, 271
Common iliac veins, 157
Complement cascade, 240
Conceptus
defined, 33
during implantation, 93, *94*
after implantation, *95*
viability of, 46
Conducting airway, 225
Cones, 337, 338, 340, 342
Congenital adrenal hyperplasia, 297, 330, 332Q, 334E
Congenital aganglionic megacolon, 221
Congenital anomalies, 1
antenatal diagnosis of, 361, 362, 381
see also Birth defects, congenital; specific types
Congenital birth defects, 1, 385–396
see also Congenital anomalies; specific types
of cardiovascular system, 160–161, 162Q, 164E
causes of, 385
of central nervous system, 185–186
correction of, 395–396
diagnosis of, 385
of ear, 356–357
etiology of, 369–381
of eye, 347
in facial development, 352
of gastrointestinal tract, 219–221
of head and neck, 315–317
incidence of, 369–370, 370(t), 385
infectious agents and, 373, 375, 377

from in vitro fertilization, 56
in mammary glands, 202
of musculoskeletal system, 137–139
of skin, 202
in teeth, 202
of urinary system, 272–274
Congenital corneal opacities, 347
Congenital cystic disease of kidneys, 273
Congenital diaphragmatic hernia, 121, *121*, 122Q, 124E
Congenital ectodermal dysplasia, 202, 204Q, 205E
Congenital herpes infection, 377
Congenital ichthyosis, 202, 204Q, 205E
Congenital inguinal hernia, 290
Congenital lens opacities, 347
Congenital metabolic disorders, 362–363
Congenital X-linked hypogammaglobulinemia, 256, 259Q, 261E
Congestive heart failure, 161
Conjunctiva, 337
Connecting stalk, 54, 55, 82, 87, 90E, 104, 112Q, 114E
Connective tissue domain, 353, 354
Contractions, uterine, 363, 364, 367Q
Conus medullaris, 175
Copula, 309
Cord prolapse, 366
Corium, 192
Cornea, 337, 338, 345, 348Q, 349E
Coronal plane, 2
Corona radiata, 22, 24, 31E, 46, 47
Coronary sinus, 151
Corpora cavernosa, 11
Corpus callosum, 186, 188Q, 190E
Corpus luteum, 13, 23, 25, 26, 326, 329
Corpus spongiosum, 11
Corpus striatum, 179, 180
Corticopontine tracts, 182
Corticospinal tracts, 182
Corticosterone, 326
Cortisol, 326, 330
Costal processes, 132
Counseling, genetic, 1, 386, 394
Cowper's glands, 10, 16E
Cranial, 1
Cranial nerve II, 182
Cranial nerve IV, 182
Cranial nerve V, 310, 313
Cranial nerve VII, 313
Cranial nerve VIII, 354, 356, 357
Cranial nerve IX, 183, 315
Cranial nerve X, 183, 310, 315
Cranial nerve XI, 183
Cranial nerve XII, 183, 310
Cranial pole, 62
Craniofacial defects, 256
Craniosynostosis, 139
Cribriform plate, 309
Cri du chat syndrome, 373, 384E, 389
Crista ampullaris, 355, 356
Crista dividens, 158
Crista terminalis, 151
Crown–heel length, 37, 361
Crown–rump length, 37, 39, 361
Crura cerebri, 182
Cryptorchidism, 290, 295, 395
Crystallins, 345
Cumulus oophorus, 22
Cupula, 355
Cyclopia, 347, 372
Cystic duct, 214
Cystic fibrosis, 393
Cystic hygroma, 257, *257*, *258*
Cysts, bladder, 274
Cytogenetic screening, 394
Cytokinesis, 20, 21, *21*
Cytomegalic inclusion disease, 377
Cytomegalovirus, 369, 377
Cytomorphogenesis, 8
Cytoplasmic ribosomes, 387

Cytosine, 386
Cytotoxic T cells, 248
Cytotrophoblast, 52, 54, 93, 94, 112Q, 114E
Cytotrophoblastic cell columns, 96, 98
Cytotrophoblastic cells, 95
Cytotrophoblastic shell, 96, 98

D

Dartos muscle, 289
Deafness, 357
Decidua, 93, 99–100, *101*
Decidua basalis, 99, 100
Decidua capsularis, 99
Decidual cells, 99, *100*
Decidual plate, 111Q, 114E
Decidual septa, 101, 111Q, 114E
Decidua parietalis, 99
Decidua vera, 99
Dehydroepiandrosterone sulfate, 326, 330
Deletions, chromosome, 385, 389
Delivery, see Labor and delivery
Delta cells, 327, 328
Dendrites, 170, 171, 175, 178
Dental lamina, 199
Dental papilla, 199–200
Dentate nucleus, 184
Dentin, 200, 201
Dentinal tubules, 201
11-Deoxycortisol, 330
Deoxyribonucleic acid, see DNA
Deoxyribose, 386
Dermal bones, 128
Dermal papillae, 192
Dermatomes, 132, 192
Dermis, 35, 191, 192
Dermomyotome, 81
Dermomyotomes, 81, 126
DES, see Diethylstilbestrol
Descending colon, 156, 217, 219
Desmosomes, 99
Development
 basic concepts of, 3, 5–6, 8–9
 fetal, assessment of, 361
 general aspects of, 1–13
 normal female, 298Q, 301E
 periods of, 33, *34*
Developmental age, 361
DHEAS, see Dehydroepiandrosterone sulfate
Diabetes mellitus, during pregnancy, 233, 369
Diagnostic ultrasound, see Sonography
Diaphragm, 118–119, *118*, 120–121, 122Q
Diarthroses, 135
Diazepam, 379
Diencephalon, 167, 176, 180–181, 338
Diethylstilbestrol, 379
Differential gene activity, 3
Differentiation, 3, 5, 6, 14Q
Digastric muscle, 313
DiGeorge syndrome, 256–257, *256*, 260Q, 261E, 317
Digestive system, 207–221, *208*, *209*, 327, 328
Digits, 36
 abnormalities of, 139
Dilator muscles, 67
Diphenylhydantoin, 379
Diploidy, 389
Diploid zygote nucleus, 45
Distal, 2
DNA, 19, 24, 292, 369, 386–387
Dorsal, 2
Dorsal aortas, 153, 155, 156
Dorsal ganglia, 167
Dorsal gastric mesentery, 210–211
Dorsal horns, 174, 175
Dorsal median septa, 174
Dorsal mesentery, 119, 207, 215, 218, 219

Dorsal mesocardium, 148
Dorsal mesogastrium, 223Q, 224E, 251
Dorsal root ganglia, 173, 174, 175–176
Dorsolateral hernias, 121, *121*
Down syndrome, 26, 139, 186, 357, 362, 370, 377, 381, 382Q, 384E, 385, 386, 389, 393, 398Q, 399E
 see also Translocation Down syndrome; Trisomy 21
 clinical features of, *372*
 frequency of, 371(t)
 karyotype of, *371*
 recurrence risk in, 394
Drugs, see also specific names
 teratogenic effects of, 369, 378–380, 382Q, 384E
Duct of epididymis, 285
Ductus arteriosus, 156, 158, 160, 163Q, 164E
Ductus deferens, 9, 10, 271, 282, 285
Ductus epididymidis, see Epididymis
Ductus venosus, 157, 158, 160, 163Q, 164E
Duodenal atresia, 220
Duodenal stenosis, 219, 220
Duodenum, 156, 208, 212, 218, 328
Dura mater, 172
Dwarfs, achondroplastic, 138, 139

E

Ear, 37, 351–357, *351*
 congenital anomalies of, 356–357, 358Q, 359E
Ear canal, 351
Eardrum, 351, 353
Ear rudiments, 35
Eccrine sweat glands, 191, 196, 199
Ectoderm, 6, 9, 33, 35, 54, 61, 64, 67, 74Q, 75Q, 76E, 77E, 168, 191, 192, 196, 227, 304, 321
Ectomeninx, 172, 175
Ectopic kidney, 273
Ectopic pregnancy, 1, 52, 104, 105(t)
Edema, fetal, 254, *255*
Edinger-Westphal nucleus, 182
Edwards syndrome, 26, 357, *357*, 370–372, 383Q, 384E, 389, 393
 see also Trisomy 18
 clinical features of, *374*
 frequency of, 371(t)
 recurrence risk in, 394
Efferent ductules, 10, 282, 283, 285
Efferent neurons, 174
Efferent nuclei, 183
Ehlers-Danlos syndrome, 202, 204Q, 205E
Ejaculatory duct, 10, 285
Elastic tissue, 68
Elbow, 36
Embryo
 blood vessel formation in, 82
 components of, 89Q
 defined, 61
 at 5 weeks, *135*
 growth of, 3
 increase in length of, 44E
 at mid-gastrula stage, *64*
 morphogenesis of, 6
 morphologic changes in, *36*
 during neurulation, *66*
 transfer of, 55–56
Embryoblast, 33, 50, 59E
Embryonic period, 33–37, 41Q
Enamel, 67, 200, 202
Enamel organ, 199, 200
Encephalocele, 378
Endocardial cushions, 149, 151, 153
Endocardial heart tubes, 147
Endocardium, 148
Endocrine glands, 321, *322*
Endocrine hormones, 103

Endocrine system, 68, 321–330
Endoderm, 6, 33, 35, 54, 61, 64, 68–69, 74Q, 76E, 207, 219, 223Q, 224E, 227, 321
Endolymph, 354, 355
Endolymphatic duct, 355
Endolymphatic sac, 355
Endomeninx, 172, 175
Endometrium, 13, 16E, 26, 33, 93
Endoplasmic reticulum, 136
Endothelium, 145, 345, 346
Enteric nervous system, 207
Enterochromaffin cells, 68, 328
Ependymal cells, 170, 342
Ependymal layer, of neural tube, 67, 171
Epiblast, 54, 54, 55, 62
Epicardium, 148
Epidermis, 67, 191, 192, *192*, 196
Epididymis, 9, 10, 16E, 282, 285
Epilepsy, 379
Epiphyseal plate, 8, 129, 130, 134
Epiphysis cerebri, 180
Epiploic foramen, 211
Epithalamus, 180
Epithelial-mesenchymal interactions, 8–9
Epithelium
 alveolar, 231, 233
 amniotic, 104
 ciliary, 338
 coelomic, 282, 283, 284, 300Q, 302E
 corneal, 345
 cuboidal, 231
 of digestive system, 207
 duodenal, 212
 of ear, 352, 353, 354, 358Q, 359E
 endometrial, 93
 esophageal, 209
 of fetal skin, 192
 of foregut, 208
 formed from endoderm, 69
 for gas exchange, 225
 gingival, 67
 labial, 67
 in nasal cavities, 227
 in neural tube, 67
 ocular, 67
 olfactory, 67, 226, 228, 303, 309
 oral, 199, 227
 in penile urethra, 11
 pigmented, in iris, 344
 respiratory, 225, 226, 228, 229
 seminiferous, 30Q, 32E
 squamous, 82, 145
Epitrichium, 192
Epoophoron, 288
Erectile tissue, 11
Erection, 11
Erythroblastosis fetalis, 242, 254, 255
Erythroblasts, 251
Erythrocytes, 83
Erythropoiesis, 82, 251
Esophageal atresia, 220, 272
Esophageal stenosis, 219, 220
Esophagotracheal septum, 228
Esophagus, 69, 207, 208, 209–210, *210*
Estrogen, 13, 23, 25, 197, 202, 254, 326, 327, 329, 330
Ethics, and genetic engineering, 396
Ethmoid bone, 134, 309
Eustachian tube, 69, 351, 352
Exophthalmia, 139
External auditory meatus, 351, 352, 358Q, 359E
External cephalic conversion, 366
External ear, 351, 352
 anomalies of, 356–357
Extraembryonic coelom, 54, 116, 215
Extraembryonic membranes, 50
Extraembryonic mesoderm, 54–55, 58Q, 96
Eye, 37, 67, 182, 305, 306, 337–346, *337*, *339*, *341*
 congenital anomalies of, 347

Eyelids, 36, 37, 346
Eye rudiments, 35

F

Face, 37, 303, 304–306, *304*, *305*
 congenital anomalies of, 352
Facial nerve, 313
Falciform ligament, 120, 212
Fallopian tubes, see Oviducts
False labor, 364
Fascia, 8, 68
Female pronucleus, 21
Fertility, and descent of testes, 290
Fertility drugs, 20, 56, 109
Fertilization, 12, 13, 21, 23, 26, 33, 45–46, 47–49, 57Q, 59E
 determination of genetic sex during, 18
 events of, 48, *48*
 first week after, 57Q, 59E
Fetal-maternal interaction, immunologic aspects of, 253–255
Fetal alcohol syndrome, 379, 383Q, 384E
Fetal circulation, 102, 157–160, *159*
Fetal development, clinical assessment of, 361
Fetal distress, 364
Fetal lung maturity, 232, 233, 235, 362
Fetal membranes, 93
Fetal period, 37–40, *38*
Fetal urine production, 272, 275Q, 277E
Fetal waste elimination, 272
α-Fetoprotein, 71, 220, 362, 381
Fetus, 33, 55
 in abnormal implantation site, 1
 with congenital anomaly, 1
 descent of, in uterus, 364
 injury to, from amniocentesis, 362
 interruption of blood flow to, 102
 length of, 37, 44E, 361
 maternal IgG protection of, 242
 maternal immunologic aids for, 252–253
 passive immunity to, 103
 at 17 weeks, *39*
 at 29 weeks, *40*
 weight of, 40
Fibrils, 345
Fibroblasts, 8, 133, 135, 345
Fibrous coat, of eye, 337
Fila olfactoria, 309
Filum terminale, 175
Fimbria, 13
Fingers, 37
First arch syndrome, 316–317, *317*, 318Q, 320E, 357
First pharyngeal arch, 303, 309, 318Q, 320E
First pharyngeal cleft, 352, 358Q, 359E
First pharyngeal membrane, 354
First pharyngeal pouch, 353, *353*
Fistula, 221, 274, 395
Flagellum, 8
Flexion, 35, 81, 84–85, *86*, 87, 88Q
Folia, 184
Follicle, 21–22, *22*, 29Q
Follicle-stimulating hormone, 21, 25, 329
Follicular phase, of endometrium, 13
Foramen cecum, 324
Foramen of Bochdalek, 121
Foramen of Magendie, 185
Foramen of Monro, 178
Foramen ovale, 150, 158, 160, 163Q, 164E
Foramina of Luschka, 185
Forebrain, 84, 167, 176
Foregut, 69, 87, 90E, 124E, 207, 208–212, 222Q, 224E
Foregut atresia, 220
Forelimbs, 36, 38, 43E, 80, 134
Fossa navicularis, 11
Fossa ovalis, 150

Fovea centralis, 342, *344*
Fractures, 130
Frontal bone, 134
Frontalis muscle, 313
Frontal lobes, 180
Frontal plane, 2
Frontal prominence, 303, 304
Frontonasal process, 304
Functionalis, 13

G

Galactosemia, 347
Gallbladder, 207, 208, *212*, 213, 214, *215*
GALT, see Gut-associated lymphoid tissue
Gametes
 haploid, 17, 18, 20
 male, 10
 sexually dimorphic, 17
 transport of, in female reproductive tract, 45
Gametogenesis, 17–27
 abnormalities of, 26, 27
 behavior of sex chromosomes in, 18
 features of, 17–18
 female, 20–23
 hormonal control of, 25–26
 male, 23–25
Ganglion cells, 342
Gartner's cysts, 288
Gartner's duct, 288
Gas exchange, 84, 225, 226
Gastric mesenteries, 210–212, *211*
Gastrin, 328
Gastroenteropancreatic cells, 328
Gastrointestinal tract, 91E, 126
 congenital malformations of, 219–221, 371
Gastrolienal ligament, 211
Gastroschisis, 220, 221, 362
Gastrosplenic omentum, 120
Gastrula, 61, 63, *63*
Gastrulation, 6, 35, 54, 61–64, 79, 80, 81, 167, 377
G-banding, 388
G-C base pairs, 386
Gender, see Genetic sex; Sexual differentiation
Genes
 and DNA structure, 386
 differential activity of, 3
 dominant, 390
 recessive, 390
 for sexual differentiation, 290, 292
Genetic counseling, 1, 386, 394
Genetic diversity, 17–18
Genetic engineering, ethical problems of, 396
Genetic manipulation, 395–396
Genetic sex, 279, 290–291
 see also Sexual differentiation
Genital ducts, 279, 280, 284–286, *285*, *286*, 288
Genitalia, external, 12, 37, 67, 279, 280, 288–289, *288*
 ambiguous, 330
 in indifferent stage, 288
 masculinization of, 330, *330*
 normal male, 298Q, 301E
 sexual dimorphism of, 38, 43E
Genital ridge mesenchyme, 300Q, 302E
Genital tubercle, 288, 289
Genome, 3
German measles, 373
Germ cells
 diploid, 17
 primordial, 18–19, 20, 23, 28Q
Germinal epithelium, 12
Germinal epithelium, 12
Germ layers, 61, 64, 67–69, 74Q, 76E, 79

Gestation, 41Q, 42Q
Gestational age, 33, 361
Glands
  see also specific names
  endometrial, 25
  skin, 191
Glandular stage, of pulmonary development, 230, 231, 232
Glans penis, 289
Glaucoma, 338
Glia, 5, 169, 170
Glia limitans, 170, 187Q, 190E
Glioblasts, 5, 169, 170, 178, 187Q, 190E
Glisson's capsule, 212
Glossopharyngeal nerve, 183, 315
Glucagon, 327
Glucose, 103
Glycoproteins, 5, 48, 148, 201, 239
Glycosaminoglycan macromolecules, 57Q
GnRH, see Gonadotropin-releasing hormone
Golgi apparatus, 5, 25, 31E, 99
Golgi neurons, 184
Gonadal agenesis, 292, 293(t), 294
Gonadal ducts, 68
Gonadal dysgenesis, 293(t), 294-295
Gonadal veins, 157
Gonadotropin-releasing hormone, 324
Gonadotropins, 26, 290, 324
Gonads, 38, 43E, 68, 156, 269, 279, 280-284, 281, 321, 326, 327
Gonococcal infections, 104
Granulosa cells, 12, 21, 22, 28Q, 284
Gray matter, 171
Greater omentum, 120, 211, 217
Growth hormone, 138, 324
Guanine, 386
Gubernaculum testis, 289
Gut-associated lymphoid tissue, 239, 252
Gut rotation, abnormalities of, 220-221
Gut tube, 35, 69, 156, 207
Gynecoid pelvis, 295
Gynecomastia, 295

H

Hair, 9, 67, 191, 196, 197
Hair buds, 197, 197
Hair cells, 355, 356
Hair follicles, 38, 197, 198, 203Q, 205E
Hair papilla, 197
Haploid pronuclei, 45
Hard palate, 309
Hay fever, 242
hCG, see Chorionic gonadotropin; Human chorionic gonadotropin
Head, 36, 37, 43E
Head and neck, 68, 303
  congenital anomalies of, 315-317
Hearing, 351
  congenital deficits in, 357, 375
Heart, 68, 83-84, 88Q, 116, 145, 146-149, 147
  defects of, 120, 121, 160-161
  incidence of malformations of, 370(t)
Heart loop, 148
Heart murmurs, 160, 161
Heart tubes, 84
Helper T cells, 248
Hematopoiesis, 146, 243-245, 251
Hematopoietic cells, 213, 243, 244, 245
Hemiazygos vein, 157
Hemidesmosomes, 99
Hemochorial placenta, 53, 93, 98, 254
Hemocytoblasts, 83, 249
Hemoglobin, 83, 392
Hemoglobin A, 392
Hemoglobinopathies, 392
Hemolytic anemia, 254, 255
Hemothorax, 115

Hensen's node, 63, 63
Hepatic duct, 213, 214
Hepatic sinusoids, 157
Hepatogastric ligament, 212
Hepatomegaly, 377
Hermaphroditism, 295-296
Hernia, see Congenital diaphragmatic hernia; Congenital inguinal hernia; Dorsolateral hernias
Herniation of midgut loop, 37
Heroin, 380
Herpes simplex virus, 377
Heterozygotes, 390
Hindbrain, 167, 176, 182
Hindgut, 69, 87, 207, 218-219
  congenital anomalies of, 221
Hindlimbs, 36, 38, 80, 134
Hip dysplasia, 395
Hippocampus, 180
Hirschsprung's disease, 221, 223Q, 224E
Histocompatibility antigens, 253
Homozygotes, mutant, 390
Hormone-secreting cells, 327-329
Hormones
  see also specific types
  for cryptorchidism, 290
  in development of skin appendages, 197
  for establishing gender, 279
  gonadotropic, 25
  mammary glands under control of, 202
  placental, 93, 329
  steroidal sex, 25-26
Horseshoe kidney, 273, 273, 395
Human chorionic gonadotropin, 26
Human placental lactogen, 99, 202, 329
Humoral immunity, 247
Hurler syndrome, 347, 363
Hyaline cartilage, 135
Hyaline membrane disease, see Respiratory distress syndrome
Hyalocytes, 346
Hyaloid artery, 339, 345
Hyaloid vein, 339
Hyaloid vessels, 342, 345
Hyaluronic acid, 5, 104
Hyaluronidase, 47, 59E
H-Y antigen, 291, 292, 299Q, 302E
Hydatidiform mole, 106, 110Q, 113E
Hydrocephalus, 185, 362, 377
Hydrops fetalis, 254
Hydroxyapatite, 201
21-Hydroxylase, 330
3-β-Hydroxysteroid dehydrogenase, 326, 329
Hymen, 271, 289
Hyoid arch, 313
Hyoid artery, 155
Hyoid bone, 134, 313
Hyperkeratinization, 202
Hypertension, in pregnant women, 233
Hypoblast, 54, 55, 62
Hypobranchial eminence, 309
Hypocalcemia, 256
Hypoglossal nerve, 183, 310
Hypophysis, 321
Hypophysis cerebri, 181
Hypoplasia, of lung, 121
Hypothalamus, 180, 321, 323, 325

I

Ichthyosis, 202, 204Q, 205E
IgA, 239, 242, 243, 249, 252
IgD, 239, 242
IgE, 239, 242
IgG, 103, 239, 241, 241, 242, 249, 252
IgM, 239, 242, 249
Ileum, 156, 218
Ilioinguinal lymph sacs, 249

Immune system, 68, 239-258, 240, 244
Immunodeficiency disorders, 1, 256-257
Immunoglobulins, 99, 239-242, 247, 249, 252, 254
  see also IgA; IgD; IgE; IgG; IgM
Immunosuppression, 253-254
Immunosuppressive drugs, 253
Imperforate anus, 221
Implantation, 46, 50, 51, 52-53, 61, 93-94, 94, 95, 104, 106, 377
Inbreeding, mutations from, 17
Incisive foramen, 308-309
Incisors, 308
Inclusion bodies, 231
Incus, 313, 352, 353, 354
Indomethacin, 161
Infants
  immature vision in, 342
  premature, 40, 236Q, 238E
  respiratory distress syndrome in, 232, 233
Infections
  from amniocentesis, 362
  from congenital defects, 1
  fungal, 246, 253, 256
  gonococcal, 104
  herpes, 377
  intrauterine, 249
  kidney, 273
  parasitic, 242
  Pneumocystis carinii, 256
  Treponema pallidum, 249
  viral, 160, 246, 253
  yeast, 256
Inferior, 1
Inferior colliculus, 182
Inferior mesenteric arteries, 156, 219
Inferior vena cava, 151, 157
Infertility
  anovulatory, 20
  in vitro fertilization for, 55-56
  multiple pregnancies from treatment for, 109
Infundibular process, 322, 323
Infundibular stem, 322, 323
Infundibulum, 12-13, 181, 323, 324
Inner cell mass, 93
Inner ear, 351, 353, 354-356
Insula, 180
Insulin, 327
Integument, see Skin
Interatrial septum, 149, 150, 162Q, 164E
Interatrial valve, 145-146
Intercostal muscles, 156
Interkinetic nuclear migration, 169, 169
Intermaxillary segment, 306, 308, 308
Intermediate horns, 174
Intermediate mesoderm, 79, 80, 81, 88Q, 90E, 91E, 125, 126
Intermeningeal spaces, 172
Intersegmental arteries, 153, 156
Interstitial-cell-stimulating hormone, 25
Interstitial implantation, 93
Interstitial uterine tube, 12
Interventricular foramen, 152
Interventricular septum, 152, 162Q, 164E
Intervertebral disks, 132, 133, 135, 141Q, 144E
Intervillous space, 101, 111Q, 114E
Intestinal obstruction, 362
Intraembryonic coelom, 35, 81, 82, 115-116, 116, 117, 122Q, 123Q, 124E, 147, 230, 326
Intraembryonic mesoderm, 54, 61-63, 65, 79, 80-82, 125-126, 131
Intrahepatic biliary apparatus, 214
Intraretinal space, 340, 345
Intrauterine growth retardation, from rubella virus, 375
Invasive mole, 106
In vitro fertilization, 55-56, 57Q, 59E, 109, 395
Ionizing radiation, see Radiation, ionizing

Iris, 337, 338, 344, 346
Ischemia, retinal, 338
Islets of Langerhans, 215, 327, 328
Isthmus, 12

J

Jaundice, 104, 254, 377
Jejunum, 218
Joints, 134–135
Jugular lymph sacs, 249

K

Karyotype, 291, 387
 abnormalities of, 385
 analysis of, 381, 385, 387–388, 394
 nomenclature for, 388–389, 389(t)
 of normal human male, *388*
 of trisomy 13, *375*
 of trisomy 18, *373*
 of trisomy 21, *371*
 of Turner syndrome, 257, 295
Keratin, 195
Keratinization, 191, 193–195, 203Q, 205E
Keratinized cells, 191
Keratohyalin granules, 195
Kidneys, 8, 68, 156, 217, 263–264, *263*, *264*
 anomalies of, 272–273
Kidney stones, 273
Kleeblattschädel anomaly, 139
Klinefelter syndrome, 293(t), 295, *296*, *298*, 299Q, 301E, 362, 371(t), 388, 389
Kupffer cells, 213

L

Labia majora, 12, 289
Labia minora, 12, 289
Labioscrotal swellings, 288, 289
Labor
 early signs of, 363–364
 false, 364
 premature, from amniocentesis, 362
 stages of, 364, 367Q, 368E
Labor and delivery
 complications of, 366
 normal, 363–366, *365*
Labor pain, 364
Lacrimal glands, 67, 346
Lactation, 202, 242
Lactiferous ducts, 201
Lactoferrin, 252
Lactoperoxidase, 252
Lacunae, 53, 94, 112Q, 114E
Lamina propria, 13, 68
Langhans' cells, 99
Lanugo, 38, 43E, 197
Large intestines, 69, 207
Laryngeal bones, 134
Laryngeal cartilage, 319Q, 320E
Larynx, 225, 226
Last menstrual period, 33, 361
Lateral, 2
Lateral geniculate nucleus, 343
Lateral palatine process, 226, 238E, 306, 308
Lateral plate mesoderm, 79, 80, 81–82, 115–116, 126
Lateral splanchnic arteries, 156
Lateral ventricles, 178, 179
Lecithin, 232, 233, 235
Lecithin/sphingomyelin ratio, 233, 235
Left brachiocephalic vein, 157
Lens, 67, 305, 338, 346, 348Q, 349E

Lens fibers, 345
Lens placode, 305, 339, 345
Lens vesicle, 36, 339, *340*, 345, 348Q, 349E
Leptomeninges, 172
Lesch-Nyhan syndrome, 363
Lesser omentum, 120, 212
Lesser peritoneal sac, 211
Leukocytes, granular, 68
Leydig cells, 10, 25, 26, 282, 284, 327
Libido, 10, 26
Lienorenal ligament, 120, 211
Ligaments, 8, 12, 68
 see also specific names
Ligamentum arteriosum, 156, 160
Ligamentum teres hepatis, 120, 160
Ligamentum venosum, 160
Limb bud mesenchyme, 8, 9
Limb buds, 35, 36, 134, *137*, 141Q, 144E
Limbs, 6, 7, 8–9, 156
 defects in, 138–139, 362, 379
Limbus, 338
Lip, upper, 312
Liquor folliculi, 22, 47
Lithium, 379
Liver, 36, 37, 69, 83, 104, 157, 207, 208, 212–214, *212*, 215, 217, 222Q, 224E, 243, 244, *245*, 248, 249, 254, 326, 330
Liver diverticulum, 120, 212–213, 214
Lobar bronchi, 228
Longitudinal plane, 2
Loop of Henle, 264, 265, 267, 268
LSD, 380
Lumbar puncture, 175
Lumbar vertebrae, 133
Lung buds, 117–118, 228–229, *228*, *229*, *230*
Lungs, 8, 40, 69, 80, 126, 159–160, 208, 225, 228–232
 anomalies of, 120
 hypoplasia of, 121
Luteinizing hormone, 22, 25, 329
Lymphatic valves, 249
Lymphatic vessels, 68, 239, 249
Lymph nodes, 68, 239, 248, 249, *250*
Lymphoblasts, 248, 251, 252
Lymphocyte differentiation, 246–249, *246*
Lymphocytes, 68, 239, 248, 249, 252
Lysozyme, 252

M

Macrophages, 68, 239
Maculae, 355
Macula sacculi, 356, 357
Macula utriculi, 356
Malleus, 313, 352, *353*, 354, 358Q, 359E
Malrotation of gut, 121
Mammary glands, 9, 67, 191, 201–202, 203Q, 329
 absence of, 202
 anomalies in, 202
 hormonal control of, 202, 205E
 supernumerary, 202
Mammary ridge, 201
Mandible, 134, 143Q, 144E, 199, 200, 306, 312, 319Q, 320E
Mandibular swellings, 304, 306
Mandibulofacial dysostosis, 316–317, *317*, 318Q, 320E, 357
Mantle layer
 of central nervous system, 170–171, 173, 178
 of neural tube, 189Q, 190E, 341
Marfan syndrome, 393
Marginal layer
 of central nervous system, 171, 173, 178
 of neural tube, 189Q, 190E, 341
Marrow cavity, 129, 142Q, 144E
Masseter muscle, 313
Mastication, muscles of, 313

Maternal-fetal barrier, 93, 94, 98
Maternal blood, circulation of, 101–102
Maternal serum α-fetoprotein screening, 71
Maxilla, 134, 143Q, 144E, 199, 200, 306, 312
Maxillary artery, 155
Maxillary bone, 308
Maxillary processes, 226, 306
Maxillary swellings, 304, 305–306
Meatal plug, 352
Mechanoreceptors, of ear, 351
Meckel's cartilage, 306, *311*, 313, 319Q, 320E, 354
Meckel's diverticulum, 220
Meconium, 364
Medial, 2
Medial umbilical ligaments, 160
Median eminence, 322, 323
Median palatine process, 308
Median plane, 2
Median sulcus, 309
Mediastinum testis, 10
Medulla
 of ovary, 12
 thymic, 248
Medulla oblongata, 167, 178, 182, 183, 188Q, 190E
Megakaryocytes, 251
Meibomian glands, 346
Meiosis, 19, *19*
 compared with mitosis, 18
 in females, 21
 in males, 24
 phases of, 19–20
 reduction division of, 17
Meiotic nondisjunction, 389
Melanin granules, 193
Melanoblasts, 193
Melanocytes, 61, 68, 191, 193
Melanosomes, 340
Membrane bones, 128
Membranous labyrinth, 354, *355*, 355–356
Menarche, 20, 21
Mendelian disorders, 392–393
Mendelian transmission, 390–392
Meningeal cells, 168
Meninges, 172, 175
Meningocele, 70, 71
Meningomyelocele, 70, 71, 73, *73*
Menopause, 20
Menstrual cycle, 13, 20, 26, 29Q, 31E
 anovulatory, 26
 hormonal control of, *25*
 pregnancy occurrence during, *51*
Mental retardation, 139, 185, 186, 295, 370, 371, 372, 375, 377, 378, 379, 390, 392
Mesaxon, 172, 173
Mesencephalon, 167, 176, 181–182
Mesenchymal cells, 83, 84, 127, *128*, 192, 196, 304
Mesenchymal tissue, in lung formation, 8
Mesenchyme, 3, *4*, 8, 9, 14Q, 68, 191, 199, 200, 201, 345
Mesenteries, 119–120
 abdominal, 120, *120*
 of female reproductive system, 12
 hindgut, 219
Mesocardium, 123Q, 124E
Mesocolon, 119
Mesoderm, 6, 35, 61, 64, 68, 74Q, 75Q, 76E, 77E, 168, 191, 196, 321
Mesoduodenum, 119, 123Q, 124E
Mesogastrium, 119, 120, 123Q, 124E, 210, 211, 212
Mesonephric duct, 264, 265, 266, 271, 276Q, 277E, 284, 286, 298Q, 299Q, 301E, 302E
Mesonephric tubules, 266, 284, 285, 288
Mesonephric vesicles, 265, 266
Mesonephron, 272
Mesonephros, 265–267, *267*, *268*, 269, 275Q, 277E, 276Q, 277E, 284, 285

Mesorchium, 282
Mesosalpinx, 12
Mesothelium, 82, 115, 117, 119, 122Q, 124E, 148, 230
Mesovarium, 12
Messenger RNA molecule, 386
Metabolism, disorders of, 347, 362–363, 380(t), 381
Metanephric blastema, 8, 264, 267, 268, 276Q, 277E
Metanephros, 265, 267–269, *268*, *269*, 275Q, 277E
Metastasis, 106
Metencephalon, 167, 178, 182, 183
Microcephaly, 362, 373, 377, 378, 379
Microencephaly, 392
Microglia, 170
Microorganisms, 382Q, 384E
Microphthalmia, 347, 372, 377
Microvilli, 52, 53, 94, 98
Midbrain, 167
Midbrain flexure, 176
Midbrain ventricle, 181–182
Middle ear, 69, 351, 352–354, *353*
Middle ear ossicle, 134
Midgut, 36, 87, 207, 215, 217–218, 223Q, 224E
derivatives of, 222Q, 224E
herniation of, into umbilical cord, 215, *216*, 217, *217*
rotation of, *218*
Midgut loop, 44E, 220–221, 223Q, 224E
Midsagittal plane, 2
Mitochondria, 99, 137
Mitosis, 18, 46
Mitotic cells, 378
Mitral valves, 153
Mittelschmerz, 23
Modiolus, 354
Monomers, 242
Monosomy, 26, 369, 389
Morphogenesis, 5, 6, 7, 8, 33
Morula, 33, *34*, 46, 49, *50*
Mosaicism, 138, 389
Motor neurons, 16E, 174
mRNA, *see* Messenger RNA molecule
Müllerian-inhibiting substance, 290, 292, 299Q, 302E
Müllerian duct, 284, 290, 292
Müllerian tubercle, 284
Multifactorial inheritance, 395, 397Q, 399E
Multifactorial lesions, 385
Multiple pregnancies, 56, 107–109, *107*, 362
Muscle, 68
see also Cardiac muscle; Skeletal muscle; Smooth muscle
Muscle cells, 5, 141Q, 144E
Musculoskeletal system, 125–137
congenital abnormalities of, 137–139, 369, 371
Mutations, 17, 369, 390–391
autosomal dominant, 138, 202, 316, 317, 390, 397Q, 399E
autosomal recessive, *391*, 393, 397Q, 399E, 357
and hormonal control, 292
X-linked, *392*
Myelencephalon, 167, 178, 182, 183
Myelin, 172, 173
Myelination, 172–173, 187Q, 190E
Myelin sheath, 173
Myeloblasts, 251
Myelomeningocele, 70, 370(t), 394
Myelopoiesis, 251
Myenteric plexus, 221
Mylohyoid muscle, 313
Myoblasts, 8, 136
Myocardium, 148, 153
Myocoele, 80, 131
Myocytes, 8, 148
Myoepicardial mantle, 147, 148
Myoepithelial cells, 201

Myometrium, 13
Myosin, 5, 136
Myotubes, 136, *138*

N

Nails, 9, 67, 191, 196, 202
Nasal cavities, 225, 226–228, *227*, 237Q, 238E, 303, 305, 306, *307*, 309, 318Q, 320E
Nasal conchae, 227, 238E, 303, 309
Nasal pits, 36, 226, 305, 306
Nasal placodes, 226, 305, 306
Nasal sacs, 226, 306, 308
Nasal septum, 226, 238E, 303, 306, 308
Nasal sinuses, 303
Nasal structures, 303
Nasal swellings, 226, 305, 306
Nasolacrimal duct, 306, 346
Nasolacrimal groove, 306
Nasopharynx, 225, 227, 303
Neck, *see* Head and neck
Nephrogenic cord, 265
Nephrons, 264, 266, 268, *270*, *271*
Nerve fibers, 343–344
Nervous system, *see* Autonomic nervous system; Central nervous system; Enteric nervous system; Peripheral nervous system; Primordial nervous system
Nervous tissue, differentiation of, 5
Neural cells, 80
Neural crest, 67–68, 75Q, 76E, 151, 167–168, 193, 200, 207, 321, 327, 329
Neural crest cells, 61, 65, 167, 172, 173, 175, 191, 221, 257, 311, 326, *327*
Neural fold, 61, 65
Neural groove, 61, 65
Neural plate, 6, 35, 61, 64, 65, 167
Neural retina, 337, 340, 341–342, 345, 346
Neural tube, 6, 35, 61, 65, 67, 84, 167, 171, *171*, *172*, 173
mantle layer of, 189Q, 190E, 341
marginal layer of, 189Q, 190E, 341
Neural tube defects, 69–71, 72, 73, 74Q, 76E, 75Q, 77E, 185, 362, 370, 381, 398Q, 399E
diagnosis of, in utero, 71, *72*, 73
incidence of, 394–395
recurrence risk of, 395
Neuraminic acid, 47
Neuraminidase, 47
Neuraxis, 167–168
Neuroblasts, 5, 169, 170, 178, 187Q, 190E, 341, 356
Neurocranium, 134
Neuroectoderm, 64, 65
Neuroepithelium, 5, 168, *168*, 178, 187Q, 190E
of inner ear, 354, 355, 356, 357
Neuroglia, 170
Neurohypophysis, 181, 321, 322, 323
Neurons, 5, 6, 16E, 68, 169–170, 175, 176, *176*, 178
Neuropore, 67
Neurulation, 6, 8, 35, 61, 64–67, *66*, 75Q, 76E, 79, 80, 83, 84, 167
Newborn, maternal immunologic aids for, 252–253
Nicotine, 379
Nipples, 37, 201
supernumerary, 202
Nondisjunction, 26, *27*, 29Q, 31E
Nose, 305–306, *307*
Notochord, 55, 61, 62, 63, 64, *65*, 69, 75Q, 77E, 79, 80, 131, 132, 133
Notochordal canal, 63
Notochordal cells, 133
Nucleated cells, 83
Nucleus pulposus, 69, 133
Nutrient transport, 84

O

Obstetrics, knowledge of embryology in, 1
Occipital bone, 134, 143Q, 144E
Occipital lobes, 180
Ocular adnexa, 346
Oculomotor nerve, 182
Odontoblast processes, 200
Odontoblasts, 68, 200–201
Olfaction, 226
Olfactory bulb, 309
Olfactory cilia, 228
Oligodendroblasts, 170
Oligodendrocytes, 170
Oligodendroglia, 170, 173
Oligohydramnios, 272, 273
Oligospermia, 26, 56
Olivary nucleus, 182
Omphalocele, 220, 221, *221*, 223Q, 224E, 362, 395
Oocytes, 12, 18, 19, 20, 21, 28Q, 31E, 284
Oogenesis, 11, 26
see also Gametogenesis, female
Oogonia, 18, 20, 280, 284
Optic chiasm, 342
Optic cup, 338, 339, 340, *340*, 341, 344, 345, 346, 347
Optic groove, 338
Optic nerve, 167, 338, 339, 342
Optic stalk, 167, 338, 339, 341, 342
Optic vesicle, 167, 176, 338, 347, 348Q, 349E
Oral cavity, 67, 207, 226–227, *227*, 303, 304, 306, *307*, 318Q, 320E
Ora serrata, 344
Orbicularis oculi muscle, 313
Orbicularis oris muscle, 313
Organelles, 5, 8
Organ of Corti, 67, 351, 354, 355, 356, *356*, 357
Organ of olfaction, 226
Organogenesis, 8–9, 33, 80, 377
Organ transplants, 253
Oropharyngeal membrane, 55, 63, 207, 227, 304
Ossicles, 351, 352, 353, *353*, 354
Ossification
endochondral, 127, 128–129, *130*, *131*, *132*, 134, 306
of fetal skull, 364–365
intramembranous, 127, 128, *129*, 134, 306
Osteoblasts, 8, 125, 127, 128, 129
Osteoclasts, 129
Osteocytes, 3, 8, 127
Osteogenesis, 126, 127, 244
Osteogenesis imperfecta, 393
Osteoid, 127, 128, 129
Osteoprogenitor cells, 128, 129
Ostium primum, 149, 150
Ostium secundum, 150
Otic vesicle, *353*, 355
Otolithic membrane, 355
Otoliths, 355
Ova, 11
Oval window, 352, 354
Ovarian differentiation, 283–284
Ovarian follicles, 12
Ovarian ligament, 12
Ovaries, 11, 12, 16E
hormonal secretion by, 202
ligaments of, 12
in Turner syndrome, 294, *295*
Overriding aorta, 161
Oviducts, 11, 12–13
see also Uterine tubes
Ovulation, 13, 20, 21, 22–23, 25, 26, 29Q, 31E, 46
Ovum, 17
abnormal, 26
fertilized, *47*
from follicular origin to endometrial implantation, *45*

444 *Human Developmental Anatomy*

haploid, 19, 21
and menstrual cycle, 20
at ovulation, 23
transport of, 46–47

P

Palate, 226, 227, 303, *307*
  anomalies of, *316*, see also Cleft palate
Palatine bones, 134
Palatine processes, see also Lateral palatine processes; Median palatine process
Palatine tonsils, 69, 252, 313
Pancreas, 9, 69, 126, 207, 208, 214–215, *212*, 327, *328*
Pancreatic acinar cells, 215
Pancreatic buds, 214, *215*, 327
Pancreatic ducts, 214
Pancreatic islet tissues, 321
Papillae, 263
Papillary ducts, 264, 265, 267
Papillary muscles, 153
Paracrine cells, 328
Paradidymis, 285
Parafollicular cells, 68, 324
Paramesonephric duct, 284, 285, 290, 292, 300Q, 302E
Paramesonephric tubercle, 284
Paranasal air sinuses, 309
Parasagittal plane, 2
Parathyroid agenesis, 256
Parathyroid glands, 69, 251, 315, 321, 325, 331Q, 334E, 331Q, 333Q, 334E, 335E
Parenchyma, 69, 231
Parietal bone, 134, 143Q, 144E
Parietal pericardium, 148
Paroophoron, 288
Parotid salivary glands, 310
Pars ciliaris, 344, 346
Pars distalis, 322, 324
Pars intermedia, 322, 324
Pars iridica, 344, 346
Pars nervosa, 324
Pars optica, 344
Pars tuberalis, 322, 324
Passive fetal immunization, 252, 259Q, 261E
Patau syndrome, 26, 357, 372–373, 382Q, 384E, 393
  see also Trisomy 13
  clinical features of, 376
  frequency of, 371(t)
  recurrence risk in, 394
Patent ductus arteriosus, 161, 375
PCP, 380
Pediatrics, knowledge of embryology in, 1
Pedigree, 386
Pelvic inflammatory disease, 104
Pelvic kidneys, 273
Penis, 10, 11, 16E, 289
Pentamer, 242
Peptide hormones, 328
Pericardial cavity, 81, 115, 116, 122Q, 124E, 148
Pericardioperitoneal canals, 85, 116, 117, *117*, 124E, 230
Pericardium, 115, *117*, 118
Perichondrium, 129
Periderm, 192, *193*
Perilymph, 354, 356
Perilymphatic ducts, 354
Perimetrium, 13
Peripheral nervous system, 172–173
Peristalsis, in uterus and uterine tubes, 46
Peritoneal cavity, 37, 82, 115, 124E
Peritoneum, 115
Perivitelline space, 48
Pharyngeal arches, 35, 134, 311–315, 314(t), *315*
  see also First pharyngeal arch; Second pharyngeal arch; Third pharyngeal arch

Pharyngeal clefts, 311, 312, 313, *313*
Pharyngeal membrane, 311–312, 313
Pharyngeal pouches, 69, 251, 252, 311, 312, 313, *313*, 318Q, 320E
Pharyngeal tonsils, 252
Pharynx, 69, 207, 208, 308
Phenothiazines, 379
Phenotype, 390
Phenylalanine hydroxylase, 392
Phenylketonuria, 392–393, 395, 398Q, 399E
Phenytoin, 379
Philtrum, 308
Phocomelia, 139, 379
Phonation, role of larynx in, 226
Phosphate, 103
Phosphatidylcholine, 232
Phosphatidyl ethanolamine, 363
Photoreceptor pigments, 342
Phrenic nerve, *117*, 118
Phytohemagglutinin, 248
Pia-arachnoid meninges, 68, 175
Pia mater, 172
Pigmented retina, 337, 340, 345
Pineal gland, 180, 321, 324
Pinna, 313, 351, 352
Pituitary gland, 181, 202, 321, 322–324, *323*, 326, 333Q, 335E
Pituitary growth hormone, 329
Placenta, 26, 33, 50, 55, 97, 98, *102*, 110Q, 113E, 156, 158, 202, 253, 254, 326, 327, 332Q, 334E
  see also Hemochorial placenta
  abnormal location of, 1
  circulation in, 101–102
  delivery of, 366, 367Q
  as endocrine organ, 329–330
  fetal urea eliminated via, 272
  IgG transport through, 242
  injury to, from amniocentesis, 362
  during labor, 364
  steroidogenesis in, 329–330
  structure of, 100–101
Placental abruption, 102
Placental growth hormone, 329
Placental transport, 102–104, 111Q, 113E
Placenta previa, 1, 106, *106*, 110Q, 113E
Placentation, 93
  abnormalities of, 104, 106
Plasma cells, 247, 248, 249
Plasticity, 185
Platysma muscle, 313
Pleura, 115, 230
Pleural cavities, 82, 115, 116, 122Q, 230
Pleuropericardial membranes, 117, *117*, 118, 124E
Pleuroperitoneal canals, 119
Pleuroperitoneal membranes, *118*, 119, 124E
Pneumocystis carinii infections, 256
Pneumothorax, 115
Podocytes, 264
Point mutations, 385
Polycystic kidneys, 362
Polydactyly, 139, *140*, 372
Polygenic lesions, 385
Polyhydramnios, 220, 272
Polymastia, 202
Polymers, 242
Polyploidy, 385, 389
Polysomes, 387
Polyspermy, 48, 389
Polythelia, 202
Pompe disease, 363
Pons, 167, 178, 182, 184–185, 188Q, 190E
Pontine flexure, 176, 178
Pontine nuclei, 185
Posterior, 2
Posterior chamber, 337, 338
Posterior intestinal portal, 87, 207
Posterior nares, 227
Posterior rachischisis, 70, 71
Pre-embryonic period, 33

Pre-embryonic structure, layers of, 53–54
Predentin, 200, 201
Pregnancy
  and abnormal implantation site, 1
  breast duct proliferation during, 202
  calculating duration of, 33
  cytomegalovirus during, 377
  ectopic, see Ectopic pregnancy
  effect of drugs on, 297, 378–380
  effect of ionizing radiation on, 377–378
  gestational age of, 361
  herpes simplex virus during, 377
  hypertension during, 233
  infectious disease during, 347
  mammary gland development during, 329
  multiple, see Multiple pregnancies
  Rh isoimmunization during, 233
  rubella virus during, 347, 357, 375
  sickle cell disease during, 233
  smoking during, 102
  Toxoplasma infection during, 377
Premaxilla, 134
Primary embryonic induction, 6, 65
Primary palate, 226, 306, 308
Primitive atrium, 149
Primitive blood vessels, 83
Primitive circulation, 80, 82–84
Primitive circulatory system, 35, 80, *146*
Primitive erythroblasts, 83, 243
Primitive erythrocytes, 83, *83*, 146, 243
Primitive erythropoiesis, 83
Primitive great vessels, 148
Primitive gut, 87, 207
Primitive hemocytoblasts, 146
Primitive knot, 63, *63*, 79
Primitive node, 63, *63*, 75Q, 77E
Primitive rectum, 270
Primitive sex cords, 280, 282, 283
Primitive streak, 62, *62*
Primitive urogenital sinus, 270
Primordial germ cells, 280, 281, 282, 284, 298Q, 301E
Primordial nervous system, 35
Processus vaginalis, 289, 290
Prochordal plate, 55
Proctodeal membrane, 288
Proctodeum, 207, 219
Progesterone, 13, 23, 25, 26, 99, 202, 254, 326, 329
Progestin, 379
Prolactin, 202, 324
Pronephros, 265
Prosencephalon, 167, 176, 178–181, 338
Prostaglandins
  in labor, 363, *363*, 367Q, 368E
  in semen, 46
Prostaglandin synthetase, 363
Prostaglandin synthetase inhibitors, 161
Prostate gland, 10, 16E
Prostatic urethra, 285
Prostatic utricle, 285
Protein
  amino acid sequences in, 386
  cell-specific, 3
  in muscle cells, 5
  in stratum corneum, 195
Protein hormones, 99
Proteoglycans, 201
Proximal, 2, 16E
Proximal duodenum, 212
Pseudohermaphroditism, 296–297
Psychosis, 379
Ptyalin, 303
Puberty
  cortical zonation and, 326
  gametogenesis and, 23
  growth of mammary glands during, 201–202
  hair growth during, 197
  secondary sexual characteristics during, 290

spermatogenesis during, 282
testical abnormalities after, 295
Pulmonary agenesis, 8
Pulmonary arteries, 156, 158
Pulmonary artery stenosis, 161
Pulmonary development, stages of, 230–232, *231*, *232*, *233*, *234*, 236Q, 238E, 362
Pulmonary maturation, 40
Pulmonary trunk, 153, 155
Pulmonary valves, 153
Pulmonary veins, 151, 158
Pupil, 338
Pupillary membrane, 345, 347
Pupillary sphincter, 67
Pupillary sphincter muscles, 344
Purkinje cells, 184
Pyloric stenosis, 220, 370(t), 395

Q

Quadruplets, 109
Quickening, 38, 43E

R

Radiation, ionizing, teratogenic effects of, 369, 377–378, 383Q, 384E
Radioimmunoassay, 329
Rathke's pouch, 67, 181, 228, 323, 324, 331Q, 334E
Rectal atresia, 221
Rectourethral fistula, 221
Rectouterine pouch, 286, *287*
Rectovaginal fistula, 221
Rectum, 69, 156, 207, 219, 288
Recurrent laryngeal nerve, 156
Red nucleus, 182
Reichert's cartilage, 313, 319Q, 320E, 354
Releasing hormones, 181, 321
Renal agenesis, 8, 272–273, 275Q, 277E
Renal arteries, 269
Renal corpuscle, 264
Renal cysts, 273
Renal pelvis, 263
Renal pyramids, 263
Renal sinus, 263
Renal vein, 157
Reproduction, sexual, 17
Reproductive system, 279–297
female, 11–13, *11*, 14Q, 20, 45, 46–47
at indifferent stage, 279, *279*, 280(t)
male, 9–11, 15Q
Respiratory distress syndrome, 232, 233, 236Q, 238E
Respiratory diverticulum, 228, *228*, 229, 230, 236Q, 238E, 237Q, 238E
Respiratory mucosa, 226
Respiratory system, 8, 207, 225–235, *225*, 327, 328
Rete testis, 10, 282–283, 285
Reticular tissue, 68
Retina, 36, 67, 167, 337, 338, 340–345, *343*, 348Q, 349E
detached, 345
Retinal artery, 342
Retroperitoneal sacs, 249
Rh antigen, 242, 254
Rh immune globulin, 255
Rh isoimmunization, 233, 254–255, 260Q, 261E
RhoGAM, 255
Rhombencephalon, 167, 176, 178, 182–185, *183*, *184*
Rhomic lip-cerebellum, 183
Ribosomes, 99
Ribs, 130, 156

Right subclavian artery, 155
Right venous valve, 151
Right ventricular hypertrophy, 161
RNA, *see* Messenger RNA molecule; Transfer RNA
RNA polymerase, 386
Rods, 337, 338, 340, 342
Roof of mouth, 312
Rostral, 1
Rough endoplasmic reticulum, 99, 387
Round window, 354
Rubella virus, 160, 249, 347, 357, 369, 373, 375, 383Q, 384E

S

Saccular stage, of pulmonary development, 231, *231*, 234
Saccule, 352, 354, 355, 356
Sacral vertebrae, 133
Saliva, 303
Salivary duct, *311*
Salivary glands, 9, 67, 69, 207, 303, 310, *311*
Sarcomeres, 5, 136, 137
Sarcoplasmic reticulum, 136
Scala media, 354
Scala tympani, 354
Scala vestibuli, 352, 354
Scaphocephaly, 139
Schwann cells, 61, 68, 168, 170, 172, 173
Sclera, 337, 345
Sclerotome, 80, 126, 131
Scrotum, 9, 289
Sebaceous glands, 67, 191, 196, 197, 199, 202, 346
Sebum, 199
Secondary chorionic villi, 110Q, 113E
Secondary enamel organ, 201
Secondary palate, 308
Secondary sexual characteristics, *see* Sexual characteristics, secondary
Second pharyngeal arch, 36, 309, 318Q, 320E, 319Q, 320E
Secretory phase, of endometrium, 13
Semen, 46
Semicircular canals, 352, 354, 355, 358Q, 359E
Semilunar valves, 153
Seminal fluid, 10
Seminal vesicle, 10, 285
Seminiferous tubules, 10, 23, 282, 283, *283*
Seminomas, 290
Sensory neurons, 174
Septum intermedium, 151, 152
Septum primum, 149, 151
Septum secundum, 158
Septum spurium, 150
Septum transversum, 84, 85, 90E, 116, 118–119, 120, 121, 147, 212, 213
Serosa, 13
Serotonin, 328
Sertoli cells, 10, 23, 25, 282, 283
Serum proteins, 103
Sex-linked inheritance, 391, *392*
Sex chromosomes, *see* Chromosomes, sex
Sex determination, through amniocentesis, 362
Sex steroids, 25–26
Sexual characteristics, secondary, 290, 295
hair growth and, 197
male, 10, 26
Sexual differentiation, 290–292, 298Q, 301E
see also Genetic sex
atypical, 280
congenital abnormalities of, 292, 293(t), 294–297
of external genitalia, 289
Sexual dimorphism, 38, 43E, 279–280
Shrapnell's membrane, 353

Sickle cell anemia, 233, 369, 392, 395, 398Q, 399E
Single-gene defects, 397Q, 399E
Sinoatrial orifice, 150
Sinus horns, 150, 162Q, 164E
Sinus venarum, 150
Sinus venosus, 148, 150–151
Skeletal muscle, 5, 35, 68, 136, 209
Skeleton, 35, 38
Skin, 69, 191–199, *194*, *195*, 196, 203Q
anomalies of, 202
Skin color, 191
Skull, 131, 134, 364–365
defects in, 139
Small intestines, 69, 207, 215, 328
Smoking, during pregnancy, 102
Smooth endoplasmic reticulum, 99
Smooth muscle, 68, 136, 145, 209, 270, 344
contractions of, 47, 363, 364, 366
Social drugs, 379–380
Soft palate, 309
Somatic cells, diploid, 17
Somatic mesoderm, 82, 91E, 116, 126
Somatopleuric extraembryonic mesoderm, 54, 59E, 94
Somatostatin, 328
Somatotropin, 329
Somites, 35, 79, *79*, 80, 80–81, *81*, 88Q, 90E, 125, 126, *126*, 131, 132
Sonography, 71, 361–362, 366, 367Q, 368E, 394
of anencephalic fetus, 72
of cystic hygroma, 257, *258*
of ectopic pregnancy, 104, *105*
of meningomyelocele, 73
of multiple pregnancies, *107*, 362
for neural tube defects, 71, 381
of normal fetus, *70*
of omphalocele, *221*
of placenta previa, *106*
of spina bifida, *72*
Sperm, *see* Spermatozoa
Spermatids, 8, 10, 24, 25, 31E
Spermatocytes, 10, 18, 19, 23, 24
Spermatogenesis, 10, 26, 29Q, 32E, 282, 290
Spermatogenic cells, 10
Spermatogonia, 10, 18, 23, 280, 282
Spermatozoa, 8, 10, 11, 17, 19, 24, 26, 46
Sperm cell motility, 46
Sperm–egg interaction, 45
Spermiogenesis, 8, 24–25
Sphenoid bone, 134
Sphingomyelin, 233, 235
Spina bifida, 70, 71, 72, 121
Spina bifida occulta, 70, 71
Spinal cord, 64, 65, 67, 68, 84, 85, 156, 167, 173–175, *174*
central canal of, 189Q, 190E
mantle layer of, 189Q, 190E, 341
marginal layer, 189Q, 190E, 341
Spinal nerves, 175–176
Spiral arteries, 111Q, 114E
Splanchnic mesoderm, 82, 91E, 116, 117, 126, 207, 213, 219, 229, 230, *230*, 237Q, 238E, 270, 324
Splanchnic mesodermal anlage, 215
Splanchnopleuric extraembryonic mesoderm, 54, 59E
Spleen, 68, 120, 211, 239, 244, 248, 251, 254, 259Q, 260Q, 261E
Spongy bone, 129
Spontaneous abortion, 56, 106, 249, 378, 379, 389
Squamous type I cells, 231, *234*
Stapedius muscle, 313
Stapes, 313, 352, *353*, 354
Stapedial artery, 155
Stereocilia, 10
Sterility, from cryptorchidism, 290
Sternal bars, 133
Sternum, 131, 133

Steroid biosynthesis, 292, 326, 329
Steroid metabolism, 292
Steroidogenesis, 329–330
Steroids, 99, 103, 202, 254, 321, 329–330, 379
  gonadal, 327
  sex, 25–26
Stomach, 69, 120, 156, 207, 208, 210, *211*, 212, 222Q, 223Q, 224E, 328
Stomodeum, 207, 227, 304
Stratum basale, 191, 193, 194, 205E, 340
Stratum corneum, 191, 193, 194, 195
Stratum granulosum, 191
Stratum lucidum, 191
Stratum spinosum, 191, 194
Stylohyoid ligament, 313
Styloid process, 313
Subarachnoid space, 172, 175, 185
Subcardinal veins, 157
Subcutaneous fat, 40, 44E
Subdural space, 172, 175
Sublingual salivary glands, 310
Submandibular salivary glands, 310
Substantia nigra, 182
Sulcus limitans, 171, 174, 178, 182
Superior, 1
Superior colliculus, 182
Superior mesenteric arteries, 156, 215
Superior vena cava, 157, 158
Suppressor T cells, 248
Supracardinal veins, 157
Suprarenal veins, 157
Surfactant, 40, 226, 231–232, 233, 235, 362
Surfactant-secreting type II cells, 231–232
Surgery, knowledge of embryology in, 1
Surrogate parenting, ethical problems of, 396
Suspensory ligament, 12
Sutures, 139
Sweat glands, 67, 191, 196, 199, 202, 346
Sympathetic ganglia, 167, 175, 176
Symphysis pubis, 135
Synarthroses, 134–135
Syncytial giant cells, 101
Syncytiotrophoblast, 52–53, 93, 94, 95, 98–99, 111Q, 112Q, 114E, 253
Syncytium, 98, 99
Syndactyly, 139, *139*
Syngamy, 48
Synovial cells, 135
Synoviocytes, 135
Syphilis, 249

T

Tail bud, 43E
Talipes equinovarus, incidence of, 370(t)
Tarsal glands, 346
Tay-Sachs disease, 347, 363, 381
T cell differentiation, 248, 256
T cells, 246–247, 248, 251, 252, 253, 260Q, 261E
Tectum, 182
Teeth, 9, 69, 191, 199–201, *199*, 202, 203Q, 205E
  congenital anomalies in, 202
  deciduous, see Teeth, primary
  primary, 200, 201, 202
  secondary, 201, 202
Tegmentum, 182
Telencephalic vesicles, 167
Telencephalon, 176, 178–179, *180*
Temporal bone, 134
Temporalis muscle, 313
Temporal lobes, 180
Tendons, 8, 68
Teratogens, 33, 37
  see also Drugs, teratogenic effects of; Radiation, ionizing, teratogenic effects of
Terminal cellular differentiation, 193

Terminal sulcus, 309
Testes, 9, 10, 16E, *24*, 38, *282*
  abnormalities in, 295
  appendix of, 285
  descent of, 289–290, *289*
Testicular differentiation, 281–283, 292
Testicular feminization syndrome, 290, 292, 293(t), 296, *297*, 299Q, 302E
Testis-determining factor, 290, 291–292, 298Q, 301E
Testosterone, 10, 25, 26, 282, 290, 327
Testosterone receptor, 292
Testosterone receptor protein, 296
Tetralogy of Fallot, 160–161, *161*
Tetraploidy, 389
Thalamus, 180
β-Thalassemia, 398Q, 399E
Thalassemias, 392
Thalidomide, 138–139, 369, 379
Theca externa, 12
Theca interna, 12
Thecal cells, 12, 284, 327
Third pharyngeal arch, 309, 318Q, 320E
Thoracic nerves, 119
Thoracic vertebrae, 133
Thorax, cavities in, 115
Thymic agenesis, 256
Thymine, 386
Thymosin, 251
Thymus, 68, 239, 246, 248, 249, 251–252, *251*, 256, 259Q, 260Q, 261E
Thymus gland, 69, 248, 315
Thyroglossal duct, 324
Thyroid gland, 69, 315, 321, 324–325, *325*, 331Q, 333Q, 334E, 335E
Thyroid-stimulating hormone, 324, 325, 329
Thyrotropin-releasing hormone, 324, 325
Thyroxine, 325
T lymphocytes, 248, 249, 252
Toe rays, 36
Toes, 37
Tomes fibers, 200
Tongue, 67, 226, 238E, 303, 308, 309–310, *310*, 312
Tonsils, 239, 252, 259Q, 261E
Tooth roots, 200, 202
Toxoplasma, 249, 369, 377
Trabeculae, 128
Trabecular meshwork, 338, 345, 346
Trachea, 126, 208, 225, 228–230
Tracheoesophageal fistula, 395
Transcription, in DNA replication, 386–387
Transfer RNA, 387
Translation, in protein synthesis, 387
Translocation Down syndrome, 394
  see also Down syndrome; Trisomy 21
Translocations, 389
Transverse colon, 215, 217
Transverse plane, 2
Treacher Collins syndrome, 316–317, *317*, 318Q, 320E, 357
Treponema pallidum infections, 249
TRH, see Thyrotropin-releasing hormone
Tricuspid atresia, 161
Tricuspid valves, 153
Trigeminal nerve, 182, 310, 313
Trigone, 271–272
Triiodothyronine, 325
Trilaminar gastrula, 35, *35*
Triplets, 109
Triploidy, 389
Trisomies, 26, 362, 369, 370–373, 381, 389
Trisomy 13, 160, 316, 347, 372–373, *375*
  see also Patau syndrome
Trisomy 18, 160, 370–372, *373*
  see also Edwards syndrome
Trisomy 21, 160, 347, 370, *371*, 385
  see also Down syndrome; Translocation Down syndrome
tRNA, see Transfer RNA
Trochlear nerve, 182

Trophic hormone, 321
Trophoblast, 33, 50, *51*, *52*, 54, 59E, 93, 98–99, 110Q, 113E
Trophoblastic disease, 106
Tropomyosin, 5, 136
Troponin, 5
Troponin complex, 136
Truncus arteriosus, 148, 153, 154, 155(t)
Trunk, 36, 37
TSH, see Thyroid-stimulating hormone
Tubal pregnancy, 104
Tubal tonsils, 353
Tuber cinereum, 323
Tuberculum impar, 309, *310*
Tubuli recti, 10, 283
Tunica albuginea, 10, 11, 12, 281, 283
Tunica muscularis, 13
Tunica vaginalis, 290
Turner syndrome, 26, 257, 293(t), 294–295, *294*, *295*, 298Q, 299Q, 301E, 302E, 362, 388
  frequency of, 371(t)
Twins, 20, 111Q, 113E
  conjoined, 108, 362
  dizygotic, 107, *108*
  monozygotic, 107–108, *109*
Tympanic cavity, 352, 353
Tympanic membrane, 312, 351, 352, 353, *353*, 354, 358Q, 359E
Type I cells, 226, 229
Type II cells, 226, 229, 232, 233, 236Q, 238E
Tyrosinase, 202

U

Ultimobranchial bodies, 324
Ultrasonography, see Sonography
Umbilical arteries, 102, 104, 153, 156, 160
Umbilical cord, 33, 54, 55, 87, 104, 158, 160, 270, 364, 366
  herniation of midgut loop into, 37, 215, 216, 217, *217*
Umbilical veins, 102, 104, 110Q, 113E, 156, 157, *158*, 160, 163Q, 164E
Unilateral renal agenesis, 273
Upper lip, 319Q, 320E
Urachus, 219, 271
Urea, 272
Ureteric bud, 8, 264, 266, 267, 268, 276Q, 277E, 284
Ureteric duplication, 274
Ureteric obstruction, 273
Ureters, 68, 263, 267, 269
  anomalies of, 274
Urethra, 69, 263, 265, 270, 271
  obstruction of, 272
  penile, 10, 11
  prostatic, 10
Urethral folds, 289
Urinary bladder, see Bladder
Urinary system, 263, 264, 266
  anomalies of, 272–274
Urine, 263, 265, 266, 267
  fetal, 272, 275Q, 277E
Uriniferous tubules, 264
Urogenital folds, 288, 289, 299Q, 302E
Urogenital membrane, 219, 271, 288
Urogenital ridge, 266, 280, 284
Urogenital sinus, 69, 219, 265, 266, 270–271, 275Q, 277E, 276Q, 277E, 284, 288
Urogenital system
  abnormalities in, with Patau syndrome, 373
  as mesodermal derivative, 68
Uromodulin, 254
Urorectal septum, 219, 288
Uterine arteries, 112Q, 114E
Uterine tubes, 16E, 22, 23, 45, 56, 284, 285
  see also Oviducts, 11

Uterus, 12, 13, 16E, 38, 284, 285, 286, *286*, *287*, 363
Utricle, 352, 354, 355
Uvea, 337, 342
Uvula, 308, 309

V

Vagina, 11, 13, 16E, 69, 284, 285, 286, *287*
Vaginal plate, 285
Vagus nerve, 156, 183, 210, 310, 315
Vascular bud, 129
Vas deferens, 271, 285
Veins, 156–157
Vellus hairs, 197
Ventral, 2
Ventral gastric mesentery, 212
Ventral horns, 174, 176
Ventral median fissure, 175, 189Q, 190E
Ventral median septa, 174
Ventral mesentery, 207
Ventral mesogastrium, 212
Ventral pancreatic bud, 222Q, 224E
Ventral splanchnic arteries, 156
Ventricles
  of brain, 67
  of heart, 147, 148, 152–153, 158, 159
Ventricular outflow tracts, 152, *152*
Ventricular septal defect, 160, 161
Ventricular septation, 151–153, *151*
Ventricular wall, 152
Vermiform appendix, 218
Vernix caseosa, 38, 199
Vertebral arches, 132
Vertebral bodies, 131–132
Vertebral column, 130
Vesicourethral canal, 270
Vesicouterine pouch, 286, *287*
Vesicular sacs, 83
Vestibular apparatus, 67, 351–352, 354
Vestibular pouch, 355, *355*, 356
Vestibule, 354
Vestibulocochlear nerve, 182, 354
Villi, 35, 43E, 55, 94–98, 100, 101, 102
Virilizing drugs, 297
Virilizing endocrine disorder, 297
Visceral pericardium, 148
Viscerocranium, 134, 306
Vision, functional anatomy of, 338

Vitelline arteries, 153, 156
Vitelline duct, 87, 90E, 124E, 207, 217, 220, 223Q, 224E
Vitelline veins, 156, 157, *158*
Vitreous body, 337, 338, 346, 348Q, 349E
Vitreous humor, 337
Vocal cords, 226
Vomer, 134

W

Wharton's jelly, 104
White matter, 171
Wild-type allele, 390
"Witch's milk," 201
Wolffian duct, 284
Wrist, 36

X

X-irradiation, birth defects from, 377–378
Xiphoid process, 133
XO genotype, frequency of, 371(t)
XXX genotype, frequency of, 371(t)
XXY genotype, frequency of, 371(t)
XYY genotype, frequency of, 371(t)

Y

Y chromatin, *291*
Yolk sac, 33, *52*, 54, 55, 82, 83, 146, 156, 207, 243, 245, 249

Z

Zona fasciculata, 326
Zona glomerulosa, 326
Zona lysins, 48
Zona pellucida, 22, 24, 46, 49, 59E
Zona reticularis, 326
Zygomatic arch, 134, 143Q, 144E
Zygote, 3, 17, 18
Zygote nucleus, diploid, 48